ENDOPATH* TRISTAR TROCAR

THE CLEAR CHOICE

- Patented clear trocar enhances visibility in specimen removal

- Safety-shielded blade protects patients and OR staff

- Double-gasket system with 45° flapper valve reduces sprayback of fluids and smoke

- TriStar available in the efficient ENDOPATH FlexTray Delivery System

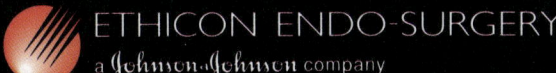

*TRADEMARK

PROCESS ENG

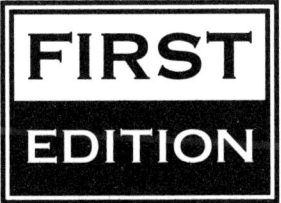

SURGEONS'
REFERENCE™

FOR MINIMALLY INVASIVE SURGERY PRODUCTS™

MEDICAL ECONOMICS

SURGEONS' REFERENCE FOR MINIMALLY INVASIVE SURGERY PRODUCTS™

PRODUCT MANAGER: Thomas G. Ferro
EDITOR: Heidi M. Siegenthaler Garrett
MANAGER, DATABASE ADMINISTRATION: Lynne Handler
DATABASE SUPERVISOR: Christine Niedermaier
DATA ANALYST: Mary Ellen Hegarty
NATIONAL SALES MANAGER: James R. Pantaleo
SENIOR ACCOUNT MANAGER: Michael S. Sarajian
ACCOUNT MANAGERS: Dik N. Barsamian; Donald V. Bruccoleri;
Lawrence C. Keary; Jeffery M. Keller; P. Anthony Pinsonault; Anthony Sorce
DIRECT MARKETING MANAGER: Robert W. Chapman
COMMERCIAL SALES MANAGER: Robin B. Bartlett
DATA SALES SUPERVISOR: Nancy E. Fagan
DIRECTOR OF PRODUCTION: Marjorie A. Duffy
PRODUCTION MANAGER: Vicky Leal
FULFILLMENT MANAGER: Roni LaVine
MEDICAL CONSULTANTS: Eddie Joe Reddick, MD; William Saye, MD

DISCLAIMER: The information in this reference was obtained from the medical device suppliers whose products appear herein, from the Food and Drug Administration (FDA), and from publicly available sources, including product literature, advertising materials, annual reports, and financial prospectuses. While every effort has been made to assure accuracy, the publisher makes no warranty that the information is free of error, and specifically disclaims liability for any inaccuracy, whether originating in one of the sources named above or inadvertently introduced during preparation of this publication.

Manufacturers' product information is subject to periodic revision. To make certain that you are following the correct instructions, manufacturers recommend that you refer to the information packed with the product when first putting a device into service.

The publisher does not warrant or guarantee any of the products described herein or perform any independent analysis in connection with the product information contained herein. The publisher does not assume, and expressly disclaims, any obligation to obtain and include any information other than that provided by the manufacturer.

Copyright© 1994 and published by Medical Economics Data Production Company at Montvale, NJ 07645-1742. All rights reserved. None of the content of this publication may be reproduced, stored in a retrieval system, resold, redistributed, or transmitted in any form or by any means (electronic, mechanical, photocopying, recording, or otherwise) without the prior written permission of the publisher. Surgeons' Reference™ and Surgeons' Reference For Minimally Invasive Surgery Products™ are trademarks of Medical Economics Data Production Company.

Officers of Medical Economics Data Production Company: **President and Chief Executive Officer:** Norman R. Snesil; **Executive Vice President:** Mark L. Weinstein; **Senior Vice President and Chief Financial Officer:** J. Crispin Ashworth; **Senior Vice President of Operations:** Curtis B. Allen; **Vice President of Product Management:** William J. Gole; **Vice President of Sales and Marketing:** Thomas F. Rice; **Vice President of Operations:** John R. Ware; **Vice President of Information Systems and Services:** Edward J. Zecchini; **Vice President of Business Development:** Raymond M. Zoeller

ISBN 1-56363-073-7
Manufactured in the United States of America

CONTENTS

Section 1: Indices .... **xi**
This section provides you with two ways of locating a product:

Trade Name Index: If you're seeking detailed information on a specific brand or product line, this convenient index will direct you to the appropriate page in the Product Directory.

Keyword Index: For those times when you're not sure of the exact title of a particular type of device, this index provides you with a way of quickly locating it based on its attributes and applications. For example, in this index you'll find needle holders listed under such headings as "Needle," "Holder," and "Suture." Under each keyword heading, all associated products are listed alphabetically along with their page location in the Product Directory.

Section 2: Product Directory **1**
The core of the book, this section lists suppliers of 274 types of instruments and equipment needed in various minimally invasive procedures. The directory is divided alphabetically into 57 major product categories. Under each major heading, you'll find the devices included in that category listed alphabetically. For each device, the listings give the names, addresses, and phone numbers of all available suppliers, both domestic and foreign, again in alphabetical order. Included in the Product Directory, if the information has been made available by the manufacturer, are specific trade names of the devices offered by the company, plus detailed descriptions of these products.

Section 3: Supplier Profiles **175**
In this section you'll find additional information on each of the suppliers—domestic and foreign alike—listed in the Product Directory. Companies are listed alphabetically. Included in each entry are toll-free, Telex, TWX, and fax numbers and, when available, information on the company's sales volume, number of employees, and size of sales and marketing staff. For publicly owned companies, annual revenues and net income are also listed. You'll find information on the company's primary method of distribution and its Federal Procurement Eligibility, plus the names of several key executives. Minimally invasive surgery products supplied by the company are also listed.

FOREWORD

The explosive growth of laparoscopic surgery has sparked a profound revolution in the field of surgical instrumentation. The upheaval began five years ago with the advent of laparoscopic cholecystectomy. Prior to that time, laparoscopy had been limited to relatively simple gynecologic surgery and, in gastroenterology, a few diagnostic procedures. But when the first cholecystectomies were undertaken in 1988, the need for more advanced instruments immediately became clear.

The initial cholecystectomies were performed with basic gynecologic instrumentation. Insufflators rated at two to three liters per minute were the norm, and most were not pressure-regulated, making it difficult for the gynecologist and anesthesiologist to monitor and maintain adequate ventilation and CO_2 levels. Fortunately, most procedures performed prior to the introduction of laparoscopic cholecystectomy were relatively brief; but the more advanced operations that followed were a different matter. It was the need to support proper monitoring in these longer operations that led to the development of today's pressure-regulated insufflators.

The new, more difficult cases also required a higher flow rate to maintain pneumoperitoneum. Multiple trocar sites and frequent instrument changes caused a loss of volume. The use of cautery and lasers created smoke that had to be suctioned frequently, also reducing pneumoperitoneum. Six-liter-per-minute insufflators were a must to maintain visualization, but even these soon gave way to 10-liter-per-minute devices as more advanced procedures such as colon resection appeared on the scene. Currently, some insufflators top out at 15 liters per minute.

With increased demand for suction, irrigation and aspiration devices also underwent a metamorphosis. Powered irrigation/aspiration units were developed, and an array of new trumpet valves and hand pieces made their appearance.

Light sources, too, were of marginal clinical quality when laparoscopic cholecystectomy first was undertaken. In gynecologic procedures, the bright peritoneal surfaces of the pelvis had reflected light well enough to allow adequate visualization. But when the laparoscope was turned towards the upper abdomen, the dark surface of the liver absorbed much of the light. To accommodate the increased need for illumination, new high-output halogen and xenon light sources were soon introduced.

In 1988, the camera resolution needed for many of the more advanced laparoscopic procedures was marginal. The one-chip cameras of the time were steadily improved, but it was not until the advent of the three-chip camera that visualization became even better than in open surgery. Along with the new cameras came new, higher-resolution monitors. Now, a three-dimensional camera system has been developed. It promises to greatly enhance the surgeon's ability to visualize anatomic structures as they are seen by the naked eye during open surgery.

Grasping and retracting instrumentation also evolved in tandem with the advances in minimally invasive surgery. At the outset, it quickly became apparent that thick-walled, inflamed organs could not be grasped with available instrumentation. This prompted development of numerous specialized instruments to hold an inflamed gallbladder, acute appendix, or large ovary. Since basic graspers also proved traumatic to the intestine, bowel-grasping forceps with atraumatic jaws made their appearance. Today, grasper technology has advanced to the point that almost any instrument used in open surgery has a laparoscopic counterpart.

As laparoscopic surgery advanced, more and more dissections were performed; and it was soon evident that scissors would be dulled by the increased demand. New designs were developed to keep the blades approximating as they became worn; and disposable scissors were introduced to assure the surgeon of a sharp instrument for each case.

The surgeon's need to cut and coagulate simultaneously prompted exploration of a wide variety of energy sources. Laser was used in most early laparoscopic procedures, but due to cost and training constraints, quickly gave way to electrical surgery. While good generators were available from the outset, appropriate handpieces had to be developed. Then, when it became apparent that monopolar current had considerable inherent dangers, engineers were forced to design better insulation and safer instruments. Attention also turned to bipolar instrumentation, including bipolar scissors. To eliminate electrical energy altogether, some manufacturers have recently introduced ultrasonic cutting and coagulation devices. At the time of this writing, they show promising results.

A noteworthy entry in the monopolar surgical field is the argon beam coagulator. This device allows the surgeon to control bleeding from large oozing surfaces by directing a superficial spray of electrical energy across the entire field. For smaller bleeding sites, pharmaceutical companies entered the market with laparoscopic applicators for the topical hemostats typically used in open surgery.

Arguably the most significant advance in recent laparoscopic history was the introduction of the multiple-load clip applier. This development eliminated much of the need for tying—a painstakingly slow procedure in even the best of hands—and enabled rapid control of bleeding vessels and open ducts. Single-handedly, it transformed laparoscopic surgery from an often cumbersome procedure into a relatively efficient one. Direct off-shoots of this device include the intestinal anastomotic staplers, hernia staplers, and thoracic linear staplers that have made possible the widespread application of colectomy and herniorrhaphy.

Even with staplers available, surgeons still must have laparoscopic suturing skills. Great advances in needle-holder technology now permit the use of curved needles in laparoscopic surgery; and the development of numerous knot-tying instruments has eased the difficult task of tying a secure knot laparoscopically.

Clinical advances in laparoscopic surgery and the technological developments that support them are inextricably intertwined. It is even suggested that the trend to laparoscopic surgery has been driven by the instrument industry. The truth of the matter is quite the opposite. Though the industry has been phenomenally quick to respond, it is the clinicians who have identified the need for each new improvement.

This brief overview has only skimmed the surface of the amazing changes that have occurred in the past five years. There have also been significant improvements in trocars, needles, catheters, sutures, delivery systems, storage systems, drapes, and more. Details of these developments can be found in the commentaries that precede many of the major sections in the Product Directory portion of this book.

Despite the tremendous progress of the past five years, it seems that we have only begun to realize the full potential of minimally invasive surgery. As surgeons develop even better techniques—and manufacturers provide the means to implement them—the laparoscopic revolution is certain to continue its rapid expansion.

This book is designed to foster the spread of minimally invasive surgery by providing practitioners with a single consolidated source of information on both standard and newly developed equipment. With the cooperation and support of key innovators in this burgeoning field, we have endeavored to provide a practical, hands-on reference of value to the surgeon, nurse, purchasing agent, and administrator alike. For more information on the various ways this book can be used, we invite you to turn to the section that follows.

Eddie Joe Reddick, MD
William Saye, MD

HOW TO USE SURGEONS' REFERENCE™

Surgeons' Reference is the first medical product reference devoted entirely to the rapidly growing discipline of minimally invasive surgery. It's designed to provide you with a convenient, one-stop source of information on the array of specialized equipment these innovative procedures demand.

The core of the book is the Product Directory, which lists suppliers of 274 types of instruments and equipment needed in various minimally invasive procedures. These listings are supplemented by the book's other major section: the Supplier Profiles, which provides you with the contact information needed to place an order. At the beginning of the book, you'll find two indices to aid in locating the product information you need. Here's a more detailed look at each of these features.

PRODUCT DIRECTORY

This section is divided alphabetically into 57 major product categories. (See the table nearby for a list.) Under each major heading, you'll find the devices included in that category listed alphabetically. For each device, the listings give the names, addresses, and phone numbers of all available suppliers, both domestic and foreign, again in alphabetical order. In a number of key categories, you'll also find a commentary from Eddie Joe Reddick, MD, and William Saye, MD, the medical consultants to *Surgeons' Reference*.

Also included in the Product Directory, if the information has been made available by the manufacturer, are specific trade names of the devices offered by the company, plus detailed descriptions of these products. This information ranges from brief summaries of product specifications to complete package-insert-style documentation, with full details on such topics as indications, contraindications, precautions, instructions for use, and sterilization and maintenance guidelines.

MAJOR DEVICE CATEGORIES IN THE PRODUCT DIRECTORY

Accessories	*Endoscope*	*Needle*
Applier	*Esophagoscope*	*Nephroscope*
Arthroscope	*Forceps*	*Power Supply*
Aspirator	*Gastroscope*	*Probe*
Bag	*Holder*	*Pump*
Bronchoscope	*Imaging*	*Regulator*
Camera	*Instrument*	*Remover*
Cannula	*Insufflator*	*Retractor*
Catheter	*Irrigator*	*Scissors*
Choledochoscope	*Kit*	*Solution*
Clamp	*Knife*	*Suture*
Clip	*Laparoscope*	*System*
Coagulator	*Laryngoscope*	*Telescope*
Controller	*Laser*	*Tip*
Cutter	*Ligature*	*Trainer*
Dilator	*Light*	*Trocar*
Dispenser	*Lithotriptor*	*Ultrasound*
Drain	*Miscellaneous*	*Videointerface*
Electrocautery	*Monitor*	*Warmer*

SUPPLIER PROFILES

In this section you'll find additional information on each of the suppliers—domestic and foreign alike—listed in the Product Directory. Companies are listed alphabetically. Included in each entry are toll-free, Telex, TWX, and fax numbers and, when available, information on the company's sales volume, number of employees, and size of sales and marketing staff. For publicly owned companies, annual revenues and net income are also listed. You can also find information on the company's primary method of distribution. The alternatives and their meaning are as follows:

■ **Manufacturer Direct:** These companies manufacture most of their products themselves, and they are interested in selling directly to the end user. Their products may also be available from distributors, but they would prefer to have new customers contact them directly, to be served either by the manufacturer's own sales staff, or by a distributor assigned by the manufacturer.

■ **Manufacturer through Distributors:** These companies manufacture most of their products themselves, but do not prefer to deal directly with the end user. Unless negotiating a volume discount, new end users who are interested in these manufacturers' products should contact a local medical products distributor.

■ **Exclusive Distributor:** While these companies may manufacture some products themselves, they are primarily distributors. Furthermore, each is the exclusive distributor of the products listed in the entry. End users should contact these firms directly for information on the devices they supply.

Also included in each supplier's profile are the names of several key executives, enabling you more easily to contact the appropriate individual or department for further information or quotations. The company's Federal Procurement Eligibility is shown as well.

Listed in the profile are all minimally invasive surgery products supplied by the company. Products from the company that fall outside the scope of minimally invasive surgery can be found in *Medical Device Register*™.

TRADE NAME INDEX

If you're seeking detailed information on a specific brand or product line, this convenient index will direct you to the appropriate page in the Product Directory.

KEYWORD INDEX

For those times when you're not sure of the exact title of a particular type of device, this index provides you with a way of quickly locating it based on its attributes and applications. For example, in this index you'll find needle holders listed under such headings as "Needle," "Holder," and "Suture." Under each keyword heading, all associated products are listed alphabetically along with their page location in the Product Directory.

1
INDICES

Trade Name Index
If you're seeking detailed information on a specific brand or product line, this convenient index will direct you to the appropriate page in the Product Directory.

Keyword Index
For those times when you're not sure of the exact title of a particular type of device, this index provides you with a way of quickly locating it based on its attributes and applications. For example, in this index you'll find needle holders listed under such headings as "Needle," "Holder," and "Suture." Under each keyword heading, all associated products are listed alphabetically along with their page location in the Product Directory.

TRADE NAME INDEX

BiCOAG Forceps 101
BiLAP 60
CLV-S2O 27
Dexon II 154
EndoLumina 136
ENDOPATH Blunt Tip Trocar 166
ENDOPATH EAS 9
ENDOPATH ELC35 42
ENDOPATH ELC60 44
ENDOPATH EMS 10
ENDOPATH EZ35 47
ENDOPATH ILS 12
ENDOPATH Probe Plus 63
ENDOPATH Probe Plus II 64
ENDOPATH TriStar 167
Endovise 105
Gleeson FloVac 119
Laparoscopic Assist Devices
   8369 Series 148
Laparoscopic Assist Devices
   8570 Series 60
Laparoscopic Assist Devices
   8571 Series 61
Laparoscopic Assist Devices
   8572 Series 121
Laparoscopic Assist Device
   8572-03 132
Laparoscopic Assist Devices
   8573 & 8576 Series 62
Laparoscopic Assist Devices
   8574 Series 121
Laparoscopic Assist Devices
   8574 & 8575 132
Laparoscopic Assist Device
   8575-01 58
Laparoscopic Assist Device
   8575-02 121
Laparoscopic Assist Devices
   8577-01/-02 122
Laparoscopic Assist Device
   8578-01/-08 Series 59
Laparoscopic Assist Devices
   8579 Series 122

Laparoscopic Assist Device
   8580-01 54
Laparoscopic Assist Device
   8580-03 123
Laparoscopic Assist Device
   8580-04 124
Laparoscopic Assist Device
   8580-05 132
Lapro-Clip 8487 Series 42
Lapro-Clip 8487-00 7
Lapro-Clip 8487-98 9
Lapro-Clip 8487-99 147
Lapro-Loop 133
LIGACLIP ERCA 4
LIGACLIP MCA 5
LaparoBag 25
LaparoLith 140
LaparoOptx 39
LaparoScan 107
Maxon 155
NuSurg Laparoscopic Dispenser 53
NuSurg Laparoscopic
   Probe/Nerve Hook 114
NuSurg Thorascopic Dispenser 53
OES Telescope 130
OEV201 31
OTV-S4 OES TV System 32
Prestige 5mm Series 111
Prestige 10mm Series 97
Prestige 8364 Series 101
Prestige 8364-21 109
Prestige 8364-22 109
Prestige 8364-23 109
Prestige 8482-00 143
Professional Line 8374 Series 151
Professional Line 8375 Series 94
Professional Line
   8375 & 8376 Series 109
Professional Line
   8375 - 8450-17 Series 99
Professional Line 8375-01 41
Professional Line
   8375-09 - 8450-11 Series 99
Professional Line
   8376 & 8390 Series 100, 110

Professional Line
   8376 - 8450-14 Series 95
Professional Line
   8376 - 8450-15 Series 95
Professional Line 8377 Series ...91, 105
Professional Line 8378-02 113
Professional Line 8379-01 3
Professional Line 8380 Series 113
Professional Line 8381 Series 36
Professional Line 8381-02 145
Professional Line 8381-05 108
Professional Line 8381-06 36
Professional Line 8381-07 144
Professional Line 8381-09 115
Professional Line 8382 Series 101
Professional Line
   8384 & 8386 Series 159
Professional Line
   8385 & 8388 Series 158
Professional Line 8389 Series 79
Professional Line 8445 Series 164
Professional Line
   8447 & 8448 Series 165
Professional Line 8449 Series 165
PROXIMATE ILS 15
PROXIMATE Linear Cutter 50
PROXIMATE RH 20
PROXIMATE RHX 148
PROXIMATE RL PLUS 18
Select One Instruments 57
Select One Modular Instruments 58
Silk Sutures 156
Taut Operative Cholangiogram
   Catheters 37
TroGARD Electronic Trocar 163
Ultracision Harmonic Scalpel 66
Universal Plus Instrument System 58
URF-P2; Translaparoscopic
   Choledochoscope 40
UroOptx 89

KEYWORD INDEX

3-DIMENSIONAL
System, Camera,
   3-Dimensional......................32-34

5MM
Choledochoscope, Mini-Diameter
   (5mm or Less) 39-40

ABDOMINAL
Trocar, Abdominal 159-160

ABSORBABLE
Suture, Laparoscopy 154-156

AC-POWERED
Endoscope And Accessories,
   AC-Powered 77-78

ACCESSORIES
Accessories, Arthroscope............22-23
Accessories, Cleaning, Endoscopic......1
Accessories, Electrical Power
   (Electrocautery)..........................54
Accessories, Photographic,
   Endoscopic...............................1-2
Accessories, Surgical Camera 27
Cannula, Drainage, Arthroscopy 36
Cannula, Suction/Irrigation,
   Laparoscopic..............................36
Coagulator, Hysteroscopic
   (With Accessories) 54
Endoscope And Accessories,
   AC-Powered 77-78
Endoscope And Accessories,
   Battery-Powered 78
Equipment/Accessories, Laser,
   Laparoscopy......................132-133
Holder, Leg, Arthroscopy..............104
Holder, Shoulder, Arthroscopy.......106

ADAPTERS
Accessories, Electrical Power
   (Electrocautery)..........................54
Adapters, Bulb, Endoscope,
   Miscellaneous..............................2

AID
Trainer, Laparoscopy 157

AIR
Pump, Air, Non-Manual,
   Endoscopic..............................119

AMNIOSCOPE
Amnioscope, Transabdominal
   (Fetoscope)................................71
Endoscope, Transcervical
   (Amnioscope) 81

AMNIOTIC
Trocar, Amniotic 161

ANALYSIS
Computer, Image, Endoscopic........107

ANASTOMOSIS
Device, Anastomosis,
   Biofragmentable 140
Holder, Ring, Anastomosis............106
Sizer, Device, Anastomosis 142

ANESTHESIOLOGY
Bronchoscope, Flexible,
   Anesthesiology...........................72

ANGIOGRAPHY
Cart, Equipment, Video 139-140
Computer, Image, Endoscopic........107

ANGIOPLASTY
Cart, Equipment, Video 139-140

ANOSCOPE
Anoscope, Non-Powered 71-72

ANTI-FOG
Solution, Instrument, Laparoscopic,
   Anti-Fog..................................153

APPENDIX
Cannula, Extraction, Appendix.........36
Extractor, Gall Bladder 108

APPLIER
Applier, Clip, Laparoscopic............3-7
Applier, Clip, Repair, Hernia,
   Laparoscopic............................7-9
Applier, Ligature Clip...................7-8
Clip, Ligature..............................42
Stapler, Laparoscopic 9-20

ARC
Light Source, Endoscope,
   Xenon Arc...............................135

ARCHIVING
Camera, Video, Endoscopic 29-30
Camera, Videotape, Surgical............30
Computer, Image, Endoscopic........107
Tape, Television & Video,
   Endoscopic 34-35

ARM
System, Traction, Arthroscopy 143

ARTHROGRAM
Arthrogram Set...........................136

ARTHROSCOPE
Accessories, Arthroscope 22-23
Arthroscope 23-24
Cannula, Drainage, Arthroscopy 36

ARTHROSCOPY
Aspirator, Arthroscopy...................24
Cannula, Drainage, Arthroscopy 36
Cart, Equipment, Video 139-140
Holder, Leg, Arthroscopy..............104
Holder, Shoulder, Arthroscopy.......106
Insufflator, Other........................118
Needle, Suture, Arthroscopy 145
System, Traction, Arthroscopy 143

ASPIRATING
Drain, Suction, Closed...................54

ASPIRATION
Cannula, Suction, Pool-Tip 36
Needle, Aspiration, Cyst,
   Laparoscopic............................143
Needle, Puncture 145
Probe, Electrosurgery,
   Endoscopy............................64-66

ASPIRATOR
Aspirator, Arthroscopy...................24
Probe, Suction, Irrigator/Aspirator,
   Laparoscopic.....................121-123

ATRAUMATIC
Forceps, Grasping,
   Atraumatic 94-96

Forceps, Grasping,
  Traumatic..........................97-101
Gauge, Thickness, Tissue.............109

ATTACHMENT
Attachment, Binocular,
  Endoscopic..................................2
Teaching Attachment, Endoscopic......3

AUDIO
Camera, Cine, Endoscopic,
  With Audio...............................27
Camera, Cine, Endoscopic,
  Without Audio..........................27
Camera, Television, Endoscopic,
  With Audio...............................28
Camera, Television, Endoscopic,
  Without Audio..........................28
Camera, Television, Microsurgical,
  With Audio...............................28
Camera, Television, Microsurgical,
  Without Audio..........................28
Camera, Television, Surgical,
  With Audio...............................29
Camera, Television, Surgical,
  Without Audio..........................29

AUTOMATIC
Insufflator, Carbon-Dioxide, Automatic
  (For Endoscope).................116-117

BAG
Bag, Specimen, Laparoscopic......25-26

BALLOON
Cannula with Inflatable Balloon
  (Distal Tip)...............................35

BATTERY
Box, Battery, Pocket
  (Endoscopic)...........................145
Box, Battery, Rechargeable
  (Endoscopic)...........................145
Endoscope And Accessories,
  Battery-Powered.......................78
Power Supply, Endoscopic,
  Battery-Operated...............146-147

BILIARY
Introducer, T-Tube......................115

BINOCULAR
Attachment, Binocular,
  Endoscopic..................................2

BIOFRAGMENTABLE
Device, Anastomosis,
  Biofragmentable......................140

BIOPSY
Brush, Cytology, Endoscopic.........108
Forceps, Biopsy........................91-92

Instrument, Dissecting,
  Laparoscopic....................109-110
Instrument, Dissecting, Myoma,
  Laparoscopic...........................111
Needle, Biopsy, Mammary............143

BIPOLAR
Coagulator/Cutter, Endoscopic,
  Bipolar................................55-56

BLADDER
Extractor, Gall Bladder................108

BLADE
Blade, Knife, Laparoscopic............127
Knife, Laparoscopic.....................127

BLOOD
Endoscope, Fetal Blood
  Sampling..................................79
Probe, Detector, Flow, Blood,
  Laparoscopy, Ultrasonic............107

BLUNT
Dilator, Blunt..............................52

BOTTLE
Bottle, Endoscopic Wash..................2

BOUGIE
Bougie, Esophageal, And
  Gastrointestinal,...............136-139
Bougie, Esophageal, ENT.............139

BOWEL
Kit, Bowel.................................124

BOX
Box, Battery, Pocket
  (Endoscopic)...........................145
Box, Battery, Rechargeable
  (Endoscopic)...........................145

BRACE
Holder, Leg, Arthroscopy..............104
Holder, Shoulder, Arthroscopy......106

BRONCHOSCOPE
Bronchoscope, Flexible..................72
Bronchoscope, Flexible,
  Anesthesiology..........................72
Bronchoscope, Rigid.................72-73
Bronchoscope, Rigid,
  Non-Ventilating.........................73
Bronchoscope, Rigid, Ventilating......73

BRUSH
Accessories, Cleaning, Endoscopic.....1
Brush, Cytology, Endoscopic.........108

BULB
Adapter, Bulb, Endoscope,
  Miscellaneous.............................2
Bulb, Inflation (Endoscope)..............2

CABINET
Cabinet, Storage, Endoscope........139

CAMERA
Accessories, Surgical Camera..........27
Camera, Cine, Endoscopic,
  With Audio...............................27

Camera, Cine, Endoscopic,
  Without Audio..........................27
Camera, Still, Endoscopic..........27-28
Camera, Television, Endoscopic,
  With Audio...............................28
Camera, Television, Endoscopic,
  Without Audio..........................28
Camera, Television, Microsurgical,
  With Audio...............................28
Camera, Television, Microsurgical,
  Without Audio..........................28
Camera, Television, Surgical,
  With Audio...............................29
Camera, Television, Surgical,
  Without Audio..........................29
Camera, Video, Endoscopic......29-30
Camera, Video, Multi-Image.........30
Camera, Videotape, Surgical..........30
System, Camera,
  3-Dimensional......................32-34
Videointerface, Laparoscopic,
  Non-Removable Rod..................35

CANNULA
Cannula with Inflatable Balloon
  (Distal Tip)...............................35
Cannula, Drainage, Arthroscopy.....36
Cannula, Extraction, Appendix......36
Cannula, Suction, Pool-Tip............36
Cannula, Suction/Irrigation,
  Laparoscopic........................36-37
Cannula, Suprapubic,
  With Trocar..............................37
Trocar, Laparoscopic............163-168

CARBON
Insufflator, Automatic Carbon-Dioxide
  For Endoscope........................116
Insufflator, Carbon-Dioxide,
  Uterotubal..............................117

CARBON-DIOXIDE
Insufflator, Carbon-Dioxide, Automatic
  (For Endoscope).................116-117
Insufflator, Carbon-Dioxide,
  Uterotubal..............................117
Needle, Insufflation,
  Laparoscopic...........................144

CARDIOVASCULAR
Trocar, Cardiovascular...........161-162

CARRIER
Carrier, Sponge, Endoscopic.........108

CART
Cart, Equipment, Video.........139-140
Cart, Instrument/Equipment,
  Laparoscopy............................140

CATHETER
Catheter, Cholangiography.......37-38

CAUTERIZATION
Laser, Nd:YAG, Laparoscopy 133
Probe, Electrocauterization,
　Multi-Use 59-60
Probe, Electrocauterization,
　Single-Use 60-64

CAUTERY
Electrocautery Unit, Endoscopic 57
Electrode, Electrosurgery,
　Laparoscopic 57
Instrument, Electrosurgery,
　Laparoscopic 111-112
Module, Control, Electrosurgery 58

CAVITY
Dispenser, Laparoscopic 53
Dispenser, Thorascopic 53

CELL
Brush, Cytology, Endoscopic 108

CHOLANGIOGRAPHY
Catheter, Cholangiography 37-38
Clamp, Fixation,
　Cholangiography 41

CHOLECYSTECTOMY
Kit, Cholecystectomy 124-126

CHOLEDOCHOSCOPE
Choledochoscope,
　Flexible Or Rigid 39-40
Choledochoscope, Mini-Diameter
　(5mm or Less) 39

CINE
Camera, Cine, Endoscopic,
　With Audio 27
Camera, Cine, Endoscopic,
　Without Audio 27

CIRCULAR
Stapler, Laparoscopic 9-20

CLAMP
Clamp, Fixation,
　Cholangiography 41
Clamp, Laparoscopy 41

CLEANER
Sterilizer/Washer, Endoscope 142

CLEANING
Accessories, Cleaning, Endoscopic 1

CLIP
Applier, Clip, Laparoscopic 3-7
Applier, Clip, Repair, Hernia,
　Laparoscopic 7-9
Applier, Ligature Clip 7-8
Clip, Ligature 42
Clip, Suture 42
Remover, Clip 147-148
Stapler, Laparoscopic 9-20

CLOSED
Drain, Suction, Closed 54

COAGULATION
Probe, Electrosurgery,
　Endoscopy 64-66
Scalpel, Ultrasonic 66-70

COAGULATOR
Coagulator, Hysteroscopic
　(With Accessories) 54
Coagulator, Laparoscopic,
　Unipolar 54-56
Coagulator/Cutter, Endoscopic,
　Bipolar 55
Coagulator/Cutter, Endoscopic,
　Unipolar 56

COAGULATOR/CUTTER
Coagulator/Cutter, Endoscopic,
　Bipolar 55
Coagulator/Cutter, Endoscopic,
　Unipolar 56

COLON
Device, Anastomosis,
　Biofragmentable 140
Holder, Ring, Anastomosis 106
Sizer, Device, Anastomosis 142

COLONOSCOPE
Colonoscope, Gastro-Urology 73
Colonoscope, General &
　Plastic Surgery 73

COLPOSCOPE
Colposcope 73-74

COMPUTER
Computer, Image, Endoscopic 107

CONNECTOR
Connector, Suction/Irrigation 119

CONTAINER
Container, Specimen,
　Laparoscopic 140
Rack, Instrument, Laparoscopy 115

CONTROL
Module, Control, Electrosurgery 58

CORD
Accessories, Electrical Power
　(Electrocautery) 54
Cord, Electric, Endoscope 146

COVER
Cover, Laparoscope 127

CULDOSCOPE
Culdoscope 74

CURVED
Holder, Needle, Curved,
　Laparoscopic 104

CUTTER
Coagulator/Cutter, Endoscopic,
　Bipolar 55-56

Coagulator/Cutter, Endoscopic,
　Unipolar 56
Cutter, Linear, Laparoscopic 42-52

CYST
Needle, Aspiration, Cyst,
　Laparoscopic 143

CYSTOSCOPE
Cystoscope 74-75

CYSTOURETHROSCOPE
Cystourethroscope 75

CYTOLOGY
Brush, Cytology, Endoscopic 108

DATA
Computer, Image, Endoscopic 107

DETECTOR
Probe, Detector, Flow, Blood,
　Laparoscopy, Ultrasonic 107

DEVICE
Device, Anastomosis,
　Biofragmentable 140
Sizer, Device, Anastomosis 142

DIAGNOSTIC
Cystoscope 74, 89

DILATOR
Bougie, Esophageal, ENT 139
Dilator, Blunt 52
Dilator, Fascia, Umbilical 52
Dilator, Port, Laparoscopic 158

DIOXIDE
Insufflator, Automatic Carbon-Dioxide
　For Endoscope 116
Insufflator, Carbon-Dioxide,
　Uterotubal 117

DIRECT
Endoscope, Direct Vision 78

DISINFECTOR
Sterilizer/Washer, Endoscope 142

DISPENSER
Dispenser, Laparoscopic 53
Dispenser, Thorascopic 53

DISSECTING
Forceps, Biopsy 91-92
Forceps, Grasping,
　Traumatic 97-101
Forceps, Laparoscopy,
　Electrosurgical 101
Instrument, Dissecting,
　Laparoscopic 109-111
Instrument, Dissecting, Myoma,
　Laparoscopic 111
Instrument, Separating, Nerve 114

DISTAL
Cannula with Inflatable Balloon
 (Distal Tip).................................35
DOPPLER
Probe, Detector, Flow, Blood,
 Laparoscopy, Ultrasonic 107
DRAIN
Drain, Suction, Closed..................54
DRAINAGE
Cannula, Drainage, Arthroscopy 36
DRAPE
Cover, Laparoscope 127
DUCT
Introducer, T-Tube.......................115
DUODENOSCOPE
Duodenoscope, Esophago/Gastro 75
EFFUSION
Dispenser, Thorascopic...................53
ELECTRIC
Cord, Electric, Endoscope 146
ELECTRICAL
Accessories, Electrical Power
 (Electrocautery)...........................54
Sigmoidoscope, Rigid, Electrical.......87
Sigmoidoscope, Rigid,
 Non-Electrical........................87-88
ELECTRICITY
Generator, Power,
 Electrosurgical 146
ELECTROCAUTERIZATION
Forceps, Grasping,
 Traumatic..............................97-101
Laser, Nd:YAG, Laparoscopy 133
Probe, Electrocauterization,
 Multi-Use...............................59-60
Probe, Electrocauterization,
 Single-Use..............................60-64
ELECTROCAUTERY
Accessories, Electrical Power
 (Electrocautery)...........................54
Electrocautery Unit, Endoscopic.......57
Electrode, Electrosurgery,
 Laparoscopic...............................57
Handle, Instrument, Laparoscopic
 (Electrocautery)...........................58
Instrument, Electrosurgery,
 Laparoscopic......................111-112
Module, Control, Electrosurgery 58
Probe, Electrosurgery,
 Endoscopy.............................64-66
Scalpel, Ultrasonic....................66-70

ELECTRODE
Electrode, Electrosurgery,
 Laparoscopic...............................57
ELECTRONIC
Endoscope, Electronic
 (Videoendoscope)...................78-79
ELECTROSURGERY
Electrode, Electrosurgery,
 Laparoscopic...............................57
Forceps, Grasping,
 Traumatic..............................97-101
Instrument, Electrosurgery,
 Laparoscopic......................111-112
Module, Control, Electrosurgery 58
Probe, Electrosurgery,
 Endoscopy.............................64-66
ELECTROSURGICAL
Coagulator, Laparoscopic,
 Unipolar 54
Coagulator/Cutter, Endoscopic,
 Bipolar 55
Coagulator/Cutter, Endoscopic,
 Unipolar 56
Forceps, Electrosurgical.............92-93
Forceps, Laparoscopy,
 Electrosurgical 101-102
Generator, Power,
 Electrosurgical 146
Scissors, Laparoscopy,
 Electrosurgical 152
ENDOSCOPE
Adapter, Bulb, Endoscope,
 Miscellaneous...............................2
Amnioscope, Transabdominal
 (Fetoscope).................................71
Anoscope, Non-Powered 71-72
Arthroscope............................23-24
Bronchoscope, Flexible 72
Bronchoscope, Flexible,
 Anesthesiology 72
Bronchoscope, Rigid 72-73
Bronchoscope, Rigid,
 Non-Ventilating 73
Bronchoscope, Rigid, Ventilating......73
Bulb, Inflation (Endoscope)..............2
Cabinet, Storage, Endoscope.........139
Choledochoscope,
 Flexible Or Rigid 39-40
Colonoscope, Gastro-Urology..........73
Colonoscope,
 General & Plastic Surgery 73
Colposcope............................73-74
Connector, Suction/Irrigation.........119
Cord, Electric, Endoscope 146
Culdoscope..................................74
Cystoscope.............................74-75
Cystourethroscope.........................75
Duodenoscope, Esophago/Gastro 75
Endoscope..............................76-77
Endoscope And Accessories,
 AC-Powered...........................77-78

Endoscope And Accessories,
 Battery-Powered...........................78
Endoscope, Direct Vision 78
Endoscope, Electronic
 (Videoendoscope)...................78-79
Endoscope, Fetal Blood Sampling.....79
Endoscope, Flexible 79
Endoscope, Neurological 79
Endoscope, Rigid 79-81
Endoscope, Transcervical
 (Amnioscope) 81
Enteroscope.................................81
Esophagoscope
 (Flexible Or Rigid).......................91
Esophagoscope, Rigid,
 Gastro-Urology...........................91
Gastroduodenoscope......................81
Gastroscope, Flexible...................102
Gastroscope, Gastro-Urology...102-103
Gastroscope, General &
 Plastic Surgery..........................103
Gastroscope, Rigid......................103
Hysteroscope...........................81-82
Illuminator, Fiberoptic
 (For Endoscope) 134
Insufflator, Carbon-Dioxide, Automatic
 (For Endoscope) 116-117
Laparoscope, General &
 Plastic Surgery..........................128
Laparoscope, Gynecologic.......129-130
Laparoscope, Semi-Flexible...........130
Laryngoscope..........................82-83
Light Source, Endoscope,
 Xenon Arc................................135
Monitor, Video, Endoscope 31-32
Nasopharyngoscope
 (Flexible Or Rigid).......................83
Nephroscope, Flexible...............83-84
Nephroscope, Rigid 84
Observerscope..............................84
Panendoscope...............................84
Peritoneoscope.............................84
Pharyngoscope..............................85
Proctoscope............................85-86
Proctosigmoidoscope......................86
Pyeloscope...................................86
Resectoscope................................87
Sigmoidoscope, Flexible.................87
Sigmoidoscope, Rigid, Electrical.......87
Sigmoidoscope, Rigid,
 Non-Electrical........................87-88
Sphincteroscope............................88
Sterilizer/Washer,
 Endoscope.........................142-143
Telescope, Rigid, Endoscopic.........130
Thoracoscope..........................88-89
Transformer, Endoscope.................89
Ureteroscope...........................89-90
Urethroscope................................90
Vaginoscope.................................90
Warmer, Endoscope.....................172

ENDOSCOPIC
Accessories, Cleaning, Endoscopic......1
Accessories, Photographic,
　Endoscopic.....................................1-2
Attachment, Binocular, Endoscopic....2
Bottle, Endoscopic Wash 2
Box, Battery, Pocket
　(Endoscopic).................................145
Box, Battery, Rechargeable
　(Endoscopic).................................145
Brush, Cytology, Endoscopic 108
Camera, Cine, Endoscopic,
　With Audio 27
Camera, Cine, Endoscopic,
　Without Audio 27
Camera, Still, Endoscopic............27-28
Camera, Television, Endoscopic,
　With Audio 28
Camera, Television, Endoscopic,
　Without Audio 28
Camera, Video, Endoscopic 29-30
Carrier, Sponge, Endoscopic 108
Coagulator/Cutter, Endoscopic,
　Bipolar..55-56
Coagulator/Cutter, Endoscopic,
　Unipolar...56
Computer, Image, Endoscopic........107
Electrocautery Unit, Endoscopic.......57
Eyepiece, Lens, Non-Prescription,
　Endoscopic..2
Eyepiece, Lens, Prescription,
　Endoscopic..3
Forceps, Endoscopic 93-94
Forceps, Grasping, Flexible
　Endoscopic..................................96-97
Kit, Gastrostomy, Endoscopic,
　Percutaneous.................................125
Lamp, Endoscopic,
　Incandescent..........................134-135
Light, Surgical, Endoscopic 135-136
Mirror, Endoscopic 115
Needle, Endoscopic..................143-144
Obturator, Endoscopic 159
Power Supply, Endoscopic,
　Battery Operated 146
Power Supply, Endoscopic,
　Line Operated.......................146-147
Pump, Air, Non-Manual,
　Endoscopic....................................119
Sheath, Endoscopic 142
Snare, Endoscopic.....................115-116
Tape, Television & Video,
　Endoscopic................................34-35
Teaching Attachment, Endoscopic......3
Telescope, Rigid,
　Endoscopic............................130-131
Tube, Smoke Removal,
　Endoscopic..3

ENDOSCOPY
Cart, Equipment, Video 139-140
Generator, Power, Electrosurgical...146
Probe, Electrosurgery,
　Endoscopy..................................64-66

ENT
Bougie, Esophageal, ENT 139

ENTEROSCOPE
Enteroscope..81

EQUIPMENT
Cart, Equipment, Video 139-140
Cart, Instrument/Equipment,
　Laparoscopy..................................140
Equipment/Accessories, Laser,
　Laparoscopy..........................132-133
Equipment, Suction/Irrigation,
　Laparoscopic..........................119-120

ESOPHAGEAL
Bougie, Esophageal, And
　Gastrointestinal.....................136-139
Bougie, Esophageal, ENT 139
Prosthesis, Esophageal 141

ESOPHAGO/GASTRO
Duodenoscope, Esophago/Gastro 75

ESOPHAGOSCOPE
Esophagoscope
　(Flexible Or Rigid)..........................91
Esophagoscope, Rigid,
　Gastro-Urology...............................91

EXCISION
Forceps, Biopsy..........................91-92

EXTENSION
Dilator, Port, Laparoscopic............158

EXTRACTION
Cannula, Extraction, Appendix........36

EXTRACTOR
Extractor, Gall Bladder..................108

EYEPIECE
Eyepiece, Lens, Non-Prescription,
　Endoscopic..2
Eyepiece, Lens, Prescription,
　Endoscopic..3

FAN-TYPE
Retractor, Fan-Type,
　Laparoscopy..........................148-149

FASCIA
Dilator, Fascia, Umbilical.................52

FETAL
Endoscope, Fetal Blood Sampling.....79

FETOSCOPE
Amnioscope, Transabdominal
　(Fetoscope).....................................71

FIBEROPTIC
Illuminator, Fiberoptic
　(For Endoscope) 134

FIXATION
Clamp, Fixation,
　Cholangiography............................41
Clamp, Laparoscopy 41

FLEXIBLE
Bronchoscope, Flexible 72
Bronchoscope, Flexible,
　Anesthesiology................................72
Cabinet, Storage, Endoscope..........139
Choledochoscope,
　Flexible Or Rigid 39-40
Cystoscope...................................74-75
Endoscope, Flexible 79
Esophagoscope
　(Flexible Or Rigid)..........................91
Forceps, Grasping,
　Flexible Endoscopic..................96-97
Gastroscope, Flexible......................102
Laparoscope, Flexible 127
Nasopharyngoscope
　(Flexible Or Rigid)..........................83
Nephroscope, Flexible................83-84
Sigmoidoscope, Flexible 87
Sterilizer/Washer, Endoscope...142-143

FLOW
Probe, Detector, Flow, Blood,
　Laparoscopy, Ultrasonic 107

FLUID
Probe, Suction, Irrigator/Aspirator,
　Laparoscopic..................................121

FORCEPS
Extractor, Gall Bladder..................108
Forceps, Biopsy..........................91-92
Forceps, Electrosurgical..............92-93
Forceps, Endoscopic 93-94
Forceps, Grasping,
　Atraumatic 94-96
Forceps, Grasping, Flexible
　Endoscopic.................................96-97
Forceps, Grasping,
　Traumatic 97-101
Forceps, Laparoscopy,
　Electrosurgical 101-102

FURNITURE
Cabinet, Storage, Endoscope..........139

GALL
Extractor, Gall Bladder..................108

GALLBLADDER
Trocar, Gallbladder 162-163

GAS
Needle, Insufflation,
　Laparoscopic..................................144

GASTRO-UROLOGY
Bougie, Esophageal, And
　Gastrointestinal.....................136-139
Colonoscope, Gastro-Urology..........73
Esophagoscope, Rigid,
　Gastro-Urology...............................91
Gastroscope, Gastro-Urology........102
Trocar, Gastro-Urology 163

GASTRODUODENOSCOPE
Gastroduodenoscope......................81

GASTROESOPHAGEAL
Duodenoscope, Esophago/Gastro 75

GASTROINTESTINAL
Bougie, Esophageal, And
    Gastrointestinal..................136-139

GASTROSCOPE
Gastroscope, Flexible....................102
Gastroscope,
    Gastro-Urology..................102-103
Gastroscope,
    General & Plastic Surgery..........103
Gastroscope, Rigid......................103

GASTROSTOMY
Kit, Gastrostomy, Endoscopic,
    Percutaneous............................125

GAUGE
Gauge, Thickness, Tissue...............109

GENERAL
Colonoscope,
    General & Plastic Surgery............73
Gastroscope,
    General & Plastic Surgery..........103
Laparoscope,
    General & Plastic Surgery....128-129

GENERATOR
Generator, Power,
    Electrosurgical.........................146

GRASPING
Extractor, Gall Bladder.................108
Forceps, Grasping,
    Atraumatic..........................94-96
Forceps, Grasping,
    Flexible Endoscopic...............96-97
Forceps, Grasping,
    Traumatic..........................97-101

GRIP
Handle, Instrument, Laparoscopic
    (Electrocautery)..........................58

GYNECOLOGIC
Laparoscope, Gynecologic........129-130

HANDLE
Blade, Knife, Laparoscopic............127
Handle, Instrument, Laparoscopic
    (Electrocautery)..........................58
Handle, Instrument,
    Laparoscopic (Irrigation)............121
Knife, Laparoscopic......................127

HERNIA
Applier, Clip, Repair, Hernia,
    Laparoscopic............................7-9

HOLDER
Holder, Instrument,
    Laparoscopic..........................103
Holder, Laparoscope............103-104
Holder, Leg, Arthroscopy..............104
Holder, Needle, Curved,
    Laparoscopic..........................104
Holder, Needle,
    Laparoscopic...................105-106

Holder, Ring, Anastomosis............106
Holder, Shoulder, Arthroscopy.......106
Holder/Scissors, Needle,
    Laparoscopic..........................106
Instrument, Knot Tying, Suture,
    Laparoscopic..........................113
Instrument, Needle
    Holder/Knot Tying...............113-114
Instrument, Passing, Suture,
    Laparoscopic..........................114
Retractor, Fan-Type,
    Laparoscopy............................148
Retractor, Laparoscopy, Other.......149

HOLDER/SCISSORS
Holder/Scissors, Needle,
    Laparoscopic..........................106

HYSTEROSCOPE
Hysteroscope..........................81-82

HYSTEROSCOPIC
Coagulator, Hysteroscopic
    (With Accessories).....................54
Insufflator, Hysteroscopic.............117

ILLUMINATOR
Illuminator, Fiberoptic
    (For Endoscope)......................134

IMAGE
Computer, Image, Endoscopic........107

IMAGING
System, Imaging, Laparoscopy,
    Ultrasonic..............................107

IMPLANT
Prosthesis, Esophageal.................141

INCANDESCENT
Lamp, Endoscopic,
    Incandescent....................134-135

INFLATABLE
Cannula with Inflatable Balloon
    (Distal Tip)................................35

INFLATION
Bulb, Inflation (Endoscope)...............2

INSTRUMENT
Cart, Instrument/Equipment,
    Laparoscopy............................140
Handle, Instrument, Laparoscopic
    (Electrocautery)..........................58
Handle, Instrument,
    Laparoscopic (Irrigation)............121
Holder, Instrument, Laparoscopic...103
Instrument, Dissecting,
    Laparoscopic....................109-111
Instrument, Dissecting, Myoma,
    Laparoscopic..........................111
Instrument, Electrosurgery,
    Laparoscopic....................111-112
Instrument, Knot Tying, Suture,
    Laparoscopic..........................113
Instrument, Needle
    Holder/Knot Tying...............113-114

Instrument, Passing, Suture,
    Laparoscopic..........................114
Instrument, Separating,
    Nerve................................114-115
Knob, Instrument, Rotating...........140
Rack, Instrument, Laparoscopy......115
Solution, Instrument, Laparoscopic,
    Anti-Fog.................................153
Tray, Sterilization, Instrument........143

INSTRUMENT/EQUIPMENT
Cart, Instrument/Equipment,
    Laparoscopy............................140

INSUFFLATION
Needle, Insufflation,
    Laparoscopic....................144-145

INSUFFLATOR
Insufflator, Carbon-Dioxide, Automatic
    (For Endoscope)................116-117
Insufflator, Carbon-Dioxide,
    Uterotubal..............................117
Insufflator, Hysteroscopic.............117
Insufflator, Laparoscopic.........117-118
Insufflator, Other..................118-119
Insufflator, Vaginal......................119

INTRODUCER
Introducer, T-Tube......................115

IRRIGATION
Aspirator, Arthroscopy...................24
Cannula, Suction/Irrigation,
    Laparoscopic........................36-37
Connector, Suction/Irrigation.........119
Handle, Instrument,
    Laparoscopic (Irrigation)............121
Probe, Electrosurgery,
    Endoscopy...........................64-66
Tubing, Irrigation...................123-124

IRRIGATOR
Probe, Suction, Irrigator/Aspirator,
    Laparoscopic....................121-123

IRRIGATOR/ASPIRATOR
Probe, Suction, Irrigator/Aspirator,
    Laparoscopic....................121-123

KIDNEY
Nephroscope, Flexible...............83-84
Nephroscope, Rigid.......................84

KIT
Kit, Bowel................................124
Kit, Cholecystectomy.............124-125
Kit, Gastrostomy, Endoscopic,
    Percutaneous..........................125
Kit, Laparoscopy..................125-126
Kit, Pelviscopy...........................126
Kit, Trocar................................126

KNIFE
Blade, Knife, Laparoscopic 127
Cutter, Linear, Laparoscopic.......42-52
Instrument, Dissecting,
    Laparoscopic 109-110
Instrument, Dissecting, Myoma,
    Laparoscopic 111
Knife, Laparoscopic 127
Scalpel, Ultrasonic...................66-70
Scissors with Removable Tips,
    Laparoscopy 151
Scissors, Laparoscopy............151-152

KNOB
Knob, Instrument, Rotating 140

KNOT
Holder, Needle, Curved,
    Laparoscopic 104
Holder, Needle, Laparoscopic........105
Holder/Scissors, Needle,
    Laparoscopic 106
Instrument, Knot Tying, Suture,
    Laparoscopic 113
Instrument, Needle
    Holder/Knot Tying 113-114

LAMP
Lamp, Endoscopic,
    Incandescent..................134-135

LAPAROSCOPE
Connector, Suction/Irrigation.........119
Cover, Laparoscope 127
Holder, Laparoscope.............103-104
Laparoscope, Flexible 127
Laparoscope,
    General & Plastic Surgery 128-129
Laparoscope, Gynecologic.......129-130
Laparoscope, Semi-Flexible...........130

LAPAROSCOPIC
Applier, Clip, Laparoscopic............3-7
Applier, Clip, Repair, Hernia,
    Laparoscopic 7-9
Bag, Specimen, Laparoscopic 25-26
Blade, Knife, Laparoscopic 127
Cannula, Suction/Irrigation,
    Laparoscopic.....................36-37
Coagulator, Laparoscopic,
    Unipolar............................54-55
Container, Specimen,
    Laparoscopic 140
Cutter, Linear, Laparoscopic.......42-52
Dilator, Port, Laparoscopic 158-159
Dispenser, Laparoscopic 53
Electrode, Electrosurgery,
    Laparoscopic 57
Equipment, Suction/Irrigation,
    Laparoscopic 119-120
Handle, Instrument, Laparoscopic
    (Electrocautery)........................58
Handle, Instrument, Laparoscopic
    (Irrigation).............................121

Holder, Instrument,
    Laparoscopic 103
Holder, Needle, Curved,
    Laparoscopic 104
Holder, Needle,
    Laparoscopic 105-106
Holder/Scissors, Needle,
    Laparoscopic 106
Instrument, Dissecting,
    Laparoscopic 109-110
Instrument, Dissecting, Myoma,
    Laparoscopic 111
Instrument, Electrosurgery,
    Laparoscopic 111-112
Instrument, Knot Tying, Suture,
    Laparoscopic 113
Instrument, Passing, Suture,
    Laparoscopic 114
Insufflator, Laparoscopic 117-118
Knife, Laparoscopic 127
Ligature, Laparoscopic 133
Lithotriptor, Laparoscopic 140-141
Needle, Aspiration, Cyst,
    Laparoscopic 143
Needle, Insufflation,
    Laparoscopic 144-145
Probe, Suction, Irrigator/Aspirator,
    Laparoscopic 121
Solution, Instrument, Laparoscopic,
    Anti-Fog..............................153
Stapler, Laparoscopic 9-20
Trocar,
    Laparoscopic 163-168
Videointerface, Laparoscopic,
    Non-Removable Rod 35

LAPAROSCOPY
Cart, Instrument/Equipment,
    Laparoscopy 140
Clamp, Laparoscopy 41
Equipment/Accessories, Laser,
    Laparoscopy 132-133
Forceps, Laparoscopy,
    Electrosurgical 101-102
Kit, Laparoscopy 125-126
Laser, Nd:YAG, Laparoscopy 133
Probe, Detector, Flow, Blood,
    Laparoscopy, Ultrasonic 107
Rack, Instrument, Laparoscopy......115
Retractor, Fan-Type,
    Laparoscopy.....................148-149
Retractor, Laparoscopy, Other.......149
Scissors with Removable Tips,
    Laparoscopy 151
Scissors, Laparoscopy............151-152
Scissors, Laparoscopy,
    Electrosurgical 152
Suture, Laparoscopy 154-156
System, Imaging, Laparoscopy,
    Ultrasonic..............................107
Trainer, Laparoscopy 157

LARYNGEAL
Trocar, Laryngeal 169

LARYNGOSCOPE
Laryngoscope...........................82-83

LASER
Equipment/Accessories, Laser,
    Laparoscopy 132-133
Laser, Nd:YAG, Laparoscopy 133

LEG
Holder, Leg, Arthroscopy..............104

LENS
Eyepiece, Lens, Non-Prescription,
    Endoscopic................................2
Eyepiece, Lens, Prescription,
    Endoscopic................................3

LESS
Choledochoscope, Mini-Diameter
    (5mm or Less)..........................39

LIGATURE
Applier, Clip, Laparoscopic............3-7
Applier, Ligature Clip..................7-8
Clip, Ligature................................42
Ligature, Laparoscopic 133

LIGHT
Illuminator, Fiberoptic
    (For Endoscope) 134
Lamp, Endoscopic,
    Incandescent 134
Light Source, Endoscope,
    Xenon Arc............................135
Light, Surgical, Endoscopic 135-136

LINE
Power Supply, Endoscopic,
    Line Operated 146

LINEAR
Cutter, Linear, Laparoscopic.......42-52
Stapler, Laparoscopic 9-20

LITHOSCOPE
Cystoscope...............................74-75

LITHOTRIPTOR
Lithotriptor, Laparoscopic 140-141

LIVER
Retractor, Fan-Type,
    Laparoscopy 148

MAMMARY
Needle, Biopsy, Mammary 143

MAMMOGRAPHY
Needle, Biopsy, Mammary 143

MANUAL
Pump, Air, Non-Manual,
    Endoscopic 119

MEDICATION
Dispenser, Laparoscopic 53

MICROSCOPE
Colposcope...............................73-74

MICROSURGICAL
Camera, Television, Microsurgical,
    With Audio 28
Camera, Television, Microsurgical,
    Without Audio 28

MINI-DIAMETER
Choledochoscope, Mini-Diameter
    (5mm or Less) 39-40

MIRROR
Mirror, Endoscopic 115

MISCELLANEOUS
Adapter, Bulb, Endoscope,
    Miscellaneous 2

MODULE
Module, Control, Electrosurgery 58

MONITOR
Cart, Equipment, Video 139-140
Monitor, Video, Endoscope 31-32

MULTI-IMAGE
Camera, Video, Multi-Image 30

MULTI-USE
Probe, Electrocauterization,
    Multi-Use 59-60

MYOMA
Instrument, Dissecting, Myoma,
    Laparoscopic 111

NASOPHARYNGOSCOPE
Nasopharyngoscope
    (Flexible Or Rigid) 83

ND:YAG
Equipment/Accessories, Laser,
    Laparoscopy 132-133
Laser, Nd:YAG, Laparoscopy 133

NEEDLE
Gauge, Thickness, Tissue 109
Holder, Needle, Curved,
    Laparoscopic 104
Holder, Needle,
    Laparoscopic 105-106
Holder/Scissors, Needle,
    Laparoscopic 106
Instrument, Knot Tying, Suture,
    Laparoscopic 113
Instrument, Needle
    Holder/Knot Tying 113-114
Instrument, Passing, Suture,
    Laparoscopic 114
Needle, Aspiration, Cyst,
    Laparoscopic 143
Needle, Biopsy, Mammary 143
Needle, Endoscopic 143-144
Needle, Insufflation,
    Laparoscopic 144-145
Needle, Puncture 145
Needle, Suture, Arthroscopy 145
Trocar, Amniotic 161
Trocar, Cardiovascular 161-162
Trocar, Other 169-170

NEODYMIUM
Equipment/Accessories, Laser,
    Laparoscopy 5
Laser, Nd:YAG, Laparoscopy 133

NEPHROSCOPE
Cystoscope 74-75
Nephroscope, Flexible 83-84
Nephroscope, Rigid 84
Pyeloscope 86

NERVE
Instrument, Separating,
    Nerve 114-115

NEUROLOGICAL
Endoscope, Neurological 79

NON-ABSORBABLE
Suture, Laparoscopy 154-156

NON-ELECTRICAL
Sigmoidoscope, Rigid,
    Non-Electrical 87-88

NON-MANUAL
Pump, Air, Non-Manual,
    Endoscopic 119

NON-POWERED
Anoscope, Non-Powered 71-72

NON-PRESCRIPTION
Eyepiece, Lens, Non-Prescription,
    Endoscopic 2

NON-REMOVABLE
Videointerface, Laparoscopic,
    Non-Removable Rod 35

NON-TRAUMATIC
Forceps, Grasping,
    Atraumatic 94-96
Forceps, Grasping,
    Traumatic 97-101
Gauge, Thickness, Tissue 109

NON-VENTILATING
Bronchoscope, Rigid,
    Non-Ventilating 73

OBSERVERSCOPE
Observerscope 84

OBTURATOR
Obturator, Endoscopic 159

OPERATED
Power Supply, Endoscopic,
    Battery Operated 146
Power Supply, Endoscopic,
    Line Operated 146

OPHTHALMIC
Eyepiece, Lens, Prescription,
    Endoscopic 3

ORGAN
Retractor, Laparoscopy, Other 149

OTHER
Insufflator, Other 118-119
Retractor, Laparoscopy, Other 149
Trocar, Other 169-170

PANENDOSCOPE
Panendoscope 84

PASSING
Instrument, Passing, Suture,
    Laparoscopic 114

PEG
Kit, Gastrostomy, Endoscopic,
    Percutaneous 125

PELVISCOPY
Kit, Pelviscopy 126

PERCUTANEOUS
Kit, Gastrostomy, Endoscopic,
    Percutaneous 125

PERITONEOSCOPE
Peritoneoscope 84

PHARYNGOSCOPE
Pharyngoscope 85

PHOTOGRAPHIC
Accessories, Photographic,
    Endoscopic 1-2
Accessories, Surgical Camera 27
Camera, Cine, Endoscopic,
    With Audio 27
Camera, Cine, Endoscopic,
    Without Audio 27
Camera, Still, Endoscopic 27-28
Camera, Television, Endoscopic,
    With Audio 28
Camera, Television, Endoscopic,
    Without Audio 28
Camera, Television, Microsurgical,
    With Audio 28
Camera, Television, Microsurgical,
    Without Audio 28
Camera, Television, Surgical,
    With Audio 29
Camera, Television, Surgical,
    Without Audio 29
Camera, Videotape, Surgical 30

PLASTIC
Colonoscope,
    General & Plastic Surgery 73
Gastroscope,
    General & Plastic Surgery 103
Laparoscope,
    General & Plastic Surgery ...128-129

PLEURAL
Dispenser, Thorascopic 53

PNEUMOPERITONEUM
Needle, Insufflation,
    Laparoscopic 144

POCKET
Box, Battery, Pocket
    (Endoscopic) 145

POOL-TIP
Cannula, Suction, Pool-Tip 36

PORT
Dilator, Port, Laparoscopic 158-159
Kit, Trocar 126
Sleeve, Trocar 159
Trocar, Abdominal 159-160
Trocar, Laparoscopic 163-168
Trocar, Other 169-170
Trocar, Short 170
Trocar, Thoracic 170

POWER
Accessories, Electrical Power
 (Electrocautery) 54
Generator, Power,
 Electrosurgical 146
Power Supply, Endoscopic,
 Battery Operated 146
Power Supply, Endoscopic,
 Line Operated 146-147

POWERED
Anoscope, Non-Powered 71-72
Endoscope And Accessories,
 AC-Powered 77-78
Endoscope And Accessories,
 Battery-Powered 78

PRE-TIED
Suture, Laparoscopy 154-156

PRESCRIPTION
Eyepiece, Lens, Prescription,
 Endoscopic 3

PROBE
Probe, Detector, Flow, Blood,
 Laparoscopy, Ultrasonic 107
Probe, Electrocauterization,
 Multi-Use 59-60
Probe, Electrocauterization,
 Single-Use 60-64
Probe, Electrosurgery,
 Endoscopy 64-66
Probe, Suction, Irrigator/Aspirator,
 Laparoscopic 121-123
System, Imaging, Laparoscopy,
 Ultrasonic 107

PROCESSOR
Sterilizer/Washer, Endoscope 142

PROCTOSCOPE
Proctoscope 85-86

PROCTOSIGMOIDOSCOPE
Proctosigmoidoscope 86

PROSTHESIS
Prosthesis, Esophageal 141

PUMP
Aspirator, Arthroscopy 24
Pump, Air, Non-Manual,
 Endoscopic 119

PUNCTURE
Needle, Puncture 145

PYELOSCOPE
Pyeloscope 86

RACK
Rack, Instrument, Laparoscopy 115

REAL-TIME
System, Imaging, Laparoscopy,
 Ultrasonic 107

RECHARGEABLE
Box, Battery, Rechargeable
 (Endoscopic) 145

REMOVABLE
Scissors with Removable Tips,
 Laparoscopy 151

REMOVAL
Remover, Staple, Surgical 148
Tube, Smoke Removal,
 Endoscopic 3

REMOVER
Remover, Clip 147-148
Remover, Staple, Surgical 148

REPAIR
Applier, Clip, Repair, Hernia,
 Laparoscopic 7-9

RESECTOSCOPE
Resectoscope 87

REST
Holder, Leg, Arthroscopy 104
Holder, Shoulder, Arthroscopy 106

RETAINER
Holder, Instrument,
 Laparoscopic 103

RETRACTOR
Retractor, Fan-Type,
 Laparoscopy 148-149
Retractor, Laparoscopy, Other 149

RIGID
Bronchoscope, Rigid 72-73
Bronchoscope, Rigid,
 Non-Ventilating 73
Bronchoscope, Rigid, Ventilating ... 73
Choledochoscope,
 Flexible Or Rigid 39-40
Cystoscope 74-75
Endoscope, Rigid 79-81
Esophagoscope
 (Flexible Or Rigid) 91
Esophagoscope, Rigid,
 Gastro-Urology 91
Gastroscope, Rigid 103
Nasopharyngoscope
 (Flexible Or Rigid) 83
Nephroscope, Rigid 84
Sigmoidoscope, Rigid, Electrical 87
Sigmoidoscope, Rigid,
 Non-Electrical 87-88
Sterilizer/Washer, Endoscope 142
Telescope, Rigid, Endoscopic ... 130-131

RING
Holder, Ring, Anastomosis 106

ROD
Videointerface, Laparoscopic,
 Non-Removable Rod 35

ROTATING
Knob, Instrument, Rotating 140

SAMPLE
Bag, Specimen, Laparoscopic ... 25-26
Instrument, Dissecting,
 Laparoscopic 109-110
Instrument, Dissecting, Myoma,
 Laparoscopic 111

SAMPLER
Brush, Cytology, Endoscopic 108

SAMPLING
Endoscope, Fetal Blood Sampling 79

SANITIZER
Sterilizer/Washer, Endoscope 142

SCALPEL
Blade, Knife, Laparoscopic 127
Knife, Laparoscopic 127
Scalpel, Ultrasonic 66-70
Scissors with Removable Tips,
 Laparoscopy 151
Scissors, Laparoscopy 151-152

SCISSORS
Blade, Knife, Laparoscopic 127
Holder/Scissors, Needle,
 Laparoscopic 106
Instrument, Dissecting,
 Laparoscopic 109-110
Instrument, Dissecting, Myoma,
 Laparoscopic 111
Knife, Laparoscopic 127
Scissors with Removable Tips,
 Laparoscopy 151
Scissors, Laparoscopy 151-152
Scissors, Laparoscopy,
 Electrosurgical 152

SCOPE
Pyeloscope 86

SEMI-FLEXIBLE
Laparoscope, Semi-Flexible 130

SEPARATING
Instrument, Separating,
 Nerve 114-115

SHEATH
Sheath, Endoscopic 142

SHORT
Trocar, Short 170

SHOULDER
Holder, Shoulder, Arthroscopy 106
System, Traction, Arthroscopy 143

SIGMOIDOSCOPE
Sigmoidoscope, Flexible 87
Sigmoidoscope, Rigid, Electrical 87

Sigmoidoscope, Rigid,
 Non-Electrical 87-88
SIMULATION
Trainer, Laparoscopy 157
SINGLE-USE
Probe, Electrocauterization,
 Single-Use 60-64
SINUS
Trocar, Sinus 170
SIZER
Sizer, Device, Anastomosis 142
SLEEVE
Dilator, Port, Laparoscopic 158
Sleeve, Trocar 159
SMOKE
Tube, Smoke Removal,
 Endoscopic 3
SNARE
Snare, Endoscopic 115-116
SOLUTION
Solution, Instrument, Laparoscopic,
 Anti-Fog 153
SOURCE
Light Source, Endoscope,
 Xenon Arc 135
SPECIMEN
Bag, Specimen, Laparoscopic 25-26
Container, Specimen,
 Laparoscopic 140
SPHINCTEROSCOPE
Sphincteroscope 88
SPONGE
Carrier, Sponge, Endoscopic 108
STAPLE
Remover, Staple, Surgical 148
Stapler, Surgical 20-22
STAPLER
Applier, Clip, Laparoscopic 3-7
Applier, Clip, Repair, Hernia,
 Laparoscopic 7
Applier, Ligature Clip 7-8
Stapler, Laparoscopic 9-20
Stapler, Surgical 20-22
STERILIZATION
Cover, Laparoscope 127
Rack, Instrument, Laparoscopy 115
Tray, Sterilization, Instrument 143
STERILIZER/WASHER
Sterilizer/Washer,
 Endoscope 142-143
STILL
Camera, Still, Endoscopic 27-28

STORAGE
Cabinet, Storage, Endoscope 139
Computer, Image, Endoscopic 107
Rack, Instrument, Laparoscopy 115
STRUCTURE
Instrument, Separating, Nerve 114
SUCTION
Aspirator, Arthroscopy 24
Cannula, Suction, Pool-Tip 36
Cannula, Suction/Irrigation,
 Laparoscopic 36
Connector, Suction/Irrigation 119
Drain, Suction, Closed 54
Handle, Instrument, Laparoscopic
 (Irrigation) 121
Needle, Puncture 145
Probe, Electrosurgery,
 Endoscopy 64-66
Probe, Suction, Irrigator/Aspirator,
 Laparoscopic 121-123
Tubing, Irrigation 123-124
SUCTION/IRRIGATION
Cannula, Suction/Irrigation,
 Laparoscopic 36-37
Connector, Suction/Irrigation 119
Equipment, Suction/Irrigation,
 Laparoscopic 119-120
SUPPLY
Power Supply, Endoscopic,
 Battery Operated 146
Power Supply, Endoscopic,
 Line Operated 146-147
SUPPORT
Holder, Leg, Arthroscopy 104
Holder, Shoulder, Arthroscopy 106
SUPRAPUBIC
Cannula, Suprapubic, With Trocar ... 37
SURGERY
Cart, Equipment, Video 139-140
Colonoscope,
 General & Plastic Surgery 73
Computer, Image, Endoscopic 107
Gastroscope,
 General & Plastic Surgery 103
Holder, Leg, Arthroscopy 104
Holder, Shoulder, Arthroscopy 106
Laparoscope,
 General & Plastic Surgery 128-129
SURGICAL
Accessories, Surgical Camera 27
Aspirator, Arthroscopy 24
Camera, Television, Surgical,
 With Audio 29
Camera, Television, Surgical,
 Without Audio 29
Camera, Videotape, Surgical 30
Electrocautery Unit, Endoscopic 57
Light, Surgical, Endoscopic 135-136
Remover, Staple, Surgical 148
Stapler, Surgical 20-22
Trocar, Surgical 170

SUTURE
Applier, Clip, Laparoscopic 3-7
Applier, Clip, Repair, Hernia,
 Laparoscopic 7
Applier, Ligature Clip 7-8
Clip, Ligature 42
Clip, Suture 42
Gauge, Thickness, Tissue 109
Holder, Needle, Curved,
 Laparoscopic 104
Holder, Needle,
 Laparoscopic 105-106
Holder/Scissors, Needle,
 Laparoscopic 106
Instrument, Knot Tying, Suture,
 Laparoscopic 113
Instrument, Needle
 Holder/Knot Tying 113-114
Instrument, Passing, Suture,
 Laparoscopic 114
Needle, Suture, Arthroscopy 145
Remover, Staple, Surgical 148
Stapler, Laparoscopic 9-20
Stapler, Surgical 20-22
Suture, Laparoscopy 154-156
SYSTEM
System, Camera,
 3-Dimensional 32-34
System, Imaging, Laparoscopy,
 Ultrasonic 107
System, Traction, Arthroscopy 143
T-TUBE
Introducer, T-Tube 115
TAPE
Tape, Television & Video,
 Endoscopic 34-35
TEACHING
Observerscope 84
Teaching Attachment, Endoscopic 3
Trainer, Laparoscopy 157
TELESCOPE
Telescope, Rigid,
 Endoscopic 130-131
TELEVISION
Camera, Television, Endoscopic,
 With Audio 28
Camera, Television, Endoscopic,
 Without Audio 28
Camera, Television, Microsurgical,
 With Audio 28
Camera, Television, Microsurgical,
 Without Audio 28
Camera, Television, Surgical,
 With Audio 29
Camera, Television, Surgical,
 Without Audio 29
Tape, Television & Video,
 Endoscopic 34-35

THERMAL
Electrocautery Unit, Endoscopic 57
THICKNESS
Gauge, Thickness, Tissue 109
THORACIC
Trocar, Thoracic 170-171
THORACOSCOPE
Thoracoscope 88-89
THORASCOPIC
Dispenser, Thorascopic 53
TIP
Cannula with Inflatable Balloon
    (Distal Tip) 35
Probe, Electrocauterization,
    Multi-Use 59-60
Probe, Electrocauterization,
    Single-Use 60-64
Probe, Suction, Irrigator/Aspirator,
    Laparoscopic 121
TIPS
Scissors with Removable Tips,
    Laparoscopy 151
TISSUE
Gauge, Thickness, Tissue 109
Retractor, Laparoscopy, Other 149
TRACHEAL
Trocar, Tracheal 171-172
TRACTION
System, Traction, Arthroscopy 143
TRAINER
Teaching Attachment, Endoscopic 3
Trainer, Laparoscopy 157
TRAINING
Observerscope 84
Teaching Attachment, Endoscopic 3
TRANSABDOMINAL
Amnioscope, Transabdominal
    (Fetoscope) 71
TRANSCERVICAL
Endoscope, Transcervical
    (Amnioscope) 81
TRANSFORMER
Transformer, Endoscope 89
TRAUMATIC
Forceps, Grasping,
    Atraumatic 94-96
Forceps, Grasping,
    Traumatic 97-101
Gauge, Thickness, Tissue 109
TRAY
Rack, Instrument, Laparoscopy 115
Tray, Sterilization, Instrument 143
TROCAR
Cannula, Suprapubic, With Trocar ... 37
Dilator, Port, Laparoscopic 158-159
Kit, Trocar 126
Sleeve, Trocar 159

Trocar, Abdominal 159-160
Trocar, Amniotic 161
Trocar, Cardiovascular 161-162
Trocar, Gallbladder 162-163
Trocar, Gastro-Urology 163
Trocar, Laparoscopic 163-168
Trocar, Laryngeal 169
Trocar, Other 169-170
Trocar, Short 170
Trocar, Sinus 170
Trocar, Surgical 170
Trocar, Thoracic 170-171
Trocar, Tracheal 171-172
TUBE
Trocar, Other 169-170
Tube, Smoke Removal, Endoscopic 3
TUBING
Tubing, Irrigation 123-124
TUMOR
Needle, Biopsy, Mammary 143
TYING
Holder, Needle, Curved,
    Laparoscopic 104
Holder, Needle, Laparoscopic 105
Holder/Scissors, Needle,
    Laparoscopic 106
Instrument, Knot Tying, Suture,
    Laparoscopic 113
Instrument, Needle
    Holder/Knot Tying 113-114
ULTRASONIC
Probe, Detector, Flow, Blood,
    Laparoscopy, Ultrasonic 107
Scalpel, Ultrasonic 66-70
System, Imaging, Laparoscopy,
    Ultrasonic 107
UMBILICAL
Dilator, Fascia, Umbilical 52
UNIPOLAR
Coagulator, Laparoscopic,
    Unipolar 54-55
Coagulator/Cutter, Endoscopic,
    Unipolar 56
UNIT
Electrocautery Unit, Endoscopic 57
URETEROSCOPE
Ureteroscope 89-90
URETHROSCOPE
Urethroscope 90
UROGRAPHY
Pyeloscope 86

UROLOGY
Bougie, Esophageal, And
    Gastrointestinal 136-139
Colonoscope, Gastro-Urology 73
Esophagoscope, Rigid,
    Gastro-Urology 91
Gastroscope, Gastro-Urology 102
Trocar, Gastro-Urology 163
UTEROTUBAL
Insufflator, Carbon-Dioxide,
    Uterotubal 117
VAGINAL
Insufflator, Vaginal 119
VAGINOSCOPE
Esophagoscope
    (Flexible Or Rigid) 91
Vaginoscope 90
VENTILATING
Bronchoscope, Rigid,
    Ventilating 73
VESSEL
Instrument, Separating, Nerve 114
VIDEO
Camera, Video, Endoscopic 29-30
Camera, Video, Multi-Image 30
Cart, Equipment, Video 139-140
Monitor, Video, Endoscope 31-32
System, Camera, 3-Dimensional 32
Tape, Television & Video,
    Endoscopic 34-35
VIDEOENDOSCOPE
Endoscope, Electronic
    (Videoendoscope) 78-79
VIDEOINTERFACE
Videointerface, Laparoscopic,
    Non-Removable Rod 35
VIDEOTAPE
Camera, Videotape, Surgical 30
VISION
Endoscope, Direct Vision 78
Eyepiece, Lens, Prescription,
    Endoscopic 3
WARMER
Warmer, Endoscope 172
WASH
Bottle, Endoscopic Wash 2
WASHER
Sterilizer/Washer,
    Endoscope 142-143
WRIST
System, Traction, Arthroscopy 143
XENON
Light Source, Endoscope,
    Xenon Arc 135
YAG
Equipment/Accessories, Laser,
    Laparoscopy 5
Laser, Nd:YAG, Laparoscopy 133

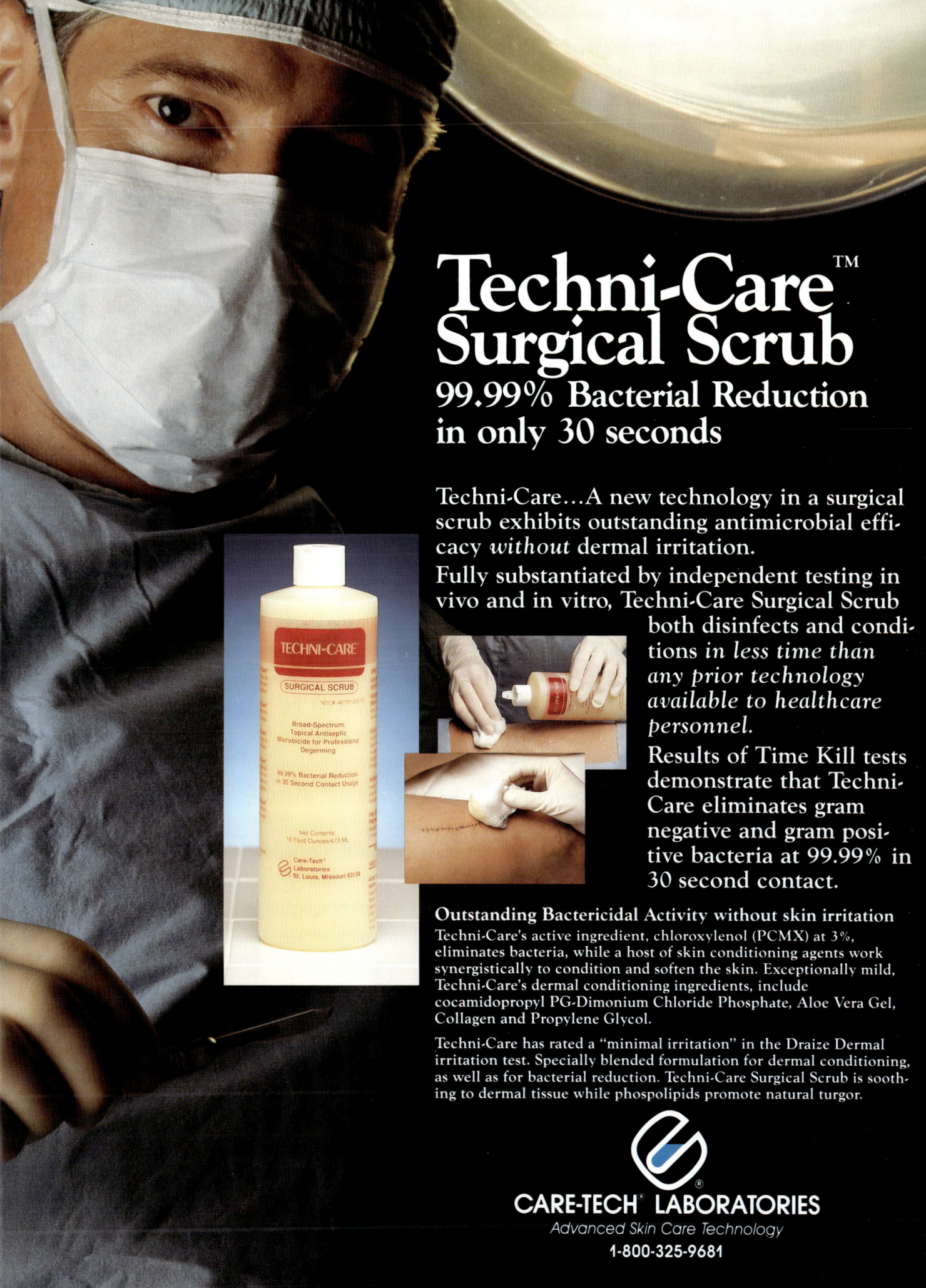

FOR THE ADVANCED SURGEON...

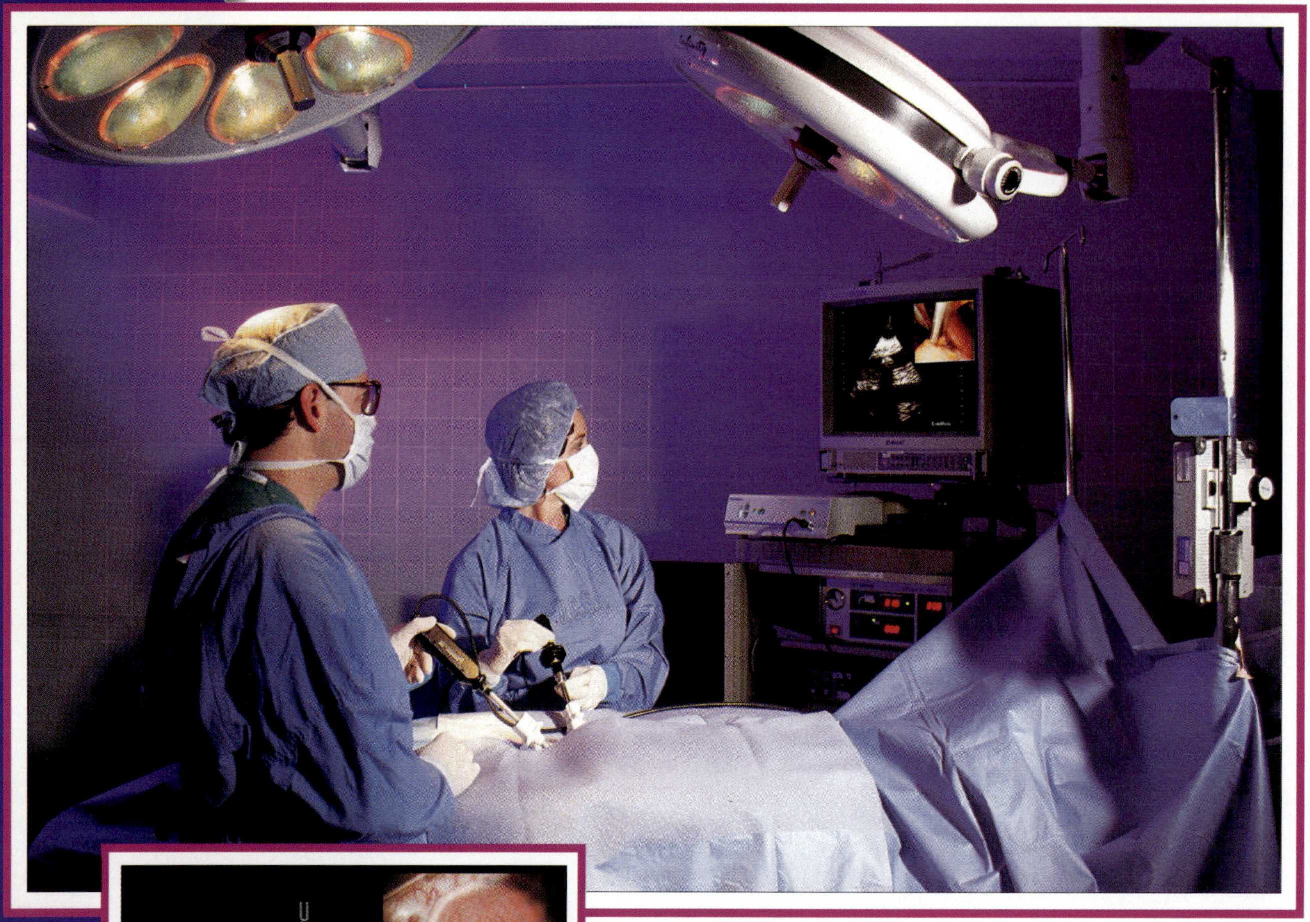

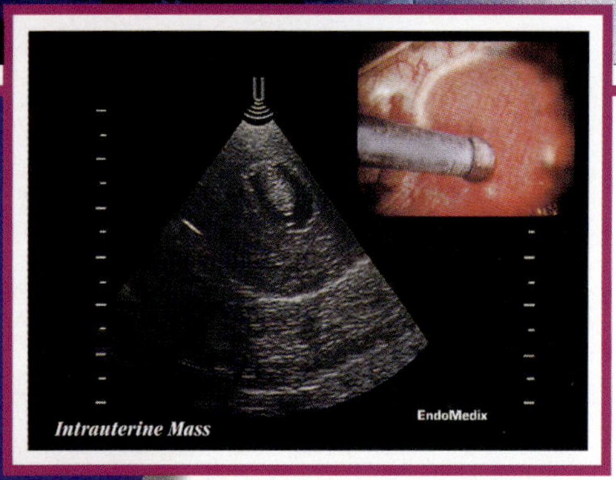

THE NEXT STEP...
LAPAROSCOPIC ULTRASOUND IMAGING

LOCALIZATION OF MASSES

INFERTILITY EVALUATION

EXPLORATORY & DIAGNOSTIC LAPAROSCOPY

LAPAROSCAN™
Dedicated Laparoscopic Ultrasound Imaging

ENDOMEDIX

EndoMedix Corporation
2162 Michelson Drive
Irvine, CA 92715 (USA)
(714) 253-1050 • (800) 553-6361

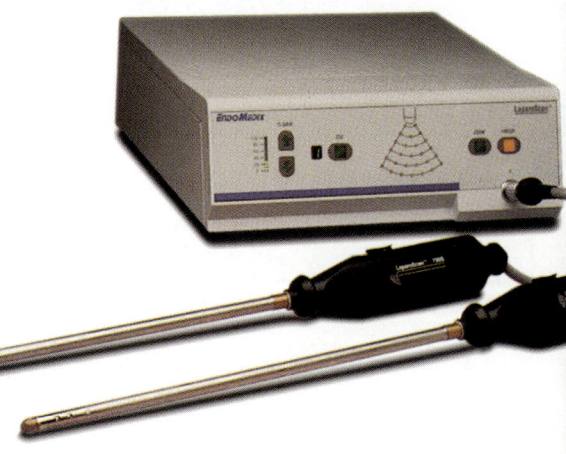

Ask us about our laparoscopic ultrasound training programs.

2
PRODUCT DIRECTORY

Listed in this section are suppliers of 274 types of instruments and equipment needed in various minimally invasive surgical procedures. The directory is divided alphabetically into 57 major product categories. Under each major heading, you'll find the devices included in that category listed alphabetically. For each device, the listings give the names, addresses, and phone numbers of all available suppliers, both domestic and foreign, again in alphabetical order. In a number of key categories, you'll also find an overview of the available equipment. Also included, if the information has been made available by the manufacturer, are specific trade names of the devices offered by the company, plus detailed descriptions of these products. This information ranges from brief summaries of product specifications to complete package-insert-style documentation, with full details on such topics as indications, contraindications, precautions, instructions for use, and sterilization and maintenance guidelines.

MAJOR DEVICE CATEGORIES IN THE PRODUCT DIRECTORY

Accessories	*Endoscope*	*Needle*
Applier	*Esophagoscope*	*Nephroscope*
Arthroscope	*Forceps*	*Power Supply*
Aspirator	*Gastroscope*	*Probe*
Bag	*Holder*	*Pump*
Bronchoscope	*Imaging*	*Regulator*
Camera	*Instrument*	*Remover*
Cannula	*Insufflator*	*Retractor*
Catheter	*Irrigator*	*Scissors*
Choledochoscope	*Kit*	*Solution*
Clamp	*Knife*	*Suture*
Clip	*Laparoscope*	*System*
Coagulator	*Laryngoscope*	*Telescope*
Controller	*Laser*	*Tip*
Cutter	*Ligature*	*Trainer*
Dilator	*Light*	*Trocar*
Dispenser	*Lithotriptor*	*Ultrasound*
Drain	*Miscellaneous*	*Videointerface*
Electrocautery	*Monitor*	*Warmer*

Accessories

ACCESSORIES, CLEANING, ENDOSCOPIC

Aesculap
1000 Gateway Blvd.
South San Francisco, CA 94080-7030
415-876-7000

Amsco
2424 West 23rd Street
P.O. Box 620
Erie, PA 16506
814-452-3100

Annex Medical, Inc.
7098 Shady Oak Rd.
Eden Prairie, MN 55344-3505
612-942-7576

Bard Ventures
1200 Technology Park Dr.
Billerica, MA 01821
508-667-1300

Cabot Medical Corp.
2021 Cabot Blvd. West
Langhorne, PA 19047-1875
215-752-8300

Coopersurgical, Inc.
15 Forest Pkwy.
Shelton, CT 06484-5458
203-929-6321

Davis & Geck Div.
American Cyanamid Company
One Cyanamid Plaza
Wayne, NJ 07470-2012
201-831-2000

Depuy, Inc.
700 Orthopaedic Dr.
P.O. Box 988
Warsaw, IN 46581-0988
219-267-8143

Encompas Unlimited, Inc.
1110 Pinellas Bayway, Ste. 104
Tierra Verde, FL 33715-8281
813-867-7701

Endoflush, Inc.
6420 Carter
Shawnee Mission, KS 66203
913-432-7200

Justman Brush Co.
P.O. Box 12364
Omaha, NE 68112-2216
402-451-4420

Keymed Medical & Industrial Equipment Ltd.
Keymed House, Stock Rd., Southend-on-Sea
Essex SS2 5QH
United Kingdom
0702/616333

Keymed, Inc.
400 Airport Executive Park
Spring Valley, NY 10977-7404
914-425-3100

Leisegang Medical, Inc.
6401 Congress Ave.
Boca Raton, FL 33487-2883
407-994-0202

Machida, Inc.
40 Ramland Rd. South
Orangeburg, NY 10962-2617
914-365-0600

Marlow Surgical Technologies, Inc.
1810 Joseph Lloyd Pkwy.
Willoughby, OH 44094-8030
216-946-2453

Miele Professional Products Group
22D Worlds Fair Dr.
Somerset, NJ 08873
908-560-0899

Mill-Rose Laboratories
7310 Corporate Blvd.
Mentor, OH 44060-4856
216-255-7995

Pentax Precision Instrument Corp.
30 Ramland Rd.
Orangeburg, NY 10962-2699
914-365-0700

Pilling-Rusch
420 Delaware Dr.
Fort Washington, PA 19034-2711
215-643-2600

R-Group International
2321 N.W. 66th Court, Ste. W4
Gainesville, FL 32606
904-378-3633

Richmond Products, Inc.
1021 S. Rogers Circle, Ste. 6
Boca Raton, FL 33487-2894
407-994-2112

Riwoplan Medizin-Techn. Einrichtungen GmbH
Postfach 80
D-75438 Knittlingen Baden-Wurttemberg
Germany
07043/3031

Shoei Industries Co. Ltd.
3-30-5, Hongo, Bunkyo-Ku
Tokyo 113
Japan
03/8140321

Storz Endoscopy-America Inc., Karl
10111 W. Jefferson Blvd.
Culver City, CA 90232-3509
310-558-1500

Storz GmbH & Co., Karl
Mittelstr. 8
Postfach 230
D-78532 Tuttlingen
Germany
07461/7080

Weck & Co. Inc., Edward
1 Weck Dr.
P.O. Box 12600
Research Triangle Park, NC 27709
919-544-8000

Welch Allyn, Inc.
4341 State Street Rd.
P.O. Box 220
Skaneateles Falls, NY 13153-0220
315-685-4100

Wolf Medical Instruments Corp., Richard
353 Corporate Woods Pkwy.
Vernon Hills, IL 60061-3110
708-913-1113

ACCESSORIES, PHOTOGRAPHIC, ENDOSCOPIC

Arthrotek, Inc.
4861 E. Airport Dr.
Ontario, CA 91761
909-988-5595

Cabot Medical Corp.
2021 Cabot Blvd. West
Langhorne, PA 19047-1875
215-752-8300

Coopersurgical, Inc.
15 Forest Pkwy.
Shelton, CT 06484-5458
203-929-6321

Electro Fiberoptics Corporation
56 Hudson St.
Northborough, MA 01532-1922
508-393-3753

Heraeus Surgical, Inc.
575 Cottonwood Dr.
Milpitas, CA 95035-7402
408-954-4000

ACCESSORIES, PHOTOGRAPHIC, ENDOSCOPIC (cont'd)

Leisegang Medical, Inc.
6401 Congress Ave.
Boca Raton, FL 33487-2883
407-994-0202

Linvatec Corporation
11311 Concept Blvd.
Largo, FL 34643-4908
813-399-5344

MP Video, Inc.
63 South St.
Hopkinton, MA 01748-2212
508-435-2131

Storz Endoscopy-America Inc., Karl
10111 W. Jefferson Blvd.
Culver City, CA 90232-3509
310-558-1500

Storz GmbH & Co., Karl
Mittelstr. 8
Postfach 230
D-78532 Tuttlingen
Germany
07461/7080

Transamerican Technologies International
7026 Koll Center Pkwy., Ste. 207
Pleasanton, CA 94566-3108
510-484-0700

Treier Endoscopie AG
Sonnrain
CH-6215 Beromunster
Switzerland
045/512323

Wect Instrument Company, Inc.
5645 N. Ravenswood
Chicago, IL 60660-3922
312-769-1944

Wolf Medical Instruments Corp., Richard
353 Corporate Woods Pkwy.
Vernon Hills, IL 60061-3110
708-913-1113

ADAPTERS, BULB, ENDOSCOPE, MISCELLANEOUS

Bard Ventures
1200 Technology Park Dr.
Billerica, MA 01821
508-667-1300

Cabot Medical Corp.
2021 Cabot Blvd. West
Langhorne, PA 19047-1875
215-752-8300

Coopersurgical, Inc.
15 Forest Pkwy.
Shelton, CT 06484-5458
203-929-6321

Pentax Precision Instrument Corp.
30 Ramland Rd.
Orangeburg, NY 10962-2699
914-365-0700

Wect Instrument Company, Inc.
5645 N. Ravenswood
Chicago, IL 60660-3922
312-769-1944

ATTACHMENT, BINOCULAR, ENDOSCOPIC

Bard Ventures
1200 Technology Park Dr.
Billerica, MA 01821
508-667-1300

Metallisation Et Traitemens Optiques
11 Rue Ampere Bp 6
F-91301 Massy/Cedex
France
6/9206307

BOTTLE, ENDOSCOPIC WASH

Bard Ventures
1200 Technology Park Dr.
Billerica, MA 01821
508-667-1300

Fujinon (Europe) GmbH
Heerdter Lohweg 89
D-40549 Duesseldorf 11
Germany
0211/52050

Fujinon, Inc.
10 High Point Dr.
Wayne, NJ 07470-7434
201-633-5600

BULB, INFLATION (ENDOSCOPE)

Bard Ventures
1200 Technology Park Dr.
Billerica, MA 01821
508-667-1300

Graham-Field, Inc.
400 Rabro Dr. East
Hauppauge, NY 11788-4226
516-582-5900

Wolf Medical Instruments Corp., Richard
353 Corporate Woods Pkwy.
Vernon Hills, IL 60061-3110
708-913-1113

EYEPIECE, LENS, NON-PRESCRIPTION, ENDOSCOPIC

Coopersurgical, Inc.
15 Forest Pkwy.
Shelton, CT 06484-5458
203-929-6321

Leisegang Medical, Inc.
6401 Congress Ave.
Boca Raton, FL 33487-2883
407-994-0202

Pilling-Rusch
420 Delaware Dr.
Fort Washington, PA 19034-2711
215-643-2600

Storz Endoscopy-America Inc., Karl
10111 W. Jefferson Blvd.
Culver City, CA 90232-3509
310-558-1500

Storz GmbH & Co., Karl
Mittelstr. 8
Postfach 230
D-78532 Tuttlingen
Germany
07461/7080

EYEPIECE, LENS, PRESCRIPTION, ENDOSCOPIC

Life Medical Technologies, Inc.
3649 W. 1987 S.
Salt Lake City, UT 84104
801-972-1900

Storz Endoscopy-America Inc., Karl
10111 W. Jefferson Blvd.
Culver City, CA 90232-3509
310-558-1500

Storz GmbH & Co., Karl
Mittelstr. 8
Postfach 230
D-78532 Tuttlingen
Germany
07461/7080

Wolf Medical Instruments Corp., Richard
353 Corporate Woods Pkwy.
Vernon Hills, IL 60061-3110
708-913-1113

TEACHING ATTACHMENT, ENDOSCOPIC

Circon Acmi
300 Stillwater Ave.
Stamford, CT 06902-3640
203-328-8689

Cory Brothers Co.
4 Dollis Pk.
London, N3 1HG
United Kingdom
081/349/1081

Ethicon Endo-Surgery
4545 Creek Road
Cincinnati, OH 45242
513-786-7000

Pentax Precision Instrument Corp.
30 Ramland Rd.
Orangeburg, NY 10962-2699
914-365-0700

Storz Endoscopy-America Inc., Karl
10111 W. Jefferson Blvd.
Culver City, CA 90232-3509
310-558-1500

Storz GmbH & Co., Karl
Mittelstr. 8
Postfach 230
D-78532 Tuttlingen
Germany
07461/7080

Wect Instrument Company, Inc.
5645 N. Ravenswood
Chicago, IL 60660-3922
312-769-1944

Wisap Gesellschaft
Rudolf Diesel Ring 20
D-82054 Sauerlach
Germany
08104/1067

Wolf Medical Instruments Corp., Richard
353 Corporate Woods Pkwy.
Vernon Hills, IL 60061-3110
708-913-1113

Yagami International Trading Co. Ltd.
3-2-29, Marunouchi, Naka-Ku
Nagoya 460
Japan
052/9623811

TUBE, SMOKE REMOVAL, ENDOSCOPIC

Conmed Corp.
310 Broad Street
Utica, NY 13501
315-797-8375

Electro Surgical Instrument Co.
37 Centennial St.
Rochester, NY 14611-1732
716-235-1430

I.C. Medical, Inc.
2340 W. Shangri-La, Ste. 202
Phoenix, AZ 85029-4746
602-943-6162

Laser Technologies Group
6606 Bryant Ave. N.
Minneapolis, MN 55430-1805
612-560-0433

Leisegang Medical, Inc.
6401 Congress Ave.
Boca Raton, FL 33487-2883
407-994-0202

M.D. Engineering
3464 Depot Rd.
Hayward, CA 94545-2714
510-732-9950

Northgate Technologies, Inc.
3930 Ventura Dr., Ste. 150
Arlington Heights, IL 60004
708-506-9872

Stackhouse Inc.
2059 Atlanta Ave.
Riverside, CA 92507-2439
909-276-4600

Wolf Medical Instruments Corp., Richard
353 Corporate Woods Pkwy.
Vernon Hills, IL 60061-3110
708-913-1113

Applier

APPLIER, CLIP, LAPAROSCOPIC

Davis & Geck Endosurgery
1 Casper St.
Danbury, CT 06810
203-743-4451

PROFESSIONAL LINE 8379-01

DESCRIPTION: Clip Applicator for titanium clips (order number 8379-01):
  10mm diameter, non-insulated, working length 38cm. For ligation of structures and vessels using Ethicon style LC/TI 300 clips:

CLIP APPLICATOR FOR TITANIUM CLIPS

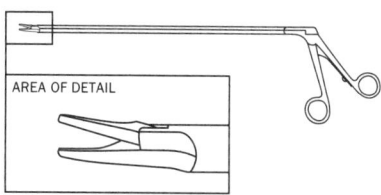

INDICATIONS: The DAVIS & GECK endoscopic manual instruments are designed to perform cutting, grasping, dissecting, perforating, and/or cauterizing functions through long mechanisms to delicate working tips. These instruments are introduced through a trocar/sheath.
  The use of these endoscopic instruments for a task other than for which it is intended will usually result in a damaged or broken instrument.

CARE & MAINTENANCE: Inspect instruments before each use for bent, broken, cracked, or worn parts.
  Use caution and make sure the jaw is closed when inserting or removing instruments through cannulas.
  Do not apply lateral pressure on the instruments, as this will damage the working tip.
  To avoid overstressing the ratchet or spring mechanisms of instruments, grip and maneuver the instrument properly during surgery.
  When not in use, store endoscopic instruments in a clean, dry environment taking care to protect the instrument.
  Instruments must be properly cleaned after each use.
  1. After each use in surgery, disassemble instrument (e.g. trocars), if possible, before cleaning.
  2. Clean instruments thoroughly with a soft brush (or appropriate devices) using warm water and a non-abrasive cleansing agent. Flush interior channels (sheaths, trocar, sleeves, and irrigation ports) with a

APPLIER, CLIP, LAPAROSCOPIC *(cont'd)*

cleaning device, or clean with an appropriately sized brush.

3. Rinse thoroughly in distilled water after cleaning to remove residual debris and/or cleansing agent.

4. Soak the clean instrument in a high level disinfectant following the manufacturer's directions. Ensure that all surfaces are exposed to the disinfectant solution, including interior channels, lumens, and irrigation ports.

5. Thoroughly rinse the disinfectant. Use distilled water on the final rinse.

6. Thoroughly dry the lumens, channels, and irrigation ports of each instrument, using compressed air or a 70% alcohol rinse.

7. Lubricate the instrument after every cleaning, and prior to sterilization, with a steam-permeable lubricant. Open the stop cock of the instruments for best penetration and protection.

STERILIZATION GUIDELINES: Sterilize product before use. Steam sterilize at a minimum temperature of 250°F (121°C).

1. Do not disinfect or sterilize in EtO/Freon.

2. Do not disinfect or sterilize in liquid solutions.

3. Do not sterilize at temperatures greater than 275°F (135°C).

SERVICE REQUIREMENTS & CONTACTS:

1) Repair of the instruments by parties other than DAVIS & GECK will void the warranty.

2) If the instrument requires repair or maintenance, return the instrument to the attention of the DAVIS & GECK Repair Services Department.

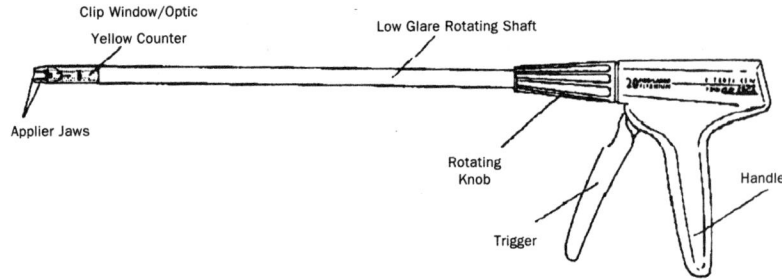

LIGACLIP ERCA

Ethicon Endo-Surgery
4545 Creek Rd.
Cincinnati, OH 45242
513-786-7000

LIGACLIP ERCA

DESCRIPTION:

The LIGACLIP* ERCA Applier is a sterile, disposable instrument. The instrument is preloaded and delivers 20 titanium LIGACLIP Extra Clips that individually advance after each firing. The instrument and clips are designed to offer a rapid, efficient means of ligation through ENDOPATH* Disposable Surgical Trocars. The clips are applied by positioning the clip around the tissue structure and applying pressure to the trigger. The shaft of the instrument is designed to rotate 360° in either direction to accommodate a one-handed technique and is also low-glare to minimize reflective distortion during the procedure.

INDICATIONS: The LIGACLIP ERCA Applier is intended for use on tubular structures or vessels. The tissue being ligated should be consistent with the size of the clip.

CONTRAINDICATIONS: The LIGACLIP ERCA Applier is not intended for contraceptive tubal occlusion.

Do not use the LIGACLIP ERCA Applier on vessels upon which metal ligating clips would not normally be used.

WARNINGS: To avoid damage, do not flip the LIGACLIP ERCA Applier onto the Mayo stand.

Prior to each clip application, the jaw tips should be inspected to ensure the clip is fully advanced to the end of the applier jaws.

Check to ensure that each clip has been securely placed around the tissue being ligated.

If a clip is dislodged prematurely from the jaw tip or fails to advance, the instrument may be recycled by fully squeezing the trigger until halted and fully released to advance the next clip into the jaws of the instrument.

Dispose of all fired instruments. DO NOT RESTERILIZE the LIGACLIP ERCA Applier. Resterilization may compromise the integrity of the applier, which may result in its malfunctioning.

Instrument should be *fully squeezed* on each firing.

Read all instructions carefully. Failure to properly follow the instructions may lead to the improper formation of clips and, therefore, unsatisfactory ligation of tissue.

INSTRUCTIONS FOR USE:

IMPORTANT: This insert is designed to provide instructions for the use of the LIGACLIP ERCA Endoscopic Rotating Multiple Clip Applier and is not intended as a guide to ligating techniques.

DELIVERY:

1. Using sterile technique, remove the applier from the blister package.

2. Fully squeeze the trigger until the motion is halted. Releasing the trigger advances the first clip into the jaws of the instrument. Failure to completely squeeze the trigger can result in clip misloading.

NOTE: The applier may be introduced through the appropriate diameter trocar sleeve with or without a clip in the jaw. The ratchet mechanism in the handle facilitates a one-way firing stroke and provides clip security in the jaws.

FIRING:

1. Introduce the jaws of the applier centered through the appropriate diameter ENDOPATH Trocar (see table under Specifications/How Supplied).

LIGACLIP ERCA

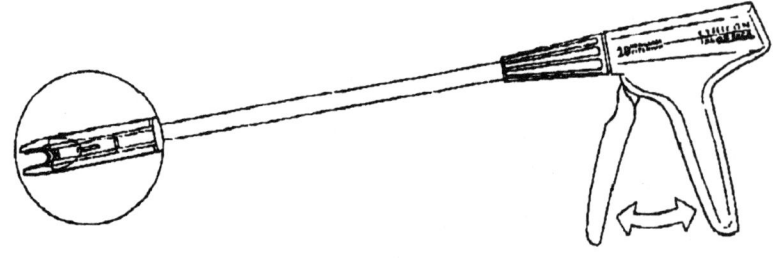

APPLIER/5

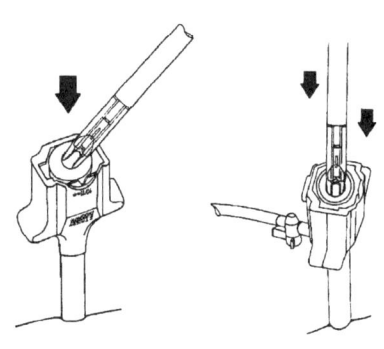

2. Position the jaws with the clip completely around the vessel to be ligated.

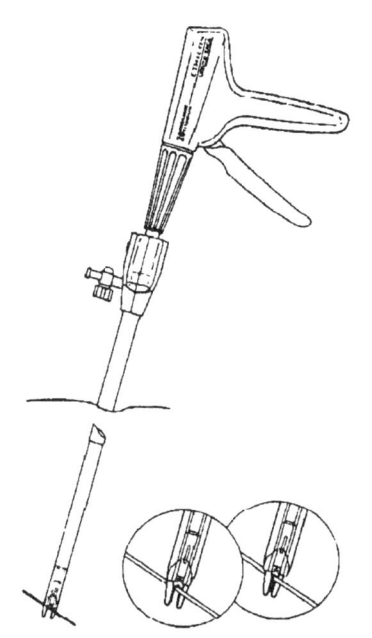

3. Fully squeeze the trigger until it stops and the firing cycle is complete. The next clip is automatically advanced as the trigger is released. Instrument jaw tips should be inspected after each use to ensure a new clip is present before the next firing.

CAUTION: Check to ensure that each clip has been securely placed around the tissue being ligated.

4. When there are only 3 clips remaining in the applier, an optic yellow clip counter bar will appear in the window.

Please read all information carefully. Failure to properly follow the instructions may lead to serious surgical consequences.

STERILIZATION GUIDELINES: Sterility is guaranteed unless the package is opened or damaged. DO NOT RESTERILIZE.

SPECIFICATIONS/HOW SUPPLIED: The instruments are designated by the following product codes.

CAUTION: Federal (USA) law restricts this device to sale by or on the order of a physician.

Ethicon Endo-surgery
4545 Creek Rd.
Cincinnati, OH 45242
513-786-7000

LIGACLIP MCA

DESCRIPTION:

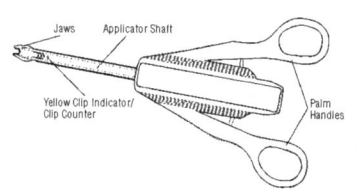

The LIGACLIP* MCA is a sterile, disposable, automatic, ligating clip applier that delivers titanium ligating clips. The instrument is preloaded with either 20 or 30 clips that individually advance after each clip application. The instrument and clips are designed to offer a fast, efficient means of ligation. The clips are applied to the vessel or other tubular structure by positioning the jaws with the clip around the vessel and fully squeezing the handles of the applier. When the handles are completely released, a new clip is automatically advanced into the jaws of the instrument. After the last clip has been used, the instrument is designed to lock out, preventing the handles from being squeezed.

INDICATIONS: The LIGACLIP MCA is intended for use in vessels or other tubular structures whenever the surgeon decides a metallic ligating clip is indicated. The tissue being ligated should be consistent with the size of the clip.

CONTRAINDICATIONS:

1. The LIGACLIP MCA is not intended for contraceptive tubal occlusion.

2. Do not use the LIGACLIP MCA on tissues upon which metal ligating clips would not normally be used.

WARNINGS: To avoid damage to the LIGACLIP MCA, do not flip it into the sterile field.

Ensure that the clip is the correct size for the vessel or tubular structure being ligated.

Upon each clip application, fully squeeze the handles of the instrument until they come to a stop. Failure to fully squeeze the handles can result in improper formation of clips and, therefore, unsatisfactory ligation of tissue.

Ensure that each clip has been securely and completely positioned around the tissue being ligated.

Prior to each clip application, inspect the jaws of the instrument to ensure the clip is fully advanced to the end of the instrument jaws. If a clip is dislodged prematurely from the jaws or fails to advance, refire the instrument by fully squeezing the handles until they come to a stop and fully releasing to advance the next clip into the jaws of the instrument.

During the release cycle, a clip may be forcibly ejected from the instrument jaws if not fired in tissue.

PRODUCT SPECIFICATIONS

Product Code	Clip Size/Qty	Clip Dimension (mm)	Overall Shaft Length (approx.)	Cannula Diameter
ER220	Medium/20		11.20 inches (28.5cm)	10/11mm
ER320	Med.-Large/20		11.39 inches (28.9cm)	10/11mm
ER420	Large/20		13.43 inches (34.1cm)	12mm

APPLIER, CLIP, LAPAROSCOPIC (cont'd)

Do not close the jaws of the instrument over other surgical instruments.

Dispose of all fired instruments. DO NOT RESTERILIZE the LIGACLIP MCA. Resterilization may compromise the integrity of the instrument, which may result in its malfunctioning.

INSTRUCTIONS FOR USE: Read all instructions carefully. Failure to properly follow the instructions may lead to improper formation of clips and, therefore, unsatisfactory ligation of tissue.

IMPORTANT: This package insert is designed to provide instructions for the use of the LIGACLIP MCA Multiple Clip Applier. It is not a reference to ligation techniques.

1. Using sterile technique, remove the instrument from the blister package. To avoid damage to the instrument, do not flip it into the sterile field.

2. Ensure that a clip is in the jaws of the instrument.

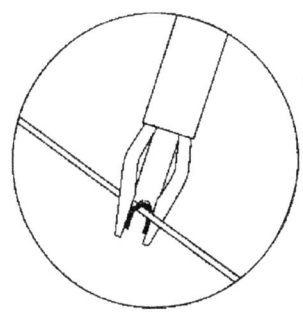

3. Position the jaws with the clip completely around the vessel to be ligated.

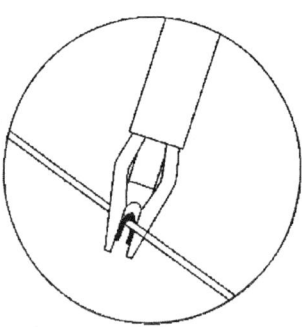

4. Fully squeeze the handles together until they come to a stop. As the handles are squeezed, the clip is closing and occluding the vessel or tubular structure.

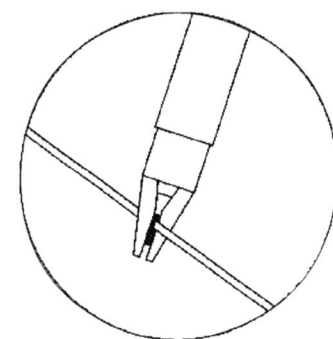

5. Fully release the handles to return the instrument to its original, open position. The next clip is automatically advanced. Inspect the jaw tips after each clip application to ensure a new clip is present before the next clip application.

CAUTION: Ensure that each clip has been securely and completely placed around the tissue being ligated.

6. Repeat steps as necessary to continue ligation of tissue.

NOTE: The back of the shaft permits visibility of the remaining clips. A yellow clip indicator follows the last clip down the shaft. When the instrument has five clips remaining, the clip counter will be visible (5, 4, 3, 2, 1). When there are no clips remaining in the instrument, the safety interlock mechanism prevents the handles from being squeezed.

STERILIZATION GUIDELINES: Sterility is guaranteed unless the package is opened or damaged. DO NOT RESTERILIZE.

SPECIFICATIONS/HOW SUPPLIED: The LIGACLIP MCA is supplied as a sterile, disposable instrument with 20 or 30 titanium ligating clips per instrument as listed below and is for single-patient use. Discard after use.

CAUTION: Federal (USA) law restricts this device to sale by or on the order of a physician.

The LIGACLIP MCA is available in the following sizes and clip counts:

Product Code	Multiple Clip Applier Description
MCS20	20 Small Clips in 9 3/8" Applier
MSM20	20 Medium Clips in 9 3/8" Applier
MCM20	20 Medium Clips in 11 1/2" Applier
MCM30	30 Medium Clips in 11 1/2" Applier
MCL20	20 Large Clips in 13 1/4" Applier

CLIP DIMENSIONS AND CLOSURES

SMALL CLIP .082 IN. (2.1 MM)   .148 IN. (3.8 MM)

MEDIUM CLIP .168 IN. (4.3 MM)   .236 IN. (6.0 MM)

LARGE CLIP .249 IN. (6.3 MM)   .425 IN. (10.8 MM)

Aesculap
1000 Gateway Blvd.
South San Francisco, CA 94080-7030
415-876-7000

Bryan Corp.
4 Plympton St.
Woburn, MA 01801-2908
617-935-0004

Cabot Medical Corp.
2021 Cabot Blvd. West
Langhorne, PA 19047-1875
215-752-8300

Davis & Geck Div.
American Cyanamid Company
One Cyanamid Plaza
Wayne, NJ 07470-2012
201-831-2000

Leisegang Medical, Inc.
6401 Congress Ave.
Boca Raton, FL 33487-2883
407-994-0202

Mist, Inc.
6307 E. Angus Dr.
Raleigh, NC 27613
919-787-8377

Origin Medsystems, Inc.
135 Constitution Dr.
Menlo Park, CA 94025
415-617-5000

Synectic Engineering, Inc.
4 Oxford Rd.
Milford, CT 06460-7007
203-877-8488

United States Surgical Corp.
150 Glover Ave.
Norwalk, CT 06856-5080
203-845-1000

APPLIER, CLIP, REPAIR, HERNIA, LAPAROSCOPIC

Ethicon Endo-surgery
4545 Creek Road
Cincinnati, OH 45242
513-786-7000

Leisegang Medical, Inc.
6401 Congress Ave.
Boca Raton, FL 33487-2883
407-994-0202

Schwarz Medical
Kirchstrasse 24
D-86935 Rott
Germany
8869/1881

Synectic Engineering, Inc.
4 Oxford Rd.
Milford, CT 06460-7007
203-877-8488

United States Surgical Corp.
150 Glover Ave.
Norwalk, CT 06856-5080
203-845-1000

APPLIER, LIGATURE CLIP

Davis & Geck Endosurgery
1 Casper St.
Danbury, CT 06810
203-743-4451

LAPRO-CLIP 8487-00

DESCRIPTION: LAPRO-CLIP* Reusable Single Ligating Clip Applier:

SINGLE LIGATING CLIP APPLIER

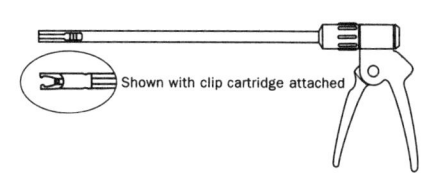

Shown with clip cartridge attached

LAPRO-CLIP ligating clips are molded from two polymers: polyglycolic acid and polyglyconate. Polyglycolic acid is used in DEXON sutures. Polyglyconate is used in MAXON sutures. The outer body is polyglycolic acid and slides over an inner track that is polyglyconate. LAPRO-CLIP ligating clips are sterile. The polymers are nonantigenic and nonpyrogenic.

All LAPRO-CLIP ligating clip appliers are designed to be used through a 10mm trocar.

The LAPRO-CLIP ligating clip is delivered by a single-use cartridge and actuated by a reusable applier. The applier is stainless steel and is supplied non-sterile. The cartridge delivers one LAPRO-CLIP ligating clip. The cartridges are ethylene oxide sterilized, and are for single use only.

SINGLE LIGATING CLIP APPLIER
CARTRIDGE   APPLIER   END CAP
INTERLOCK GROOVE
ROTATING SHAFT
HANDLE

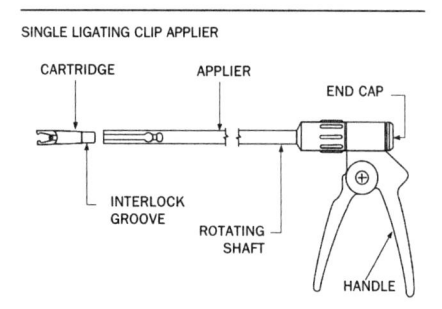

ACTIONS: A single-use cartridge is loaded onto the applier and the instrument is actuated by firmly squeezing the handle. This causes the rigid outer body to slide over and compress the flexible inner track to securely ligate tissue enclosed within the track (see diagram "A" below). The clip is released by releasing the handle. As a fail-safe mechanism, additional force on the handle will also release the clip.

The absorption characteristics of polyglycolic acid and polyglyconate have been extensively studied and documented for DEXON and MAXON sutures and additionally for LAPRO-CLIP ligating clips. The breakdown of these two polymers in the body occurs by hydrolysis.

Animal studies show that the clips retained their strength longer than necessary for complete healing to occur in the vessel.

CLOSURE SEQUENCE OF A CLIP

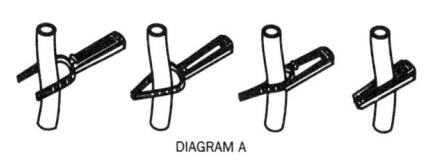

DIAGRAM A

INDICATIONS: LAPRO-CLIP ligating clips are intended for use as absorbable ligatures. LAPRO-CLIP ligating clips are radiotransparent and will not interfere with interpretations of post operative X-ray, CT or MRI scans. LAPRO-CLIP ligating clips can be used for ligation of the cystic artery and cystic duct, and other general ligation.

CONTRAINDICATIONS: LAPRO-CLIP ligating clips should not be used where prolonged or permanent ligation of tissues or vessels is required. This device is not intended for contraceptive tubal ligation, but may be used to achieve hemostasis following transection of the fallopian tube.

WARNINGS:

1. The cartridges and the LAPRO-CLIP ligating clips are ethylene oxide sterilized and supplied sterile. Once the package has been opened, all cartridges should be used immediately. THE CLIP CARTRIDGES SHOULD NOT BE RESTERILIZED.

2. The reusable applier is not electrically insulated and care should be taken to avoid contact with electrosurgical devices.

3. The tissue to be ligated should be located completely within the closed clip.

4. LAPRO-CLIP ligating clips are a secure means of ligation. Prior to closure, all tissues within the clip should be inspected to assure that the correct tissues will be ligated. It may be difficult to remove a fully closed clip.

INSTRUCTIONS FOR USE:

1. Cartridge should be removed from package prior to attachment to instrument.

Insert the cartridge module into the instrument until the latch closes and locks in place.

INSTRUCTIONS FOR USE, STEP 1

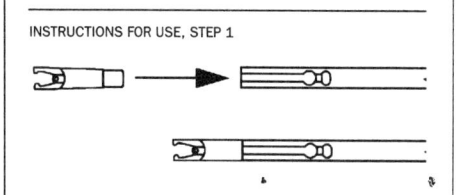

APPLIER, LIGATURE CLIP, *(cont'd)*

2. Place vessel or duct within the jaws of the cartridge until both legs of the aperture opening can be seen coming around the vessel or duct. Rotation of the instrument barrel will facilitate placement of the clip cartridge around the vessel.

INSTRUCTIONS FOR USE, STEP 2

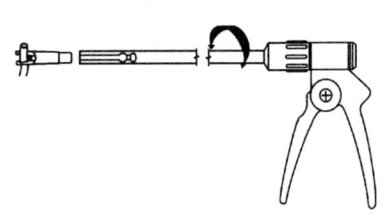

3. The handle should be firmly squeezed until it will not move further without excessive force.

INSTRUCTIONS FOR USE, STEP 3

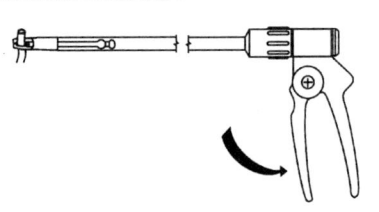

4. The clip will be held by the instrument until released. This is accomplished by allowing the handle to spring back into the original position.

INSTRUCTIONS FOR USE, STEP 4

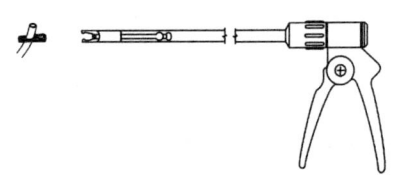

5. The clip should be inspected to assure closure and adequate ligation.

INSTRUCTIONS FOR USE, STEP 5

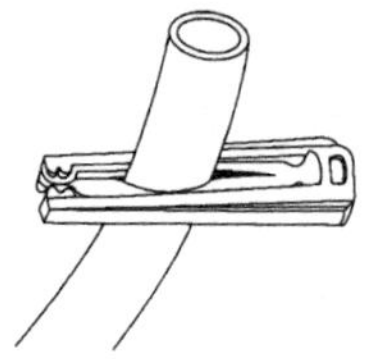

CARE & MAINTENANCE: After each use, the reusable applier should be dismantled, cleaned, reassembled and sterilized. Clean the parts of the applier (end cap, outer body and inner shaft assembly) using normal methods for stainless steel instruments.

Dismantle LAPRO-CLIP Single Ligating Clip Applier as follows:
1. Unscrew the end cap.

DISASSEMBLY, STEP 1

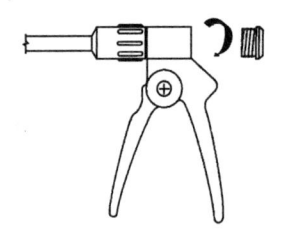

2. Push handle forward.

DISASSEMBLY, STEP 2

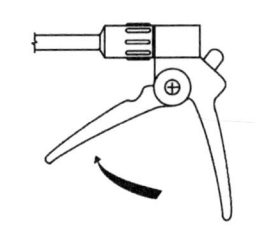

3. Remove inner shaft assembly.

DISASSEMBLY, STEP 3

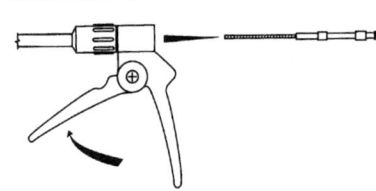

Reassemble LAPRO-CLIP Single Ligating Clip Applier:
1. Push the handle forward.

REASSEMBLY, STEP 1

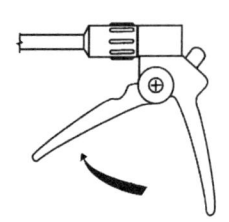

2. Replace the inner shaft assembly, taking care that all grooves are aligned between the handle, inner shaft and rotating shaft.

REASSEMBLY, STEP 2

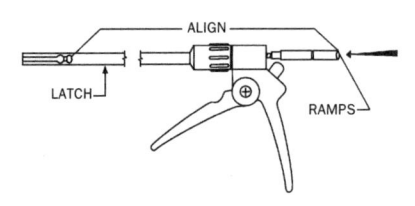

3. Pull the handle back and replace the end cap.

REASSEMBLY, STEP 3

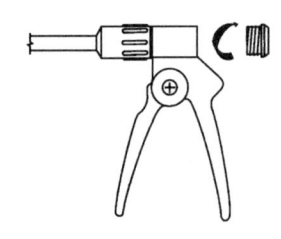

4. After each cleaning, it is recommended to use a surgical instrument lubricant (such as Instrument Milk) prior to autoclaving.

STERILIZATION GUIDELINES: The reusable applier should be autoclave sterilized prior to each use.

SPECIFICATIONS/HOW SUPPLIED: The LAPRO-CLIP ligating clips are supplied sterile and undyed in two sizes: large and medium/large. Clips are supplied one clip per single-use cartridge. The LAPRO-CLIP Single Ligating Clip Applier is sold separately.

Product Codes:
8487-00 LAPRO-CLIP
  Single Ligating Clip Applier
8487-08 Medium/Large LAPRO-CLIP
  Ligating Clip (6 clips per sterile package)
8487-12 Large LAPRO-CLIP
  Ligating Clip (6 clips per sterile package)
8487-13 Large LAPRO-CLIP
  Ligating Clip (2 clips per sterile package)
8487-82 Medium/Large LAPRO-CLIP
  Ligating Clip (2 clips per sterile package).

Davis & Geck Endosurgery
1 Casper St.
Danbury, CT 06810
203-743-4451

LAPRO-CLIP 8487-98

DESCRIPTION: Lapro-Clip Ligating Clip Short Clip Applier (order number 8487-98):

LAPRO-CLIP LIGATING CLIP APPLIER (SHORT, REUSABLE)

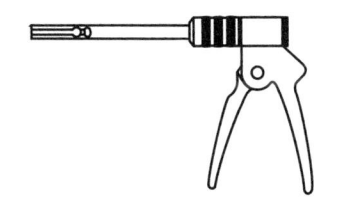

10mm diameter, short 12.2cm working length. For conventional surgery.

Davis & Geck Div.
American Cyanamid Company
One Cyanamid Plaza
Wayne, NJ 07470-2012
201-831-2000

STAPLER, LAPAROSCOPIC

Ethicon Endo-surgery
4545 Creek Rd.
Cincinnati, OH 45242
513-786-7000

ENDOPATH EAS

DESCRIPTION: The ENDOPATH* EAS Endoscopic 60° Stapler is a disposable endoscopic stapler designed for use with the 10/11mm diameter ENDOPATH Disposable Surgical Trocar. The instrument is packaged sterile and is designed to deliver 20 titanium staples. The instrument applies rectangular staples which close to approximately 4.4mm x 3.7mm (.172in. x .144in.).

The instrument is intended for single use only. Discard after use.

ENDOPATH EAS LAPAROSCOPIC STAPLER

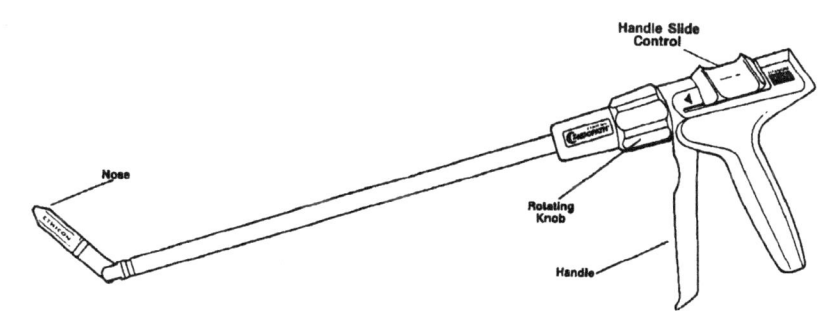

INDICATIONS: The ENDOPATH EAS Endoscopic 60° Stapler may be used to approximate tissue or affix prosthetic material in a variety of endoscopic or other surgical procedures.

CONTRAINDICATIONS: These staples are not intended for use in vascular or neural tissue, or in solid organs.

These staples are not hemostatic.

WARNINGS: Endoscopic procedures should be performed only by persons having adequate training and familiarity with endoscopic techniques. Consult medical literature relative to techniques, complications, and hazards prior to performance of any endoscopic procedure.

When endoscopic instruments and accessories from different manufacturers are employed together in a procedure, ensure that electrical isolation or grounding is not compromised.

Dispose of all fired instruments. DO NOT RESTERILIZE the ENDOPATH EAS stapler. Resterilization may compromise the integrity of the product, which may result in its malfunctioning.

Read all instructions carefully. Failure to properly follow the instructions may lead to the improper formation of staples and, therefore, unsatisfactory stapling of tissue.

INSTRUCTIONS FOR USE: IMPORTANT: This insert is designed to provide instructions for use of the ENDOPATH EAS Endoscopic 60° Articulating Stapler and is not intended as a guide to stapling techniques.

1. Introduce instrument through a 10/11mm diameter ENDOPATH Trocar in the nonarticulated mode. (See Fig. 1)

Fig. 1

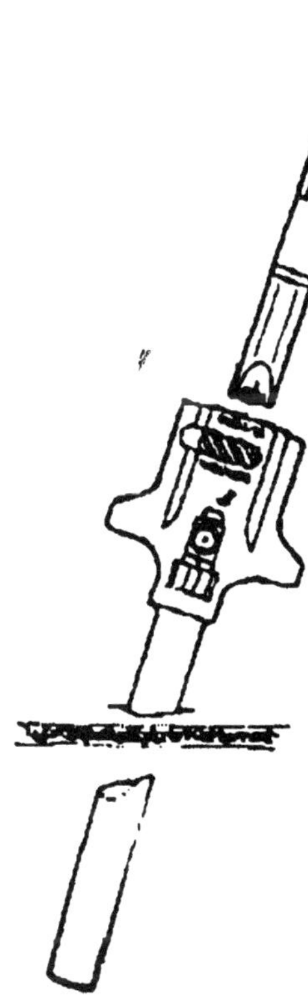

2. Under direct visualization, locate site to be stapled.
NOTE: Avoid using excessive force when externally palpating with the stapler perpendicular to the desired location. This may damage the articulating joint.
3. Use rotating knob to position the instrument over location to be stapled.
NOTE: If manual rotation of the nose is desired (See Fig. 2), position the nose to the nonarticulated mode and remove the instrument from the trocar.

Fig. 2

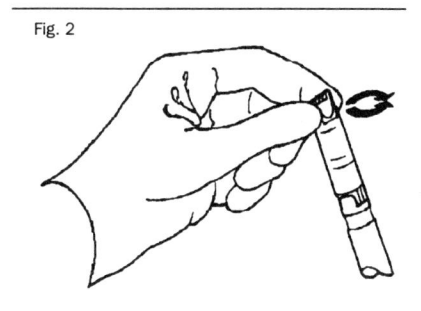

Reintroduce the instrument through the trocar in nonarticulated mode.

STAPLER, LAPAROSCOPIC
(cont'd)

4. The nose may be articulated to four stop positions, approximately 15°, 30°, 45°, and 60°, by pulling back on the handle slide control. (See Fig. 3)

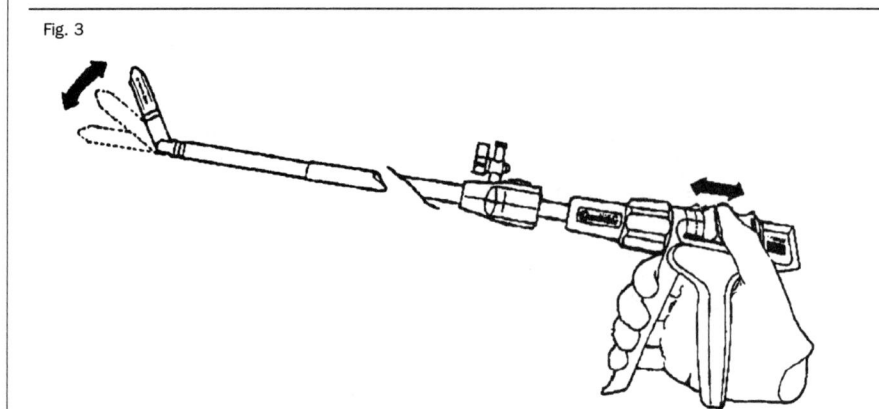

Fig. 3

5. For staple formation, squeeze the handle until reaching a full stop. (See Fig. 4)

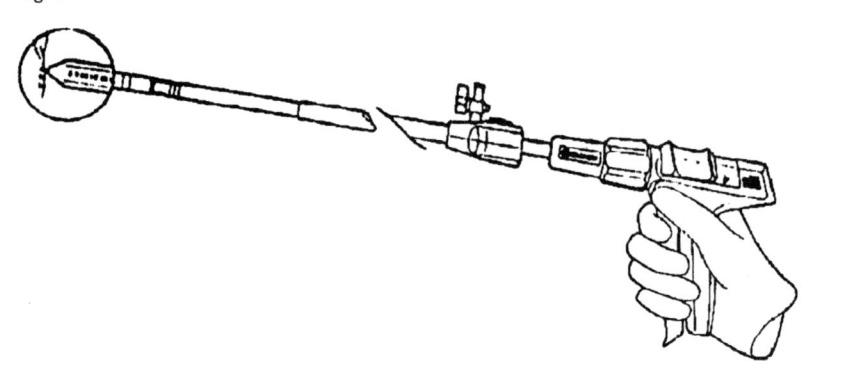

Fig. 4

6. Release the handle completely to place staple. (See Fig. 5)

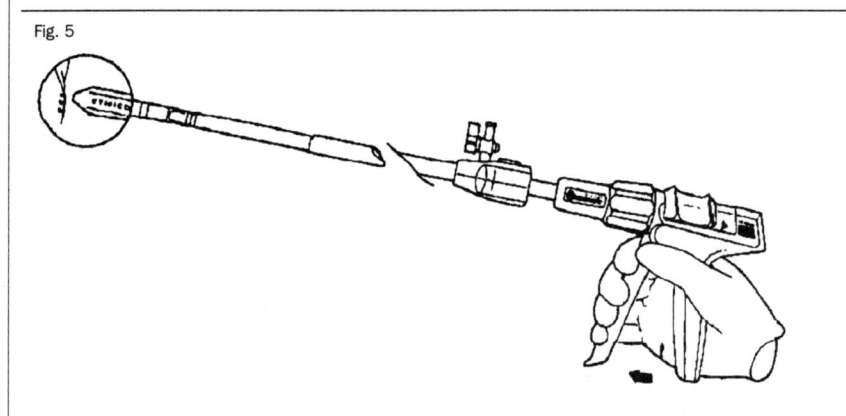

Fig. 5

7. Inspect site of staple placement to ensure complete staple formation and placement.
8. Repeat steps 2-7 to place next staple.
NOTE: The instrument can be fired in a nonarticulated mode or fired in the articulated mode, at stop positions at 15°, 30°, 45°, and 60°.

Please read all information carefully. Failure to properly follow the instructions may lead to serious surgical consequences.

STERILIZATION GUIDELINES: Sterility is guaranteed unless package is damaged or opened. DO NOT RESTERILIZE.

SPECIFICATIONS/HOW SUPPLIED:
CAUTION: Federal (USA) law restricts this device to sale by or on the order of a physician.

Ethicon Endo-Surgery
4545 Creek Rd.
Cincinnati, OH 45242
513-786-7000

ENDOPATH EMS
DESCRIPTION:

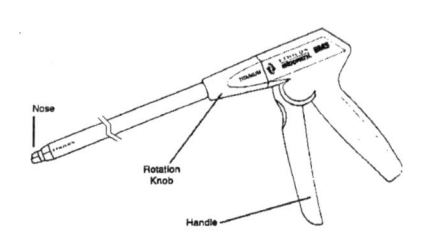

The ENDOPATH* EMS Endoscopic Multifeed Stapler is a disposable endoscopic stapler designed for use with the 10/11mm diameter ENDOPATH Disposable Surgical Trocar. The device places rectangular titanium staples. Closed staple dimensions are approximately 5.3mm x 3.7mm (.210in. x .143in.); contains 20+ staples.

INDICATIONS: The ENDOPATH EMS Endoscopic Multifeed Stapler may be used to approximate tissue or affix prosthetic material in a variety of endoscopic or other surgical procedures.

CONTRAINDICATIONS:
1. These staples are not intended for use in vascular or neural tissue, or in solid organs.
2. These staples are not hemostatic.

WARNINGS:

1. Endoscopic procedures should be performed only by persons having adequate training and familiarity with endoscopic techniques. Consult medical literature relative to techniques, complications, and hazards prior to performance of any endoscopic procedure.

2. When endoscopic instruments and accessories from different manufacturers are employed together in a procedure, ensure that electrical isolation or grounding is not compromised.

3. Dispose of all fired instruments. DO NOT RESTERILIZE the ENDOPATH EMS Stapler. Resterilization may compromise the integrity of the product, which may result in its malfunctioning.

Read all instructions carefully. Failure to properly follow the instructions may lead to improper formation of staples and, therefore, unsatisfactory stapling of tissue.

INSTRUCTIONS FOR USE:

IMPORTANT: This insert is designed to provide instructions for use of the ENDOPATH EMS Endoscopic Multifeed Stapler and is not intended as a guide to stapling techniques.

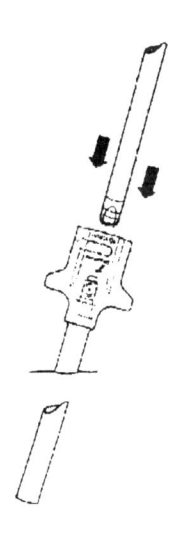

1. Introduce instrument through a 10/11mm diameter ENDOPATH Trocar.
2. Under direct visualization, locate site to be stapled.

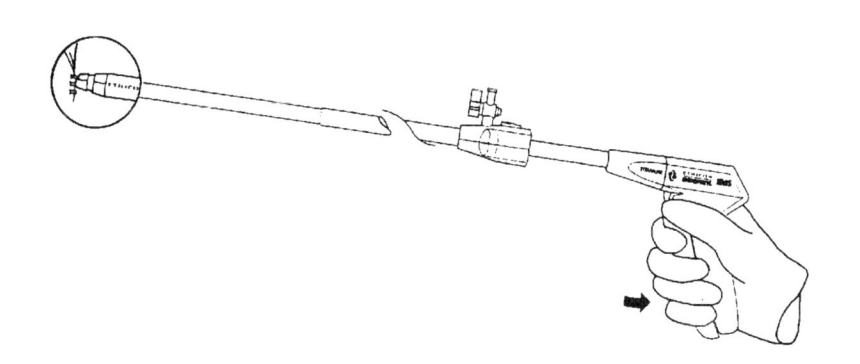

3. Using rotation knob, position the instrument over desired location to be stapled. For staple formation, squeeze the handle until reaching a full stop.

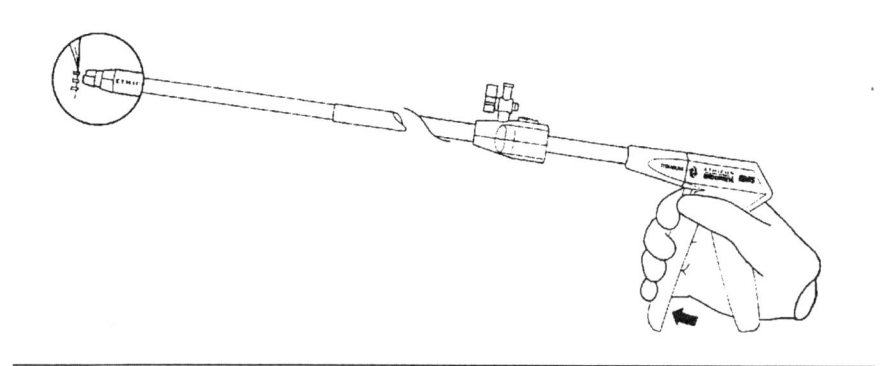

4. Release the handle completely to place staple.
5. Inspect site of staple placement to ensure complete staple formation and placement.
6. Repeat Steps 2-5 to place next staple.
Please read all information carefully.
Failure to properly follow the instructions may lead to serious surgical consequences.

STERILIZATION GUIDELINES: Sterility is guaranteed unless package is damaged or opened. DO NOT RESTERILIZE.

SPECIFICATIONS/HOW SUPPLIED: The ENDOPATH EMS Endoscopic Multifeed Stapler is designed as a disposable, sterile instrument to deliver 20 titanium staples per instrument and is for single-patient use. Discard after use.

CAUTION: Federal (USA) law restricts this device to sale by or on the order of a physician.

STAPLER, LAPAROSCOPIC
(cont'd)

Ethicon Endo-Surgery
4545 Creek Rd.
Cincinnati, OH 45242
513-786-7000

ENDOPATH ILS

DESCRIPTION: The ENDOPATH* ILS Endoscopic Circular Stapler (ECS) is a sealed-shaft, low-reflective anastomotic stapler available in three sizes to permit matching of instrument to diameter of the lumen. The instrument is identified as follows:

The ECS, with longer sealed shaft, low-profile anvil, and low-reflective surfaces facilitates endoscopic use where maintaining pneumoperitoneum, improved access, and visibility are necessary. The instrument provides for tissue attachment to the anvil in a location remote from the main body of the instrument. The instrument allows the surgeon to control tissue compression by varying the height of the closed staple. The instrument has been designed to improve insertion, operation, and ease of removal, while providing the largest knife blade diameter resulting in a larger lumen. It is disposable and is intended for single-use only. Therefore, no cleaning, maintenance or repair is required.

INDICATIONS: The ENDOPATH ILS Endoscopic Circular Stapler has applications throughout the alimentary tract for end-to-end, end-to-side, and side-to-side anastomoses.

CONTRAINDICATIONS: Do not use where the combined tissue thickness is less than 1.0mm or greater than 2.5mm or where the internal diameter of the structure is less than 21mm. If the instrument is used on tissue less than 1.0mm or greater than 2.5mm in thickness, an inadequate anastomosis could be formed, resulting in leakage, inadequate hemostasis, or improper healing.

WARNINGS: Endoscopic procedures should be performed only by persons having adequate training and familiarity with endoscopic techniques. Consult medical literature relative to techniques, complications, and hazards prior to performance of any endoscopic procedure.

Do not force safety open until instrument is ready to be fired. (Safety cannot be released until the orange indicator is within green range.)

Always check the security of the detachable head assembly prior to firing.

Do not immerse the ENDOPATH ILS Stapler in alcohol or any quaternary ammonium solutions.

Always inspect the anastomotic staple line for hemostasis and check the completed anastomosis for integrity and leakage. Metal clips, staples, or sutures contained in the area to be stapled may affect the integrity of the anastomosis. Corrective action, if required, may include the use of sutures or electrocautery.

Make certain purse-string sutures are tied snugly against the anvil shaft and trocar shaft and that no redundant tissue is present.

Make certain that the tissue thickness is within the indicated range, and that it is evenly distributed in the instrument. Excess tissue on one side may result in unacceptable staple formation and can result in staple line leakage.

BEFORE FIRING, MAKE CERTAIN THE ORANGE INDICATOR IS FULLY WITHIN THE GREEN RANGE OF THE GAP SETTING SCALE.

Make certain that the firing handle is fully squeezed to ensure proper staple formation and cutting of tissue.

Keep the trocar visible at all times to prevent personal injury or inadvertent trauma to adjacent structures. DO NOT use the anvil shaft to assist in piercing the tissue by placing it over the unexposed trocar. To avoid inclusion of tissue within the anvil shaft, DO NOT use it for piercing.

DO NOT clamp across or grip on the locking springs when attempting to reattach the detachable head assembly.

Squeezing the firing handle will expose the knife. Engage the red safety prior to removing washer and donuts from within the circular knife.

Dispose of all fired instruments. Assure safety is engaged prior to disposing. DO NOT RESTERILIZE. Resterilization may compromise the integrity of the stapler, which may result in wound leakage or disruption.

Endoscopic instruments may vary in diameter from manufacturer to manufacturer. When endoscopic instruments and accessories from different manufacturers are employed together in a procedure, verify compatibility prior to initiation of procedure and ensure that electrical isolation or grounding is not compromised.

A thorough understanding of the principles and techniques involved in laparoscopic laser and electrosurgical procedures is essential to avoid shock and burn hazards to both patient and medical personnel and damage to the device or other medical instruments.

Read all instructions carefully. Failure to properly follow the instructions may lead to serious surgical consequences such as leakage or disruption.

INSTRUCTIONS FOR USE: Descriptions and usage of the circular stapler are detailed in the following pages.

Read all information carefully.

Endoscopic procedures should be performed only by persons having adequate training and familiarity with endoscopic techniques. Consult medical literature relative to techniques, complications, and hazards prior to performance of any endoscopic procedure.

For endoscopic procedures, the ENDOPATH Disposable Surgical Transparent 33mm Diameter Trocar Sleeve Kit is available for the transabdominal instrument or detachable head insertion. The 33mm Diameter Trocar Sleeve and longer, non-reflective, sealed shaft of the Endoscopic Circular Stapler are designed to provide improved access and visibility, and to maintain pneumoperitoneum.

1. To remove the spacer tab, open the instrument by turning the adjusting knob counterclockwise two revolutions. (See Fig. 1.)

ENDOPATH ILS ENDOSCOPIC CIRCULAR STAPLER

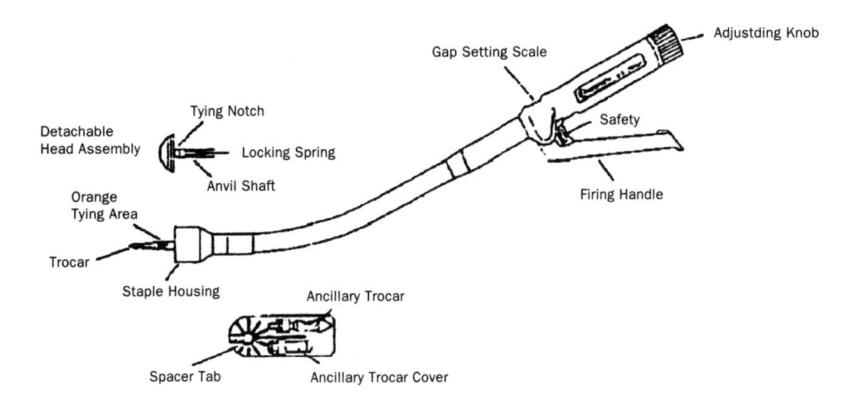

PRODUCT CODE	HEAD COLOR	KNIFE DIAMETER	NUMBER TITANIUM STAPLES[1]
ECS21 (21mm diameter head)	Light Green	12.4mm	16
ECS25 (25mm diameter head)	White	16.4mm	20
ECS29 (29mm diameter head)	Blue	20.4mm	24
ECS33 (33mm diameter head)	Dark Green	24.4mm	28

[1] Staple dimension before closure 4.0mm x 5.5mm (0.157 in. x 0.217 in.)

Fig. 1

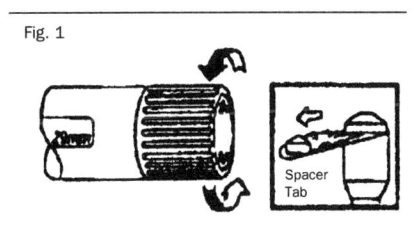

NOTE: If use of the Ancillary Trocar and/or Ancillary Trocar Cover are anticipated, do not discard the spacer tab. See section for "Required Ancillary Products."

2. Place purse-string sutures in the organs to be anastomosed. (See Fig. 2a.)

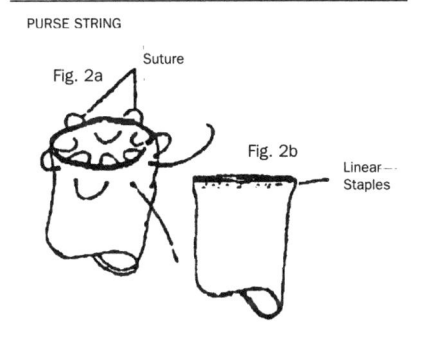

PURSE STRING

Fig. 2a — Suture

Fig. 2b — Linear Staples

Based on surgeon experience and judgement, a closed lumen technique (double or triple stapling technique) may be employed as an alternative to a purse-string technique. (See Fig. 2b.)

3. For a double stapling technique, open the instrument using the adjusting knob until the orange tying area is visible. Remove the detachable head assembly to expose the trocar. (See Fig. 3a.)

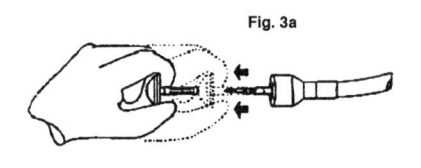

Fig. 3a

Retract the trocar by rotating the adjusting knob clockwise until a stop is reached. Check trocar to verify that it is fully retracted before proceeding. (See Fig. 3b.)

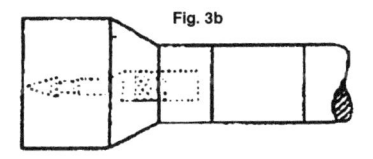

Fig. 3b

NOTE: The instrument may also be inserted without removing the detachable head assembly if the preferred application is a sutured purse-string technique. In this case, however, prior to insertion, the detachable head assembly and the staple housing must be closed by rotating the adjusting knob clockwise. (See Fig. 3c.)

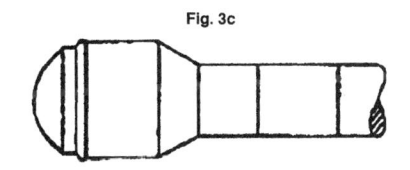

Fig. 3c

4. Insert the detachable head assembly into the lumen and secure the purse-string onto the anvil shaft above the tying notch. (See Fig. 4.)

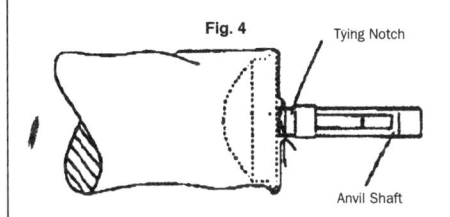

Fig. 4 — Tying Notch, Anvil Shaft

5. Insert the instrument up to the closed lumen with the detachable head assembly removed and the trocar fully retracted. Fully extend the trocar and pierce tissue by rotating the adjusting knob counterclockwise. Push the tissue down to where the orange tying area is visible. (See Fig. 5.)

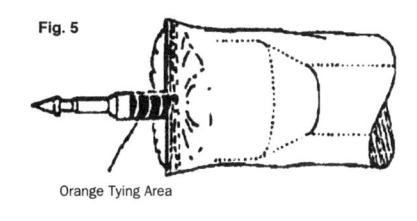

Fig. 5 — Orange Tying Area

CAUTION: Keep the trocar visible at all times to prevent personal injury or inadvertent trauma to adjacent structures.

6. Reattach the detachable head assembly by sliding the anvil shaft over the trocar and pushing until the detachable head assembly snaps into its fully seated position. (See Fig. 6.)

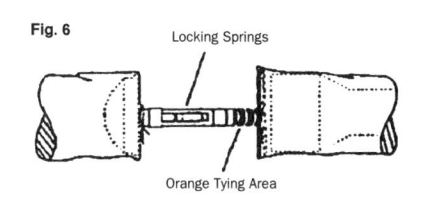

Fig. 6 — Locking Springs, Orange Tying Area

CAUTION: DO NOT clamp across or grip on the locking springs when attempting to reattach the detachable head assembly.

To avoid inclusion of tissue within the anvil shaft, DO NOT use it for piercing. Instead, insert the Ancillary Trocar (included with stapler) into the anvil shaft as described in the section on "Use of Ancillary Trocar."

7. While closing the instrument, keep the organ segments in proper orientation. Inspect to ensure extraneous tissue is excluded. Turn the adjusting knob clockwise to close the instrument. (See Fig. 7a.)

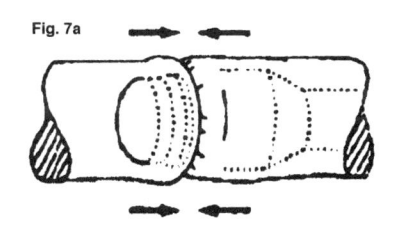

Fig. 7a

As the final adjusting revolution is approached, the orange indicator will move into the green range of the gap setting scale. (See Fig. 7b.)

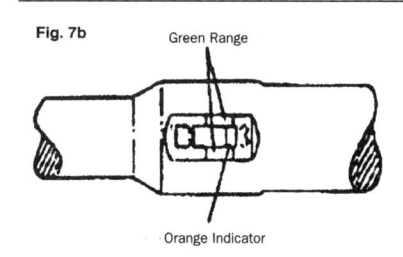

Fig. 7b — Green Range, Orange Indicator

Should the tissue segments to be anastomosed appear unusually thick or thin, the surgeon should adjust the instrument until, in his/her judgement, the tissue is adequately compressed for proper anastomosis. This adjustment may occur providing the orange indicator falls fully within the green range of the gap setting scale. This allows the surgeon to place staples at the height required for desired tissue compression.

STAPLER, LAPAROSCOPIC
(cont'd)

CAUTION: DO NOT fire the instrument if the orange indicator is not fully within the green range of the gap setting scale.

8. Prefire checklist:
Orange indicator is fully within green range.
Check for secure attachment of the head assembly.
To fire the instrument, draw the red safety back toward the adjusting knob until it seats into the body of the instrument. If the safety cannot be released, the instrument is not in the safe firing range. Once released, squeeze the firing handle with a firm, steady pressure. (See Fig. 8.)

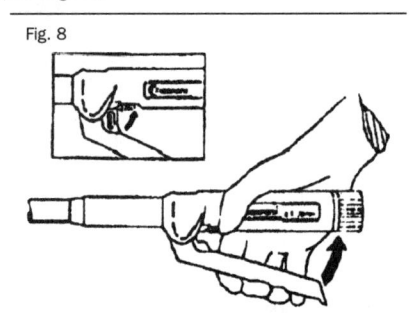

Fig. 8

The surgeon will feel reduced trigger pressure and hear a "crunch" as the instrument completes the firing cycle. After firing, release the firing handle, allowing it to return to its original position, and re-engage the safety. To reset the safety, pull the firing handle back to its original position, if necessary.

9. Open the instrument by turning the adjusting knob counterclockwise as indicated on the end of the knob. For easy removal, open the instrument only one half to three-fourths of a revolution. (See Fig. 9.)

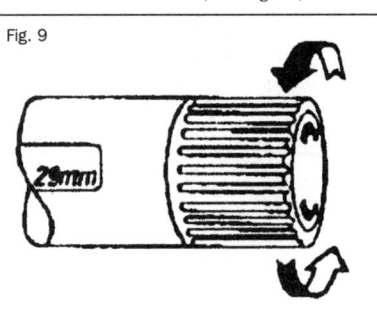

Fig. 9

10. To assure the anvil is free from tissue, rotate the instrument 90° in both directions. To withdraw the open instrument, gently apply rearward traction while simultaneously rotating it. (See Fig. 10.)

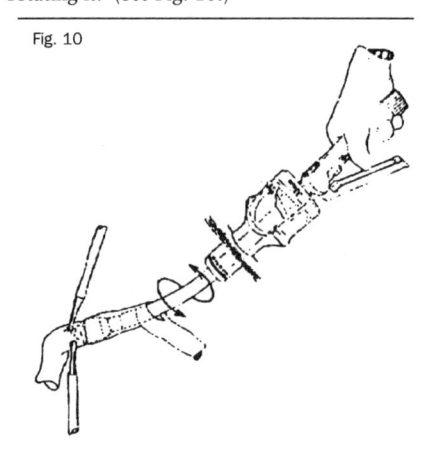

Fig. 10

11. To inspect the donuts, remove the detachable head assembly, washer (if present), and donuts from within the circular knife. (See Fig. 11a and 11b.)

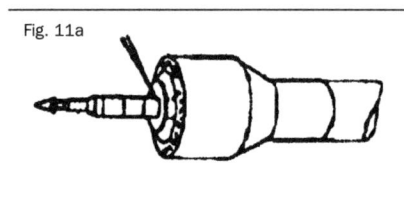

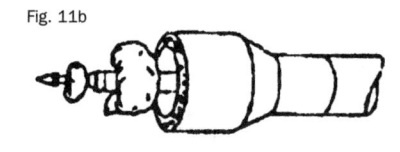

Fig. 11a

Fig. 11b

Examine the integrity of the donuts. Donuts should be intact and include all tissue layers. If donuts are not complete, the anastomosis should be carefully checked for leakage and appropriate repairs made.

CAUTION: Squeezing the firing handle will expose the knife. Engage the red safety prior to removing the washer and donuts from within the circular knife.

REQUIRED ANCILLARY PRODUCTS:
Use of Ancillary Trocar:
The Ancillary Trocar is designed to facilitate controlled penetration through tissue selected by the surgeon. For example, a surgeon may elect to use the Ancillary Trocar to perform a triple stapling technique or end-to-side anastomosis.

NOTE: Keep the trocar visible at all times to prevent personal injury or inadvertent trauma to adjacent structures.

Attaching the Ancillary Trocar to the detachable head assembly:
1. The Ancillary Trocar is shipped in the spacer tab of each ILS instrument.
2. To remove the Ancillary Trocar, grasp the finger notches and pull outward. (See Fig. a.)

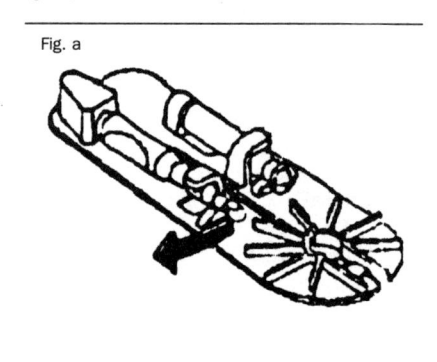

Fig. a

3. Place the blunt end of the Ancillary Trocar into the anvil shaft of the detachable head assembly. Be certain that the finger notches on the Ancillary Trocar are aligned as in Fig. b. This is the unlocked position and will ensure ease of attachment. (See Fig. b.)

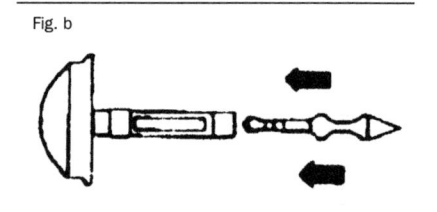

Fig. b

4. Rotate the Ancillary Trocar 90° in the anvil shaft so that the finger notches are in line with the locking springs. This is the locked position. (See Fig. c.)

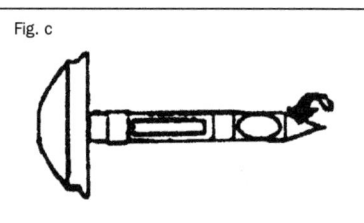

Fig. c

Ensure the locked position is achieved by pulling the Trocar and the detachable head assembly in opposite directions.

Detaching the Ancillary Trocar from the detachable head assembly:

1. Rotate the Ancillary Trocar 90° in the anvil shaft so that the finger notches are perpendicular to the locking springs (unlocked position).

2. Utilizing the finger notches, pull the Ancillary Trocar out of the anvil shaft.

3. Discard the Ancillary Trocar in a sharps disposal.

NOTE: Both the Ancillary Trocar and the Ancillary Trocar Cover are radiopaque. The Ancillary Trocar and the Ancillary Trocar Cover are intended for use with the endoscopic circular stapler only. Product codes that are intended for use are ECS21, ECS25, ECS29, ECS33.

Use of the Ancillary Trocar Cover:
Whenever additional protection of surrounding viscera is desired, the Ancillary Trocar Cover may be used. For example, it may be desired when the ILS is being used intra-abdominally for double stapling technique.

Attaching the Ancillary Trocar Cover to the Integral Trocar:

1. The Ancillary Trocar Cover is shipped in the spacer tab of the ILS instrument.

2. To remove the Ancillary Trocar Cover, grasp the cover and pull outward.

3. Place the cover over the Integral Trocar of the ILS.

Detaching the Ancillary Trocar Cover from the Integral Trocar:

1. When Trocar protection is no longer necessary, remove the cover by pulling upwards until the cover is separated from the Integral Trocar.

NOTE: The Ancillary Trocar Cover must be removed in order to reattach the detachable head assembly. The detachable head assembly will not connect with the Integral Trocar while the Ancillary Trocar Cover is in place.

2. Discard the Ancillary Trocar Cover.

STERILIZATION GUIDELINES: Sterility is guaranteed unless the package is opened or damaged. DO NOT RESTERILIZE.

SPECIFICATIONS/HOW SUPPLIED: The ENDOPATH ILS Endoscopic Circular Stapler with Low-Profile Anvil is designed for single-patient use only. Discard after use. CAUTION: Federal (USA) law restricts this device to sale by or on the order of a physician.

Ethicon Endo-Surgery
4545 Creek Rd.
Cincinnati, OH 45242
513-786-7000

PROXIMATE ILS
DESCRIPTION:

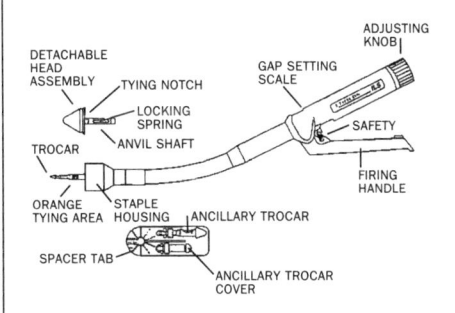

The PROXIMATE* ILS Curved Intraluminal Stapler (CDH) is an anastomotic stapler available in four sizes to permit proper matching of instrument to diameter of the lumen.

The instruments are identified as follows:

PRODUCT CODE	HEAD COLOR
CDH21 (21mm diameter head)	Lt. Green
CDH25 (25mm diameter head)	White
CDH29 (29mm diameter head)	Blue
CDH33 (33mm diameter head)	Dk. Green

The CDH permits tissue attachment to the anvil shaft in a location remote from the main body of the instrument to improve access and visibility. The instrument allows the surgeon to control tissue compression by varying the height of the closed staple. The instrument has been designed to facilitate insertion, operation, and removal. It is disposable and is intended for single-patient use. Therefore, no cleaning, maintenance, or repair is required.

INDICATIONS: The Curved Intraluminal Stapler has applications throughout the alimentary tract for end-to-end, end-to-side, and side-to-side anastomoses.

CONTRAINDICATIONS: Do not use where the combined tissue thickness is less than 1.0mm or greater than 2.5mm or where the internal diameter of the structure is less than 21mm.

WARNINGS:

1. When using the Curved Intraluminal Stapler, Ancillary Trocar, and Ancillary Trocar Cover, please contact an Ethicon Endo-Surgery sales representative first for a demonstration.

2. Do not force safety open until instrument is ready to be fired. (Safety cannot be released until the orange indicator is within green range.)

3. Always check the security of the detachable head assembly prior to firing.

4. Do not immerse the PROXIMATE ILS stapler in an alcoholic solution or any quaternary ammonium solutions.

5. Always inspect the anastomotic staple line for hemostasis and check the completed anastomosis for integrity and leakage. Metal clips, staples, or sutures contained in the area to be stapled may affect the integrity of the anastomosis. Corrective action, if required, may include the use of sutures or electrocautery.

6. Make certain purse-string sutures are tied snugly against the anvil shaft and trocar shaft and that no redundant tissue is present.

7. Make certain that the tissue thickness is within the indicated range, and that it is evenly distributed in the instrument. Excess tissue on one side may result in unacceptable staple formation and can result in staple line leakage.

8. BEFORE FIRING MAKE CERTAIN THE ORANGE INDICATOR IS FULLY WITHIN THE GREEN RANGE OF THE GAP SETTING SCALE.

9. Make certain that the firing handle is fully squeezed to ensure proper staple formation and cutting of tissue.

10. Keep the trocar visible at all times to prevent personal injury or inadvertent trauma to adjacent structures. DO NOT use the anvil shaft to assist in piercing the tissue by placing it over the unexposed trocar. To avoid inclusion of tissue within the anvil shaft, DO NOT use it for piercing.

11. DO NOT clamp across or grip on the locking springs when attempting to reattach the detachable head assembly.

12. Squeezing the firing handle will expose the knife. Engage the red safety prior to removing washer and donuts from within the circular knife.

13. Dispose of all fired instruments. Assure safety is engaged prior to disposing. DO NOT RESTERILIZE. Resterilization may compromise the integrity of the stapler, which may result in wound leakage or disruption.

Read all instructions carefully. Failure to properly follow the instructions may lead to serious surgical consequences, such as leakage or disruption.

INSTRUCTIONS FOR USE: Read all information carefully. Descriptions and usage of the Circular Stapler are detailed in the following pages.

It is suggested that first-time users of the Curved (CDH) Intraluminal Stapler review the operation of the Instrument, Ancillary Trocar, and Ancillary Trocar Cover with an Ethicon Endo-Surgery representative prior to use.

STAPLER, LAPAROSCOPIC (cont'd)

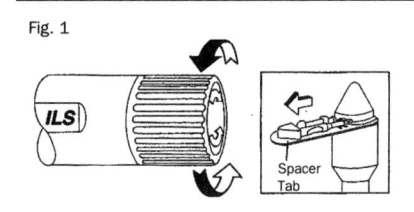

Fig. 1

1. To remove the spacer tab, open the instrument by turning the adjusting knob counterclockwise two revolutions (see Fig. 1).

NOTE: If use of the Ancillary Trocar and/or Ancillary Trocar Cover is anticipated, DO NOT discard the spacer tab. See section for "Use of the Ancillary Trocar," and/or section for "Use of the Ancillary Trocar Cover."

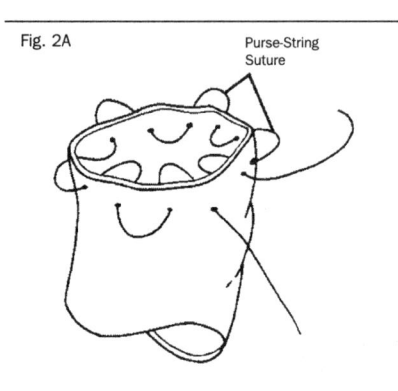

Fig. 2A

2. Place purse-string sutures in the organs to be anastomosed (see Fig. 2A).

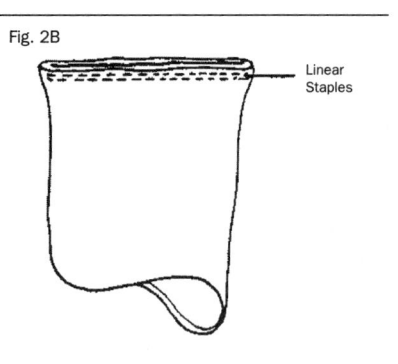

Fig. 2B

On the basis of surgeon experience and judgment, a closed lumen technique (double or triple stapling technique) may be employed as an alternative to a purse-string technique (see Fig. 2B).

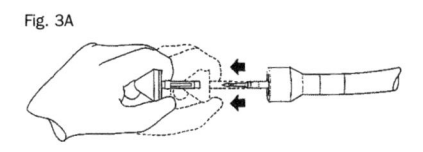

Fig. 3A

3. For a double stapling technique, open the instrument using the adjusting knob until the orange tying area is visible. Remove the detachable head assembly to expose the trocar (see Fig. 3A).

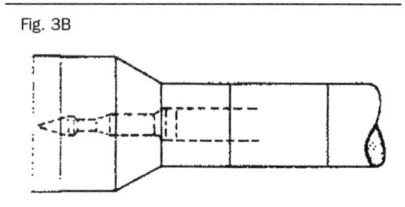

Fig. 3B

Retract the trocar by rotating the adjusting knob clockwise until a stop is reached. Check trocar to verify that it is fully retracted before proceeding (see Fig. 3B).

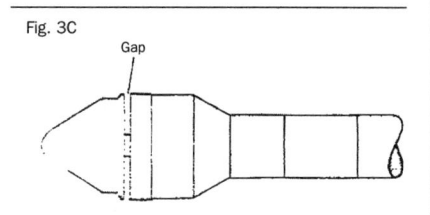

Fig. 3C

NOTE: The instrument may also be inserted without removing the detachable head assembly if the preferred application is a sutured purse-string technique. In this case however, prior to insertion, the detachable head assembly and the staple housing must be closed by rotating the adjusting knob clockwise (see Fig. 3C).

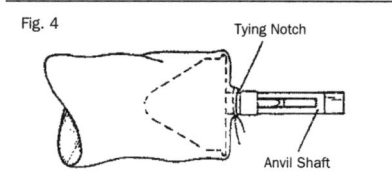

Fig. 4

4. Insert the detachable head assembly into the lumen and secure the purse-string onto the anvil shaft above the tying notch (see Fig. 4).

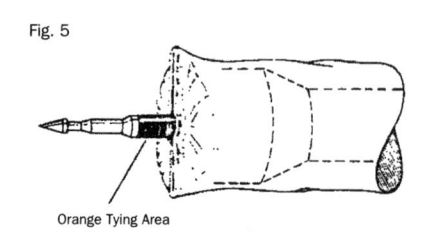

Fig. 5

5. Insert the instrument up to the closed lumen with the detached head assembly removed and the trocar fully retracted. Fully extend the trocar and pierce tissue by rotating the adjusting knob counterclockwise. Push the tissue down to where the orange tying area is visible (see Fig. 5).

CAUTION: Keep the trocar visible at all times to prevent personal injury or inadvertent trauma to adjacent structures.

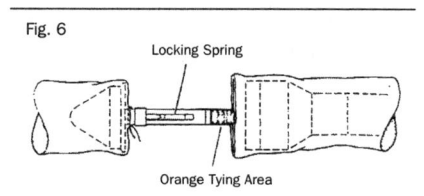

Fig. 6

6. Reattach the detachable head assembly by sliding the anvil shaft over the trocar and pushing until the detachable head assembly snaps into its fully seated position (see Fig. 6).

CAUTION: DO NOT clamp across or grip on the locking springs when attempting to reattach the detachable head assembly.

To avoid inclusion of tissue within the anvil shaft, DO NOT use it for piercing. Instead, insert the Ancillary Trocar (included with stapler) into the anvil shaft as described in the section on "Use of Ancillary Trocar."

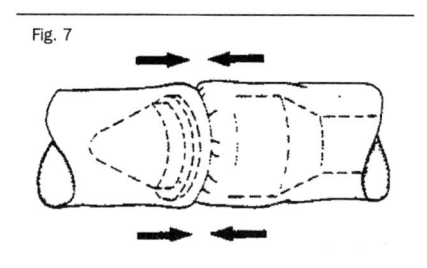

Fig. 7

7. While closing the instrument, keep the organ segments in proper orientation. Inspect to ensure extraneous tissue is excluded. Turn the adjusting knob clockwise to close the instrument (see Fig. 7A).

Fig. 7B
Green Range
Orange Indicator

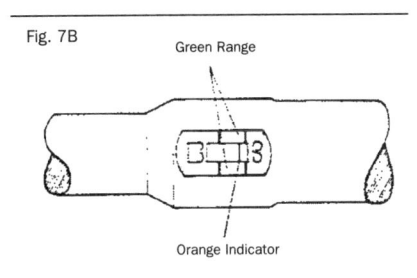

As the final adjusting revolution is approached, the orange indicator will move into the green range of the gap setting scale (see Fig. 7B).

Should the tissue segments to be anastomosed appear unusually thick or thin, the surgeon should adjust the instrument until, in his/her judgment, the tissue is adequately compressed for proper anastomosis. This adjustment may occur providing the orange indicator falls fully within the green range of the gap setting scale. This allows the surgeon to place staples at the height required for desired tissue compression.

CAUTION: DO NOT fire the instrument if the orange indicator is not fully within the green range of the gap setting scale.

8. Prefire checklist:
– Orange indicator is fully within green range
– Check for secure attachment of the head assembly

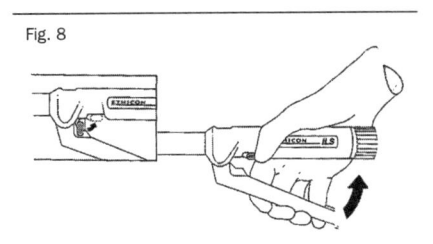

Fig. 8

To fire the instrument draw the red safety back toward the adjusting knob until it seats into the body of the instrument. If the safety cannot be released, the instrument is not in the safe firing range. Once released, squeeze the firing handle with a firm, steady pressure (see Fig. 8).

The surgeon will feel reduced trigger pressure and hear a "crunch" as the instrument completes the firing cycle.

After firing, release the firing handle, allowing it to return to its original position, and re-engage the safety. To reset the safety, pull the firing handle back to its original position if necessary.

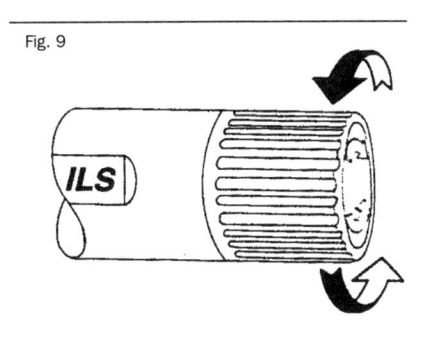

Fig. 9

9. Open the instrument by turning the adjusting knob counterclockwise as indicated on the end of the knob. For easy removal, open the instrument only one half to three-fourths of a revolution (see Fig. 9).

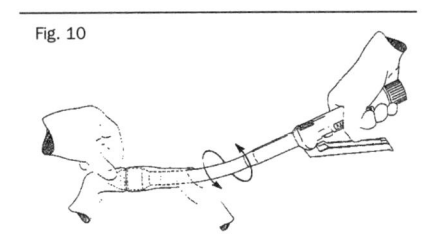

Fig. 10

10. To ensure the anvil is free from tissue, rotate the instrument 90° in both directions. To withdraw the open instrument, gently apply rearward traction while simultaneously rotating it (see Fig. 10).

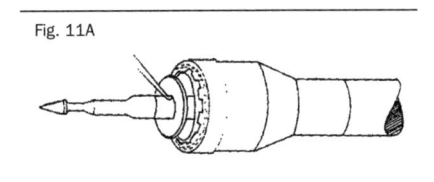

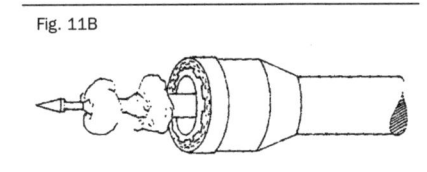

Fig. 11A

Fig. 11B

11. To inspect the donuts, remove the detachable head assembly, washer (if present), and donuts from within the circular knife (see Fig. 11A and 11B). Examine the integrity of the donuts. Donuts should be intact and include all tissue layers. If donuts are not complete, the anastomosis should be carefully checked for leakage and appropriate repairs made.

CAUTION: Squeezing the firing handle will expose the knife. Engage the red safety prior to removing the washer and donuts from within the circular knife.

REQUIRED ANCILLARY PRODUCTS:
Use of the Ancillary Trocar:

The Ancillary Trocar is designed to facilitate controlled penetration through tissue selected by the surgeon. For example, a surgeon may elect to use the Ancillary Trocar to perform a triple stapling technique or end-to-side anastomosis.

NOTE: Keep the trocar visible at all times to prevent personal injury or inadvertent trauma to adjacent structures.

Attaching the Ancillary Trocar to the detachable head assembly:

1. The Ancillary Trocar is shipped in the spacer tab of each ILS instrument.

2. To remove the Ancillary Trocar, grasp the finger notches and pull outwards (see Fig. A).

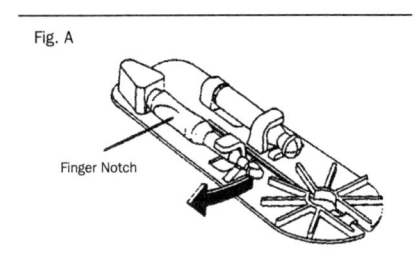

Fig. A
Finger Notch

3. Place the blunt end of the Ancillary Trocar into the anvil shaft of the detachable head assembly. Be certain that the finger notches on the Ancillary Trocar are aligned as in Fig. B. This is the unlocked position and will ensure ease of attachment (see Fig. B).

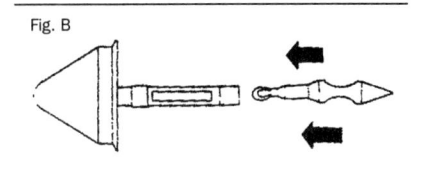

Fig. B

4. Rotate the Ancillary Trocar 90° in the anvil shaft so that the finger notches are in line with the locking springs. This is the locked position (see Fig. C). Ensure the locked position is achieved by pulling the Trocar and the detachable head assembly in opposite directions.

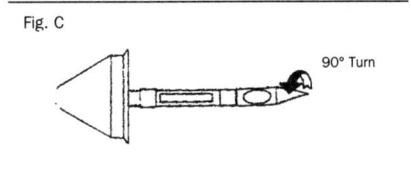

Fig. C
90° Turn

STAPLER, LAPAROSCOPIC
(cont'd)

Detaching the Ancillary Trocar from the detachable head assembly:

1. Rotate the Ancillary Trocar 90° in the anvil shaft so that the finger notches are perpendicular to the locking springs (unlocked position).

2. Utilizing the finger notches, pull the Ancillary Trocar out of the anvil shaft.

3. Discard the Ancillary Trocar in a sharps disposal.

NOTE: Both the Ancillary Trocar and the Ancillary Trocar Cover are radiopaque. The Ancillary Trocar and the Ancillary Trocar Cover are intended for use with the curved and straight ILS only. Product codes that are intended for use are: CDH21, SDH21, CDH29, SDH29, CDH25, SDH25, CDH33, and SDH33.

Use of the Ancillary Trocar Cover:
Whenever additional protection of surrounding viscera is desired, the Ancillary Trocar Cover may be used. For example, it may be desired when the ILS is being used intra-abdominally for double stapling technique.

Attaching the Ancillary Trocar Cover to the Integral Trocar:

1. The Ancillary Trocar Cover is shipped in the spacer tab of the ILS instrument.

2. To remove the Ancillary Trocar Cover, grasp the cover and pull outwards.

3. Place the cover over the Integral Trocar of the ILS.

Detaching the Ancillary Trocar Cover from the Integral Trocar:

1. When trocar protection is no longer necessary, remove the cover by pulling upwards until the cover is separated from the Integral Trocar.

NOTE: The Ancillary Trocar Cover must be removed in order to reattach the detachable head assembly. The detachable head assembly will not connect with the Integral Trocar while the Ancillary Trocar Cover is in place.

2. Discard the Ancillary Trocar Cover.

STERILIZATION GUIDELINES: Sterility is guaranteed unless the package is opened or damaged. DO NOT RESTERILIZE.

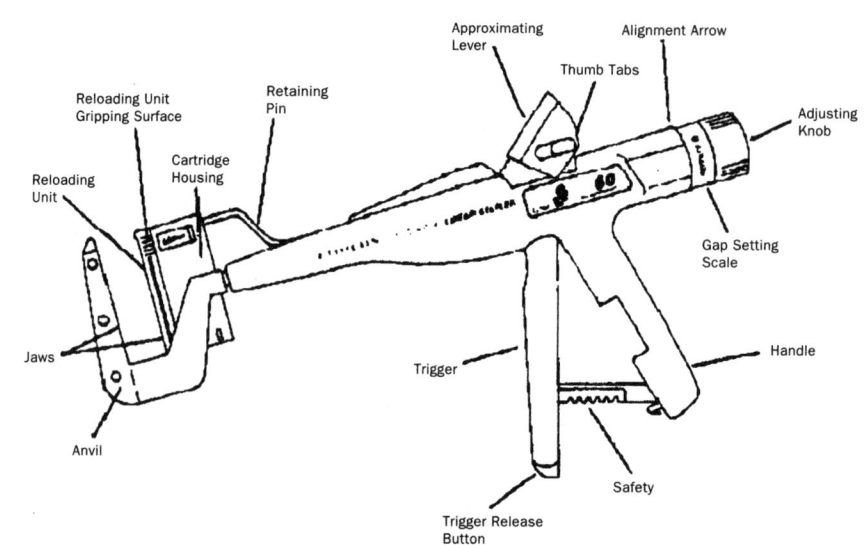

PROXMATE RL PLUS RELOADABLE LINEAR STAPLER

Ethicon Endo-Surgery
4545 Creek Rd.
Cincinnati, OH 45242
513-786-7000

PROXIMATE RL PLUS

DESCRIPTION:

The PROXIMATE* RL PLUS Reloadable Linear Stapler delivers a double staggered row of titanium staples in order to approximate internal tissues. The instrument is available in three sizes to accommodate different tissue. They are identified by the following codes:

TP30 (applies 11 staples in a double staggered line of approximately 30mm)
TP60 (applies 21 staples in a double staggered line of approximately 60mm)
TP90 (applies 33 staples in a double staggered line of approximately 90mm)

Closed staple height is adjustable to compensate for various tissue thicknesses. The RL PLUS Reloadable Linear Stapler is disposable and is intended for single-patient use, therefore, no cleaning, maintenance, or repair is required.

The PROXIMATE RL PLUS Reloadable Linear Stapler may be reloaded during a single procedure by using the appropriate reloading unit:

TR30 (reloads the TP30 with 11 staples)
TR60 (reloads the TP60 with 21 staples)
TR90 (reloads the TP90 with 33 staples)

It is suggested that the PROXIMATE Reloadable Linear Stapler be reloaded no more than three times per case for a maximum of four firings per instrument.

INDICATIONS: The TP30, TP60, and TP90 RL PLUS Reloadable Linear Staplers have application throughout the alimentary tract and in thoracic surgery for transection and resection of internal tissues.

CONTRAINDICATIONS: Do not use on tissue in the alimentary tract with a thickness that requires an instrument setting outside of the white gap setting scale.

Do not use on ischemic or necrotic tissue.
Do not use on pulmonary vessels.

WARNINGS:

1. Before firing, verify that the tissue retaining pin is in proper position in the distal jaw. This is critical for correct staple formation.

2. Do not release the safety until the instrument is ready to be fired.

3. The trigger must be pulled back completely to the handle and locked.

4. Inspect for hemostasis and integrity of the staple line after removal of the linear stapler. Corrective action, if required, may include the use of sutures or electrocautery.

5. Dispose of all fired instruments and used reloading units. DO NOT RESTERILIZE the linear stapler or the reloading unit. Resterilization may compromise the integrity of the linear stapler or the reloading unit, which may result in wound leakage or disruption.

Read all instructions carefully. Failure to properly follow the instructions may lead to serious surgical consequences such as leakage or disruption.

INSTRUCTIONS FOR USE: Please Read All Information Carefully.

The description and use of the PROXIMATE Reloadable Linear RL PLUS Staplers are described in the following pages.

This information is designed to provide instructions for the use of the PROXIMATE Reloadable Linear RL PLUS Stapler. It is not intended as a guide to surgical stapling techniques.

1. The RL PLUS is delivered to the surgeon in the open position. The tissue to be transected or resected is positioned in the jaws of the instrument.

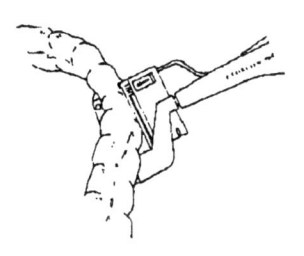

The TP30, TP60, and TP90 are available to permit selection of an appropriate staple line length for the specific tissue. The instruments allow the surgeon to adjust the height of the closed staple for different tissue thicknesses.

2. To close the RL PLUS, push the approximating lever down until the lever is flush with the instrument and the lever is locked. The retaining pin automatically advances into the distal jaw of the instrument. This aligns the anvil and cartridge housing to provide the correct staple formation and also prevents compressed tissue from slipping from the jaws.

CAUTION: Make sure that the pin is seated correctly in the anvil hole; this is critical for correct staple formation.

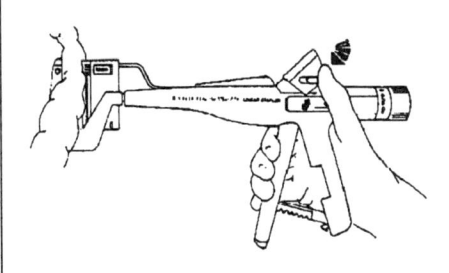

3. The surgeon adjusts the gap between the jaws by rotating the adjusting knob clockwise until the proper reading is indicated on the white gap setting scale. The final setting may be determined based upon the surgeon's own experience, or discrete settings are provided on the scale which correspond to a 1.5 (blue zone) and 2.0 (green zone) closed staple height.

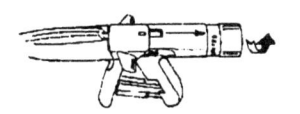

These settings form staples to the predetermined heights of linear staplers of other manufacturers and may be used to guide the surgeon in gap setting.

Tissue blanching and resistance to closing may be observed as the final gap setting is achieved. The instrument is now ready for "firing."

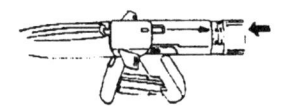

4. The instrument is actuated ("fired") in the following manner:
  a. The safety is drawn back toward the handle. (NOTE: The instrument is designed to inhibit release of the safety unless the gap is set in the appropriate range and the approximating lever is closed.)

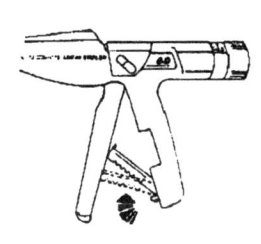

  b. Pull the trigger back firmly until it locks into the handle. The trigger will remain in the "fired" position.

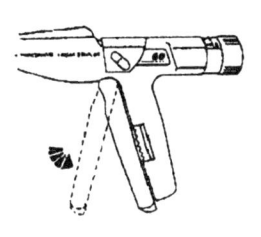

  c. Prior to removal, the instrument edge may be used as a cutting guide to transect the tissue, or to excise any margin of tissue protruding through the jaws. This will aid in cutting at a proper distance from the staple line.

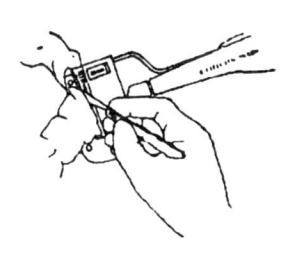

  d. Open the instrument by pushing upward on the approximating lever. Both the instrument jaws and the retaining pin will return to their original positions.

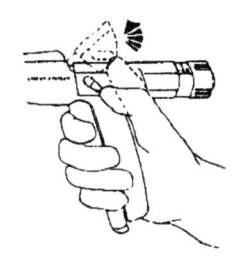

  e. Examine the staple line for hemostasis and complete closure. Corrective action, if required, may include the use of sutures or electrocautery.

NOTE: The instrument may be preset to a desired height before placing the instrument on tissue by turning the adjustment knob clockwise and aligning the instrument arrow with the desired staple heights on the white gap setting scale.

SUMMARY OF OPERATING INSTRUCTIONS for PROXIMATE RL PLUS Reloadable Linear Stapler:
  1. Insert tissue into jaws.
  2. Close approximating lever and ensure pin is seated into the anvil.
  3. Set the gap by turning the adjusting knob clockwise.
  4. Release the safety.
  5. Fire the instrument by squeezing the trigger firmly back to the handle.
  6. Use instrument as cutting guide if so desired.
  7. Push up on thumb tabs to open jaws and release retaining pin.
  8. Remove instrument.
  9. Reload for subsequent firing, if desired.

SUMMARY OF OPERATING INSTRUCTIONS FOR PROXIMATE RL PLUS Linear Reloading Unit:
  1. Release the trigger.
  2. Reset the safety.
  3. Return adjustment knob to fully opened position.
  4. Slide the empty reloading unit from the cartridge.
  5. Remove and discard the staple retaining cap from a new reloading unit.
  6. Insert the new reloading unit into the cartridge housing.

NOTE: The reloading units will only fit and operate properly in the linear stapler for which they have been designed.

For further description, see the appropriate sections.

STAPLER, LAPAROSCOPIC
(cont'd)

ASSEMBLY GUIDELINES: Reloading PROXIMATE RL PLUS Reloadable Linear Stapler:

1. Press the trigger release button. The trigger will spring back to its original position.

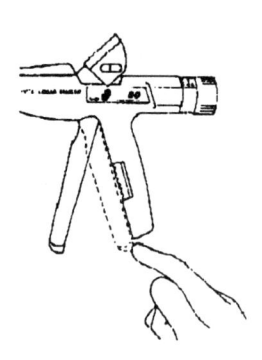

2. Reset the safety.

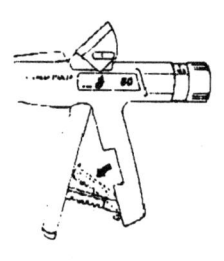

3. Return the adjustment knob to its fully opened position by turning the knob counter-clockwise.

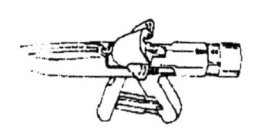

4. Grasp the gripping surface of the empty reloading unit and slide it from the cartridge housing. Discard the used reloading unit. Any formed but unused staples should be cleaned from the instrument by rinsing in sterile solution.

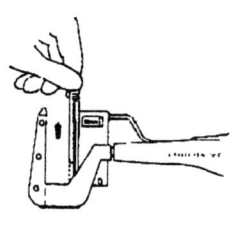

NOTE: The reloading unit will not slide out of the instrument unless the trigger is reset.

5. Remove and discard the staple retaining cap from a new Reloading Unit.

NOTE: The reloading units will only fit and operate properly in the linear stapler for which they have been designed.

TR30 reloads the TP30 (30mm linear)
TR60 reloads the TP60 (60mm linear)
TR90 reloads the TP90 (90mm linear)
TRV30 reloads the TPV30 (30mm linear-vascular)
TRH30 reloads the TPH30 (30mm linear-heavy wire)
TRH60 reloads the TPH60 (60mm linear-heavy wire)
TRH90 reloads the TPH90 (90mm linear-heavy wire)

6. Insert the new reloading unit into the cartridge housing. The reloading unit will snap into position. The instrument is now ready for use.

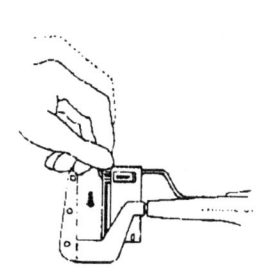

STERILIZATION GUIDELINES: Sterility is guaranteed unless the package is opened or damaged. DO NOT RESTERILIZE.

3M Health Care
3M Center,
Bldg. 275-4E-01
St. Paul, MN 55144-1000
612-733-1110

Davis & Geck Endosurgery
1 Casper Street
Danbury, CT 06810
203-743-4451

Design Standards Corp.
643 North Ave.
Bridgeport, CT 06606-5745
203-366-7046

United States Surgical Corp.
150 Glover Ave.
Norwalk, CT 06856-5080
203-845-1000

STAPLER, SURGICAL

Ethicon Endo-Surgery
4545 Creek Rd.
Cincinnati, OH 45242
513-786-7000

PROXIMATE RH

INDICATIONS: The PROXIMATE* RH Skin Stapler may be employed for routine skin closure in a wide variety of surgical procedures.

CONTRAINDICATIONS: When it is not possible to maintain at least a 5mm distance from the stapled skin to underlying bones, vessels, or internal organs, the use of staples for skin closure is contraindicated.

WARNINGS: Dispose of all fired instruments. DO NOT RESTERILIZE PROXIMATE RH Skin Staplers. Resterilization may compromise the integrity of the instrument.

Read all instructions carefully. Failure to properly follow the instructions may lead to serious surgical consequences such as staple line disruption.

INSTRUCTIONS FOR USE: Use of Skin Stapler: Suggested Eversion Techniques:

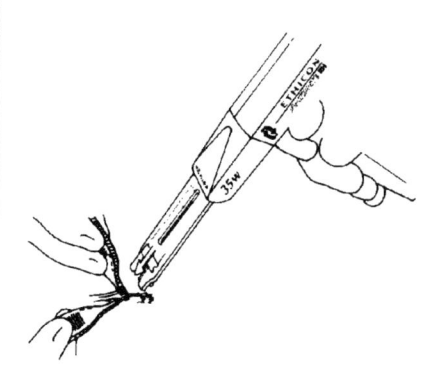

1. With two tissue forceps, pick up each wound edge individually and approximate the edges.
OR

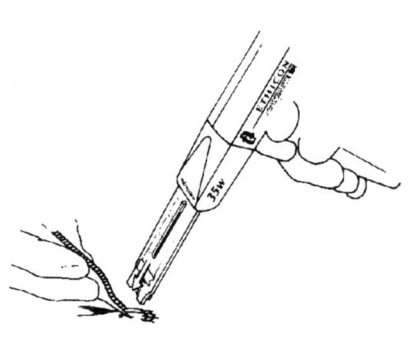

2. With one tissue forceps, force skin edges together until edges evert.

OR

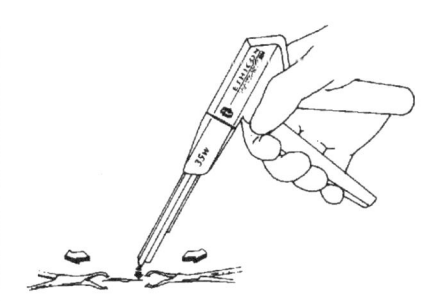

3. Apply tension to either end of the incision, such that the tissue edges begin to approximate themselves. One forceps can be used to ensure that the edges are everted.

Position:

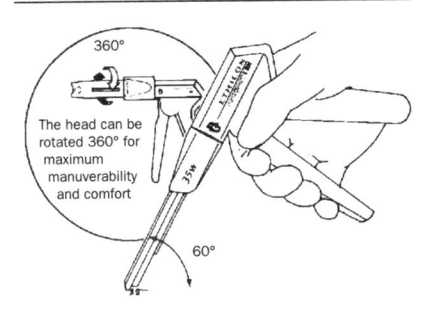

4. Position the instrument very lightly over the everted skin edges. Instrument should be held at a 60° angle to the skin.

Fire/Release:

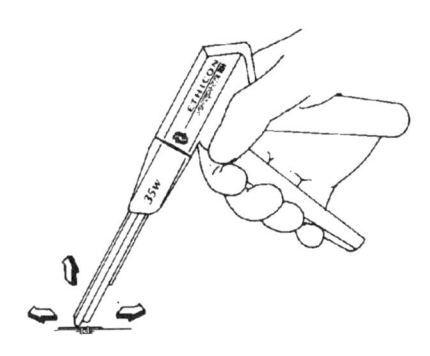

5. Squeeze the trigger until the trigger motion is halted, then release the trigger and move the instrument off the incision in any direction.

Alternate Release:

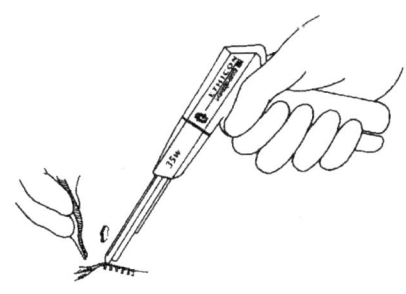

6. If desired, before releasing the trigger, lift up on the instrument. This will help to evert the skin edges, which can then be more easily grasped with the tissue forceps. Release the trigger after the forceps are in place, and repeat the sequence to fire the next staple.

Alternate Technique:

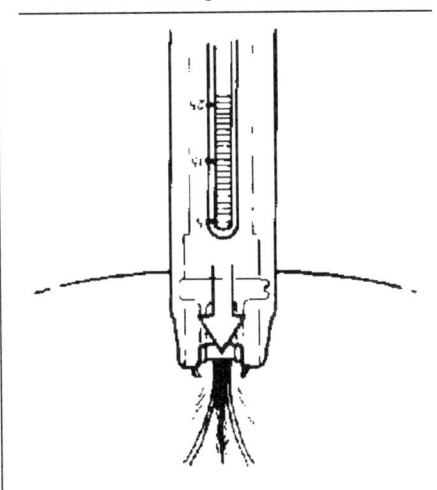

7a. The instrument can also be precocked (partially fired) so that the staple points are visible at the nose of the instrument. This feature, in conjunction with the clear nose and the alignment arrow, ensures precise staple placement in the skin.

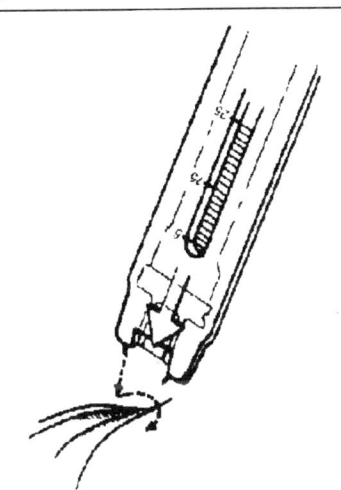

7b. If desired, after the instrument has been precocked, one leg of the staple can be hooked on to one side of the tissue.

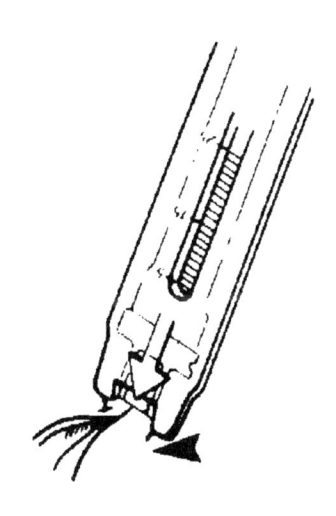

7c. This will aid in drawing the tissue together. This technique may be suitable for attaching skin grafts under moderate tension.

STERILIZATION GUIDELINES: Sterility is guaranteed unless the package is opened or damaged. DO NOT RESTERILIZE.

SPECIFICATIONS/HOW SUPPLIED: Formed Staple Dimensions:

Regular staples are formed from 0.53mm diameter wire and have the approximate dimensions shown below.

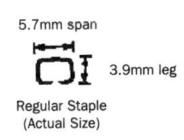

5.7mm span
3.9mm leg
Regular Staple
(Actual Size)

Wide staples are formed from 0.58mm diameter wire and have the approximate dimensions shown below.

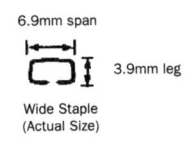

6.9mm span
3.9mm leg
Wide Staple
(Actual Size)

PROXIMATE skin staples have a rectangular configuration for greater stability in tissue. Rotation of staples, which results in painful extraction, is minimized by the stabilized rectangular design.

STAPLER, SURGICAL (cont'd)

3M Health Care
3M Center,
Bldg. 275-4E-01
St. Paul, MN 55144-1000
612-733-1110

Davis & Geck Endosurgery
1 Casper Street
Danbury, CT 06810
203-743-4451

Design Standards Corp.
643 North Ave.
Bridgeport, CT 06606-5745
203-366-7046

Ethicon, Inc.
U.S. Route 22
P.O. Box 151
Somerville, NJ 08876
908-218-0707

Ethnor
192 Ave. Charles De Gaulle
F-92523 Neuilly S/Seine Cedex
France
1/47382233

I.S.I. Manufacturing, Inc.
1947 Ivanhoe Dr.
Irwin, PA 15642-4454
412-863-4911

Martin, Gebr. GmbH & Co. KG
Ludwigstaler Str. 132
Postf. 60
D-78532 Tuttlingen
Germany
07461/7060

Richard-Allan Medical Industries, Inc.
8850 M-89
P.O. Box 351
Richland, MI 49083-0351
616-629-5811

Synectic Engineering, Inc.
4 Oxford Rd.
Milford, CT 06460-7007
203-877-8488

Technalytics, Inc.
210 Summit Ave.
Montvale, NJ 07645-1526
201-391-0494

United States Surgical Corp.
150 Glover Ave.
Norwalk, CT 06856-5080
203-845-1000

Arthroscope

ACCESSORIES, ARTHROSCOPE

Acufex Microsurgical, Inc.
130 Forbes Blvd.
Mansfield, MA 02048
508-339-9700

Anspach Effort, Inc.
4500 Riverside Dr.
Palm Beach Gardens, FL 33410
407-627-1080

Arthrex Arthroscopy Instrument
3050 North Horseshoe Dr., Ste. 168
Naples, FL 33942-7909
813-643-5553

Arthrex Medical Instrument Gmbh
Von Kahr Str. 2
D-80997 Muenchen 50
Germany
89/142257

Arthro-Medic, Inc.
4203 Belfort Rd., Ste. 150
Jacksonville, FL 32216-5896
904-296-1188

Citation Medical Corp.
230 Edison Way
Reno, NV 89502
702-324-1212

Clarus Medical Systems, Inc.
2605 Fernbrook Lane
Minneapolis, MN 55447-4736
612-559-8640

Cuda Products Corporation
6000 Powers Ave.
Jacksonville, FL 32217-2212
904-737-7611

Depuy, Inc.
700 Orthopaedic Dr.
P.O. Box 988
Warsaw, IN 46581-0988
219-267-8143

Dufner Instrumente
Foehrenstr. 9 - Postfach 4149
D-78532 Tuttlingen
Germany
07461/3697

Dyonics Video Division
4533 Enterprise Drive
Oklahoma City, OK 73128
405-949-0171

Hall Surgical
1170 Mark Ave.
Carpinteria, CA 93013-2918
805-684-0456

Instrument Makar, Inc.
2950 E. Mt. Hope
Okemos, MI 48864-1910
517-332-3593

Leibinger GmbH
Botzinger Strasse 41
D-70437 Freiburg
Germany
0761/49058-0

Leibinger L.P.
14540 Beltwood Pkwy. E., Ste. 1
Dallas, TX 75244
214-392-3636

Linvatec Corporation
11311 Concept Blvd.
Largo, FL 34643-4908
813-399-5344

Linvatec, Div. of Zimmer of Canada Ltd.
2323 Argentia Rd.
Mississauga, ONT L5N 5N3
Canada
905-858-8588

Lorenz Surgical, Walter
1520 Tradeport Dr.
Jacksonville, FL 32229-8009
904-741-4400

Microlux, Inc.
6000-1 Powers Ave., Medical Bldg.
Jacksonville, FL 32217
904-737-9660

Nextec Surgical Corp.
2629 South Horseshoe Dr.
Naples, FL 33942-6122
813-643-2553

O.R. Surgical Co., Inc.
120 Montlieu Ave.
Greensboro, NC 27409-2620
919-855-6714

Olsen Electrosurgical Inc.
2100 Meridian Park Blvd.
Concord, CA 94520-5709
510-825-8151

Optical Resources, Inc.
15 Harriman Ave.
Sloatsburg, NY 10974-2628
914-753-5309

Optik, Inc.
1370 Blair Dr.
Odenton, MD 21113
410-551-9700

Orthopedic Systems, Inc.
1897 National Ave.
Hayward, CA 94545-1794
510-785-1020

Portlyn Medical Products
Route 25
Moultonboro, NH 03254
603-476-5538

Questus Corp.
Lime St.
P.O. Box 9
Marblehead, MA 01945-0009
617-639-1900

Smith & Nephew Dyonics, Inc.
160 Dascomb Rd.
Andover, MA 01810-5893
508-470-2800

Sodem Systems
110, Chemin du Pont du Centenaire
Pont-du-Centenaire
CH-1228 Plan-les-Quates/Geneva
Switzerland
22/794-9696

Tnco, Inc.
P.O. Box 231
Whitman, MA 02382-0231
617-447-6661

W.J. Medical Instruments, Inc.
3537 Old Conejo Rd.
Newbury Park, CA 91320
805-499-8676

WM Instrumente GmbH
Panoramastr. 6
D-78604 Rietheim 1
Germany
07424/501310

Wolf Medical Instruments Corp., Richard
353 Corporate Woods Pkwy.
Vernon Hills, IL 60061-3110
708-913-1113

ARTHROSCOPE

Acufex Microsurgical, Inc.
130 Forbes Blvd.
Mansfield, MA 02048
508-339-9700

Arthrex Arthroscopy Instrument
3050 North Horseshoe Dr., Ste. 168
Naples, FL 33942-7909
813-643-5553

Arthrex Medical Instrument GmbH
Von Kahr Str. 2
D-80997 Muenchen 50
Germany
89/142257

Carsen Group Inc.
151 Telson Rd.
Markham, ONT L3R 1E7
Canada
416-479-4100

Chakoff Endoscopy
15405 SW 72 Ct.
Miami, FL 33157
305-253-0321

Chirurgische Instrumente
Hauptstrasse 18
D-78582 Balgheim
Germany
7424/501319

Citation Medical Corp.
230 Edison Way
Reno, NV 89502
702-324-1212

Clarus Medical Systems, Inc.
2605 Fernbrook Lane
Minneapolis, MN 55447-4736
612-559-8640

Comeg GmbH
Dornierstr. 55
D-78532 Tuttlingen 14
Germany
07461/8036

Contec Medical Ltd.
11 Haroshet Street
P.O. Box 1400
Ramat Hasharon 47113
Israel
03/5491153

Danek Medical, Inc.
3092 Directors Row
Memphis, TN 38131-0401
901-396-3133

Depuy, Inc.
700 Orthopaedic Dr.
P.O. Box 988
Warsaw, IN 46581-0988
219-267-8143

Electro Fiberoptics Corporation
56 Hudson St.
Northborough, MA 01532-1922
508-393-3753

Expanded Optics, Inc.
7382 Bolsa Ave.
Westminster, CA 92683-5212
714-891-3996

Hipp GmbH, Anton
Annastr. 25/1
Postfach 80
D-78567 Fridingen
Germany
07463/7776-5088

Horizon Medical
324 State St.
St. Paul, MN 55107-1608
612-298-0843

Innovasive Devices, Inc.
100B South St.
Hopkinton, MA 01748
508-435-6000

Instrument Makar, Inc.
2950 E. Mt. Hope
Okemos, MI 48864-1910
517-332-3593

Keymed Medical & Industrial Equipment Ltd.
Keymed House, Stock Rd., Southend-on-Sea
Essex SS2 5QH
United Kingdom
0702/616333

Linvatec Corporation
11311 Concept Blvd.
Largo, FL 34643-4908
813-399-5344

Linvatec, Div. of Zimmer of Canada Ltd.
2323 Argentia Rd.
Mississauga, ONT L5N 5N3
Canada
905-858-8588

Machida Endoscope Co. Ltd.
6-13-8, Honkomagome, Bunkyo-Ku
Tokyo 113
Japan
03/946-2151

Medizintechnik
Wurttemberger Str. 26
D-78567 Fridingen
Germany
07/463-8076

Medmetric Corp.
7542 Trade St.
San Diego, CA 92121-2412
619-536-9122

Midas Rex Institute
3000 Race Street
Fort Worth, TX 76111
817-831-2604

Nextec Surgical Corp.
2629 South Horseshoe Dr.
Naples, FL 33942-6122
813-643-2553

ARTHROSCOPE (cont'd)

O.R. Surgical Co., Inc.
120 Montlieu Ave.
Greensboro, NC 27409-2620
919-855-6714

Olympus America, Inc.
4 Nevada Drive
Lake Success, NY 11042-1179
516-488-3880

Olympus Optical Co. Ltd.
San-Ei Bldg.
1-22-2, Nishi-Shinjuku
Shinjuku-Ku, Tokyo 163-91
Japan
03/3402111

Olympus Winter & Ibe GmbH
Kuehnstrasse 61, Postf. 701709
D-22045 Hamburg 70
Germany
040/66966-0

Optical Resources, Inc.
15 Harriman Ave.
Sloatsburg, NY 10974-2628
914-753-5309

Questus Corp.
Lime St.
P.O. Box 9
Marblehead, MA 01945-0009
617-639-1900

Rema Medizintechnik GmbH
In Breiten 10
D-78589 Duerbheim-Tuttlingen
Germany
07424-4064

RFQ Medizintechnik GmbH & Co. KG
Bruderhofstr. 10-12
Postfach 4652
D-78532 Tuttlingen
Germany
07461/4066

Rx Honing Machine Corporation
1301 East Fifth St.
Mishawaka, IN 46544-2827
219-259-1606

Schoelly Fiberoptic GmbH
Robert Bosch Str. 1-3
Postfach 1280
D-79211 Denzlingen
Germany
07666/1018/1019

Shinko Optical Co. Ltd.
3-13-4, Hongo, Bunkyo-Ku
Tokyo 113
Japan
03/8114194

Simal Belgium Instrument Co.
2131 Espey Court, Suite 7
Crofton, MD 21114-2424

Smith & Nephew Dyonics, Inc.
160 Dascomb Rd.
Andover, MA 01810-5893
508-470-2800

Storz Endoscopy-America Inc., Karl
10111 W. Jefferson Blvd.
Culver City, CA 90232-3509
310-558-1500

Storz GmbH & Co., Karl
Mittelstr. 8
Postfach 230
D-78532 Tuttlingen
Germany
07461/7080

Stryker B.V.
Industrielaan 1 - Postbox 118
NL-5400 AC Uden
Netherlands
4132-61555

Stryker Corp., Surgical Div.
4100 E. Milham Ave.
Kalamazoo, MI 49003-6197
616-323-7700

Stryker Pacific
53 Wong Chuk Hang Rd
Sungib Ind Ctr. 7th
Aberdeen,
Hong Kong
852/5/538165

Surgical Instrument Co. of America
1185 Edgewater Ave.
Ridgefield, NJ 07657-2102
201-941-6500

Wect Instrument Company, Inc.
5645 N. Ravenswood
Chicago, IL 60660-3922
312-769-1944

Wisap USA
P.O. Box 324
Tomball, TX 77377-0324
713-351-2629

WM Instrumente GmbH
Panoramastr. 6
D-78604 Rietheim 1
Germany
07424/501310

Wolf Medical Instruments Corp., Richard
353 Corporate Woods Pkwy.
Vernon Hills, IL 60061-3110
708-913-1113

Aspirator

ASPIRATOR, ARTHROSCOPY

Contec Medical Ltd.
11 Haroshet Street
P.O. Box 1400
Ramat Hasharon 47113
Israel
03/5491153

Davol, Inc.
100 Sockanossett
P.O. Box 8500
Cranston, RI 02920-0500
401-463-7000

O.R. Surgical Co., Inc.
120 Montlieu Ave.
Greensboro, NC 27409-2620
919-855-6714

Simal Belgium Instrument Co.
2131 Espey Court, Suite 7
Crofton, MD 21114-2424

Smith & Nephew Dyonics, Inc.
160 Dascomb Rd.
Andover, MA 01810-5893
508-470-2800

Bag

BAG, SPECIMEN, LAPAROSCOPIC

Endomedix Corp.
2162 Michelson Dr.
Irvine, CA 92715
714-253-1000

LAPAROBAG

DESCRIPTION: The LaparoBag™ Tissue Retrieval System is a sterile, single-use system designed to temporarily contain tissue or stones within a patient's body for removal during laparoscopic surgery. The main component of this system is a disposable, flexible, plastic Holding Bag which can be used to contain a variety of tissue, organs or stones to isolate them from the patient's body. The LaparoBag System may be used in conjunction with a variety of applications including debulking gallstone-laden gallbladders, reducing the size of tissue/organs, containing fragile tissue, collecting small pieces or fragments of tissue/organs, etc., in order to facilitate their removal through a small laparoscopic incision. The Holding Bag Assembly consists of the flexible, plastic Holding Bag and a Hoop around the bag opening that assures the mouth of the bag is open during use. At one point on the Hoop, there is a plastic Bag Tag where the Holding Bag Assembly is grasped by grasping forceps. There is a Tether attached to the Bag Tag that can also be grasped by grasping forceps or pulled by hand to withdraw the Holding Bag into the Introducer. The entire assembly is preloaded into the Introducer. The Introducer consists of a plastic tube with a Valve Assembly on one end. The Valve Assembly contains a flexible valve that allows passage of grasping forceps. During a procedure, the Introducer is inserted into a 10mm or larger portal. The Introducer also facilitates bag extraction.

WARNINGS: Do not use an extraction pull-force on the Holding Bag Assembly greater than 10 pounds.

INSTRUCTIONS FOR USE: Open the "peel-open" pouch and remove the entire LaparoBag unit within the sterile field. Grasp the Bag Tag located at the Valve Assembly end of the Introducer with grasping forceps and slide the Introducer loaded with the Holding Bag Assembly into a 10mm or larger laparoscopic portal until its tip enters the peritoneal cavity as viewed on the video monitor.

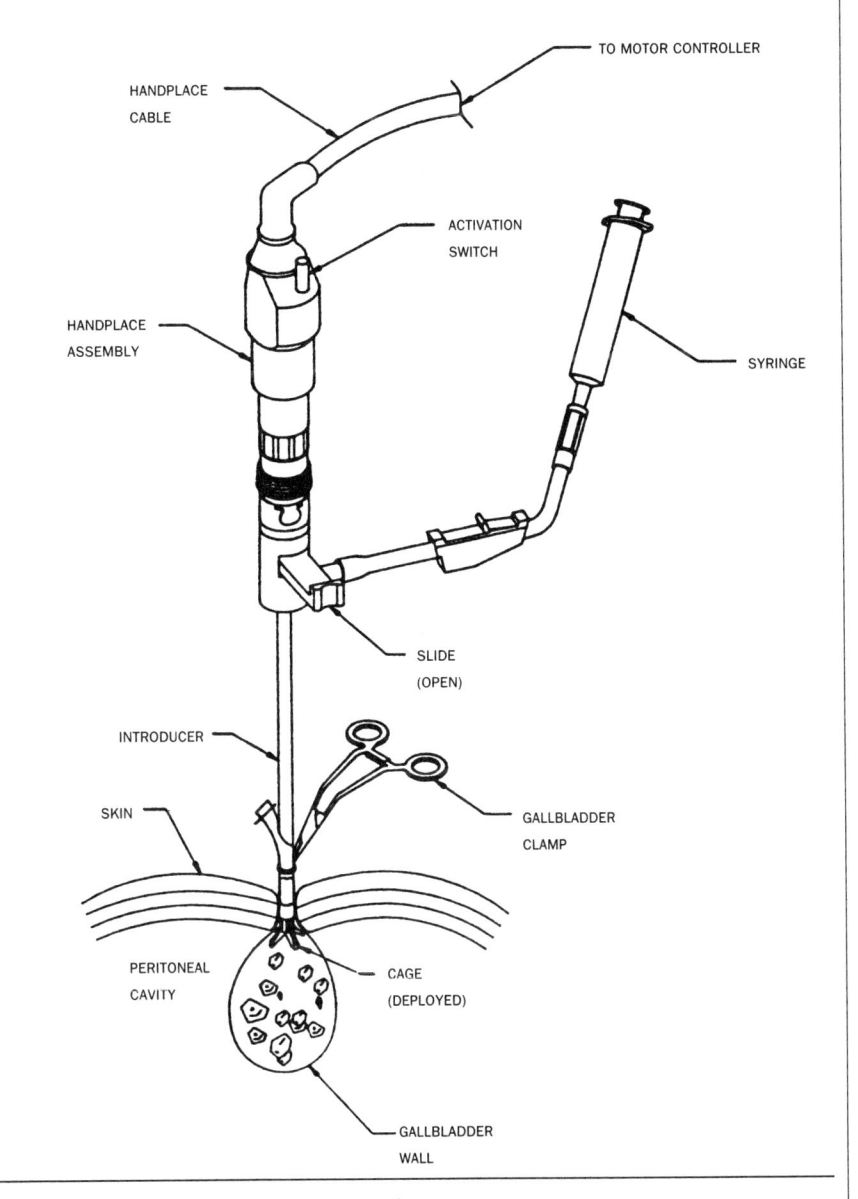

Deploy the Holding Bag Assembly by pushing it out of the Introducer and into the peritoneal cavity with the grasping forceps. Insert tissue or stones into the Holding Bag opening. Perform tissue manipulations as appropriate. When ready to remove the Holding Bag Assembly from the peritoneal cavity, smoothly and steadily pull on the grasping forceps attached to the Bag Tag or the Tether itself until the Hoop of the Holding Bag is inside the Introducer. Once the Hoop of the Holding Bag is entirely enclosed inside the Introducer, simultaneously pull the Introducer, the grasping forceps and the laparoscopic portal from the peritoneal cavity, thus externalizing the neck of the Holding Bag outside the laparoscopic incision. When the tissue manipulations, dissection, fragmentation, debulking, etc., have been completed, smoothly and steadily pull the Holding Bag and its contents out through the laparoscopic incision.

STERILIZATION GUIDELINES: Do not resterilize or reuse this device.

SPECIFICATIONS/HOW SUPPLIED: The LaparoBag Tissue Retrieval System (Model B9350D case of 8) is supplied ready for use as a single, sterile unit in a "peel-open" Tyvek® pouch. A standard 5mm atraumatic laparoscopic grasping forceps with locking mechanism is required for use of the LaparoBag System, but not supplied with this system.

SPECIFICATIONS:
Size of Bag (Flat): Approx. 15.8 by 7.6cm, Max. Bag Opening: Approx. 6.4cm diameter, Bag Volume: Approx. 275ml, Introducer Outside Diameter: 9.8mm, Introducer Inside Diameter: 8.3mm, Portal Compatibility: 10mm and larger, Length: 23.6cm.

BAG, SPECIMEN, LAPAROSCOPIC *(cont'd)*

Advanced Surgical, Inc.
305 College Rd. East
Princeton, NJ 08540
609-987-2340

Cabot Medical Corp.
2021 Cabot Blvd. West
Langhorne, PA 19047-1875
215-752-8300

Dexide, Inc.
7509 Flagstone Dr.
P.O. Box 185789
Fort Worth, TX 76118-6953
817-589-1454

Ethicon Endo-Surgery
4545 Creek Road
Cincinnati, OH 45242
513-786-7000

Marlow Surgical Technologies, Inc.
1810 Joseph Lloyd Pkwy.
Willoughby, OH 44094-8030
216-946-2453

Synectic Engineering, Inc.
4 Oxford Rd.
Milford, CT 06460-7007
203-877-8488

U.s. Endoscopy Group
7123 Industrial Park Blvd.
Mentor, OH 44060
216-269-8226

Uniflex Inc., Medical Packaging Division
383 W. John St.
P.O. Box 96
Hicksville, NY 11802
516-932-2000

United States Surgical Corp.
150 Glover Ave.
Norwalk, CT 06856-5080
203-845-1000

Ximed Medical Systems
2195 Trade Zone Blvd.
San Jose, CA 95131
408-945-4040

Zenith Medical Inc.
10064 Mesa Ridge Ct., Ste. 218
San Diego, CA 92121
619-535-0216

Camera

The video camera, coupled with the laparoscope and monitors, is the most important component of the laparoscopic system. Indeed, without the visualization that the camera provides, the entire field of laparoscopic surgery would not exist.

While all cameras on the market have similar functional characteristics, their image quality may vary considerably. To be sure you have the best camera for a particular application, it is important to evaluate several systems prior to purchase.

Most cameras currently in use employ a single imaging chip. Once balanced to a white background, they automatically equilibrate all other colors. They generally give good color definition; and all provide 250 lines of resolution or better. Three-chip cameras, which were introduced several years ago, have only recently come into widespread use. These cameras provide better color definition and usually more lines of resolution than their one-chip counterparts. With the introduction of more difficult procedures requiring greater visibility, the three-chip model may become the camera of choice.

Cameras can be coupled with the laparoscope in several ways; and each has its advantages and drawbacks. If the camera is attached to the eyepiece of the scope with a coupling device, it can easily be removed for use with a variety of scopes. However, this configuration creates an air pocket between the camera and the scope which can cause a slight decrease in the quality of the image or even lead to fogging.

Alternatively, the eyepiece of the laparoscope can be removed and the camera attached directly to its lens system. This arrangement tends to improve image quality. However, fogging can still be a problem if the camera is not cleaned and warmed prior to coupling.

Finally, there's the sealed camera/scope system. This approach eliminates all interface problems, but precludes use of the camera with interchangeable scopes, requiring the purchase of a complete system for each purpose. It's worth remembering, too, that if any part of the combined system malfunctions, all the other elements will be out of commission as well.

Cameras come in many sizes and weights. Assuming that image quality stays up to par, the smaller and lighter the camera the better. For instance, many cameras now include VCR connections and zoom capabilities. While these features are advantageous in certain circumstances, they do add to the weight and cost of the camera, and can lead to greater fatigue for the camera operator.

Be careful, also, to examine the camera's focus ring. If too loose, it will be continually knocked out of focus; if too tight, focusing will prove difficult.

Just beginning to enter the market is the three-dimensional camera. Although considerably more expensive than two-dimensional systems, these cameras provide a more realistic view of the anatomy. Glasses are required; but when the surgeon looks away from the screen, a sensor turns them 'off,' returning the user to normal vision.

ACCESSORIES, SURGICAL CAMERA

Olympus America, Inc.
4 Nevada Dr.
Lake Success, NY 11042-1179
516-488-3880

CLV-S20
DESCRIPTION:

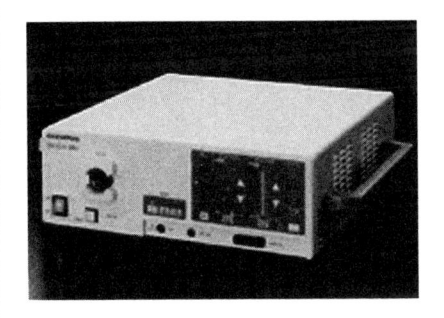

The new CLV-S20 delivers high-power illumination required for today's advanced endoscopic surgical techniques. Incorporating a powerful 300W xenon lamp, the CLV-S20 provides clear, bright, high-contrast video images for accurate observation. Variable illumination is available with the automatic High-Intensity mode and automatic brightness control. Built to meet the rigorous safety requirements of hospital operating rooms and endoscopy suites, the CLV-S20 features an easy-to-clean flush surface control panel, as well as an emergency halogen lamp and lamp life meter to ensure smooth, safe operation.

Cabot Medical Corp.
2021 Cabot Blvd. West
Langhorne, PA 19047-1875
215-752-8300

Kelleher Medical, Inc.
9710 Farrar Court, Suite N
Richmond, VA 23236
804-323-4040

Linvatec Corporation
11311 Concept Blvd.
Largo, FL 34643-4908
813-399-5344

Medical Dynamics, Inc.
99 Inverness Dr. E.
Englewood, CO 80112-5115
303-790-2990

Microtek Medical, Inc.
602 Lehmberg Rd.
P.O. Box 2487
Columbus, MS 39702-2487
601-327-1863

Schwarz Medical
Kirchstrasse 24
D-86935 Rott
Germany
8869/1881

CAMERA, CINE, ENDOSCOPIC, WITH AUDIO

Cine Graphics Inc.
933 Egyptian Way
Grand Prairie, TX 75050
214-264-5212

Pioneer Medical, Inc.
34 Laurelcrest Rd.
Madison, CT 06443
203-245-9337

Smith & Nephew Dyonics, Inc.
160 Dascomb Rd.
Andover, MA 01810-5893
508-470-2800

CAMERA, CINE, ENDOSCOPIC, WITHOUT AUDIO

Coopersurgical, Inc.
15 Forest Pkwy.
Shelton, CT 06484-5458
203-929-6321

JVC Professional Products Co.
41 Slater Dr.
Elmwood Park, NJ 07407-1348
201-794-3900

Origin Medsystems, Inc.
135 Constitution Dr.
Menlo Park, CA 94025
415-617-5000

Smith & Nephew Dyonics, Inc.
160 Dascomb Rd.
Andover, MA 01810-5893
508-470-2800

CAMERA, STILL, ENDOSCOPIC

Contec Medical Ltd.
11 Haroshet Street
P.O. Box 1400
Ramat Hasharon 47113
Israel
03/5491153

Coopersurgical, Inc.
15 Forest Pkwy.
Shelton, CT 06484-5458
203-929-6321

Fujinon (Europe) GmbH
Heerdter Lohweg 89
D-40549 Duesseldorf 11
Germany
0211/52050

Fujinon, Inc.
10 High Point Dr.
Wayne, NJ 07470-7434
201-633-5600

Kelleher Medical, Inc.
9710 Farrar Court, Suite N
Richmond, VA 23236
804-323-4040

Leisegang Medical, Inc.
6401 Congress Ave.
Boca Raton, FL 33487-2883
407-994-0202

Machida, Inc.
40 Ramland Rd. South
Orangeburg, NY 10962-2617
914-365-0600

Medical Dynamics, Inc.
99 Inverness Dr. E.
Englewood, CO 80112-5115
303-790-2990

Nikon Inc., Instrument Group
1300 Walt Whitman Rd.
P.O. Box 9050
Melville, NY 11747-3012
516-547-8500

CAMERA, STILL, ENDOSCOPIC (cont'd)

Pentax Precision Instrument Corp.
30 Ramland Rd.
Orangeburg, NY 10962-2699
914-365-0700

Smith & Nephew Dyonics, Inc.
160 Dascomb Rd.
Andover, MA 01810-5893
508-470-2800

Storz Endoscopy-America Inc., Karl
10111 W. Jefferson Blvd.
Culver City, CA 90232-3509
310-558-1500

Storz GmbH & Co., Karl
Mittelstr. 8
Postfach 230
D-78532 Tuttlingen
Germany
07461/7080

Treier Endoscopie AG
Sonnrain
CH-6215 Beromunster
Switzerland
045/512323

Wild Microscopes
24 Link Drive
Rockleigh, NJ 07647-2504
201-767-1100

Wolf Medical Instruments Corp., Richard
353 Corporate Woods Pkwy.
Vernon Hills, IL 60061-3110
708-913-1113

CAMERA, TELEVISION, ENDOSCOPIC, WITH AUDIO

Hitachi Denshi Ltd.
1-23-2, Kanda Suda-Cho
Chiyoda-Ku
Tokyo 101
Japan
03/2558411

Keymed Medical & Industrial Equipment Ltd.
Keymed House, Stock Rd., Southend-on-Sea
Essex SS2 5QH
United Kingdom
0702/616333

Smith & Nephew Dyonics, Inc.
160 Dascomb Rd.
Andover, MA 01810-5893
508-470-2800

Wolf Medical Instruments Corp., Richard
353 Corporate Woods Pkwy.
Vernon Hills, IL 60061-3110
708-913-1113

Zinnanti Surgical Instruments
21540 B Prairie St.
Chatsworth, CA 91311-5886
818-700-0090

CAMERA, TELEVISION, ENDOSCOPIC, WITHOUT AUDIO

Cabot Medical Corp.
2021 Cabot Blvd. West
Langhorne, PA 19047-1875
215-752-8300

Coopersurgical, Inc.
15 Forest Pkwy.
Shelton, CT 06484-5458
203-929-6321

Electro Fiberoptics Corporation
56 Hudson St.
Northborough, MA 01532-1922
508-393-3753

Hitachi Denshi Ltd.
1-23-2, Kanda Suda-Cho
Chiyoda-Ku
Tokyo 101
Japan
03/2558411

Mediflex Surgical Products
250 Gibbs Rd.
Islandia, NY 11722-2697
516-582-8440

Mist, Inc.
6307 E. Angus Dr.
Raleigh, NC 27613
919-787-8377

Origin Medsystems, Inc.
135 Constitution Dr.
Menlo Park, CA 94025
415-617-5000

Pentax Precision Instrument Corp.
30 Ramland Rd.
Orangeburg, NY 10962-2699
914-365-0700

Seitz Technical Products, Inc.
111-C Newark Rd.
P.O. Box 338
Avondale, PA 19311-0338
215-268-2228

Smith & Nephew Dyonics, Inc.
160 Dascomb Rd.
Andover, MA 01810-5893
508-470-2800

Welch Allyn, Inc.
4341 State Street Rd.
P.O. Box 220
Skaneateles Falls, NY 13153-0220
315-685-4100

Wells Johnson Co.
8075 E. Research Ct., Ste. 101
Tucson, AZ 85710-6714
602-298-6069

Wolf Medical Instruments Corp., Richard
353 Corporate Woods Pkwy.
Vernon Hills, IL 60061-3110
708-913-1113

CAMERA, TELEVISION, MICROSURGICAL, WITH AUDIO

Hitachi Denshi Ltd.
1-23-2, Kanda Suda-Cho
Chiyoda-Ku
Tokyo 101
Japan
03/2558411

Siemens Medical Corp.
186 Wood Ave. South
Iselin, NJ 08830-2704
908-321-4500

Smith & Nephew Dyonics, Inc.
160 Dascomb Rd.
Andover, MA 01810-5893
508-470-2800

CAMERA, TELEVISION, MICROSURGICAL, WITHOUT AUDIO

Coopersurgical, Inc.
15 Forest Pkwy.
Shelton, CT 06484-5458
203-929-6321

Hitachi Denshi Ltd.
1-23-2, Kanda Suda-Cho
Chiyoda-Ku
Tokyo 101
Japan
03/2558411

Leisegang Medical, Inc.
6401 Congress Ave.
Boca Raton, FL 33487-2883
407-994-0202

Seitz Technical Products, Inc.
111-C Newark Rd.
P.O. Box 338
Avondale, PA 19311-0338
215-268-2228

Siemens Medical Corp.
186 Wood Ave. South
Iselin, NJ 08830-2704
908-321-4500

Smith & Nephew Dyonics, Inc.
160 Dascomb Rd.
Andover, MA 01810-5893
508-470-2800

Smith & Nephew Richards Inc.
1450 Brooks Road
Memphis, TN 38116
901-396-2121

Transamerican Technologies International
7026 Koll Center Pkwy., Ste. 207
Pleasanton, CA 94566-3108
510-484-0700

CAMERA, TELEVISION, SURGICAL, WITH AUDIO

Carsen Group Inc.
151 Telson Rd.
Markham, ONT L3R 1E7
Canada
416-479-4100

Helio Co. Ltd.
3-37-8, Hongo, Bunkyo-Ku
Tokyo 113
Japan
03/8143611

Hitachi Denshi America, Ltd.
150 Crossways Park Drive
Woodbury, NY 11797-2028
516-921-7200

Hitachi Denshi Ltd.
1-23-2, Kanda Suda-Cho
Chiyoda-Ku
Tokyo 101
Japan
03/2558411

Smith & Nephew Dyonics, Inc.
160 Dascomb Rd.
Andover, MA 01810-5893
508-470-2800

Storz Endoscopy-America Inc., Karl
10111 W. Jefferson Blvd.
Culver City, CA 90232-3509
310-558-1500

Storz GmbH & Co., Karl
Mittelstr. 8
Postfach 230
D-78532 Tuttlingen
Germany
07461/7080

Stryker Endoscopy
210 Baypointe Pkwy.
San Jose, CA 95134
408-435-0220

Wolf Medical Instruments Corp., Richard
353 Corporate Woods Pkwy.
Vernon Hills, IL 60061-3110
708-913-1113

CAMERA, TELEVISION, SURGICAL, WITHOUT AUDIO

Bosch GmbH, Robert
Postfach 50
D-70192 Stuttgart 1
Germany
0711/811-1

Coopersurgical, Inc.
15 Forest Pkwy.
Shelton, CT 06484-5458
203-929-6321

Faro Technologies, Inc.
125 Technology Park
Lake Mary, FL 32746-6204
407-333-9911

Hitachi Denshi Ltd.
1-23-2, Kanda Suda-Cho
Chiyoda-Ku
Tokyo 101
Japan
03/2558411

Komamura Photographic Co. Ltd.
2-12-11, Kyobashi, Chuo-Ku
Tokyo 104
Japan
03/5618591

Leisegang Medical, Inc.
6401 Congress Ave.
Boca Raton, FL 33487-2883
407-994-0202

Smith & Nephew Dyonics, Inc.
160 Dascomb Rd.
Andover, MA 01810-5893
508-470-2800

Welch Allyn, Inc.
4341 State Street Rd.
P.O. Box 220
Skaneateles Falls, NY 13153-0220
315-685-4100

CAMERA, VIDEO, ENDOSCOPIC

Amtronics, Inc.
P.O. Box 24190
New Orleans, LA 70184-4190
504-831-0691

Automation SA
Bevrijdingslaan 86
B-1640 St-Genesius-Rode
Belgium
02/358-3575

Birtcher Medical Systems, Inc.
50 Technology Dr.
Irvine, CA 92718-2301
714-753-9400

Bryan Corp.
4 Plympton St.
Woburn, MA 01801-2908
617-935-0004

Cabot Medical Corp.
2021 Cabot Blvd. West
Langhorne, PA 19047-1875
215-752-8300

Circon Corporation
460 Ward Drive
Santa Barbara, CA 93111-2310
805-967-0404

Coopersurgical, Inc.
15 Forest Pkwy.
Shelton, CT 06484-5458
203-929-6321

Electro Fiberoptics Corporation
56 Hudson St.
Northborough, MA 01532-1922
508-393-3753

Elmed, Inc.
60 W. Fay Ave.
Addison, IL 60101-5198
708-543-2792

Endo Image Corporation
1370 Blair Dr.
Odenton, MD 21113
410-551-9700

Endomedix Corp.
2162 Michelson Drive
Irvine, CA 92715
714-253-1000

Endotec, Inc.
2225 Skyland Ct.
Norcross, GA 30071
404-840-1883

Expanded Optics, Inc.
7382 Bolsa Ave.
Westminster, CA 92683-5212
714-891-3996

CAMERA, VIDEO, ENDOSCOPIC *(cont'd)*

Geister Medizintechnik GmbH
Foehrenstr. 2
Postfach 4228
D-78532 Tuttlingen
Germany
7461-8084

Heraeus Surgical, Inc.
575 Cottonwood Dr.
Milpitas, CA 95035-7402
408-954-4000

Imagyn Medical, Inc.
27651 La Paz Rd.
Laguna Beach, CA 92656
714-362-2500

Javelin Electronics
19831 Magellan Dr.
Torrance, CA 90502
310-327-7440

Karindo Alkestron P.T.
17 Tomang Raya
Jakarta 11440
Indonesia
021/5600896

Karlheinz Hinze
Endo-Engineering
Elbgaustr. 112
D-22532 Hamburg
Germany
40/842510

Leisegang Medical, Inc.
6401 Congress Ave.
Boca Raton, FL 33487-2883
407-994-0202

Linvatec Corporation
11311 Concept Blvd.
Largo, FL 34643-4908
813-399-5344

M.D. Engineering
3464 Depot Rd.
Hayward, CA 94545-2714
510-732-9950

Medical Concepts, Inc.
175 B Cremona Dr.
Goleta, CA 93117-5502
805-968-5563

Medical Dynamics, Inc.
99 Inverness Dr. E.
Englewood, CO 80112-5115
303-790-2990

Mist, Inc.
6307 E. Angus Dr.
Raleigh, NC 27613
919-787-8377

MP Video, Inc.
63 South St.
Hopkinton, MA 01748-2212
508-435-2131

Olympus America, Inc.
4 Nevada Drive
Lake Success, NY 11042-1179
516-488-3880

Origin Medsystems, Inc.
135 Constitution Dr.
Menlo Park, CA 94025
415-617-5000

Smith & Nephew Dyonics, Inc.
160 Dascomb Rd.
Andover, MA 01810-5893
508-470-2800

Smith & Nephew Richards Inc.
1450 Brooks Road
Memphis, TN 38116
901-396-2121

Storz Endoscopy-America Inc., Karl
10111 W. Jefferson Blvd.
Culver City, CA 90232-3509
310-558-1500

Surgical Technologies International, Inc.
4715 NW 157th St., #212
Miami, FL 33014
305-623-0363

Thompson Surgical Instruments, Inc.
10170 E. Cherry Bend Rd.
P.O. Box 1051
Traverse City, MI 49685
616-922-0177

Transamerican Technologies International
7026 Koll Center Pkwy., Ste. 207
Pleasanton, CA 94566-3108
510-484-0700

Welch Allyn, Inc.
4341 State Street Rd.
P.O. Box 220
Skaneateles Falls, NY 13153-0220
315-685-4100

Wolf Medical Instruments Corp., Richard
353 Corporate Woods Pkwy.
Vernon Hills, IL 60061-3110
708-913-1113

CAMERA, VIDEO, MULTI-IMAGE

Birtcher Medical Systems, Inc.
50 Technology Dr.
Irvine, CA 92718-2301
714-753-9400

Heraeus Surgical, Inc.
575 Cottonwood Dr.
Milpitas, CA 95035-7402
408-954-4000

Mist, Inc.
6307 E. Angus Dr.
Raleigh, NC 27613
919-787-8377

Smith & Nephew Dyonics, Inc.
160 Dascomb Rd.
Andover, MA 01810-5893
508-470-2800

Welch Allyn, Inc.
4341 State Street Rd.
P.O. Box 220
Skaneateles Falls, NY 13153-0220
315-685-4100

CAMERA, VIDEOTAPE, SURGICAL

Aran Technology Inc.
23061 La Cadena Dr.
Laguna Hills, CA 92653
714-951-7750

Biomedical Exports, Inc.
8002 California Ave.
P.O. Box 740
Fair Oaks, CA 95628-7506
916-967-4917

Bosch GmbH, Robert
Postfach 50
D-70192 Stuttgart 1
Germany
0711/811-1

Cabot Medical Corp.
2021 Cabot Blvd. West
Langhorne, PA 19047-1875
215-752-8300

Cory Brothers Co.
4 Dollis Pk.
London, N3 1HG
United Kingdom
081/349/1081

Heraeus Surgical, Inc.
575 Cottonwood Dr.
Milpitas, CA 95035-7402
408-954-4000

Hitachi Denshi America, Ltd.
150 Crossways Park Drive
Woodbury, NY 11797-2028
516-921-7200

Ibiom Instruments Ltd.
6640 Rue Barry
Brossard, QUE J4Z 1T8
Canada
514-678-5468

JVC Professional Products Co.
41 Slater Dr.
Elmwood Park, NJ 07407-1348
201-794-3900

Medical Dynamics, Inc.
99 Inverness Dr. E.
Englewood, CO 80112-5115
303-790-2990

Pentax Precision Instrument Corp.
30 Ramland Rd.
Orangeburg, NY 10962-2699
914-365-0700

Siemens Medical Corp.
186 Wood Ave. South
Iselin, NJ 08830-2704
908-321-4500

Stryker Endoscopy
210 Baypointe Pkwy.
San Jose, CA 95134
408-435-0220

WM Instrumente GmbH
Panoramastr. 6
D-78604 Rietheim 1
Germany
07424/501310

MONITOR, VIDEO, ENDOSCOPE

Olympus America, Inc.
4 Nevada Dr.
Lake Success, NY 11042-1179
516-488-3880

OEV201

DESCRIPTION: With over 700 lines of horizontal resolution, the OEV201 yields high-definition images with optimum clarity and true color reproduction.

Fingertip controls allow adjustment of the picture-size from NORMAL to OVERSCAN (enlargement up to 117%).

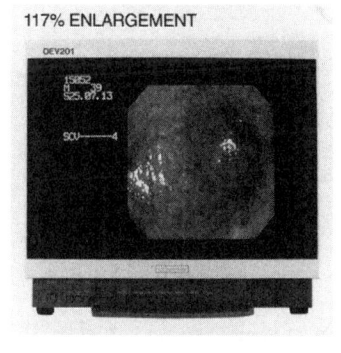

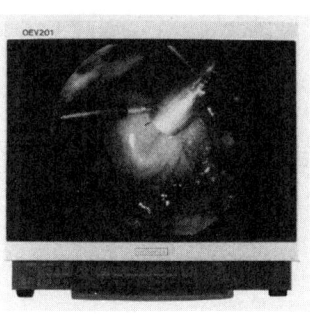

Features uncluttered, covered front panel with minimum number of controls as well as a commercial-grade comb filter to further enhance video image quality.

Includes RGB, S-VHS (Y/C), Composite Video, and loop-through terminals for connection to additional monitors to allow for maximum viewing flexibility plus automatic detection and switching of NTSC, PAL, SECAM, and M-NTSC color systems.

Automatic white balance for consistent, realistic color reproduction and cable protection to prevent damage to plugs when forced against a wall are also provided.

The OEV201 is U/L 544 listed and meets all operating safety requirements for hospitals and endoscopy suites.

SPECIFICATIONS/HOW SUPPLIED:
Horizontal resolution: More than 700 lines.
Color temperature: 9300K, 6500K switchable.
Chroma: To adjust color saturation.
Phase: To adjust hue (only valid for NTSC, Y/C signals).
Brightness: To adjust brightness of monitor.
Contrast: To adjust contrast.
Aperture: To adjust resolution.
RGB Contrast: To adjust contrast of RGB image.
Picture size overscan: To increase display size.
Color system: NTSC, M-NTSC, PAL, SECAM with complete auto-switch.
Input video signal: Composite signal, Y/C signal, RGB signal; all switchable on front panel.
Intended application: As part of endoscopic system/equipment, for use with Olympus manufactured systems and equipment.
Type of protection against electric shock: Class 1 (3-pin power plug).
Degree of protection against electric shock: Type B equipment. Direct application to heart should not be attempted.
Degree of protection against explosion: Never use OEV201 where there is a risk of flammable gases.

Power requirements:
Voltage: 120V AC, 220V-240V AC. Frequency: 50/60 Hz. Input: 1.8A. Allowable voltage fluctuation: +/- 10%.
Ambient temperature: 10-40°C (50-104°F).
Relative humidity: 30-85%.
Atmospheric pressure: 70-106 kPa (700-1060 mb).
Dimensions: 414mm (H) x 448mm (W) x 532mm (D).
Weight: 27.5 kg (60.5 lb).

MONITOR, VIDEO, ENDOSCOPE (cont'd)

Bryan Corp.
4 Plympton St.
Woburn, MA 01801-2908
617-935-0004

Cabot Medical Corp.
2021 Cabot Blvd. West
Langhorne, PA 19047-1875
215-752-8300

Carsen Group Inc.
151 Telson Rd.
Markham, ONT L3R 1E7
Canada
416-479-4100

Conrac Display Products, Inc.
1724 S. Mountain Ave.
Duarte, CA 91010-2746
818-303-0095

Coopersurgical, Inc.
15 Forest Pkwy.
Shelton, CT 06484-5458
203-929-6321

Diefenbach Ing. Buero
Am Saaelnbusch 24-26
D-60386 Frankfurt 61
Germany
069/412950

Elmed, Inc.
60 W. Fay Ave.
Addison, IL 60101-5198
708-543-2792

Fujinon (Europe) GmbH
Heerdter Lohweg 89
D-40549 Duesseldorf 11
Germany
0211/52050

Fujinon, Inc.
10 High Point Dr.
Wayne, NJ 07470-7434
201-633-5600

Heraeus Surgical, Inc.
575 Cottonwood Dr.
Milpitas, CA 95035-7402
408-954-4000

Hitachi Denshi America, Ltd.
150 Crossways Park Drive
Woodbury, NY 11797-2028
516-921-7200

Hitachi Denshi Ltd.
1-23-2, Kanda Suda-Cho
Chiyoda-Ku
Tokyo 101
Japan
03/2558411

Leisegang Medical, Inc.
6401 Congress Ave.
Boca Raton, FL 33487-2883
407-994-0202

Medical Dynamics, Inc.
99 Inverness Dr. E.
Englewood, CO 80112-5115
303-790-2990

Mist, Inc.
6307 E. Angus Dr.
Raleigh, NC 27613
919-787-8377

Mitsubishi Electronics of America
800 Cottontail Lane
Somerset, NJ 08873-6759
908-563-9889

MP Video, Inc.
63 South St.
Hopkinton, MA 01748-2212
508-435-2131

Smith & Nephew Dyonics, Inc.
160 Dascomb Rd.
Andover, MA 01810-5893
508-470-2800

Storz Endoscopy-America Inc., Karl
10111 W. Jefferson Blvd.
Culver City, CA 90232-3509
310-558-1500

Storz GmbH & Co., Karl
Mittelstr. 8
Postfach 230
D-78532 Tuttlingen
Germany
07461/7080

Stryker Corp., Surgical Div.
4100 E. Milham Ave.
Kalamazoo, MI 49003-6197
616-323-7700

Stryker Endoscopy
210 Baypointe Pkwy.
San Jose, CA 95134
408-435-0220

Welch Allyn, Inc.
4341 State Street Rd.
P.O. Box 220
Skaneateles Falls, NY 13153-0220
315-685-4100

Wisap Gesellschaft
Rudolf Diesel Ring 20
D-82054 Sauerlach
Germany
08104/1067

Wolf Medical Instruments Corp., Richard
353 Corporate Woods Pkwy.
Vernon Hills, IL 60061-3110
708-913-1113

SYSTEM, CAMERA, 3-DIMENSIONAL

Olympus America, Inc.
4 Nevada Dr.
Lake Success, NY 11042-1179
516-488-3880

OTV-S4 OES TV SYSTEM
DESCRIPTION:

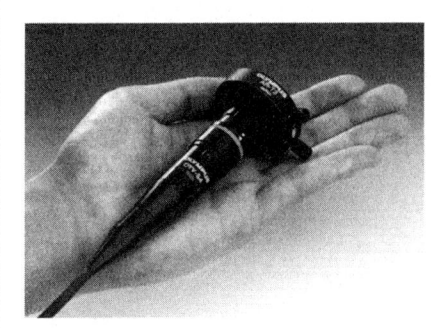

The OTV-S4 with Digital Signal Processing incorporates the latest in video imaging technology to eliminate image noise, provide sharper, clearer images, and guarantee consistent image control and brightness.

The OTV-S4 also incorporates Olympus' newest CCD image sensor with "Micro-lens" CCD technology to ensure true color reproduction, increase horizontal resolution 30% for greater detail, and provide maximum light sensitivity.

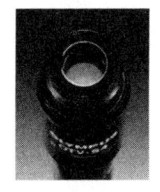

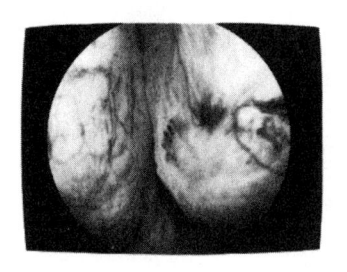

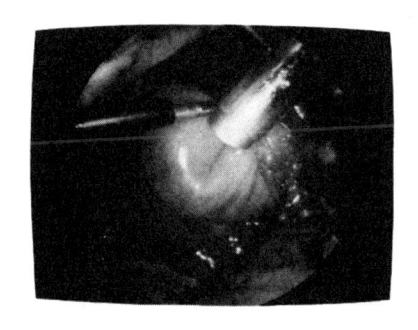

The OTV-S4 Camera Head weighs only 55 grams (1.94 ounces) and lets physicians work with minimal fatigue. The slim profile eliminates awkward protrusions for natural maneuvering.

Because fiberscopes and rigid endoscopes involve very different engineering, two camera heads are provided to extract the very best views from either type of scope. Through rigid endoscopes you will see clear, color-perfect images with the MH-201, while a special moiré-reducing filter is incorporated in the MH-204 for use with fiberscopes.

The narrow lines of the casing make for an ergonomically comfortable fit in the user's hand. A new raised upward indicator lets you confirm by touch that the image being viewed is properly oriented.

To add to the versatility of the system, Olympus has developed four different adapters to connect the camera head to the scope. These adapters are all easy to attach and use. Depending on which adapter is used, a physician can view procedures via an eyepiece, a monitor or both, without compromise in image quality.

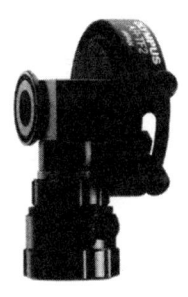

AR-TF2: Allows the operator to look through the eyepiece while others view the procedure on the monitor.

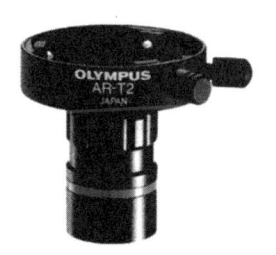

AR-T2: A direct link from the camera head to the monitor, for use when an eyepiece is unnecessary.

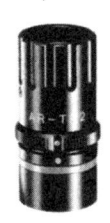

AR-TD2: An ultra-slim, compact adapter which connects directly to a telescope without an eyepiece for improved operability.

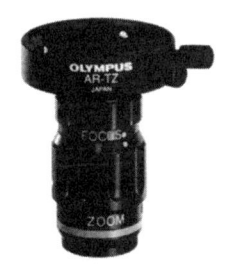

AR-TZ: A built-in zoom allows enlargement and reduction of images during observation to maintain desired image size on the monitor.

Certain tissues are notorious for their reflective properties. With the high-intensity light sources involved in endoscopy, glare from these tissues can cause video cameras to obscure vital sections of the view, drastically reducing the physician's potential for diagnosis or treatment. The AGC (Auto Gain Control) mechanism employed in the OTV-S4 senses the reflections and maintains even lighting throughout the viewfield.

The panel of the control unit is laid out simply, with large, easily identifiable switches and features touch-sensitive control keys as well.

The optional MH-199 Character Generator can be connected to the camera control unit for on-screen display and recording of comments, dates, times, and other necessary data on a VCR.

ASSEMBLY GUIDELINES: The simple "one-action system" facilitates the mounting of scopes. The pointers, which appear on the screen or in the viewfinder, offer immediate visual confirmation of orientation.

CARE & MAINTENANCE: A leakage tester is available as a safe means of discovering potential for leaks into the camera head before damage occurs.

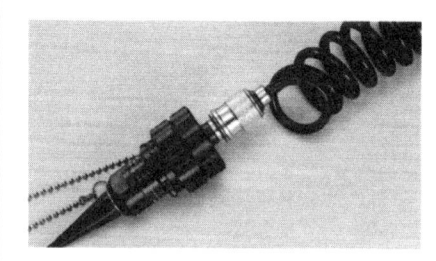

STERILIZATION GUIDELINES: The entire camera head and all cables can be immersed in disinfecting solution. EtO sterilization is also possible. The front panel of the control unit is water-resistant and flush-surfaced to facilitate cleaning.

SPECIFICATIONS/HOW SUPPLIED:
Power requirements: 9V DC, 10mA,
Backup power supply: four RO3/AAA batteries
Dimensions: 227mm (W) x 23mm (H) x 108mm (D) (8-15/16in. x 7/8in. x 4-1/4in.)
Character per page: 12 characters x 4 lines ~ 20 characters x 9 lines (10 pages)
Another new feature is an optional foot switch, which lets you control the power of a connected VCR or video printer without removing your hands from other, more vital controls.

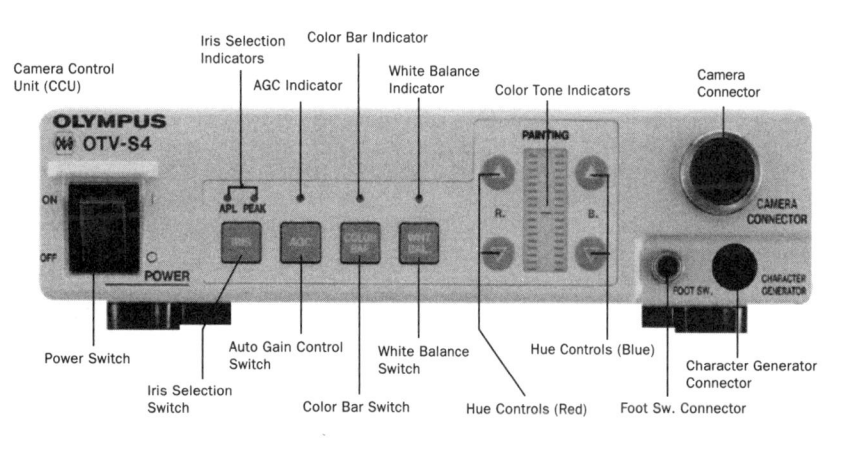

PRODUCT DIRECTORY

PRODUCT SETUP

When using the A3071 or A3072 light guide with the CLV-S, set high intensity mode to OFF.

MAIN SPECIFICATIONS

Monitor Observation:
Pickup System: Interline type CCD solid-state image pickup.
Television System: NTSC/PAL.
Video Output: V.B.S: 2 terminals, Y/C: 1 terminal.
Resolution (at center): Over 430 lines horizontally; Over 350 lines vertically.
Sensitivity: Standard: 1400 lux (F5.6); Minimum: 3 lux (F1.4/AGC: ON).
S/N: Better than 46 dB (AGC off).
Iris: Peak/average measurement.
Automatic Light Intensity Adjustment: Light reflected from subject is measured by camera head in combination with CLV-U20, CLV-10, CLV-F10 or CLV-S.
Auto White Balance: Automatically adjusted with WHITE BALANCE switch.
Color Adjustment: Red +/-8 steps; blue +/-8 steps (by control switches).
Color Bar Output: Full-field color bar.

Operating Environment:
Power Requirements: 120, 220, 240 V AC; 50/60 Hz frequency; 20 VA consumption. Allowable voltage fluctuation: +/-10%.
Ambient Temperature: 10 ~ 40°C (50 ~ 104°F).
Relative Humidity: 30 ~ 85%.
Atmospheric Pressure: 70 ~ 106 kPa (700 ~ 1060 mb).

Recording:
VTR Remote Control: Remote Control of VTR recording start/stop possible by connecting optional foot release.

Connections:
Adapter Connection: Threaded mount.
Endoscope Connection: AR-T2, AR-TF2, AR-TZ with lock-ring mount for "one-action" connection; AR-TD2 with threaded mount.

Cleaning/Disinfection:
Camera Head: Immersible in disinfectant solution, provided video adapter is attached to camera head and water-resistant cap (MH-051) to camera plug. Formalin and ethylene oxide gas sterilization possible.
CCU: May be wiped with disinfectant alcohol (glutaraldehyde).

Dimensions & Weight:
Camera Head Diameter: 20 x 48mm (13/16 x 1-7/8in.) (from mount surface), 55g (1.94oz.) (excluding cable).
CCU: 295mm (W) x 72mm (H) x 315mm (L) (11-5/8in. x 2-13/16in. x 12-3/8in.), 4kg (8.8 lbs).

Classified as Electromedical Equipment:
Type of protection against electric shock: Class 1 (3-pin power plug).
Degree of protection against electric shock: Type BF equipment. Applied part (camera head) isolated from all other parts of equipment. Direct application to heart prohibited.
Degree of protection against explosion: Never use OTV-S4 where there is risk of flammable gases.

Wolf Medical Instruments Corp., Richard
353 Corporate Woods Pkwy.
Vernon Hills, IL 60061-3110
708-913-1113

TAPE, TELEVISION & VIDEO, ENDOSCOPIC

Access Surgical International, Inc.
15 Caswell Ln.
Boat Yard Square
Plymouth, MA 02360
508-747-6006

Bryan Corp.
4 Plympton St.
Woburn, MA 01801-2908
617-935-0004

Glaser & Co. GmbH Medizintechnik
Eisenbahnstrasse 61
D-82110 Germering
Germany
089/847125

Jason Marketing Co.
P.O. Box 2608
Seal Beach, CA 90740
714-891-5544

Keymed Medical & Industrial Equipment Ltd.
Keymed House, Stock Rd., Southend-on-Sea
Essex SS2 5QH
United Kingdom
0702/616333

Keymed, Inc.
400 Airport Executive Park
Spring Valley, NY 10977-7404
914-425-3100

Leisegang Medical, Inc.
6401 Congress Ave.
Boca Raton, FL 33487-2883
407-994-0202

Omikron GmbH
Hallerstr. 70
Postfach 323 263
D-20146 Hamburg 13
Germany
040/441636

Pentax Precision Instrument Corp.
30 Ramland Rd.
Orangeburg, NY 10962-2699
914-365-0700

Stryker Endoscopy
210 Baypointe Pkwy.
San Jose, CA 95134
408-435-0220

Toshiba Medical Systems Europe B.V.
Schieweg 1
NL 2627 An Delft, AN
Netherlands
015/610121

Wolf Medical Instruments Corp., Richard
353 Corporate Woods Pkwy.
Vernon Hills, IL 60061-3110
708-913-1113

VIDEOINTERFACE, LAPAROSCOPIC, NON-REMOVABLE ROD

Coopersurgical, Inc.
15 Forest Pkwy.
Shelton, CT 06484-5458
203-929-6321

Cannula

In laparoscopy, catheters are used primarily for intraoperative cholangiography.

Some are little more than a flexible plastic tube; but most have special design features to aid insertion and anchoring. Many types are available, including rigid all-metal catheters, flexible plastic catheters with a variety of tip designs, catheters with an expandable tip area or inflatable balloon near the end, and flexible plastic catheters with a metal-reinforced tip zone. Catheters typically range in size from 3 to 5 French.

Most catheters come with an introducer for use either through a trocar sleeve or through a separate puncture. Introducers designed for the trocar are available in curved and straight models; but even the straight ones can easily be bent to the angle needed for insertion of the catheter in the cystic duct. To maintain pneumoperitoneum, the introducer should seal in the trocar sleeve and provide an airtight seal around the catheter. Although some of these introducers can be quite intricate, the simplest are usually the best, as well as being more economical. Cholangiogram clamps can also be used to introduce and manipulate the catheters within the abdominal cavity.

Needle introducers allow the surgeon to place a catheter without occupying a trocar sleeve, leaving all existing ports available for other instrumentation. This method also allows the surgeon to strategically position the catheter for introduction to the cystic ducts. To maintain pneumoperitoneum during manipulation of the needle and the catheter, the sheath should have an airtight valve.

Catheters are usually anchored in the cystic duct with sutures or clips. Sutures can be placed through a trocar or a Grice introduction needle. Most clip appliers close the tip of the clip first, then flatten the remainder until it is tight around the object. This allows the surgeon to place a clip around the cystic duct and catheter, then close it slowly. Over-tightening of the clip can cause obstruction of some catheters; but injecting saline through the catheter during closure of the clip will help prevent this problem. Balloon catheters are anchored by inflating the balloon. Similarly, catheters with an expandable tip are secured by expanding the tip zone.

CANNULA WITH INFLATABLE BALLOON (DISTAL TIP)

Marlow Surgical Technologies, Inc.
1810 Joseph Lloyd Pkwy.
Willoughby, OH 44094-8030
216-946-2453

Origin Medsystems, Inc.
135 Constitution Dr.
Menlo Park, CA 94025
415-617-5000

United States Surgical Corp.
150 Glover Ave.
Norwalk, CT 06856-5080
203-845-1000

CANNULA, DRAINAGE, ARTHROSCOPY

Arthrex Arthroscopy Instrument
3050 North Horseshoe Dr., Ste. 168
Naples, FL 33942-7909
813-643-5553

Arthrex Medical Instrument GmbH
Von Kahr Str. 2
D-80997 Muenchen 50
Germany
89/142257

Contec Medical Ltd.
11 Haroshet Street
P.O. Box 1400
Ramat Hasharon 47113
Israel
03/5491153

Davol, Inc.
100 Sockanossett
P.O. Box 8500
Cranston, RI 02920-0500
401-463-7000

Herger AG
Dornacherstr. 89, Postfach 80
CH-4008 Basel
Switzerland
61/354060

Instrument Makar, Inc.
2950 E. Mt. Hope
Okemos, MI 48864-1910
517-332-3593

Linvatec Corporation
11311 Concept Blvd.
Largo, FL 34643-4908
813-399-5344

Rovers B.V.
Lekstraat 10
NL-5347 KV - Oss
Netherlands
04120 - 48870

Scherzer Medical Program
Franz Petterstr. 18
A-2560 Berndorf
Austria
2672/7953-13

Simal Belgium Instrument Co.
2131 Espey Court, Suite 7
Crofton, MD 21114-2424

Smith & Nephew Dyonics, Inc.
160 Dascomb Rd.
Andover, MA 01810-5893
508-470-2800

Storz Endoscopy-America Inc., Karl
10111 W. Jefferson Blvd.
Culver City, CA 90232-3509
310-558-1500

Storz GmbH & Co., Karl
Mittelstr. 8
Postfach 230
D-78532 Tuttlingen
Germany
07461/7080

WM Instrumente GmbH
Panoramastr. 6
D-78604 Rietheim 1
Germany
07424/501310

Wolf Medical Instruments Corp., Richard
353 Corporate Woods Pkwy.
Vernon Hills, IL 60061-3110
708-913-1113

CANNULA, EXTRACTION, APPENDIX

Access Surgical International, Inc.
15 Caswell Ln.
Boat Yard Square
Plymouth, MA 02360
508-747-6006

Boss Instruments, Ltd.
1310 Central Ct.
Hermitage, TN 37076
615-885-2231

Ethicon Endo-Surgery
4545 Creek Road
Cincinnati, OH 45242
513-786-7000

Wolf Medical Instruments Corp., Richard
353 Corporate Woods Pkwy.
Vernon Hills, IL 60061-3110
708-913-1113

CANNULA, SUCTION, POOL-TIP

Elmed, Inc.
60 W. Fay Ave.
Addison, IL 60101-5198
708-543-2792

Ethicon Endo-Surgery
4545 Creek Road
Cincinnati, OH 45242
513-786-7000

Surgin, Inc.
14762 Bentley Circle
Tustin, CA 92680
714-832-6300

Transamerican Technologies International
7026 Koll Center Pkwy., Ste. 207
Pleasanton, CA 94566-3108
510-484-0700

CANNULA, SUCTION/IRRIGATION, LAPAROSCOPIC

Davis & Geck Endosurgery
1 Casper St.
Danbury, CT 06810
203-743-4451

PROFESSIONAL LINE 8381 SERIES
DESCRIPTION:
Suction Tube (order number 8381-03):
With luer lock connection and finger valve, 5mm diameter, working length 33cm. Can be used with Y-Connector (8381-06).

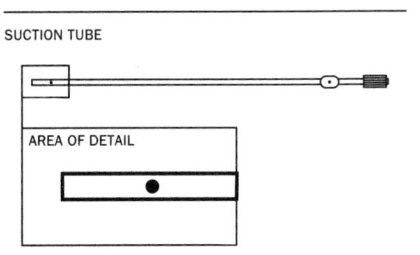

SUCTION TUBE

AREA OF DETAIL

Suction/Irrigation Tube (order number 8381-04):
With luer lock connection, 5mm diameter, working length 33cm. Can be used with Y-Connector (8381-06):

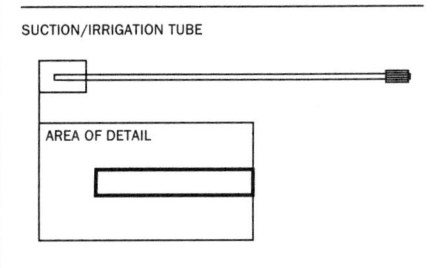

SUCTION/IRRIGATION TUBE

AREA OF DETAIL

Davis & Geck Endosurgery
1 Casper St.
Danbury, CT 06810
203-743-4451

PROFESSIONAL LINE 8381-06
DESCRIPTION: Y-Connector (order number 8381-06):

Y-CONNECTOR

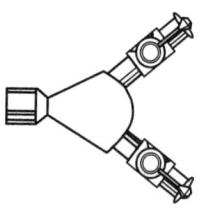

For suction and irrigation in connection with products 8381-02, 8381-03, and 8381-04.

Cabot Medical Corp.
2021 Cabot Blvd. West
Langhorne, PA 19047-1875
215-752-8300

Davis & Geck Div.
American Cyanamid Company
One Cyanamid Plaza
Wayne, NJ 07470-2012
201-831-2000

Sterling Stainless Tube
1400 W. Dartmouth Ave.
Englewood, CO 80110-1385
303-789-0528

CANNULA, SUPRAPUBIC, WITH TROCAR

Aesculap
1000 Gateway Blvd.
South San Francisco, CA 94080-7030
415-876-7000

Cal-Swiss Manufacturing Co., Inc.
390 S. Fair Oaks Ave.
P.O. Box 50430
Pasadena, CA 91105-0430
818-793-8661

Core Dynamics, Inc.
11222-4 St. Johns Indust. Pkwy.
Jacksonville, FL 32216
904-641-6611

DCG Precision Manufacturing Corp.
9 Trowbridge Dr.
Bethel, CT 06801
203-743-5525

Greenwald Surgical Co., Inc.
2688 Dekalb Street
Lake Station, IN 46405-1519
219-962-1604

Grieshaber & Co. AG
Winkelriedstr. 52
CH-8203 Schaffhausen
Switzerland
053/248121

Herger AG
Dornacherstr. 89, Postfach 80
CH-4008 Basel
Switzerland
61/354060

Kensey Nash Corporation
55 E. Uwchlan Ave., Ste. 204
Exton, PA 19341-1247
215-524-0188

Marlow Surgical Technologies, Inc.
1810 Joseph Lloyd Pkwy.
Willoughby, OH 44094-8030
216-946-2453

Martin, Gebr. GmbH & Co. KG
Ludwigstaler Str. 132
Postf. 60
D-78532 Tuttlingen
Germany
07461/7060

Mist, Inc.
6307 E. Angus Dr.
Raleigh, NC 27613
919-787-8377

Smith & Nephew Dyonics, Inc.
160 Dascomb Rd.
Andover, MA 01810-5893
508-470-2800

Star Guide Corp.
6666 Stapleton Dr. S.
Denver, CO 80216
303-333-2100

Storz Endoscopy-America Inc., Karl
10111 W. Jefferson Blvd.
Culver City, CA 90232-3509
310-558-1500

Storz GmbH & Co., Karl
Mittelstr. 8
Postfach 230
D-78532 Tuttlingen
Germany
07461/7080

Synectic Engineering, Inc.
4 Oxford Rd.
Milford, CT 06460-7007
203-877-8488

United States Surgical Corp.
150 Glover Ave.
Norwalk, CT 06856-5080
203-845-1000

Wect Instrument Company, Inc.
5645 N. Ravenswood
Chicago, IL 60660-3922
312-769-1944

Wolf Medical Instruments Corp., Richard
353 Corporate Woods Pkwy.
Vernon Hills, IL 60061-3110
708-913-1113

Catheter

CATHETER, CHOLANGIOGRAPHY

Taut, Inc.
2571 Kaneville Ct.
Geneva, IL 60134-2505
708-232-2507

TAUT OPERATIVE CHOLANGIOGRAM CATHETERS

DESCRIPTION: Taut's cholangiogram catheters consist of a length of flexible plastic catheter tubing with an integrally formed tip zone at one end and a luer lock hub affixed to the other. Catheters are available with four unique tip geometries, allowing the surgeon to choose the catheter which provides easy catheterization and assures adequate retention based on cystic duct anatomy. Three of the catheters have a metallic support tube secured within the tip of the catheter. This allows retention of the catheter in the cystic duct using surgical clips without fear of catheter collapse or occlusion.

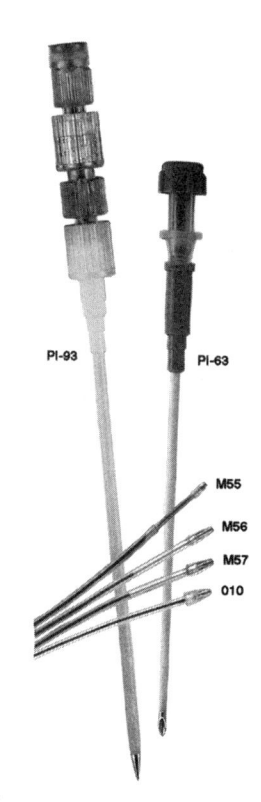

PERCUTANEOUS INTRADUCERS®

DESCRIPTION: Taut's percutaneous Intraducers are designed to provide passage of Taut's cholangiogram catheters into the peritoneal cavity, leaving all abdominal ports free to be used with other instrumentation.

CATHETER, CHOLANGIOGRAPHY (cont'd)

They are best described as miniature disposable trocars, which can be strategically inserted through the peritoneum to facilitate catheterization of the cystic duct. They are designed to prevent leakage of insufflation gas during use.

INDICATIONS: Taut's cholangiogram catheters and percutaneous Intraducers are used for performing cholangiography during either laparoscopic or open cholecystectomy. The resulting cholangiogram helps assure safe dissection of the ductal anatomy and can identify the presence of ductal stones.

PRECAUTIONS: Taut's unique catheter characteristics and tip profiles help assure safe and easy intubation of the cystic duct. Proper alignment of the catheter during intubation is important as it reduces the force necessary to insert a catheter into the duct, thus minimizing the danger of perforating the duct wall. Care should be taken to avoid inserting the catheter into the common duct.

INSTRUCTIONS FOR USE: Apply a surgical clip or clips around the cystic duct near the apex of the gallbladder. Using microscissors make a small incision in the duct near the clip. Introduce a Taut cholangiogram catheter into the abdominal cavity using one of Taut's percutaneous Intraducers, or through an existing abdominal port using a cholangiogram clamp. When using Taut's percutaneous Intraducers, choose the insertion site and angle which best facilitates alignment with, and placement of, the catheter tip through the incision and into the lumen of the cystic duct. The memory characteristics of the catheters allow the surgeon to fine tune alignment of the catheter with the axis of the cystic duct by adjusting the angle of the catheter tip zone prior to inserting the catheter into the abdominal cavity.

Using forceps through an existing abdominal port, guide the catheter tip into the cystic duct. Only minimal intubation is required. The metal support tube can be used to determine the position of the tip once it has entered the lumen of the duct. Apply a surgical clip or clips around the duct behind the catheter tip to retain it in the duct. Apply as much clip pressure as necessary to adequately retain the catheter in the duct and assure an adequate seal. The metal support tube will prevent catheter collapse or occlusion. Perform cholangiography.

STERILIZATION GUIDELINES: Taut's catheters and Intraducers are packed sterile and are intended for single use only. Resterilization is not recommended.

TAUT INC.®

(C) Taut, Inc. 1994, U.S. and Foreign Patents Pending

For more information on Taut catheters, please call 800/231-TAUT (8288) or 708/232-2507, fax to 708/232-8005, or send inquiries to: Taut, Inc., 2571 Kaneville Court, Geneva, IL 60134. All catheters are stocked and ready for immediate shipment. Order direct or call for U.S. and foreign distributors.

Tyvek® is a registered trademark of DuPont.

SPECIFICATIONS/HOW SUPPLIED

CHOLANGIOGRAM CATHETERS:

CATALOG #	CATHETER DIA.	TIP DIA.	LENGTH	TIP PROFILE	METALIC SUPPORT TUBE
20018-M55	4.5 French	4.5 French	18 in.		Yes
20018-M56	4.5 French	5.5 French	18 in.		Yes
20018-M57	4.5 French	6.5 French	18 in.		Yes
20018-010	4.5 French	7.5 French	18 in.		No

PERCUTANEOUS INTRADUCERS:

CATALOG #	DIAMETER	LENGTH	COMPATIBLE CATHETERS
PI-63	6 French	3 in.	M55 only
PI-93	9 French	3.5 in.	M55 M56 M57

Taut catheters and Intraducers are packed sterile ten units per box. Catheters are packed in clear film over Tyvek peel pouches. Intraducers are packed in Tyvek lidded blister packs.

Advanced Surgical, Inc.
305 College Rd. East
Princeton, NJ 08540
609-987-2340

Applied Medical Resources
26051 Merit Circle #104
Laguna Hills, CA 92653-7008
714-582-6120

Arrow International, Inc.
3000 Bernville Rd.
Reading, PA 19605
215-378-0131

Cook Incorporated
925 S. Curry Pike
Bloomington, IN 47403-2624
812-339-2235

Davol, Inc.
100 Sockanossett
P.O. Box 8500
Cranston, RI 02920-0500
401-463-7000

Ideas For Medicine, Inc.
12167 49th St. N
Clearwater, FL 34622-4304
813-576-2747

Laparomed Corp.
9272 Jeronimo Rd., Unit 109
Irvine, CA 92718-1914
714-768-1155

Nu Surg Medical, Inc.
4440 Glen Este-Withamsville Road
Suite 780
Cincinnati, OH 45245
513-753-3633

Origin Medsystems, Inc.
135 Constitution Dr.
Menlo Park, CA 94025
415-617-5000

Ranfac Corp.
Avon Indus. Pk./30 Doherty Ave., Box 635
Avon, MA 02322-1125
508-588-4400

Surgimedics/SLP
2828 N. Crescent Ridge Dr.
The Woodlands, TX 77381
713-363-4949

U.S. Endoscopy Group
7123 Industrial Park Blvd.
Mentor, OH 44060
216-269-8226

Uresil Corporation
5418 W. Touhy Ave.
Skokie, IL 60077-3232
708-982-0200

Wilson-Cook Medical, Inc.
4900 Bethania Station Rd.
Winston-Salem, NC 27105-1203
919-744-0157

Choledochoscope

CHOLEDOCHOSCOPE, FLEXIBLE OR RIGID

Endomedix Corp.
2162 Michelson Dr.
Irvine, CA 92715
714-253-1000

LAPAROOPTX

DESCRIPTION: The LaparoOptx™ Intraoperative Deflectable Choledochoscope is a device intended for diagnostic and therapeutic procedures within the biliary system. This Choledochoscope is a flexible, tip-deflecting, fiberoptic endoscope which can be introduced into the biliary system directly or through a cannula. The LaparoOptx Choledochoscope is nonrepairable; however, it may be reused following appropriate inspection, cleaning, and sterilization or disinfection. The small size, bi-directional deflectable tip and high level of torque make this Choledochoscope suitable for use within the biliary system. Use of the LaparoOptx Choledochoscope is limited to physicians who have been trained in the use of flexible choledochoscopes and in generally accepted techniques for performing laparoscopic cholecystectomy.

WARNINGS: Do not force the LaparoOptx Choledochoscope if it will not pass easily because this may cause trauma to the ductal tissue or damage the device.

Potential complications from use of the LaparoOptx Choledochoscope are the same as those generally associated with catheterization or endoscopy of the biliary system. They include laceration or perforation of tissues, hemorrhage, scar tissue formation, transient hyperamylasemia, infection, pancreatitis and cholangitis.

INSTRUCTIONS FOR USE: It is recommended that the LaparoOptx Choledochoscope be inserted through a cannula equipped with an appropriate reducer such as a 3.5mm reducer.

When the LaparoOptx Choledochoscope is used in conjunction with laparoscopic cholecystectomy, it may be inserted through the sub-xiphoid or other lateral cannula. The LaparoOptx Introducer (Model S200-S) should be used to aid in placement of the Choledochoscope.

Using standard operative procedures, expose the appropriate duct of the biliary system into which the LaparoOptx Choledochoscope will be inserted. Insert the LaparoOptx Introducer through an appropriate portal and advance it to the slit in the biliary duct. Insert the Soft Tip of the Choledochoscope in an undeflected position through the LaparoOptx Introducer and into the biliary duct. A guidewire also may be used through the working channel of the Choledochoscope to aid in placement. Infuse sterile saline through the working channel as necessary to maintain a clear field. Continue advancing the Choledochoscope through the biliary duct, as appropriate, until it reaches the desired end point. At the conclusion of the endoscopic procedure, withdraw the LaparoOptx Choledochoscope with the Soft Tip in an undeflected position using standard techniques.

Accessory instruments measuring 3 Fr, or smaller, are optimal for use with the LaparoOptx Choledochoscope and may be passed through the working channel. Instrument sizes should be selected to allow for sufficient irrigation. Simultaneous irrigation while using an instrument in the working channel can be achieved by connecting a Y-Adaptor (Model S160) to the Luer Hub on the Scope Handle.

CARE & MAINTENANCE: The LaparoOptx Choledochoscope must be sterilized by an ethylene oxide (EtO) gas sterilization process. If the LaparoOptx Choledochoscope is disinfected after previous sterilization (such as between consecutive cases), it may be totally immersed in a high level chemical disinfectant such as 2% alkaline glutaraldehyde. Keep the Choledochoscope and Eyepiece joined together during cleaning and disinfecting between consecutive cases, until preparation for the next sterilization cycle, at which time they should be separated for cleaning and EtO sterilizing. Do not autoclave.

The number of times the LaparoOptx Choledochoscope may be used depends upon the amount of care exerted when handling, using, cleaning, sterilizing or disinfecting, and storing this device.

SPECIFICATIONS/HOW SUPPLIED: The LaparoOptx Choledochoscope is supplied as a single nonsterile unit with the LaparoOptx Scope Sheath attached. The EndoMedix Detachable Eyepiece is required for use with the LaparoOptx Choledochoscope, but it must be procured separately. The LaparoOptx Choledochoscope (Model S760L) has a 7.6 Fr body size, 3.6 Fr working channel diameter, usable length of 40cm and a tip deflecting range of -60° to +60°.

LAPAROOPTX

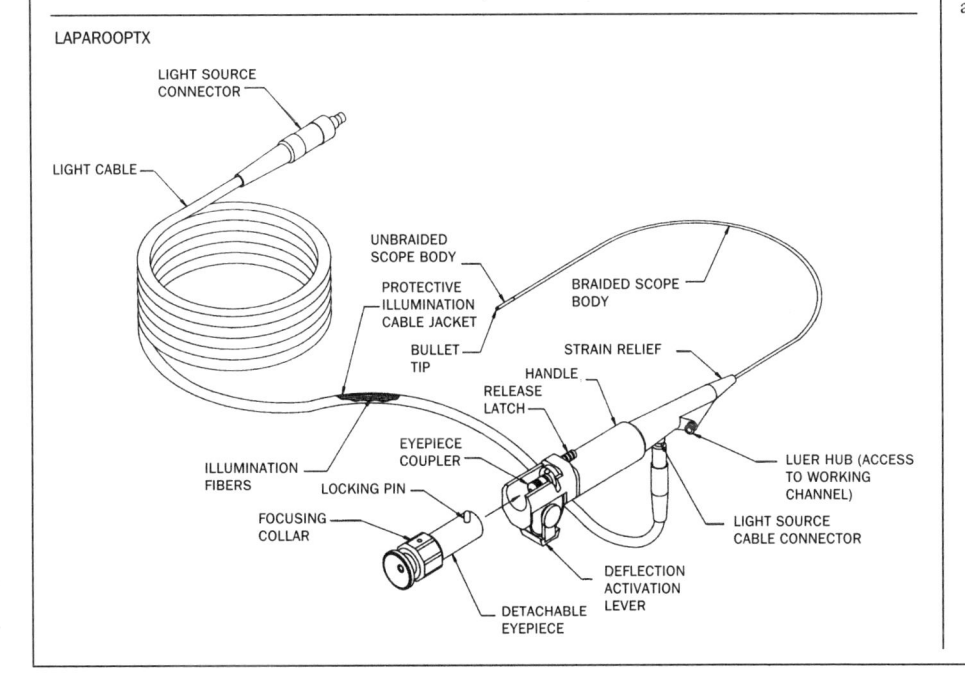

CHOLEDOCHOSCOPE, FLEXIBLE OR RIGID (cont'd)

Asahi Optical Co., Ltd.
2-36-9, Maeno-Cho, Itabashi-Ku
Tokyo 174
Japan
03/3960-5155

Carsen Group Inc.
151 Telson Rd.
Markham, ONT L3R 1E7
Canada
416-479-4100

Circon Acmi
300 Stillwater Ave.
Stamford, CT 06902-3640
203-328-8689

Electro Fiberoptics Corporation
56 Hudson St.
Northborough, MA 01532-1922
508-393-3753

Fujinon (Europe) GmbH
Heerdter Lohweg 89
D-40549 Duesseldorf 11
Germany
0211/52050

Fujinon, Inc.
10 High Point Dr.
Wayne, NJ 07470-7434
201-633-5600

Intramed Labs
11100 Roselle Street
San Diego, CA 92121-1210
619-455-5000

Life Medical Technologies, Inc.
3649 W. 1987 S.
Salt Lake City, UT 84104
801-972-1900

Linvatec Corporation
11311 Concept Blvd.
Largo, FL 34643-4908
813-399-5344

Olympus America, Inc.
4 Nevada Drive
Lake Success, NY 11042-1179
516-488-3880

Olympus Optical Co. Ltd.
San-Ei Bldg.
1-22-2, Nishi-Shinjuku
Shinjuku-Ku, Tokyo 163-91
Japan
03/3402111

Olympus Winter & Ibe GmbH
Kuehnstrasse 61, Postf. 701709
D-22045 Hamburg 70
Germany
040/66966-0

Ovamed Corporation
111 W. Evelyn Ave. Ste. #214
Sunnyvale, CA 94086-6129
408-720-9876

Pentax Precision Instrument Corp.
30 Ramland Rd.
Orangeburg, NY 10962-2699
914-365-0700

Rudolf GmbH
Tuttlinger Str. 4
Postfach 28
D-78567 Fridingen
Germany
07463/1094

Simal Belgium Instrument Co.
2131 Espey Court, Suite 7
Crofton, MD 21114-2424

Storz Endoscopy-America Inc., Karl
10111 W. Jefferson Blvd.
Culver City, CA 90232-3509
310-558-1500

Storz GmbH & Co., Karl
Mittelstr. 8
Postfach 230
D-78532 Tuttlingen
Germany
07461/7080

Treier Endoscopie AG
Sonnrain
CH-6215 Beromunster
Switzerland
045/512323

Wolf Medical Instruments Corp., Richard
353 Corporate Woods Pkwy.
Vernon Hills, IL 60061-3110
708-913-1113

CHOLEDOCHOSCOPE, MINI-DIAMETER (5MM OR LESS)

Olympus America, Inc.
4 Nevada Dr.
Lake Success, NY 11042-1179
516-488-3880

URF-P2; TRANSLAPAROSCOPIC CHOLEDOCHOSCOPE
DESCRIPTION: URF-P2

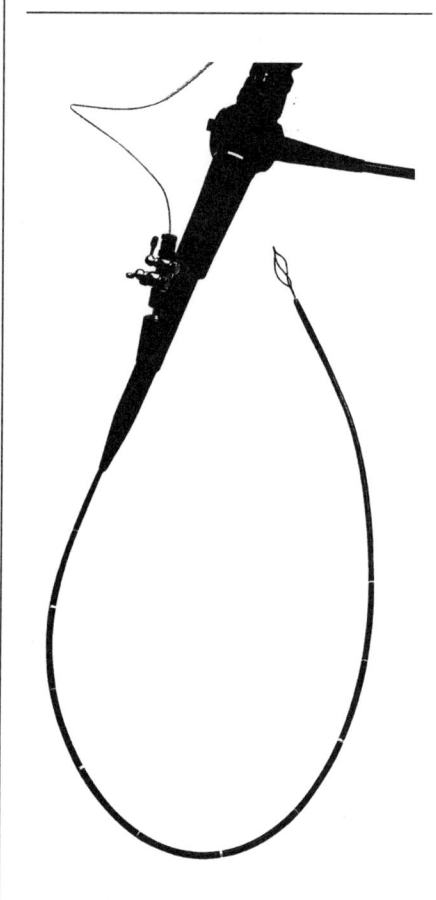

The URF-P2 has a tip tapered to 3.1mm (9.3Fr) to facilitate insertion into the cystic duct and common bile duct. The 1.2mm large working channel is designed for use with 3Fr baskets, forceps, snares, and EHL probes for gallstone extraction. The URF-P2 offers 280° of angulation and a secondary bending section, providing the angulation necessary for maneuverability and bile duct entry. Deflection also provides enhanced visibility in the common bile duct. The URF-P2 provides true-to-life, high-resolution images during translaparoscopic choledochoscopy and is fully compatible with Olympus photographic and video equipment.

STERILIZATION GUIDELINES: The URF-P2 can be disinfected through complete immersion or EtO sterilized.

SPECIFICATIONS/HOW SUPPLIED:
OPTICAL SYSTEMS
Field of view: 90°
Direction of view: 0° (forward viewing)
Depth of field: 1-50mm
DISTAL END
Outer diameter: 3.1mm (9.3Fr)
BENDING SECTION
Deflection: Up 180°, down 100°
INSERTION TUBE
Outer diameter: 3.3mm (9.9Fr)
LENGTH
Working: 700mm
Total: 1010mm
INSTRUMENT CHANNEL
Inner diameter: 1.2mm (3.6Fr)
BIOPSY FORCEPS
Minimum visible distance: 2mm from distal end
PHOTO DOCUMENTATION
Still: Olympus SC 35 (+ SM-ER3 Adapter); SC 16-10R, etc.
CCTV: Olympus OTV-S4, OTV-SX

Clarus Medical Systems, Inc.
2605 Fernbrook Lane
Minneapolis, MN 55447-4736
612-559-8640

Life Medical Technologies, Inc.
3649 W. 1987 S.
Salt Lake City, UT 84104
801-972-1900

Clamp

CLAMP, FIXATION, CHOLANGIOGRAPHY

Davis & Geck Endosurgery
1 Casper St.
Danbury, CT 06810
203-743-4451

PROFESSIONAL LINE 8375-01
DESCRIPTION: Cholangiography Clamp with Catheter Guide (order number 8375-01):

CHOLANGIOGRAPHY CLAMP WITH CATHETER GUIDE

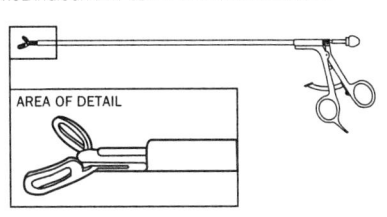

AREA OF DETAIL

5 French catheter guide, 5mm diameter, non-insulated, working length 33cm. For holding a catheter during intraoperative X-ray diagnosis.

Access Surgical International, Inc.
15 Caswell Ln.
Boat Yard Square
Plymouth, MA 02360
508-747-6006

Boss Instruments, Ltd.
1310 Central Ct.
Hermitage, TN 37076
615-885-2231

Chirurgische Instrumente
Hauptstrasse 18
D-78582 Balgheim
Germany
7424/501319

Davis & Geck Div.
American Cyanamid Company
One Cyanamid Plaza
Wayne, NJ 07470-2012
201-831-2000

Elmed, Inc.
60 W. Fay Ave.
Addison, IL 60101-5198
708-543-2792

Leisegang Medical, Inc.
6401 Congress Ave.
Boca Raton, FL 33487-2883
407-994-0202

Mist, Inc.
6307 E. Angus Dr.
Raleigh, NC 27613
919-787-8377

Schwarz Medical
Kirchstrasse 24
D-86935 Rott
Germany
8869/1881

CLAMP, LAPAROSCOPY

Access Surgical International, Inc.
15 Caswell Ln.
Boat Yard Square
Plymouth, MA 02360
508-747-6006

Aesculap
1000 Gateway Blvd.
South San Francisco, CA 94080-7030
415-876-7000

Birtcher Medical Systems, Inc.
50 Technology Dr.
Irvine, CA 92718-2301
714-753-9400

Davis & Geck Endosurgery
1 Casper Street
Danbury, CT 06810
203-743-4451

Davis & Geck Div.
American Cyanamid Company
One Cyanamid Plaza
Wayne, NJ 07470-2012
201-831-2000

Davol, Inc.
100 Sockanossett
P.O. Box 8500
Cranston, RI 02920-0500
401-463-7000

Elmed, Inc.
60 W. Fay Ave.
Addison, IL 60101-5198
708-543-2792

Leisegang Medical, Inc.
6401 Congress Ave.
Boca Raton, FL 33487-2883
407-994-0202

Performance Surgical Instruments
40 Norfolk Ave.
Easton, MA 023334
508-230-0010

Clip

CLIP, LIGATURE

Davis & Geck Endosurgery
1 Casper St.
Danbury, CT 06810
203-743-4451

LAPRO-CLIP 8487 SERIES

DESCRIPTION: LAPRO-CLIP Ligating Clip Cartridge:

LAPRO-CLIP LIGATING CLIP CARTRIDGE

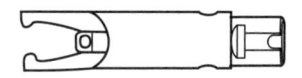

For additional information see Laparoscopic Clip Applier.

SPECIFICATIONS/HOW SUPPLIED: One clip per cartridge, six cartridges per sterile envelope, six sterile envelopes per box = 36 clips per box (order number 8487-12 for large clips and 8487-08 for medium/large clips).

One clip per cartridge, two cartridges per sterile envelope, ten sterile envelopes per box = 20 clips per box (order number 8487-13 for large clips and 8487-82 for medium/large clips).

Davis & Geck Div.
American Cyanamid Company
One Cyanamid Plaza
Wayne, NJ 07470-2012
201-831-2000

CLIP, SUTURE

Bashir, Jamil & Bros. Pvt. Ltd.
Khadim Ali Rd.
P.O. Box 7
Sialkot
Pakistan
0432-553862

Baxter Healthcare Corp.
Operating Room Div.
1500 Waukegan Rd.
McGaw Park, IL 60085-8210
708-473-1500

Davis & Geck Endosurgery
1 Casper Street
Danbury, CT 06810
203-743-4451

Davis & Geck Div.
American Cyanamid Company
One Cyanamid Plaza
Wayne, NJ 07470-2012
201-831-2000

Ethnor
192 Ave. Charles De Gaulle
F-92523 Neuilly S/Seine Cedex
France
1/47382233

Mader Instrument Corp.
25 Lamington Dr.
Succasunna, NJ 07876-2048
201-584-0816

Miltex Instrument Co., Inc.
6 Ohio Dr.
CB 5006
Lake Success, NY 11042-0006
516-775-7100

Surgical Instrument Co. Of America
1185 Edgewater Ave.
Ridgefield, NJ 07657-2102
201-941-6500

Cutter

CUTTER, LINEAR, LAPAROSCOPIC

Ethicon Endo-Surgery
4545 Creek Rd.
Cincinnati, OH 45242
513-786-7000

ENDOPATH ELC35

DESCRIPTION:

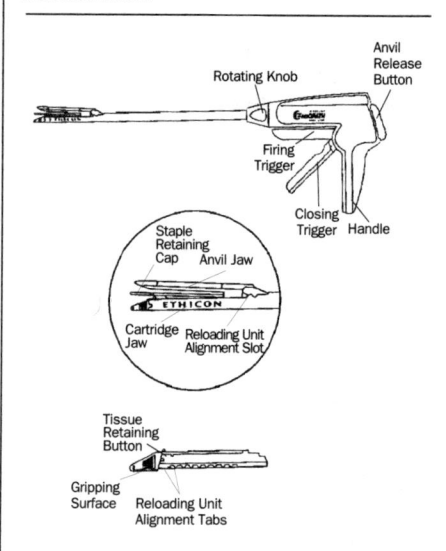

The ENDOPATH* Endoscopic Reloadable Linear Cutter with Safety Lock-Out delivers two, triple-staggered rows of staples while simultaneously dividing the tissue between the rows. The instrument's safety lock-out feature is designed to prevent firing an unloaded instrument or prevent a used cartridge from being refired. Both the standard blue cartridge and the vascular white cartridge instruments have a staple line that is approximately 37mm long and a cut line approximately 33mm long. A staple retaining cap on the cartridge protects the staple leg points during shipping and transportation.

The product codes for the ENDOPATH Endoscopic Reloadable Linear Cutter with Safety Lock-Out and their reloading units are as follows:

Both reloading units (ERU35 and EVU35) are interchangeable with the linear cutter instruments (ELC35 and EVC35). Do not reload the instrument more than seven times for a maximum of eight firings per instrument.

INDICATIONS: The ENDOPATH Endoscopic Reloadable Linear Cutter with Safety Lock-Out has applications in general, gynecologic, urologic, and thoracic surgery for transection, resection, and/or creation of anastomosis.

CUTTER/43

INSTRUMENT	RELOADING UNIT	CLOSED STAPLE HEIGHT	NUMBER OF STAPLES	CARTRIDGE COLOR	RETAINING CAP COLOR
ELC35	ERU35	1.5mm	54	Blue	Orange
EVC35	EVU35	1.0mm	54	White	Red

CONTRAINDICATIONS: DO NOT use the standard instrument with blue cartridge (ELC35) on any tissue that requires excessive force to compress to 1.5mm, or on any tissue that compresses easily to below 1.5mm.

DO NOT use the vascular instrument with white cartridge (EVC35) on any tissue that requires excessive force to compress to 1.0mm, or on any tissue that compresses to below 1.0mm.

DO NOT use any linear cutter device on ischemic or necrotic tissue.

DO NOT use the standard instrument with blue cartridge (ELC35) on pulmonary vessels.

The instrument IS NOT intended for use when surgical stapling is contraindicated.

WARNINGS: Endoscopic procedures should be performed only by persons having adequate training and familiarity with endoscopic techniques. Consult medical literature relative to techniques, complications, and hazards prior to performance of any endoscopic procedure.

Endoscopic instruments may vary in diameter from manufacturer to manufacturer. When endoscopic instruments and accessories from different manufacturers are employed together in a procedure, verify compatibility prior to initiation of procedures.

A thorough understanding of principles and techniques involved in laparoscopic laser and electrosurgical procedures is essential to avoid shock and burn hazards to both patient and medical personnel and damage to the device or other medical instruments. Refer to appropriate electrosurgical system user manual for indications and instructions to ensure that all safety precautions are followed.

Before firing, observe the surface of the reloading unit. The reloading unit must be replaced with another reloading unit if any colored drivers are visible.

Ensure that the instrument jaws are aligned and tissue is positioned properly.

The firing stroke must be completed. Do not partially fire the instrument.

After firing, completely release the firing trigger.

Before removing the instrument, be sure tissue is cleared from the jaws and then close the jaws.

After removing the instrument, examine the staple line for hemostasis and proper staple closure. If hemostasis is not present, appropriate techniques should be used to achieve hemostasis.

The ENDOPATH Endoscopic Reloadable Linear Cutter with Safety Lock-Out standard blue cartridge or vascular white cartridge instrument may be reloaded during a single procedure. Do not reload the instrument more than seven times for a total of eight firings per instrument.

The firing trigger and closing trigger must be in the open position during reloading.

Dispose of all fired instruments and used reloading units. DO NOT RESTERILIZE the ENDPATH Endoscopic Reloadable Linear Cutter with Safety Lock-Out or the Reloading Unit. Resterilization may compromise the integrity of the instrument or the reloading unit, which may result in wound leakage or disruption.

INSTRUCTIONS FOR USE: Read all instructions carefully. Failure to properly follow the instructions may lead to serious surgical consequences such as leakage or disruption.

IMPORTANT: This package insert is designed to provide instructions for the use of the ENDOPATH Endoscopic Reloadable Linear Cutter with Safety Lock-Out and Reloading Unit. It is not intended as a guide to surgical techniques.

Verify compatibility of all endoscopic instruments and accessories prior to using the ENDOPATH Endoscopic Reloadable Linear Cutter with Safety Lock-Out (refer to the second and third paragraphs under Warnings).

1. Using sterile technique, remove the instrument from the package. To avoid damage, do not flip the instrument into the sterile field.

2. Remove the staple retaining cap from the staple cartridge (Fig. 1). Discard the staple retaining cap.

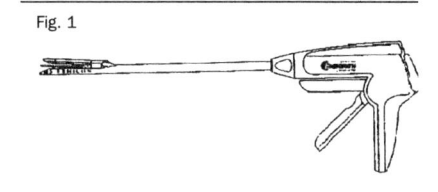

Fig. 1

NOTE: The staple retaining cap ensures proper staple orientation and protects the staple leg points during shipping and transportation.

3. Close the jaws of the instrument by squeezing the closing trigger until it locks in place (Fig. 2).

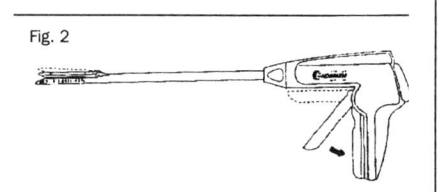

Fig. 2

CAUTION: Do not squeeze the firing trigger at this time.

4. Introduce the instrument into the body cavity through the appropriate trocar (minimum 12mm diameter trocar, Fig. 3).

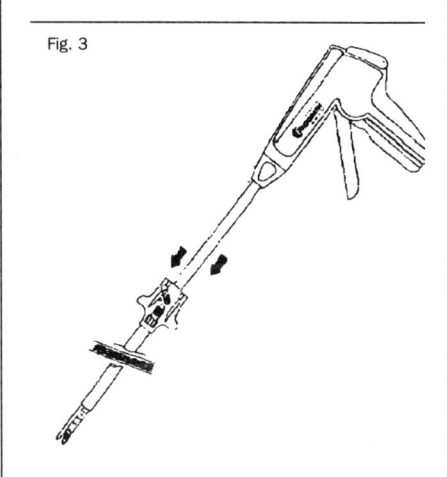

Fig. 3

CAUTION: The jaws of the instrument must be closed in order to be introduced into the cavity through the trocar. To close, squeeze the closing trigger toward the handle until it locks (Fig. 3).

5. Once it is in the cavity, reopen the instrument by pressing the release button. The closing trigger will return to its original position (Fig. 4).

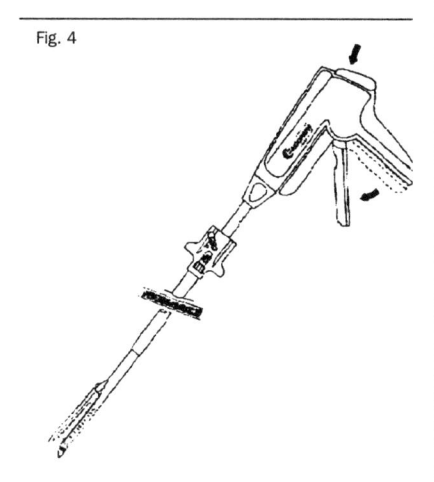

Fig. 4

NOTE: The instrument jaws can be opened manually by pulling upwards on the closing trigger until the trigger returns to its original open position.

6. After positioning the jaws of the instrument around the tissue to be stapled, close the jaws by squeezing the closing trigger

CUTTER, LINEAR, LAPAROSCOPIC (cont'd)

toward the handle until it locks. In the closed position, the firing trigger will move into grasping reach for instrument firing.

NOTE: Figures 5a. (uterus) and 5b. (appendix) are two examples of the many possible linear cutter applications.

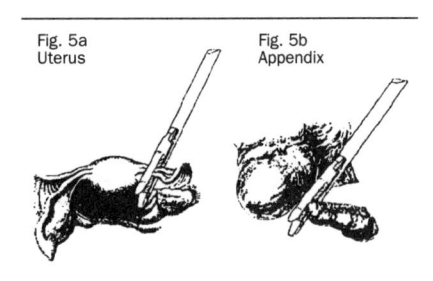

Fig. 5a Uterus

Fig. 5b Appendix

CAUTION: Ensure that the tissue lies flat between the jaws. Any "bunching" of tissue along the cartridge may result in an incomplete staple line.

CAUTION: Between firing, check to make sure that the instrument jaws are aligned.

7. Fire the instrument by squeezing the firing trigger completely until it rests on the closing trigger (Fig. 6). Release the trigger, allowing the firing trigger to return to the previous position.

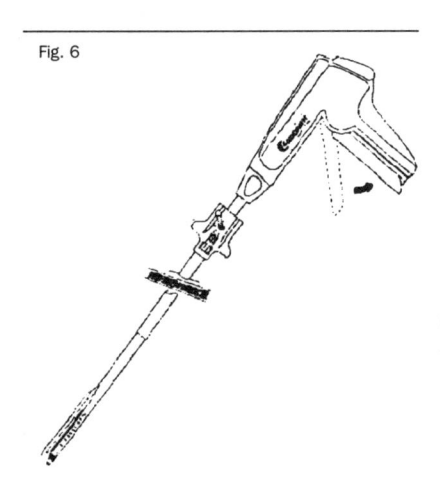

Fig. 6

CAUTION: The firing stroke must be completed. DO NOT partially fire the instrument.

8. Separate the instrument jaws by pressing the release button. Before removing the instrument from the trocar, make sure that tissue has been removed from the jaws [Fig. 7a. (uterus) and 7b. (appendix)].

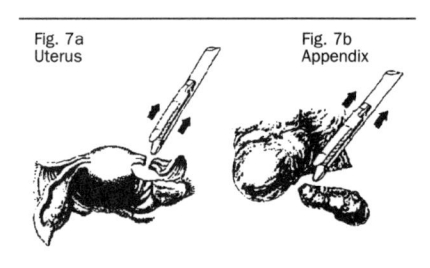

Fig. 7a Uterus

Fig. 7b Appendix

CAUTION: Examine the staple lines for hemostasis and proper staple closure. If hemostasis is not present, appropriate techniques should be used to achieve hemostasis.

9. To remove the instrument from the cavity, squeeze the closing trigger until it locks, closing the jaws of the instrument. Completely withdraw the instrument in the closed position from the trocar (Fig. 8).

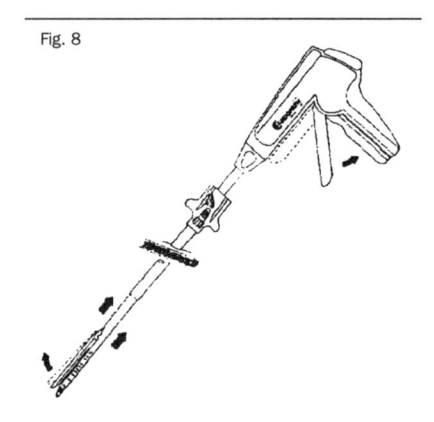

Fig. 8

ASSEMBLY GUIDELINES:
Reloading the Linear Cutter:

1. Ensure that the instrument is in the open position (Fig. 9).

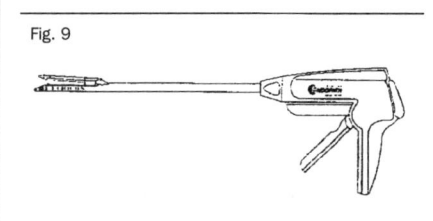

Fig. 9

NOTE: The reloading unit cannot be inserted unless the firing trigger is in its original position.

2. With an upward motion on the gripping surface, unsnap the reloading unit from the cartridge jaw (Fig. 10). Discard the used reloading unit.

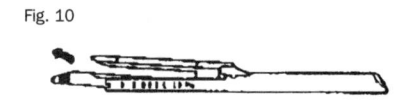

Fig. 10

CAUTION: Clean any formed but unused staples from the instrument by wiping the anvil and cartridge jaw or rinsing in sterile solution.

3. Examine the reloading unit for the presence of a staple retaining cap. If the retaining cap is not in place, discard the reloading unit.

4. Insert the new reloading unit by sliding against the bottom of the cartridge jaw until it stops in the reloading unit alignment slot. Snap the cartridge securely in place (Fig. 11a.). Remove the staple retaining cap and discard (Fig. 11b.).

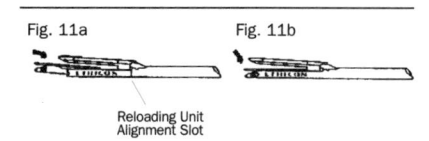

Fig. 11a   Fig. 11b

Reloading Unit Alignment Slot

5. After reloading, observe the surface of the new unit. If the colored drivers are visible, replace with another reloading unit. (The drivers are used to push the staples out of the pocket, through the tissue to be stapled and into the forming anvil.) The linear cutter is now reloaded and ready for use.

STERILIZATION GUIDELINES: Sterility is guaranteed unless the package is opened or damaged. DO NOT RESTERILIZE.

SPECIFICATIONS/HOW SUPPLIED: The ENDOPATH Endoscopic Reloadable Linear Cutter with Safety Lock-Out and Reloading Unit is for single-patient use only. The linear cutter package contains one sterile instrument per box and is preloaded, ready for use.

CAUTION: Federal (USA) law restricts this device to sale by or on the order of a physician.

Ethicon Endo-Surgery
4545 Creek Rd.
Cincinnati, OH 45242
513-786-7000

ENDOPATH ELC60

DESCRIPTION: The description and use of the ENDOPATH* Endoscopic Reloadable Linear Cutter with Safety Lock-Out and the ENDOPATH Linear Cutter Reloading Unit with Safety Lock-Out are provided in the following pages.

This package insert applies to both standard and thick-tissue linear cutter instruments.

The ENDOPATH Endoscopic Reloadable Linear Cutter with Safety Lock-Out, delivers two double staggered rows of staples while simultaneously dividing the tissue between the rows. This instrument has a safety lock-out feature which prevents a used reloading unit or an unloaded instrument from being fired. Standard and thick-tissue instruments and reloading units are designated by the following product codes:

ELC60 (Standard): applies 64 staples in two double staggered rows, approximately 63mm long, and cuts a line approximately

CUTTER / 45

ENDOPATH ELC60

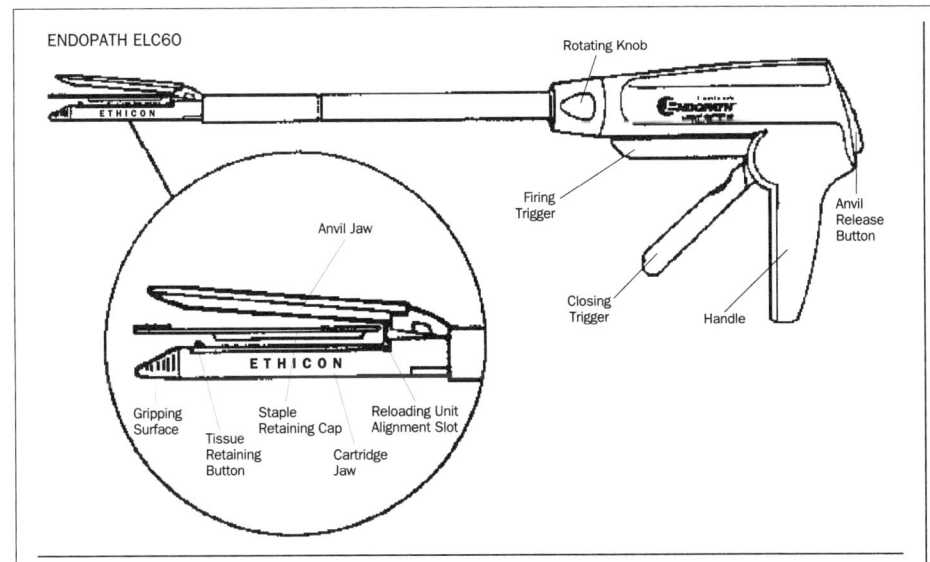

60mm long. Applies staples which close to approximately 1.5mm in height.

ETC60 (Thick Tissue): applies 64 staples in a double staggered row, approximately 63mm long, and cuts a line approximately 60mm long. Applies staples which close to approximately 2.0mm in height.

ERU60 (Standard): reloads the ELC60 with 64 staples.

ETU60 (Thick Tissue): reloads the ETC60 with 64 staples.

The ENDOPATH Endoscopic Reloadable Linear Cutter with Safety Lock-Out is packaged sterile and preloaded ready for use. The instrument is completely disposable and intended for single-patient use. Therefore, no cleaning, maintenance, or repair is required. The instrument may be reloaded during a single procedure by using the ENDOPATH Endoscopic Linear Cutter Reloading Unit with Safety Lock-Out. It is suggested that the instrument be reloaded no more than four times for a maximum of five firings per instrument.

INDICATIONS: The ENDOPATH Endoscopic Reloadable Linear Cutter with Safety Lock-Out has applications in gastro-intestinal and thoracic surgery for transection, resection, and creation of anastomosis.

CONTRAINDICATIONS: DO NOT use the standard instrument with blue cartridge (ELC60) on any tissue that requires excessive force to compress to 1.5mm or any tissue that compresses easily to below 1.5mm.

DO NOT use the thick tissue instrument with green cartridge (ETC60) on any tissue that requires excessive force to compress to 2.0mm or any tissue that compresses easily to below 2.0mm.

DO NOT use on ischemic or necrotic tissue.

DO NOT use on pulmonary vessels.

The instrument IS NOT intended for use when surgical stapling is contraindicated.

WARNINGS:

1. Before firing, observe the surface of the reloading unit. The reloading unit must be replaced with another reloading unit if any orange or yellow drivers are visible.

2. Ensure that the instrument jaws are aligned and tissue is positioned properly.

3. The firing stroke must be completed. Do not partially fire the instrument.

4. After firing, completely release the firing trigger to the previous position.

5. Before removal of the instrument, be sure tissue is cleared from the jaws and then close the jaws.

6. After removing the instrument, examine the staple line for hemostasis and proper staple closure. If hemostasis is not present, appropriate techniques should be utilized to achieve hemostasis.

7. The ENDOPATH Endoscopic Reloadable Linear Cutter with Safety Lock-Out, standard or thick-tissue instrument, may be reloaded during a single procedure. It is suggested that the instrument be reloaded no more than four times for a total of five firings per single patient.

8. The firing trigger and closing trigger must be in the open position during reloading.

9. Dispose of all fired instruments and used reloading units. DO NOT RESTERILIZE the ENDOPATH Endoscopic Reloadable Linear Cutter with Safety Lock-Out or the reloading unit. Resterilization may compromise the integrity of the instrument, or the reloading unit, which may result in wound leakage or disruption.

10. Endoscopic procedures should be performed only by persons having adequate training and familiarity with endoscopic techniques. Consult medical literature relative to techniques, complications, and hazards prior to performance of any endoscopic procedure.

11. Endoscopic instruments may vary in diameter from manufacturer to manufacturer. When endoscopic instruments and accessories from different manufacturers are employed together in a procedure, verify compatibility prior to initiation of procedures.

12. A thorough understanding of the principles and techniques involved in laparoscopic laser and electrosurgical procedures is essential to avoid shock and burn hazards to both patient and medical personnel and damage to the device or other medical instruments. Ensure proper electrical isolation or grounding if an Electrosurgical Unit is to be employed.

Read all instructions carefully. Failure to properly follow the instructions may lead to serious surgical consequences, such as leakage or disruptions.

INSTRUCTIONS FOR USE:

IMPORTANT: This package insert is intended to provide instructions for the use of the ENDOPATH Endoscopic Reloadable Linear Cutter with Safety Lock-Out and the ENDOPATH Endoscopic Linear Cutter Reloading Unit. It is not intended as a guide to surgical techniques.

1. The ENDOPATH Endoscopic Reloadable Linear Cutter with Safety Lock-Out is presterilized and packaged in the open position.

Fig. 1

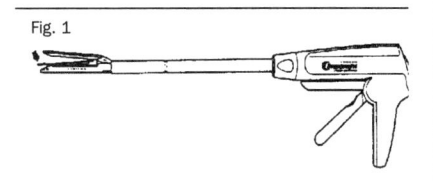

2. Remove the staple retaining cap from the reloading unit (see Fig. 1). Discard the staple retaining cap.

NOTE: The staple retaining cap ensures proper staple orientation and protects the staple leg points during shipping and transportation.

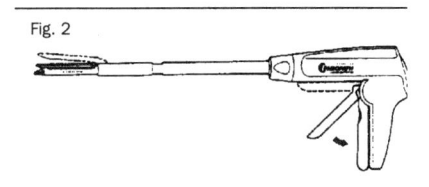

Fig. 2

3. Close the jaws of the instrument by squeezing the closing trigger until it clicks and locks in place (see Fig. 2).

CAUTION: Do not squeeze the firing trigger at this time.

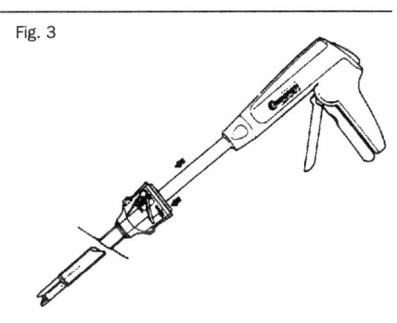

Fig. 3

4. Introduce the instrument into the abdominal or thoracic cavity through the appropriate trocar (minimum 18mm diameter trocar, see Fig. 3).

CUTTER, LINEAR, LAPAROSCOPIC (cont'd)

CAUTION: The jaws of the instrument must be closed to be introduced into the cavity through the trocar. To close, squeeze the closing trigger towards the handle, until it locks (see Fig. 3).

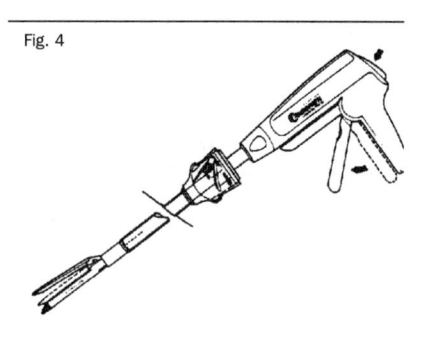

Fig. 4

5. Once it is in the cavity, reopen the instrument by depressing the release button at the proximal end of the instrument, which enables the closing trigger to return to its original position (see Fig. 4).

6. After positioning the jaws of the instrument around the tissue to be stapled, close the jaws of the instrument by squeezing the closing trigger toward the handle, until it locks. The tissue retaining button helps secure the tissue in the proper position. In the closed position, the firing trigger will move into grasping reach for instrument firing.

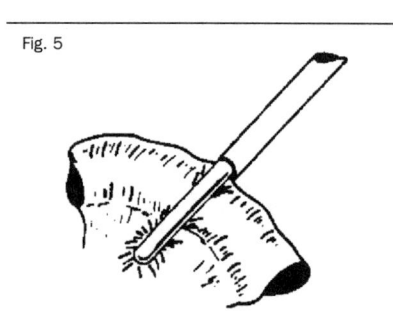

Fig. 5

CAUTION: Make sure the tissue lies flat between the jaws. Any bunching of tissue along the cartridge may result in an incomplete staple line (see Fig. 5). Also, before firing, check that the instrument jaws are aligned.

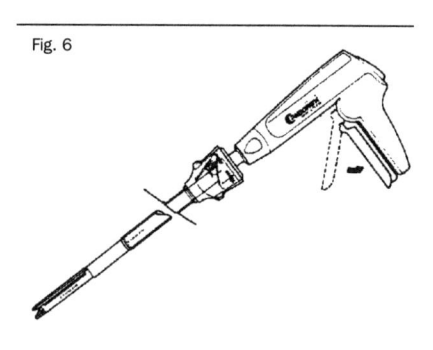

Fig. 6

7. Fire the instrument by squeezing the firing trigger completely until it comes to a stop against the closing trigger (see Fig. 6). To release, allow the firing trigger to return to the previous position.

CAUTION: The firing stroke must be completed. DO NOT partially fire the instrument.

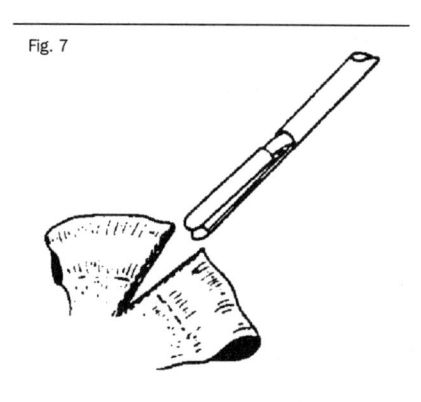

Fig. 7

8. Separate the instrument jaws by depressing the release button at the proximal end of the instrument. Before proceeding with removal of the instrument, ensure that tissue has been removed from the jaws (see Fig. 7).

CAUTION: Examine the staple lines for hemostasis and proper staple closure. If hemostasis is not present, appropriate techniques should be utilized to achieve hemostasis.

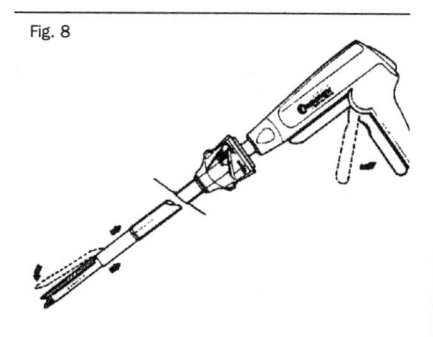

Fig. 8

9. To remove instrument from the cavity, squeeze the closing trigger until it locks, closing the jaws of the instrument. Completely withdraw the instrument, in the closed position, from the trocar (see Fig. 8).

Reloading the ENDOPATH Endoscopic Reloadable Linear Cutter with Safety Lock-Out:

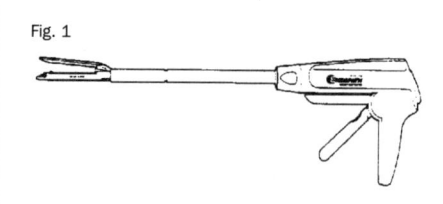

Fig. 1

1. Make sure the instrument is in the open position (see Fig. 1).

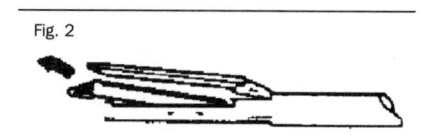

Fig. 2

2. With an upward motion on the gripping surface, unsnap the reloading unit from the cartridge jaw (see Fig. 2). Discard the used reloading unit.

3. Clean any formed but unused staples from the instrument by wiping the anvil and cartridge channel or rinsing in sterile solution.

4. Examine the reloading unit for the presence of a staple retaining cap. If the retaining cap is not in place, discard the reloading unit.

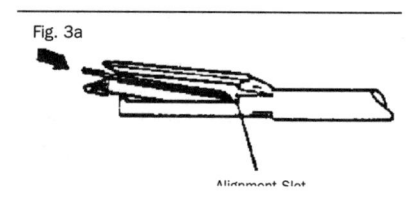

Fig. 3a

5. Insert the new ENDOPATH Endoscopic Linear Cutter Reloading Unit by placing the alignment tabs into the alignment slots and pivoting the reloading unit into the cartridge jaw (see Fig. 3a).

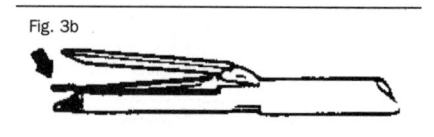

Fig. 3b

The reloading unit will snap into position. Remove staple retaining cap and discard (see Fig. 3b). After reloading, observe the surface of the reloading unit. The reloading unit must be replaced with another reloading unit if orange or yellow drivers are visible. The ENDOPATH Endoscopic Reloadable Linear Cutter with Safety Lock-Out is now reloaded and ready for use.

1. Remove the instrument from the package.
2. Remove the staple retaining cap.
3. Close the jaws of the instrument and introduce through the appropriate trocar.
4. Once in the cavity, separate the jaws of the instrument by depressing the release button at the proximal end of the instrument.
5. Position the instrument jaws on the tissue.
6. Close the instrument by squeezing the closing trigger toward handle until it locks.
7. Fire the instrument by squeezing the firing trigger completely until it comes to a stop against the closing trigger.
8. Allow the firing trigger to return to its previous position.
9. Depress the release button, allowing the closing trigger to return to the open position, which separates the instrument jaws.
10. Remove the tissue from the jaws of the instrument.
11. Close the instrument jaws by squeezing the closing trigger towards the handle.
12. Remove the instrument from the trocar.

Other:
1. Make sure the firing and closing triggers of the instrument are in the open position.
2. Remove and discard the used reloading unit.
3. Staple retaining cap must be in place when package is opened. If not, discard the reloading unit.
4. Load a new reloading unit into the cartridge jaw. After reloading, observe the surface of the reloading unit. The reloading unit must be replaced with another reloading unit if any orange or yellow drivers are visible.

STERILIZATION GUIDELINES: Sterility is guaranteed unless the package is opened or damaged. DO NOT RESTERILIZE.

SPECIFICATIONS/HOW SUPPLIED: CAUTION: Federal (USA) law restricts this device to sale by or on the order of a physician.

Ethicon Endo-surgery
4545 Creek Rd.
Cincinnati, OH 45242
513-786-7000

ENDOPATH EZ35

DESCRIPTION: The ENDOPATH* Endoscopic Reloadable Linear Cutter with Safety Lock-Out delivers two, triple-staggered rows of staples while simultaneously dividing the tissue between the rows. The instrument's safety lock-out feature is designed to prevent firing an unloaded instrument or prevent a used cartridge from being refired. Both the standard blue cartridge and the vascular white cartridge instruments have a staple line that is approximately 37mm long and a cut line approximately 33mm long. A staple retaining cap on the cartridge protects the staple leg points during shipping and transportation.

The product codes for the ENDOPATH Endoscopic Reloadable Linear Cutter with Safety Lock-Out and their reloading units are as follows:

The instrument is reloadable with either a standard blue cartridge or a vascular white cartridge. Do not reload the instrument more than seven times for a maximum of eight firings per instrument.

INDICATIONS: The ENDOPATH Endoscopic Reloadable Linear Cutter with Safety Lock-Out has applications in general, gynecologic, urologic, and thoracic surgery for transection, resection, and/or creation of anastomosis.

CONTRAINDICATIONS: DO NOT use the standard blue cartridge on any tissue that requires excessive force to compress to 1.5mm, or on any tissue that compresses easily to below 1.5mm.
DO NOT use the vascular white cartridge on any tissue that requires excessive force to compress to 1.0mm, or on any tissue that compresses easily to below 1.0mm.
DO NOT use any linear cutting device on ischemic or necrotic tissue.
DO NOT use the standard blue cartridge on pulmonary vessels.
The instrument IS NOT intended for use when surgical stapling is contraindicated.

ENDOPATH EZ35

INSTRUMENT	RELOADING UNIT	CLOSED STAPLE HEIGHT	NUMBER OF STAPLES	CARTRIDGE COLOR
EZ35B	ERU35	1.5mm	54	Blue
EZ35W	EVU35	1.0mm	54	White

ENDOPATH EZ35

1. Rotating Knob
2. Anvil Release Button
3. Handle
4. Closing Trigger
5. Firing Trigger
6. Gripping Surface
7. Tissue Retaining Button
8. Reloading Unit Alignment Tabs
9. Staple Retaining Cap
10. Anvil Jaw
11. Reloading Unit Alignment Slot
12. Cartridge Jaw
13. reloading Unit Alignment Notches

WARNINGS:
1. Endoscopic procedures should be performed only by persons having adequate training and familiarity with endoscopic techniques. Consult medical literature relative to techniques, complications, and hazards prior to performance of any endoscopic procedure.
2. Endoscopic instruments may vary in diameter from manufacturer to manufacturer. When endoscopic instruments and accessories from different manufacturers are employed together in a procedure, verify compatibility prior to initiation of procedures.
3. A thorough understanding of principles and techniques involved in laparoscopic laser and electrosurgical procedures is essential to avoid shock and burn hazards to both patient and medical personnel and damage to the device or other medical instruments. Refer to appropriate electrosurgical system user manual for indications and instructions to ensure that all safety precautions are followed.
4. Before firing, observe the surface of the reloading unit. The reloading unit must be replaced with another reloading unit if any colored drivers are visible.
5. Ensure that the instrument jaws are aligned and tissue is positioned properly.
6. The firing stroke must be completed. DO NOT partially fire the instrument.
7. After firing, completely release the firing trigger.
8. Before removing the instrument, be sure tissue is cleared from the jaws and then close the jaws.

CUTTER, LINEAR, LAPAROSCOPIC (cont'd)

9. After removing the instrument, examine the staple line for hemostasis and proper staple closure. If hemostasis is not present, appropriate techniques should be used to achieve hemostasis.

10. The ENDOPATH Endoscopic Reloadable Linear Cutter with Safety Lock-Out standard blue cartridge or vascular white cartridge may be reloaded during a single procedure. Do not reload the instrument more than seven times for a total of eight firings per instrument.

11. The firing trigger and closing trigger must be in the open position during reloading.

12. Dispose of all fired instruments and used reloading units. DO NOT RESTERILIZE the ENDOPATH Endoscopic Reloadable Linear Cutter with Safety Lock-Out or the Reloading Unit. Resterilization may compromise the integrity of the instrument or the reloading unit, which may result in wound leakage or disruption.

INSTRUCTIONS FOR USE: Read all instructions carefully. Failure to properly follow the instructions may lead to serious surgical consequences, such as leakage or disruption.

IMPORTANT: This package insert is designed to provide instructions for use of the ENDOPATH Endoscopic Reloadable Linear Cutter with Safety Lock-Out and Reloading Unit. It is not intended as a guide to surgical techniques.

Verify compatibility of all endoscopic instruments and accessories prior to using the ENDOPATH Endoscopic Reloadable Linear Cutter with Safety Lock-Out (refer to paragraphs 1 and 2 under Warnings).

1. Using sterile technique, remove the instrument from the package. To avoid damage, do not flip the instrument into the sterile field.

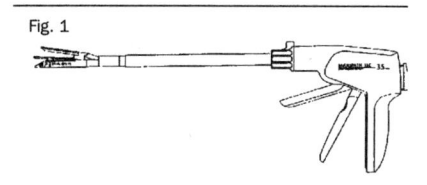

Fig. 1

2. Remove the staple retaining cap from the staple cartridge (Fig. 1). Discard the staple retaining cap.
NOTE: The staple retaining cap ensures proper staple orientation and protects the staple leg points during shipping and transportation.

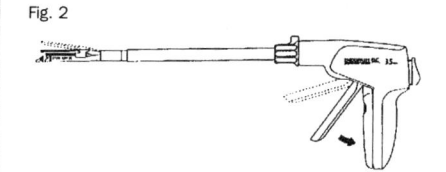

Fig. 2

3. Close the jaws of the instrument by squeezing the closing trigger until it locks in place (Fig. 2).
CAUTION: Do not squeeze the firing trigger at this time.

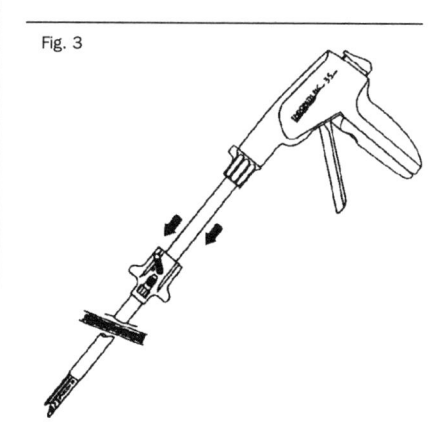

Fig. 3

4. Introduce the instrument into the body cavity through the appropriate trocar (minimum 12mm diameter (Fig. 3).
CAUTION: The jaws of the instrument must be closed to be introduced into the cavity through the trocar. To close, squeeze the closing trigger toward the handle until it locks (Fig. 3).

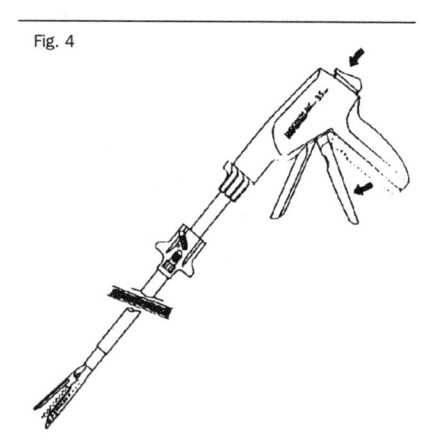

Fig. 4

5. Once in the cavity, reopen the instrument by pressing the anvil release button. The closing trigger will return to its original position (Fig. 4).
NOTE: The instrument jaws can be opened manually by pulling upwards on the closing trigger until the trigger returns to its original open position.

6. After positioning the jaws of the instrument around the tissue to be stapled, close the jaws by squeezing the closing trigger toward the handle until it locks. In the closed position, the firing trigger will move into grasping reach for instrument firing.

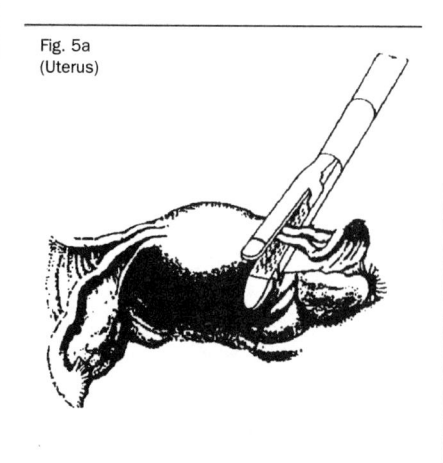

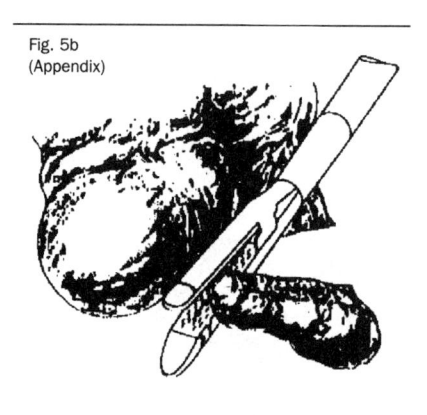

Fig. 5a (Uterus)

Fig. 5b (Appendix)

NOTE: Figure 5a (uterus) and 5b (appendix) are two examples of the many possible linear cutter applications.
CAUTION: Ensure that the tissue lies flat between the jaws. Any "bunching" of tissue along the cartridge may result in an incomplete staple line.

Before firing, check to make sure that the instrument jaws are aligned.

Fig. 6

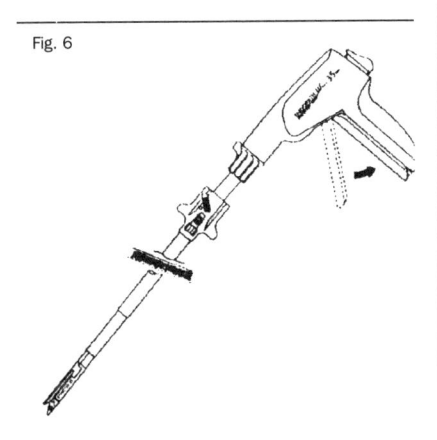

7. Fire the instrument by squeezing the firing trigger completely until it rests on the closing trigger (Fig. 6). Release the trigger, allowing the firing trigger to return to the previous position.

CAUTION: The firing stroke must be completed. DO NOT partially fire the instrument.

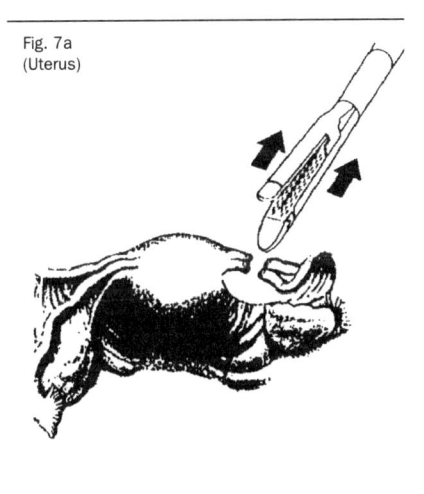

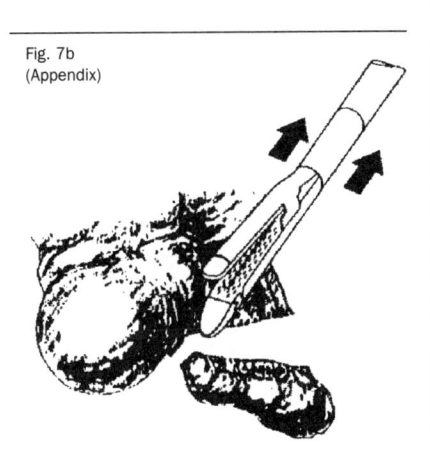

Fig. 7a (Uterus)

Fig. 7b (Appendix)

8. Separate the instrument jaws by pressing the anvil release button. Before removing the instrument from the trocar, make sure that tissue has been removed from the jaws [Fig. 7a (uterus) and 7b (appendix)].

CAUTION: Examine the staple lines for hemostasis and proper staple closure. If hemostasis is not present, appropriate techniques should be used to achieve hemostasis.

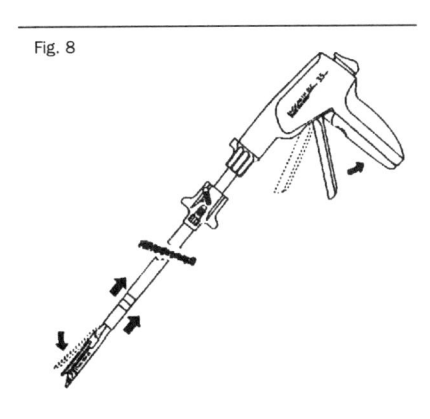

Fig. 8

9. To remove the instrument from the cavity, squeeze the closing trigger until it locks, closing the jaws of the instrument. Completely withdraw the instrument in the closed position from the trocar (Fig. 8).

Reloading the Linear Cutter:

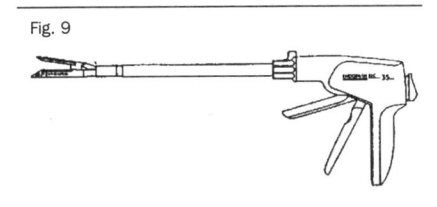

Fig. 9

1. Ensure that the instrument is in the open position (Fig. 9).
NOTE: The reloading unit cannot be inserted unless the firing trigger is in its original position.

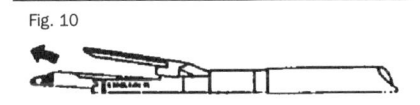

Fig. 10

2. With an upward motion on the gripping surface, unsnap the reloading unit from the cartridge jaw (Fig. 10). Discard the used reloading unit.

CAUTION: Clean any formed but unused staples from the instrument by wiping the anvil and cartridge jaw or rinsing in sterile solution.

3. Examine the reloading unit for the presence of a staple retaining cap. If the retaining cap is not in place, discard the reloading unit.

4. Insert the new reloading unit by sliding against the bottom of the cartridge jaw until it stops in the reloading unit alignment slot.

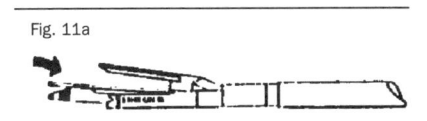

Fig. 11a

Snap the cartridge securely in place (Fig. 11a).

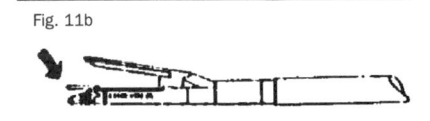

Fig. 11b

Remove the staple retaining cap and discard (Fig. 11b).

5. After reloading, observe the surface of the new unit. If the colored drivers are visible, replace with another reloading unit. (The drivers are used to push the staples out of the pocket, through the tissue to be stapled, and into the forming anvil.) The linear cutter is now reloaded and ready for use.

STERILIZATION GUIDELINES: Sterility is guaranteed unless the package is opened or damaged. **DO NOT RESTERILIZE.**

SPECIFICATIONS/HOW SUPPLIED: The ENDOPATH Endoscopic Reloadable Linear Cutter with Safety Lock-Out and Reloading Unit is for single-patient use only. The linear cutter package contains one sterile instrument which is preloaded, ready for use.

CAUTION: Federal (USA) law restricts this device to sale by or on the order of a physician.

CUTTER, LINEAR, LAPAROSCOPIC (cont'd)

Ethicon Endo-Surgery
4545 Creek Rd.
Cincinnati, OH 45242
513-786-7000

PROXIMATE LINEAR CUTTER

DESCRIPTION: The description and use of the PROXIMATE* Linear Cutter with Safety Lock-Out and the PROXIMATE Reloading Unit with Safety Lock-Out are provided in the following pages.

This package insert applies to both Standard and Thick Tissue linear cutter instruments.

The PROXIMATE Linear Cutter with Safety Lock-Out delivers two double-staggered rows of staples while simultaneously dividing the tissue between rows. This instrument has a safety lock-out feature which prevents a used cartridge from being refired or the instrument from being opened if only partially fired, thus exposing the knife. Standard instruments and reloading units are designated by the following product codes: TLC55, TCR55, TVC55, TVR55, TLC75, and TCR75. Thick Tissue instruments and reloading units are designated by the following product codes: TCT55, TRT55, TCT75, and TRT75.

TCR55 (Standard) - Reloads the TLC55 with 56 staples.
TVR55 (Vascular) - Reloads the TVC55 with 56 staples.
TRT55 (Thick Tissue) - Reloads the TCT55 with 56 staples.
TCR75 (Standard) - Reloads the TLC75 with 76 staples.
TRT75 (Thick Tissue) - Reloads the TCT75 with 76 staples.

TCR55, TRT55 and TVR55 reloading units are interchangeable with the TLC55, TCT55, and TVC55 instruments.

TCR75 and TRT75 reloading units are interchangeable with the TLC75 or TCT75 instruments.

The PROXIMATE Linear Cutter with Safety Lock-Out is packaged sterile and preloaded, ready for use. The PROXIMATE Linear Cutter with Safety Lock-Out is completely disposable and is intended for single-patient use; therefore, no cleaning, maintenance or repair is required.

The PROXIMATE Linear Cutter with Safety Lock-Out may be reloaded during a single procedure by using the PROXIMATE Linear Cutter Reloading Unit. It is suggested that the PROXIMATE Linear Cutter with Safety Lock-Out be reloaded no more than seven times for a maximum of eight firings per instrument.

PROXIMATE LINEAR CUTTER

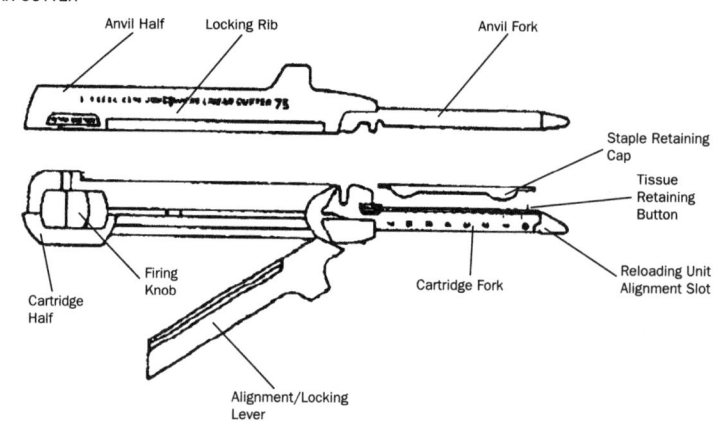

INDICATIONS: The PROXIMATE Linear Cutter with Safety Lock-Out has applications in gastrointestinal and thoracic surgery for transection, resection and the creation of anastomoses.

CONTRAINDICATIONS:
1. Do not use standard instrument with blue cartridge and orange retaining cap (TLC55, TLC75) on any tissue that requires excessive force to compress to 1.5mm or on any tissue that compresses easily to below 1.5mm.
2. Do not use thick tissue instrument with green cartridge and yellow retaining cap (TCT55, TCT75) on any tissue that requires excessive force to compress to 2.0mm or on any tissue that compresses easily to below 2.0mm.
3. Do not use Vascular instrument with white cartridge and blue retaining cap (TVC55) on any tissue that requires excessive force to compress to 1.0mm or on any tissue that compresses easily to below 1.0mm.
4. Do not use on ischemic or necrotic tissue.
5. Do not use on pulmonary vessels.

WARNINGS:
1. Before firing, ensure that the instrument halves are aligned and the tissue is positioned properly.
2. The firing stroke must be completed. The instrument cannot be opened unless the firing knob is returned to its original (Return Knob Here) position.
3. Completely return the firing knob to the original (Return Knob Here) position after firing and before separating the instrument halves.
4. Examine the staple lines for hemostasis and complete closure. Corrective action, if required, may include the use of sutures or electrocautery.
5. The PROXIMATE Linear Cutter with Safety Lock-Out may be reloaded during a single procedure. It is suggested that the instrument be reloaded no more than seven times for a maximum of eight firings per single patient.

6. Make sure that the firing knob is in the original (Return Knob Here) position during and after reloading.
7. Do not interchange instrument halves with other PROXIMATE Linear Cutter devices without safety lock-out.
8. Dispose of all fired instruments and used reloading units. DO NOT RESTERILIZE the PROXIMATE Linear Cutter with Safety Lock-Out or the PROXIMATE Linear Cutter Reloading Unit. Resterilization may compromise the integrity of the linear cutter or the reloading unit, which may result in wound leakage or disruption.

Read all instructions carefully. Failure to properly follow the instructions may lead to serious surgical consequences such as leakage or disruption.

INSTRUCTIONS FOR USE: This information is intended to provide instructions for the use of PROXIMATE Linear Cutter with Safety Lock-Out and the PROXIMATE Linear Cutter Reloading Unit. It is not intended as a guide to surgical techniques.

1. The PROXIMATE Linear Cutter with Safety Lock-Out is presterilized and packaged in the closed position.

Separate the instrument halves by completely disengaging the alignment/locking lever.

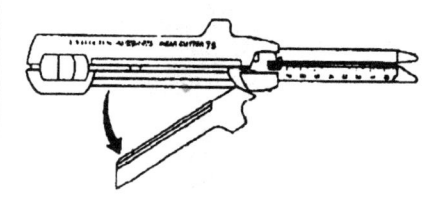

2. Remove and discard the staple retaining cap from the cartridge fork.

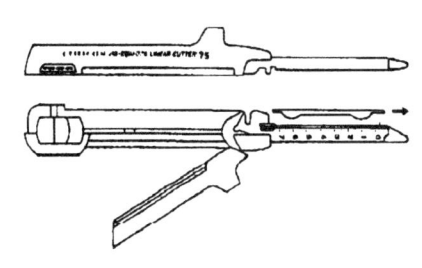

NOTE: The staple retaining cap ensures proper staple orientation and protects the staple leg points during shipping and transportation.

3. The instrument is placed across the tissue for transection or into the lumina to form an anastomosis.

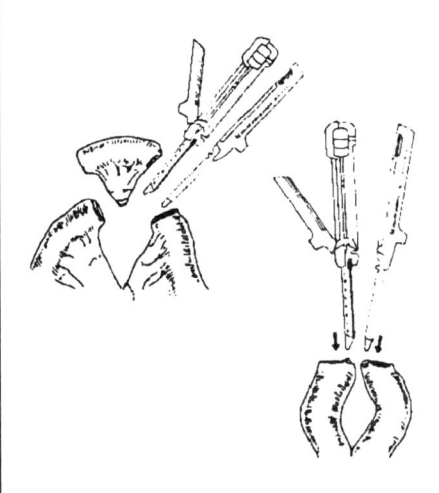

4. With the alignment/locking lever in the completely open position, join the instrument halves together. The halves may be brought together by aligning either from the center or the front or back end of the instrument.

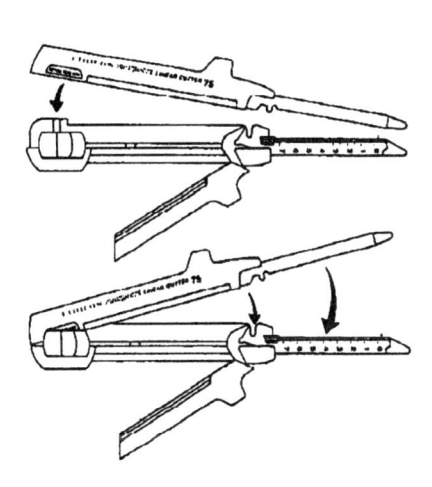

5. For final adjustment of the tissue on the forks, the alignment/locking lever may be moved to the intermediate position. This allows for maneuvering of the tissue while the instrument halves are joined.

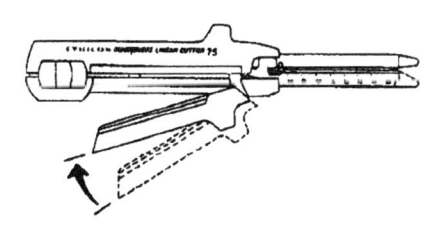

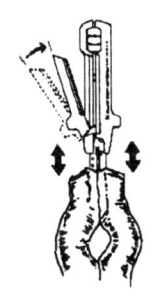

NOTE: This step is optional. The alignment/locking lever may be moved from the completely open to the completely closed position.

6. Close the alignment/locking lever completely. The tissue retaining button helps secure the tissue in the proper position.

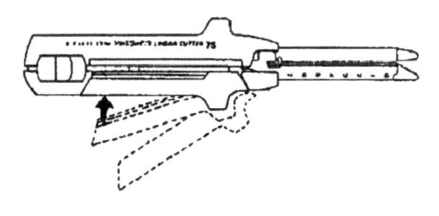

CAUTION: Make sure that the tissue lies flat between the forks. Any "bunching" of tissue at the proximal end of the forks or along the scale may result in an incomplete staple line.

7. Place the thumb on the firing knob and two fingers on the shoulders of the PROXIMATE Linear Cutter with Safety Lock-Out. Fire the device by pushing the firing knob completely forward in the same manner as firing a syringe.

CAUTION: Before firing, check to make sure that the instrument halves are aligned.

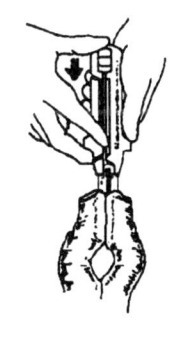

CAUTION: The firing stroke must be completed. Do not partially fire the instrument.

8a. Completely return the firing knob to the original (Return Knob Here) position.

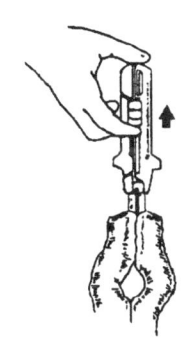

8b. Separate the instrument halves by opening the alignment/locking lever, and remove the instrument.

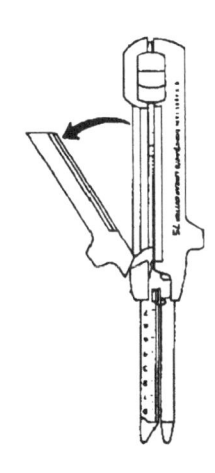

CAUTION: Examine the staple lines for proper staple closure.

Summary of operating instructions for PROXIMATE Linear Cutter with Safety Lock-Out:

1. Remove the closed instrument from the package.
2. Separate the instrument halves.
3. Remove the staple retaining cap.
4. Position the instrument halves on or in the tissue.
5. Join the instrument halves together.
6. If desired, move the alignment/locking lever to the intermediate position for final tissue adjustment.
7. Close the instrument.
8. Fire the PROXIMATE Linear Cutter with Safety Lock-Out by pushing the knob completely forward.
9. Return the firing knob to the original (Return Knob Here) position and separate the instrument halves.
10. Remove the instrument.

CUTTER, LINEAR, LAPAROSCOPIC (cont'd)

Summary of operating instructions for PROXIMATE Reloading Unit:
1. Make sure the firing knob is in the original (Return Knob Here) position.
2. Unsnap and discard the used reloading unit.
3. Staple retaining cap must be in place when package is opened or discard the cartridge.
4. Snap a new reloading unit into the cartridge fork. If orange or yellow drivers are present, reload with an unused cartridge. The instrument is now reloaded and ready for use.

ASSEMBLY GUIDELINES:
RELOADING THE LINEAR CUTTER:
1. Make sure that the firing knob is returned to the original (Return Knob Here) position.

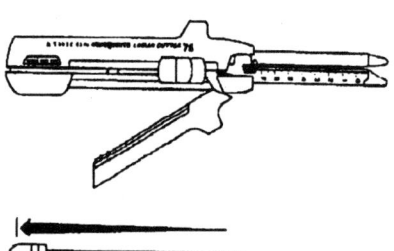

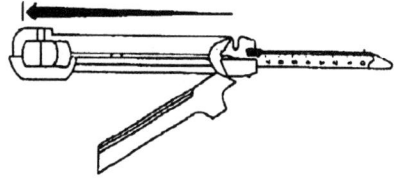

2. With an upward motion on the gripping surface, unsnap the PROXIMATE Linear Cutter Reloading Unit from the cartridge fork. Discard the used reloading unit.

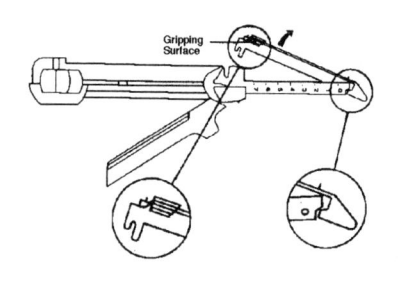

3. Any formed but unused staples should be cleaned from the instrument by wiping the anvil or rinsing in sterile solution.
CAUTION: Do not interchange instrument halves with other PROXIMATE Linear Cutter devices without safety lock-out.
4. Examine the cartridge for the presence of an orange or yellow staple retaining cap. If the retaining cap is not in place, discard cartridge. The presence of an orange or yellow colored retaining cap indicates that this reloading unit is intended to be used only with an instrument with safety lock-out.
5. Insert a new PROXIMATE Linear Cutter Reloading Unit by placing the alignment tabs into the slots and pivoting the reloading unit into the cartridge fork. The reloading unit will snap into position. Remove staple retaining cap. The PROXIMATE Linear Cutter with Safety Lock-Out is now reloaded and ready for use.

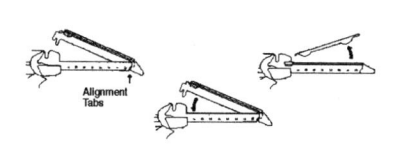

6. After reloading, observe the cartridge surface. If any orange, yellow or blue drivers are present, the cartridge has been previously fired and must be replaced before use.

STERILIZATION GUIDELINES: Sterility is guaranteed unless the package is opened or damaged. DO NOT RESTERILIZE the PROXIMATE Linear Cutter or the PROXIMATE Linear Cutter Reloading Unit.

Valleylab, Inc.
5920 Longbow Dr.
Boulder, CO 80301-3202
303-530-2300

Dilator

DILATOR, BLUNT

Boss Instruments, Ltd.
1310 Central Ct.
Hermitage, TN 37076
615-885-2231

Elmed, Inc.
60 W. Fay Ave.
Addison, IL 60101-5198
708-543-2792

Ethicon Endo-Surgery
4545 Creek Road
Cincinnati, OH 45242
513-786-7000

Leisegang Medical, Inc.
6401 Congress Ave.
Boca Raton, FL 33487-2883
407-994-0202

Wolf Medical Instruments Corp., Richard
353 Corporate Woods Pkwy.
Vernon Hills, IL 60061-3110
708-913-1113

DILATOR, FASCIA, UMBILICAL

Wolf Medical Instruments Corp., Richard
353 Corporate Woods Pkwy.
Vernon Hills, IL 60061-3110
708-913-1113

Dispenser

DISPENSER, LAPAROSCOPIC

Nu Surg Medical, Inc.
4440 Glen Este-Withamsville Rd., Ste.780
Cincinnati, OH 45245
513-753-3633

NUSURG LAPAROSCOPIC DISPENSER

DESCRIPTION:

LAPAROSCOPIC DISPENSER

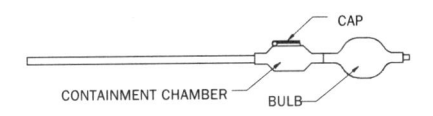

The Nu Surg Disposable Laparoscopic Dispenser is a single-use dispensing device with a bulb plunger, containment chamber, and shaft which is used in conjunction with a 10mm trocar under direct vision by endoscope. After the chamber is loaded with the material of choice, the plunger bulb is squeezed and the material dispensed.

INDICATIONS: The Nu Surg Laparoscopic Dispenser has applications in a variety of laparoscopic, gynecological, or thoracic procedures requiring the dispersion of an agent within a body cavity.

WARNINGS: Failure to read and follow the instructions furnished in this product insert may result in serious patient injury.

PRECAUTIONS: Laparoscopic procedures should be performed only by physicians having adequate training and familiarity with laparoscopic procedures. Complications include the risks associated with the medication as well as the patient's degree of tolerance. The physician is responsible for complete assessment of the complications associated with the use of this device. This device is provided sterile and is intended for multiple uses during a single laparoscopic procedure. Discard after use. Do not resterilize after use.

INSTRUCTIONS FOR USE:
1. Make sure the sterile packaging of the Laparoscopic Dispenser has not been opened or damaged.
2. Assure that both the Laparoscopic Dispenser and product of choice are within a sterile field prior to opening.
3. Surgical technician removes the Laparoscopic Dispenser from the sterile packaging and opens the Containment Chamber Cap.
4. Surgical technician then fills the Laparoscopic Dispenser Containment Chamber with the product of choice, to less than 1/2 of chambers capacity and closes Containment Chamber Cap.
5. The filled Laparoscopic Dispenser is then handed to the surgeon who places it, under direct vision through a 10mm trocar.
6. The Laparoscopic Dispenser is directed to the area of concern, the bulb is then depressed by the surgeon dispensing the product of choice.

NOTE: This is a sterile, disposable, single procedure item. Discard after use. Do not resterilize.

STERILIZATION GUIDELINES: Assure that the sterile packaging of the Laparoscopic Dispenser has not been opened or damaged. If opened, do not use and discard.

Discard after use. Do not resterilize.

SERVICE REQUIREMENTS & CONTACTS:
Nu Surg Medical, Inc.
4440 Glen Este-Withamsville Road
Suite 780
Cincinnati, OH 45245
800-225-2922

Always include the purchase order number and a written description of the problem.

DISPENSER, THORASCOPIC

Nu Surg Medical, Inc.
4440 Glen Este-Withamsville Rd., Ste.780
Cincinnati, OH 45245
513-753-3633

NUSURG THORASCOPIC DISPENSER

DESCRIPTION:

THORASCOPIC DISPENSER

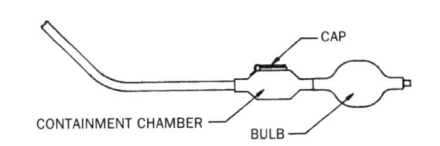

The Nu Surg Disposable Thorascopic Dispenser is a single-use dispensing device with a bulb plunger, containment chamber, and curved shaft which aids the dispensing of products into the pleural cavity. After the chamber is loaded with the material of choice, the plunger bulb is squeezed and the material dispensed.

INDICATIONS: The Nu Surg Thorascopic Dispenser is used to dispense the product of choice (preferably powder) within the Pleural Cavity under direct vision of a Thoracoscope. The mechanical device may aid in administering treatments for Pleural Effusions of Pneumothoracices.

WARNINGS: Failure to read and follow the instructions furnished in this product insert may result in serious patient injury.

PRECAUTIONS: Thorascopic procedures should be performed only by physicians having adequate training and familiarity with thorascopic procedures. Complications include the risks associated with the medication and the thorascopic procedure, as well as the patient's degree of tolerance. The physician is responsible for complete assessment of the complications associated with the use of this device. This device is provided sterile and is intended for multiple uses during a single thorascopic procedure.

INSTRUCTIONS FOR USE:
1. Make sure the sterile packaging of the Thorascopic Dispenser has not been opened or damaged.
2. Assure that both the Thorascopic Dispenser and product of choice are within a sterile field prior to opening.
3. Surgical technician removes the Thorascopic Dispenser from the sterile packaging and opens the Containment Chamber Cap.
4. Surgical technician then fills the Thorascopic Dispenser Containment Chamber with the product of choice, using a very small amount, and closes Containment Chamber Cap.
5. The filled Thorascopic Dispenser is then handed to the surgeon who places it, under direct vision of a thoracoscope.
6. The Thorascopic Dispenser is directed to the area of concern, the bulb is then depressed by the surgeon dispensing the product of choice.

NOTE: This is a sterile, disposable, single procedure item. Discard after use. Do not resterilize.

STERILIZATION GUIDELINES: Assure that the sterile packaging of the Thorascopic Dispenser has not been opened or damaged. If opened, do not use and discard.

Discard after use. Do not resterilize after use.

SERVICE REQUIREMENTS & CONTACTS:
Nu Surg Medical, Inc.
4440 Glen Este-Withamsville Road
Suite 780
Cincinnati, OH 45245
800-225-2922

Always include the purchase order number and a written descr iption of the problem.

Drain

DRAIN, SUCTION, CLOSED

Apple Medical Corp.
93 Nashaway Rd.
Bolton, MA 01740
508-779-2926

Davol, Inc.
100 Sockanossett
P.O. Box 8500
Cranston, RI 02920-0500
401-463-7000

Kensey Nash Corporation
55 E. Uwchlan Ave., Ste. 204
Exton, PA 19341-1247
215-524-0188

Electrocautery

ACCESSORIES, ELECTRICAL POWER (ELECTROCAUTERY)

Davis & Geck Endosurgery
1 Casper St.
Danbury, CT 06810
203-743-4451

LAPAROSCOPIC ASSIST DEVICE 8580-01
DESCRIPTION: Foot Switch Connection Cord for use with all Standard Banana Plug Adaptors:

FOOT SWITCH CONNECTION CORD

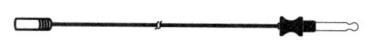

SPECIFICATIONS/HOW SUPPLIED: 5 units per box (order number 8580-01).

Davis & Geck Div.
American Cyanamid Company
One Cyanamid Plaza
Wayne, NJ 07470-2012
201-831-2000

COAGULATOR, HYSTEROSCOPIC (WITH ACCESSORIES)

Cabot Medical Corp.
2021 Cabot Blvd. West
Langhorne, PA 19047-1875
215-752-8300

Elmed, Inc.
60 W. Fay Ave.
Addison, IL 60101-5198
708-543-2792

Leisegang Medical, Inc.
6401 Congress Ave.
Boca Raton, FL 33487-2883
407-994-0202

Synectic Engineering, Inc.
4 Oxford Rd.
Milford, CT 06460-7007
203-877-8488

Wolf Medical Instruments Corp., Richard
353 Corporate Woods Pkwy.
Vernon Hills, IL 60061-3110
708-913-1113

COAGULATOR, LAPAROSCOPIC, UNIPOLAR

Aesculap
1000 Gateway Blvd.
South San Francisco, CA 94080-7030
415-876-7000

American Hydro-Surgical Instruments, Inc.
430 Commerce Dr., Ste. 50E
Delray Beach, FL 33445
407-278-5664

Berchtold KG, Gebr.
Weimarstr. 13-15
D-78532 Tuttlingen
Germany
07461/2345

Birtcher Medical Systems, Inc.
50 Technology Dr.
Irvine, CA 92718-2301
714-753-9400

Boss Instruments, Ltd.
1310 Central Ct.
Hermitage, TN 37076
615-885-2231

Bryan Corp.
4 Plympton St.
Woburn, MA 01801-2908
617-935-0004

Cabot Medical Corp.
2021 Cabot Blvd. West
Langhorne, PA 19047-1875
215-752-8300

Core Dynamics, Inc.
11222-4 St. Johns Indust. Pkwy.
Jacksonville, FL 32216
904-641-6611

Davis & Geck Endosurgery
1 Casper Street
Danbury, CT 06810
203-743-4451

Davis & Geck Div.
American Cyanamid Company
One Cyanamid Plaza
Wayne, NJ 07470-2012
201-831-2000

Davol, Inc.
100 Sockanossett
P.O. Box 8500
Cranston, RI 02920-0500
401-463-7000

Design Standards Corp.
643 North Ave.
Bridgeport, CT 06606-5745
203-366-7046

Design Standards Corp., Charlestown Div.
Ceda Industrial Park
P.O. Box 996
Charlestown, NH 03603-0996
603-826-7744

Elmed, Inc.
60 W. Fay Ave.
Addison, IL 60101-5198
708-543-2792

Erbe Elektromedizin GmbH
Waldhoernle Str. 17
D-72072 Tuebingen
Germany
07071/70010

Erbe USA, Inc.
2225 NW Parkway, Ste. 105
Marietta, GA 30067
404-955-4400

Ethicon Endo-Surgery
4545 Creek Road
Cincinnati, OH 45242
513-786-7000

Hipp GmbH, Anton
Annastr. 25/1
Postfach 80
D-78567 Fridingen
Germany
07463/7776-5088

Laparomed Corp.
9272 Jeronimo Rd., Unit 109
Irvine, CA 92718-1914
714-768-1155

Leisegang Medical, Inc.
6401 Congress Ave.
Boca Raton, FL 33487-2883
407-994-0202

Lican Medical Products Ltd.
5120 Halford Dr., R.R. 1
Windsor, ONT N9A 6J3
Canada
519-737-1142

Northgate Technologies, Inc.
3930 Ventura Dr., Ste. 150
Arlington Heights, IL 60004
708-506-9872

Redfield Corporation
210 Summit Ave.
Montvale, NJ 07645-1526
201-391-0494

Smith & Nephew Dyonics, Inc.
160 Dascomb Rd.
Andover, MA 01810-5893
508-470-2800

Synectic Engineering, Inc.
4 Oxford Rd.
Milford, CT 06460-7007
203-877-8488

Transamerican Technologies International
7026 Koll Center Pkwy., Ste. 207
Pleasanton, CA 94566-3108
510-484-0700

Valleylab, Inc.
5920 Longbow Dr.
Boulder, CO 80301-3202
303-530-2300

Wisap Gesellschaft
Rudolf Diesel Ring 20
D-82054 Sauerlach
Germany
08104/1067

Wisap USA
P.O. Box 324
Tomball, TX 77377-0324
713-351-2629

Wolf Medical Instruments Corp., Richard
353 Corporate Woods Pkwy.
Vernon Hills, IL 60061-3110
708-913-1113

Ximed Medical Systems
2195 Trade Zone Blvd.
San Jose, CA 95131
408-945-4040

COAGULATOR/CUTTER, ENDOSCOPIC, BIPOLAR

Access Surgical International, Inc.
15 Caswell Ln.
Boat Yard Square
Plymouth, MA 02360
508-747-6006

Aesculap
1000 Gateway Blvd.
South San Francisco, CA 94080-7030
415-876-7000

Birtcher Medical Systems, Inc.
50 Technology Dr.
Irvine, CA 92718-2301
714-753-9400

Bissinger, Medizintechnik GmbH
Gottlieb-Daimler Str.5
D-79331 Teningen 1
Germany
07641/8038

Cabot Medical Corp.
2021 Cabot Blvd. West
Langhorne, PA 19047-1875
215-752-8300

Cameron-Miller, Inc.
3949 S. Racine Ave.
Chicago, IL 60609-2523
312-523-6360

Davis & Geck Div.
American Cyanamid Company
One Cyanamid Plaza
Wayne, NJ 07470-2012
201-831-2000

Design Standards Corp.
643 North Ave.
Bridgeport, CT 06606-5745
203-366-7046

Elmed, Inc.
60 W. Fay Ave.
Addison, IL 60101-5198
708-543-2792

Erbe Elektromedizin GmbH
Waldhoernle Str. 17
D-72072 Tuebingen
Germany
07071/70010

Erbe USA, Inc.
2225 NW Parkway, Ste. 105
Marietta, GA 30067
404-955-4400

Ethicon Endo-Surgery
4545 Creek Road
Cincinnati, OH 45242
513-786-7000

Everest Medical Corp.
13755 First Avenue. N.
Minneapolis, MN 55441-5454
612-473-6262

Greenwald Surgical Co., Inc.
2688 Dekalb Street
Lake Station, IN 46405-1519
219-962-1604

Instrument Makar, Inc.
2950 E. Mt. Hope
Okemos, MI 48864-1910
517-332-3593

Kirwan Surgical Products, Inc.
83 East Water St.
P.O. Box 545
Rockland, MA 02370-1837
617-878-2706

Leisegang Medical, Inc.
6401 Congress Ave.
Boca Raton, FL 33487-2883
407-994-0202

COAGULATOR/CUTTER, ENDOSCOPIC, BIPOLAR
(cont'd)

Medesign GmbH
Partnachplatz 7-9
D-81373 Muenchen
Germany
089/769-5217

Olsen Electrosurgical Inc.
2100 Meridian Park Blvd.
Concord, CA 94520-5709
510-825-8151

Origin Medsystems, Inc.
135 Constitution Dr.
Menlo Park, CA 94025
415-617-5000

Scanlan International, Inc.
One Scanlan Plaza
St. Paul, MN 55107-1629
612-298-0997

Select-Sutter GmbH
Tullastr. 87
D-79108 Freiburg/Breisgau
Germany
0761/515510

Site Microsurgical Systems, Inc.
135 Gibraltar Rd.
Horsham, PA 19044-0936
215-674-5800

Storz Endoscopy-America Inc., Karl
10111 W. Jefferson Blvd.
Culver City, CA 90232-3509
310-558-1500

Storz GmbH & Co., Karl
Mittelstr. 8
Postfach 230
D-78532 Tuttlingen
Germany
07461/7080

Surgical Instrument Manufacturers, Inc.
1549 Fenpark Dr.
Fenton, MO 63026-2915
314-349-4960

Synectic Engineering, Inc.
4 Oxford Rd.
Milford, CT 06460-7007
203-877-8488

Wisap Gesellschaft
Rudolf Diesel Ring 20
D-82054 Sauerlach
Germany
08104/1067

Wisap USA
P.O. Box 324
Tomball, TX 77377-0324
713-351-2629

Wolf Medical Instruments Corp., Richard
353 Corporate Woods Pkwy.
Vernon Hills, IL 60061-3110
708-913-1113

Ximed Medical Systems
2195 Trade Zone Blvd.
San Jose, CA 95131
408-945-4040

COAGULATOR/CUTTER, ENDOSCOPIC, UNIPOLAR

Access Surgical International, Inc.
15 Caswell Ln.
Boat Yard Square
Plymouth, MA 02360
508-747-6006

Aesculap
1000 Gateway Blvd.
South San Francisco, CA 94080-7030
415-876-7000

American Hydro-Surgical Instruments, Inc.
430 Commerce Dr., Ste. 50E
Delray Beach, FL 33445
407-278-5664

Birtcher Medical Systems, Inc.
50 Technology Dr.
Irvine, CA 92718-2301
714-753-9400

Cabot Medical Corp.
2021 Cabot Blvd. West
Langhorne, PA 19047-1875
215-752-8300

Conmed Corp.
310 Broad Street
Utica, NY 13501
315-797-8375

Davis & Geck Div.
American Cyanamid Company
One Cyanamid Plaza
Wayne, NJ 07470-2012
201-831-2000

Design Standards Corp.
643 North Ave.
Bridgeport, CT 06606-5745
203-366-7046

Elmed, Inc.
60 W. Fay Ave.
Addison, IL 60101-5198
708-543-2792

Erbe Elektromedizin GmbH
Waldhoernle Str. 17
D-72072 Tuebingen
Germany
07071/70010

Erbe USA, Inc.
2225 NW Parkway, Ste. 105
Marietta, GA 30067
404-955-4400

Ethicon Endo-Surgery
4545 Creek Road
Cincinnati, OH 45242
513-786-7000

Everest Medical Corp.
13755 First Avenue. N.
Minneapolis, MN 55441-5454
612-473-6262

Laparomed Corp.
9272 Jeronimo Rd., Unit 109
Irvine, CA 92718-1914
714-768-1155

Leisegang Medical, Inc.
6401 Congress Ave.
Boca Raton, FL 33487-2883
407-994-0202

Mist, Inc.
6307 E. Angus Dr.
Raleigh, NC 27613
919-787-8377

Smith & Nephew Dyonics, Inc.
160 Dascomb Rd.
Andover, MA 01810-5893
508-470-2800

Synectic Engineering, Inc.
4 Oxford Rd.
Milford, CT 06460-7007
203-877-8488

Valleylab, Inc.
5920 Longbow Dr.
Boulder, CO 80301-3202
303-530-2300

Wisap Gesellschaft
Rudolf Diesel Ring 20
D-82054 Sauerlach
Germany
08104/1067

Wisap USA
P.O. Box 324
Tomball, TX 77377-0324
713-351-2629

Wolf Medical Instruments Corp., Richard
353 Corporate Woods Pkwy.
Vernon Hills, IL 60061-3110
708-913-1113

Ximed Medical Systems
2195 Trade Zone Blvd.
San Jose, CA 95131
408-945-4040

ELECTROCAUTERY UNIT, ENDOSCOPIC

Apple Medical Corp.
93 Nashaway Rd.
Bolton, MA 01740
508-779-2926

Birtcher Medical Systems, Inc.
50 Technology Dr.
Irvine, CA 92718-2301
714-753-9400

Cabot Medical Corp.
2021 Cabot Blvd. West
Langhorne, PA 19047-1875
215-752-8300

Cameron-Miller, Inc.
3949 S. Racine Ave.
Chicago, IL 60609-2523
312-523-6360

Conmed Corp.
310 Broad Street
Utica, NY 13501
315-797-8375

Contec Medical Ltd.
11 Haroshet Street
P.O. Box 1400
Ramat Hasharon 47113
Israel
03/5491153

Cory Brothers Co.
4 Dollis Pk.
London, N3 1HG
United Kingdom
081/349/1081

Elmed, Inc.
60 W. Fay Ave.
Addison, IL 60101-5198
708-543-2792

Erbe USA, Inc.
2225 NW Parkway, Ste. 105
Marietta, GA 30067
404-955-4400

Laserscope
3052 Orchard Dr.
San Jose, CA 95134-2011
408-943-0636

Leisegang Medical, Inc.
6401 Congress Ave.
Boca Raton, FL 33487-2883
407-994-0202

Tiemann & Co., George
25 Plant Ave.
Hauppauge, NY 11788-3804
516-273-0005

Valleylab, Inc.
5920 Longbow Dr.
Boulder, CO 80301-3202
303-530-2300

Wolf Medical Instruments Corp., Richard
353 Corporate Woods Pkwy.
Vernon Hills, IL 60061-3110
708-913-1113

ELECTRODE, ELECTROSURGERY, LAPAROSCOPIC

Conmed Corp.
310 Broad St.
Utica, NY 13501
315-797-8375

SELECT ONE INSTRUMENTS

DESCRIPTION: These are hand-held electrosurgical instruments for use in surgical endoscopic procedures, including laparoscopy, pelviscopy, thoracoscopy, et al. All are sterile, for single-patient use.

There are 3 groups:

Solid Shaft Electrosurgical Electrodes, which can be connected to the Aspen Hand-Trol, Concept Tech-Switch, and CONMED electrosurgical pencils for hand-controlled activation of the electrosurgical generator, or to a disposable electrosurgical cord for footcontrolled activation.

Hollow Shaft Electrosurgical Electrodes with suction/irrigation capability can be connected to an electrosurgical pencil or to the disposable cable for footswitch control. They have an internal channel and luer-lock connection for the stopcock, for connection to a suction/irrigation source.

Integral Handle Electrosurgical Instruments with suction/irrigation capability are connected to the footswitch accessory with the disposable cord provided in each package, together with a stopcock for connection to a suction irrigation source.

All come with a variety of electrode tips, which include spatulas, L-Hooks, J-Hooks, Ball Tips, Blades, and Hook blades in 27 & 32cm lengths, with extended insulation.

CONTRAINDICATIONS: These electrosurgical instruments should only be used by surgeons trained in surgical endoscopy according to established protocols.

See package insert for use directions, cautions, warnings and detailed product descriptions.

Access Surgical International, Inc.
15 Caswell Ln.
Boat Yard Square
Plymouth, MA 02360
508-747-6006

American Hydro-Surgical Instruments, Inc.
430 Commerce Dr., Ste. 50E
Delray Beach, FL 33445
407-278-5664

Berchtold Corp.
2050 Mabeline Rd., Ste. C
North Charlestown, SC 29418-4643
803-569-6100

Birtcher Medical Systems, Inc.
50 Technology Dr.
Irvine, CA 92718-2301
714-753-9400

Circon Acmi
300 Stillwater Ave.
Stamford, CT 06902-3640
203-328-8689

Electroscope, Inc.
4890 Sterling Dr.
Boulder, CO 80301
303-444-2600

Ethicon Endo-Surgery
4545 Creek Road
Cincinnati, OH 45242
513-786-7000

Gabris Surgical Corp.
547 Susan Constant Dr.
Virginia Beach, VA 23451
804-491-6487

Nu Surg Medical, Inc.
4440 Glen Este-Withamsville Road
Suite 780
Cincinnati, OH 45245
513-753-3633

O.R. Concepts, Inc.
12250 Nicollet Ave. South
Burnsville, MN 55337
612-894-7523

Reznik Instrument, Inc.
7337 North Lawndale
Skokie, IL 60076
708-673-3444

Sherwood Intrascopic Div.
1915 Olive St.
St. Louis, MO 63103
314-241-5700

U.S. Endoscopy Group
7123 Industrial Park Blvd.
Mentor, OH 44060
216-269-8226

Valleylab, Inc.
5920 Longbow Dr.
Boulder, CO 80301-3202
303-530-2300

HANDLE, INSTRUMENT, LAPAROSCOPIC (ELECTROCAUTERY)

Davis & Geck Endosurgery
1 Casper St.
Danbury, CT 06810
203-743-4451

LAPAROSCOPIC ASSIST DEVICE 8575-01

DESCRIPTION: Multifunction Pistol Grip Handpiece for use with 8576, 8577, 8578, 8579 - probes not included - (luer lock-type connector for irrigation; barb connector for suction).

ELECTROCAUTERY HANDPIECE

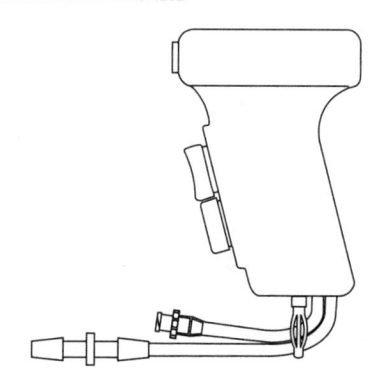

SPECIFICATIONS/HOW SUPPLIED: Supplied sterile, in boxes of 5 units (order number 8575-01).

Davis & Geck Div.
American Cyanamid Company
One Cyanamid Plaza
Wayne, NJ 07470-2012
201-831-2000

Ethicon Endo-Surgery
4545 Creek Road
Cincinnati, OH 45242
513-786-7000

Microsurge, Inc.
150 A St.
Needham, MA 02194
617-444-2300

MODULE, CONTROL, ELECTROSURGERY

Conmed Corp.
310 Broad St.
Utica, NY 13501
315-797-8375

SELECT ONE MODULAR INSTRUMENTS

DESCRIPTION: The CONMED SelectONE™ Modular Electrosurgical Instruments are sterile, single-patient use dissecting instruments with suction/irrigation channels within the instrument shaft for use in surgical endoscopic procedures such as laparoscopy, pelviscopy, and thoracoscopy, et al. This instrument system consists of a modular handle assembly and removable blades with a variety of working tips. All are sterile, for single patient use.

The Handle Modules come in four interchangeable styles allowing individual surgeon's choice of hand or off-site controls:
- Footcontrolled Electrosurgery Forward Module. No controls on the handle; CUT/COAG controls are footcontrolled.
- Handcontrolled Electrosurgery Forward Module. Offers handcontrolled activation of the electrosurgery CUT/COAG.
- Handcontrolled Suction/Irrigation Rear Module with 10ft. suction/irrigation tubing set. Offers handcontrolled activation of the suction/irrigation sources. NOTE: This module must be used with either the Footcontrolled or Handcontrolled Electrosurgery Forward Modules for connection of the Removable Blade Instruments. The module irrigation tubing should be connected to a pressurized irrigation source, such as an inflatable pressure infusion bag, mechanical pump or other source approved for laparoscopic use. Suction tubing should be connected to a high-flow, regulated suction source. This module can also be directly connected to a 5mm cannula, yielding a simple suction irrigation system.
- Rear Module. For "Off-Instrument" or remote control of suction/irrigation.

The Removable, Interchangeable Electrodes connect directly to the hand or footcontrolled electrosurgical modules by a luer-lock connection. They are available in a wide variety of tips including L-hooks, spatula, J-hook, sphere, L-hook sphere, J-hook sphere, hook blade and L-hook blade, in 27 and 32cm lengths with extended insulation.

CONTRAINDICATIONS: These electrosurgical instruments should only be used by surgeons trained in surgical endoscopy according to established protocols.
See package insert for use directions, cautions, warnings, and detailed product descriptions.

Conmed Corp.
310 Broad St.
Utica, NY 13501
315-797-8375

UNIVERSAL PLUS INSTRUMENT SYSTEM

DESCRIPTION: The sterile, single-patient use CONMED SelectOne UNIVERSAL PLUS Electrosurgical and Suction/Irrigation Instrument provides hand or footcontrolled CUT/COAG electrosurgery and high volume, handcontrolled suction/irrigation capability in one familiar pistol grip instrument. A lockout feature prevents simultaneous activation of electrosurgical current and suction/irrigation.

A variety of sterile 5mm rotatable interchangeable electrosurgical electrode tips with low volume suction/irrigation capacity AND 5mm & 10mm high volume interchangeable suction/irrigation tips also attach to the handle, thereby meeting all electrosurgical electrode and suction/irrigation needs with one instrument. 10ft. of sterile suction/irrigation tubing are attached.

The UNIVERSAL PLUS instrument should be connected to a pressurized irrigation source such as an inflatable pressure infusion bag, a mechanical pump, or other source approved for laparoscopic use. Suction tubing should be connected to a high-flow regulated suction source.

CONTRAINDICATIONS: This electrosurgical suction/irrigation instrument should only be used by surgeons trained in surgical endoscopy according to established protocols. See package insert for use directions, cautions, warnings and detailed product descriptions.

Fujinon, Inc.
10 High Point Dr.
Wayne, NJ 07470-7434
201-633-5600

PROBE, ELECTROCAUTERIZATION, MULTI-USE

Davis & Geck Endosurgery
1 Casper St.
Danbury, CT 06810
203-743-4451

LAPAROSCOPIC ASSIST DEVICE 8578-01/-08 SERIES

DESCRIPTION: Modular Suction/Irrigation/Electrocautery Probes for use with Multi-function Pistol Grip Devices 8573, 8575.

L Hook (order number 8578-01):

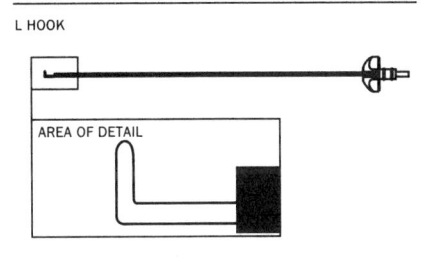

Standard Hook (order number 8578-02):

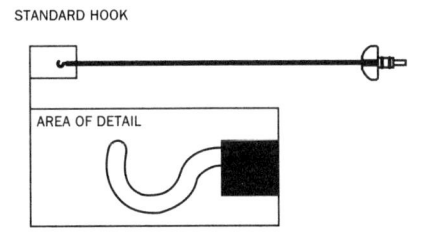

Hockey Stick Hook (order number 8578-03):

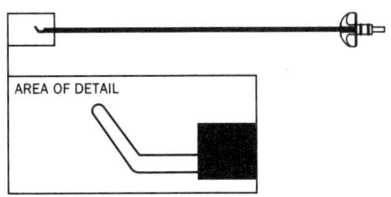

J Hook (order number 8578-04):

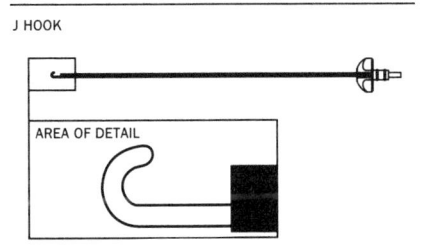

Spatula (order number 8578-05):

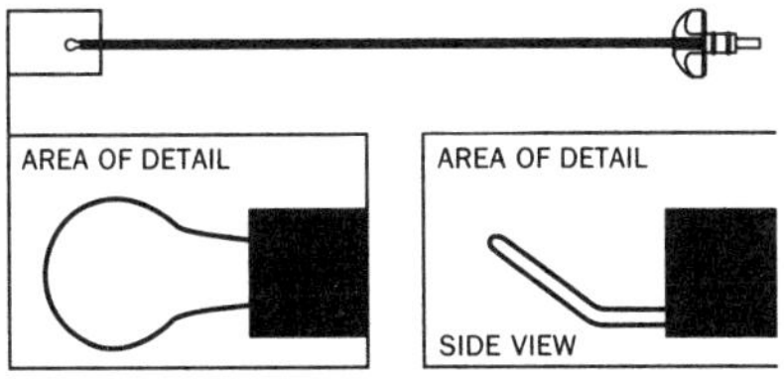

Blade (order number 8578-06):

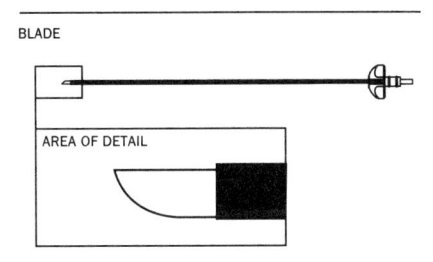

Ball (order number 8578-07):

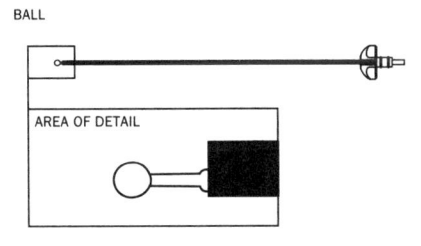

Needle (order number 8578-08):

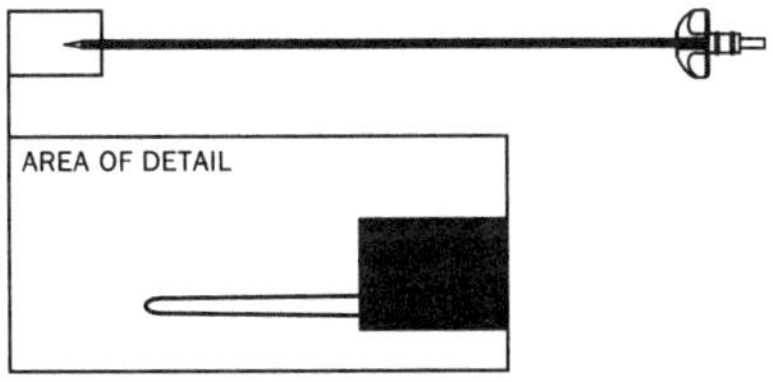

WARNINGS:

1. Do not use the electrode if the insulation appears cracked, flawed or otherwise damaged.

2. Do not use electrosurgery in the presence of flammable anesthetics or other flammable gases, near flammable fluids or objects, or in the presence of oxidizing agents, as fire could result.

3. Place active accessories in a dedicated instrument holder or in a clean, dry non-conductive and visible area, away from the patient when not in use. Inadvertent contact with the patient may result in burns. Contact with drapes may cause a fire.

INSTRUCTIONS FOR USE: All surgeons and surgical staff involved in the performance of electrosurgical procedures should read these instructions, warnings, and precautions prior to performing electrosurgery. The surgical staff and other related hospital personnel should be fully trained in this surgical technique prior to use of all electrosurgical devices.

Usage: Refer to your electrosurgical unit's operator manual for proper setup and use. Assure that all manufacturer's safety precautions are followed for both the electrosurgical generator as well as the suction/irrigation unit.

Follow all precautions normally used with electrosurgical cutting and coagulation devices.

Ensure that a proper dispersive electrode (i.e., grounding pad) is used in accordance with manufacturer's instructions for use.

Product Setup:

1. Use accepted aseptic technique when removing the single-use laparoscopic multi-function pistol grip from the sterile package.

2. Attach suction system or wall suction to the suction port (1) using tubing and the irrigation system to the irrigation port, (2) using tubing and luer lock connectors.

3. Insert the footswitch connector (3) into footswitch cord (4) for your electrosurgical unit.

4. Inspect the connection between the electrode and the footswitch cord connector for a secure fit and to ensure that no bare metal is exposed.

5. Select the coagulation or cutting power on the electrosurgical unit to obtain the desired tissue effect.

6. Before surgical use, depress each trigger valve firmly once to prime the valve.

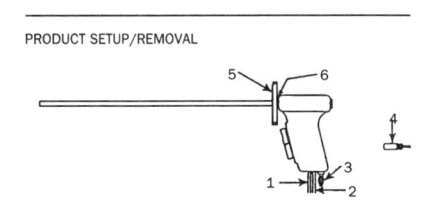

Probe Removal:

1. To remove probes from the handle, grasp the white finger wheel (5) on the reusable probe shaft and remove it from the pistol grip handpiece by gently rotating and separating the two units.

2. Install the sterile probe in similar fashion by gripping the white finger wheel on the probe shaft and insert it into the probe recess (6) on the front of the pistol grip handle.

3. You may want to lubricate the "O" rings on the finger wheel with sterile water to facilitate assembly.

4. Ensure that the probe is securely seated all the way into the probe recess prior to use.

PROBE, ELECTROCAUTERIZATION, MULTI-USE *(cont'd)*

Everest Medical Corp.
13755 First Ave. N.
Minneapolis, MN 55441-5454
612-473-6262

BILAP

DESCRIPTION: BiLAP™ bipolar electrosurgical devices from Everest Medical incorporate bipolar cut, coag and blend modes for minimally invasive surgery. These bipolar devices have been designed for greater safety to minimize lateral tissue damage and the risk of alternate site burns. The result is controlled cutting and coagulation for precise tissue dissection.

Other features of BiLAP devices include a variety of tip configurations and a 33cm working length. Suction and irrigation can also be performed with the BiLAP device. The extendible sheath, which locks into place, helps to protect the BiLAP tip during insertion through the trocar, acts as a stable device for blunt dissection, and protects tissue during suction.

Access Surgical International, Inc.
15 Caswell Ln.
Boat Yard Square
Plymouth, MA 02360
508-747-6006

Aesculap
1000 Gateway Blvd.
South San Francisco, CA 94080-7030
415-876-7000

Birtcher Medical Systems, Inc.
50 Technology Dr.
Irvine, CA 92718-2301
714-753-9400

Core Dynamics, Inc.
11222-4 St. Johns Indust. Pkwy.
Jacksonville, FL 32216
904-641-6611

Davis & Geck Endosurgery
1 Casper Street
Danbury, CT 06810
203-743-4451

Davol, Inc.
100 Sockanossett
P.O. Box 8500
Cranston, RI 02920-0500
401-463-7000

Erbe USA, Inc.
2225 NW Parkway, Ste. 105
Marietta, GA 30067
404-955-4400

Everest Medical Corp.
13755 First Avenue. N.
Minneapolis, MN 55441-5454
612-473-6262

Kensey Nash Corporation
55 E. Uwchlan Ave., Ste. 204
Exton, PA 19341-1247
215-524-0188

Laserscope
3052 Orchard Dr.
San Jose, CA 95134-2011
408-943-0636

Leisegang Medical, Inc.
6401 Congress Ave.
Boca Raton, FL 33487-2883
407-994-0202

Marlow Surgical Technologies, Inc.
1810 Joseph Lloyd Pkwy.
Willoughby, OH 44094-8030
216-946-2453

Performance Surgical Instruments
40 Norfolk Ave.
Easton, MA 023334
508-230-0010

Synectic Engineering, Inc.
4 Oxford Rd.
Milford, CT 06460-7007
203-877-8488

Unisurge, Inc.
10231 Bubb Rd.
Cupertino, CA 95014
408-996-4700

Valleylab, Inc.
5920 Longbow Dr.
Boulder, CO 80301-3202
303-530-2300

W.J. Medical Instruments, Inc.
3537 Old Conejo Rd.
Newbury Park, CA 91320
805-499-8676

Wolf Medical Instruments Corp., Richard
353 Corporate Woods Pkwy.
Vernon Hills, IL 60061-3110
708-913-1113

Ximed Medical Systems
2195 Trade Zone Blvd.
San Jose, CA 95131
408-945-4040

PROBE, ELECTROCAUTERIZATION, SINGLE-USE

Davis & Geck Endosurgery
1 Casper St.
Danbury, CT 06810
203-743-4451

LAPAROSCOPIC ASSIST DEVICES 8570 SERIES

DESCRIPTION: Standard Straight Electrodes for use with Footswitch Connection Cord (no suction or irrigation):

L Hook (order number 8570-01):

L HOOK

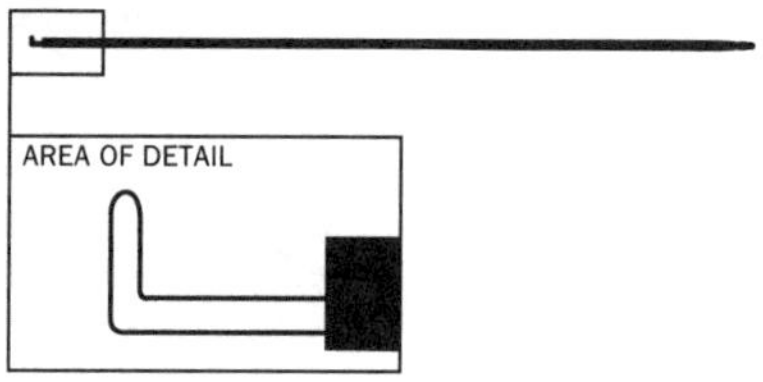

AREA OF DETAIL

Standard Hook (order number 8570-02):

STANDARD HOOK

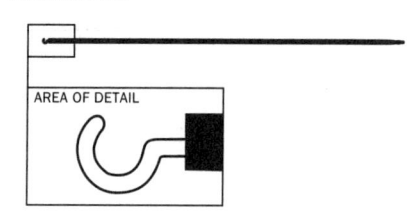

AREA OF DETAIL

Hockey Stick Hook (order number 8570-03):

HOCKEY STICK HOOK

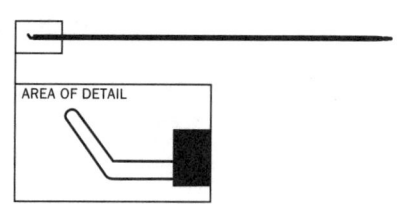

AREA OF DETAIL

J Hook (order number 8570-04):

J HOOK

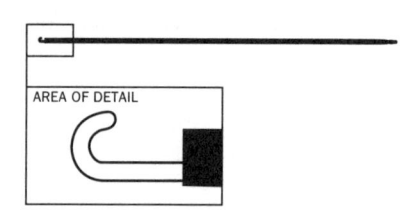

AREA OF DETAIL

Spatula (order number 8570-05):

SPATULA

AREA OF DETAIL   SIDE VIEW

Blade (order number 8570-06):

BLADE

AREA OF DETAIL

Ball (order number 8570-07):

BALL

AREA OF DETAIL

Needle (order number 8570-08):

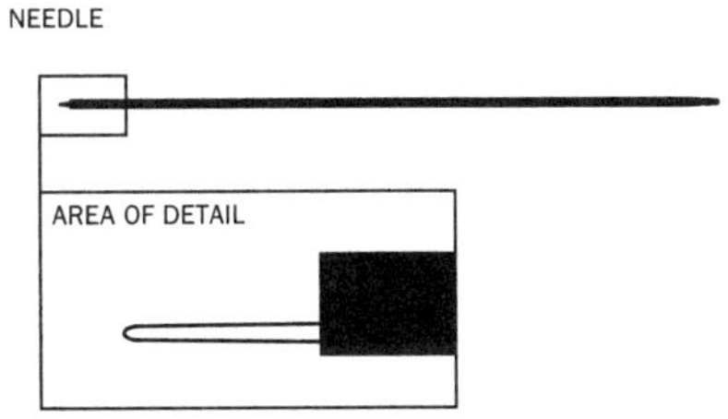

NEEDLE

AREA OF DETAIL

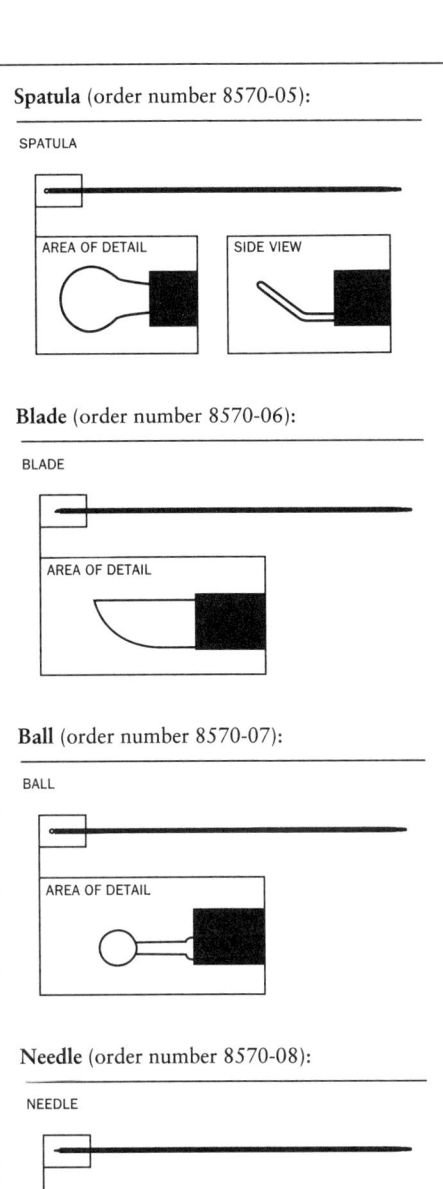

INSTRUCTIONS FOR USE: Refer to your electrosurgical unit's operator manual for proper setup and use. Assure that all manufacturer's safety precautions are followed.

Follow all precautions normally used with electrosurgical cutting and coagulation devices.

Assure that a proper dispersive electrode (i.e., grounding pad) is used in accordance with manufacturer's instructions for use.

Use accepted aseptic technique when removing the single-use standard laparoscopic electrode from the package.

Insert proximal connector (1) into footswitch cord (2) for your electrosurgical unit.

STANDARD ELECTRODE

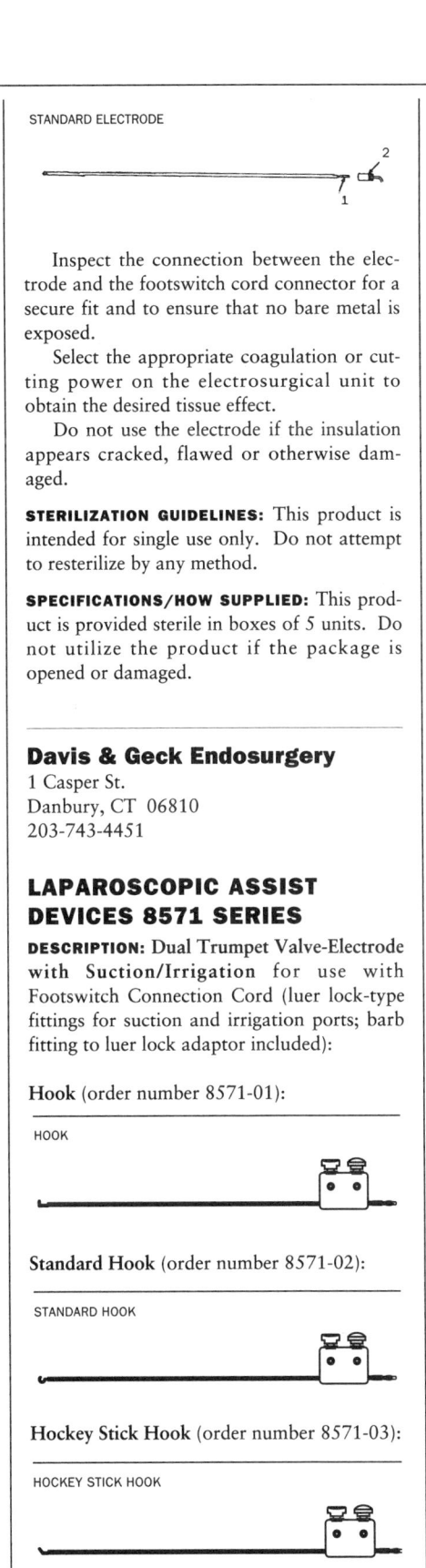

Inspect the connection between the electrode and the footswitch cord connector for a secure fit and to ensure that no bare metal is exposed.

Select the appropriate coagulation or cutting power on the electrosurgical unit to obtain the desired tissue effect.

Do not use the electrode if the insulation appears cracked, flawed or otherwise damaged.

STERILIZATION GUIDELINES: This product is intended for single use only. Do not attempt to resterilize by any method.

SPECIFICATIONS/HOW SUPPLIED: This product is provided sterile in boxes of 5 units. Do not utilize the product if the package is opened or damaged.

Davis & Geck Endosurgery
1 Casper St.
Danbury, CT 06810
203-743-4451

LAPAROSCOPIC ASSIST DEVICES 8571 SERIES

DESCRIPTION: Dual Trumpet Valve-Electrode with Suction/Irrigation for use with Footswitch Connection Cord (luer lock-type fittings for suction and irrigation ports; barb fitting to luer lock adaptor included):

Hook (order number 8571-01):

HOOK

Standard Hook (order number 8571-02):

STANDARD HOOK

Hockey Stick Hook (order number 8571-03):

HOCKEY STICK HOOK

J Hook (order number 8571-04):

J HOOK

Spatula (order number 8571-05):

SPATULA

Blade (order number 8571-06):

BLADE

Ball (order number 8571-07):

BALL

Needle (order number 8571-08):

NEEDLE

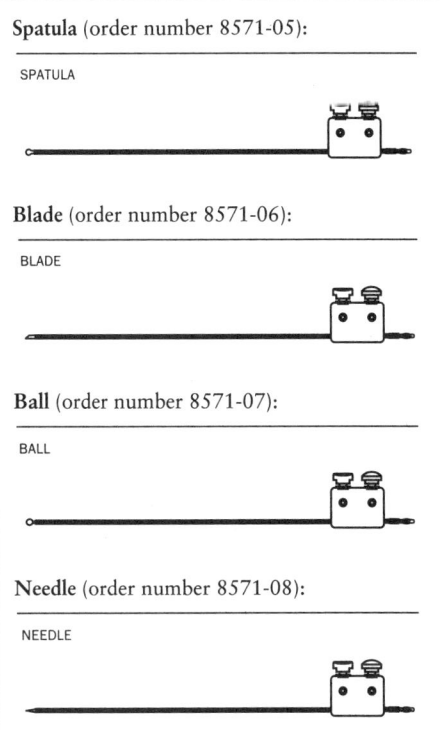

WARNINGS: Do not use the electrode if the insulation appears cracked, flawed or otherwise damaged.

INSTRUCTIONS FOR USE: Refer to your electrosurgical as well as your suction/irrigation unit manuals for proper setup and use. Assure that all manufacturers' safety precautions are followed.

Follow all precautions normally used with electrosurgical cutting and coagulation devices.

Assure that a proper dispersive electrode (i.e., grounding pad) is used in accordance with manufacturer's instructions for use.

Use accepted aseptic technique when removing the single-use Laparoscopic Electrosurgical probe from the package.

Attach suction system or wall suction to the suction port (1) and the irrigation system to the irrigation port (2) using tubing or luer lock connectors.

Insert proximal connector (3) into footswitch cord (4) for your electrosurgical unit.

Before use in surgery, depress each trumpet valve firmly to activate and prime the valve.

62/PRODUCT DIRECTORY

PROBE, ELECTROCAUTERIZATION, SINGLE-USE (cont'd)

DUAL TRUMPET VALVE ELECTRODE ASSEMBLY

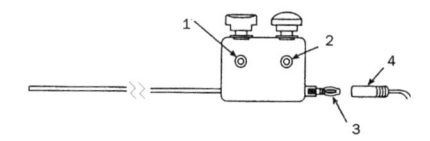

Inspect the connection between the electrode and the footswitch cord connector for a secure fit and to ensure that no bare metal is exposed.

Select the appropriate coagulation or cutting power on the electrosurgical unit to obtain the desired tissue effect.

STERILIZATION GUIDELINES: This product is intended for single use only. Do not attempt to resterilize by any method.

SPECIFICATIONS/HOW SUPPLIED: This product is provided sterile in boxes of 5 units. Do not utilize the product if the package is opened or damaged.

Davis & Geck Endosurgery
1 Casper St.
Danbury, CT 06810
203-743-4451

LAPAROSCOPIC ASSIST DEVICES 8573 & 8576 SERIES

DESCRIPTION: Modular Interchangeable Suction/Irrigation/Electrocautery Probes and Multifunction Pistol Grip Devices (luer lock-type connector for irrigation, barb connector for suction):

L Hook (order number 8576-01):
L HOOK

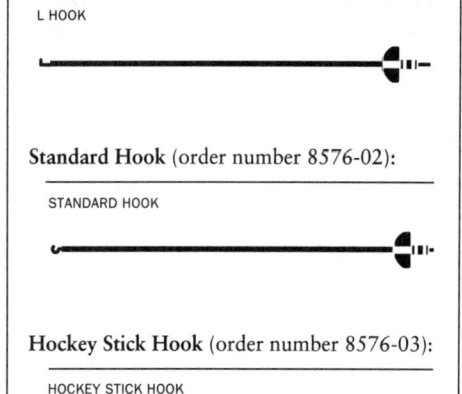

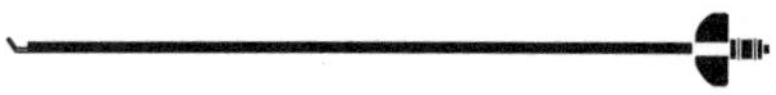

Standard Hook (order number 8576-02):
STANDARD HOOK

Hockey Stick Hook (order number 8576-03):
HOCKEY STICK HOOK

J Hook (order number 8576-04):
J HOOK

Spatula (order number 8576-05):
SPATULA

Blade (order number 8576-06):
BLADE

Ball (order number 8576-07):
BALL

Needle (order number 8576-08):
NEEDLE

L Hook (order number 8573-01):
L HOOK

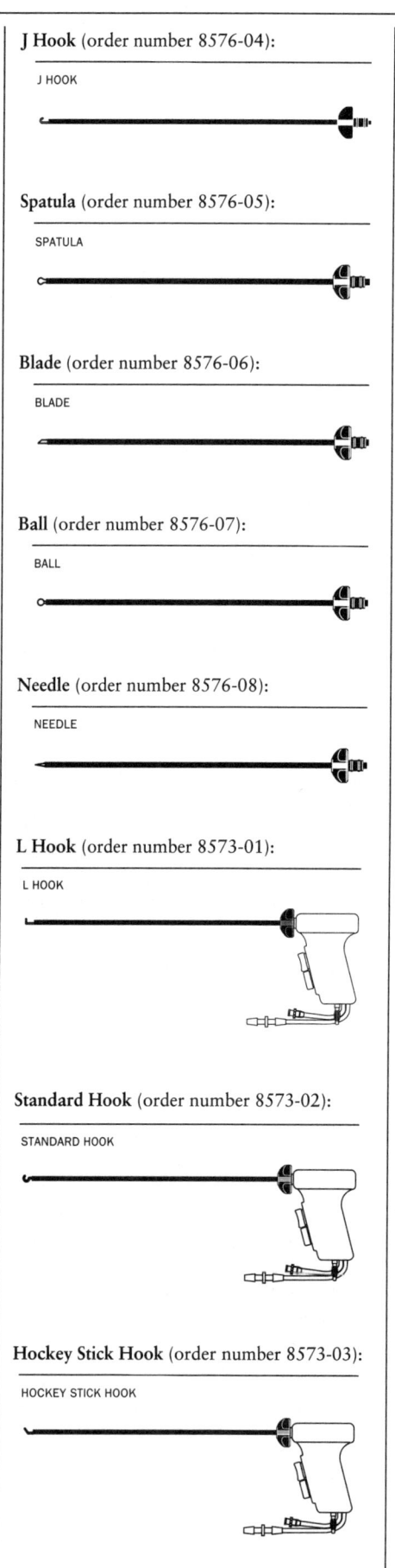

Standard Hook (order number 8573-02):
STANDARD HOOK

Hockey Stick Hook (order number 8573-03):
HOCKEY STICK HOOK

J Hook (order number 8573-04):
J HOOK

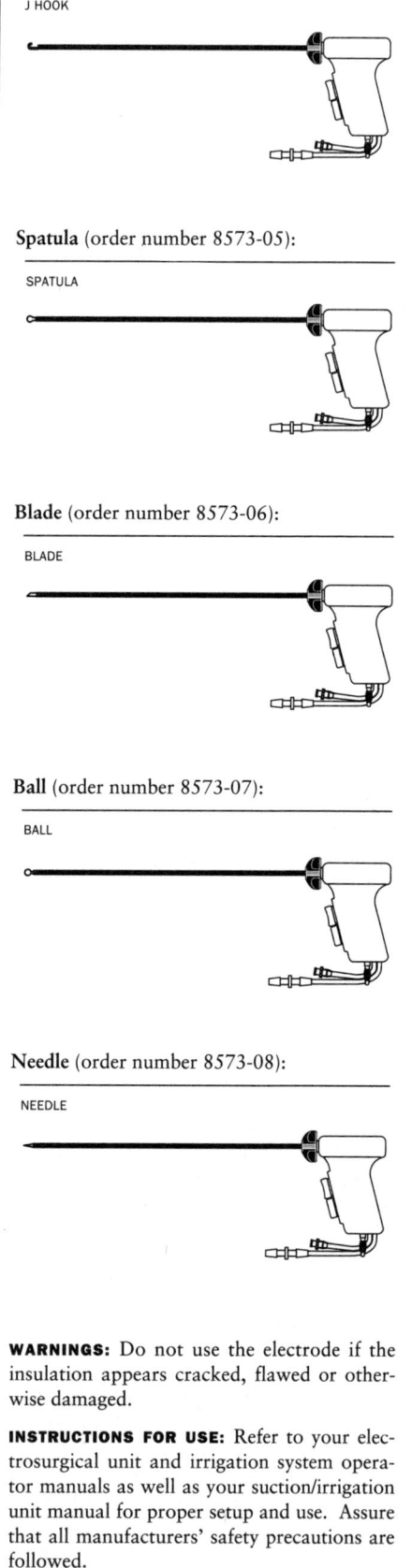

Spatula (order number 8573-05):
SPATULA

Blade (order number 8573-06):
BLADE

Ball (order number 8573-07):
BALL

Needle (order number 8573-08):
NEEDLE

WARNINGS: Do not use the electrode if the insulation appears cracked, flawed or otherwise damaged.

INSTRUCTIONS FOR USE: Refer to your electrosurgical unit and irrigation system operator manuals as well as your suction/irrigation unit manual for proper setup and use. Assure that all manufacturers' safety precautions are followed.

Follow all precautions normally used with electrosurgical cutting and coagulation devices.

Assure that a proper dispersive electrode (i.e., grounding pad) is used in accordance with manufacturer's instructions for use.

Use accepted aseptic technique when removing the single-use Laparoscopic Electrosurgical Probe and Multifunction Pistol Grip from the package.

Attach the suction system or wall suction to the suction port via universal barb attachment (1) and the irrigation system to the irrigation port (2), using tubing or luer lock connectors.

Insert proximal connector (3) into footswitch cord (4) for your electrosurgical unit.

Before surgical use, depress each trigger valve firmly once to prime the valve.

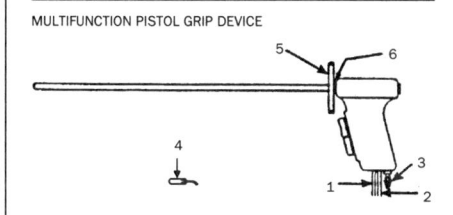

MULTIFUNCTION PISTOL GRIP DEVICE

Inspect the connection between the electrode and the footswitch cord connector for a secure fit and to ensure that no bare metal is exposed.

Select the appropriate coagulation or cutting power on the electrosurgical unit to obtain the desired tissue effect.

To change probes, grasp the black knurled knob (5) on the probe shaft and remove it from the pistol grip handpiece by gently separating the two units in a twisting motion.

Replace the probe in similar fashion. Grip the black knurled knob on the probe shaft and insert it into the probe recess (6) on the front of the pistol grip handle. Ensure that the probe is securely seated all the way into the probe recess prior to use.

STERILIZATION GUIDELINES: This product is intended for single use only. Do not attempt to resterilize by any method.

SPECIFICATIONS/HOW SUPPLIED: This product is provided sterile in boxes of 5 units. Do not utilize the product if the package is opened or damaged.

Ethicon Endo-Surgery
4545 Creek Rd.
Cincinnati, OH 45242
513-786-7000

ENDOPATH PROBE PLUS
DESCRIPTION:

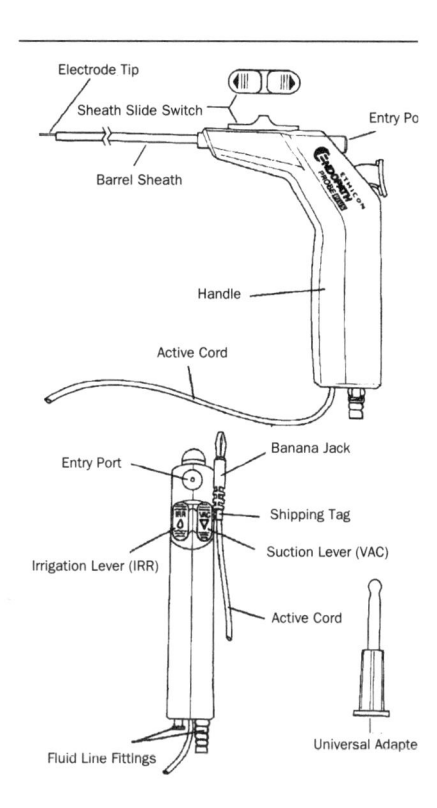

The ENDOPATH* Electrosurgery Probe Plus is a hand-held, monopolar device which offers right hook opening, left hook opening, spatula and right angle electrode tips. The device provides a port, which accommodates an electrically non-conductive fiber or implements, not greater than 0.080in. (2mm) diameter. The device is for use through a 5mm diameter ENDOPATH Disposable Surgical Trocar and is compatible with commonly used irrigation and vacuum devices and monopolar electrosurgical units.

INDICATIONS: The ENDOPATH Electrosurgery Probe Plus device has application in endoscopic procedures to facilitate tissue dissection, coagulation, irrigation, and fluid evacuation through a common cannula.

CONTRAINDICATIONS:

1. The device is not intended for contraceptive coagulation of fallopian tissue, but may be used to achieve hemostasis following transection of the fallopian tube.

2. This device is not intended for use when endoscopic techniques are contraindicated.

WARNINGS:

1. Endoscopic procedures should be performed only by persons having adequate training and familiarity with endoscopic techniques. Consult medical literature relative to techniques, complications, and hazards prior to performance of any endoscopic procedure.

2. A thorough understanding of principles and techniques involved in laparoscopic laser and electrosurgical procedures is essential to avoid shock and burn hazards to both patient and medical personnel and damage to the device or other medical instruments. Refer to appropriate laser and electrosurgical system user manuals for use indications and instructions to ensure that all safety precautions are followed.

3. When endoscopic instruments and accessories from different manufacturers are employed together in a procedure, verify compatibility prior to initiation of the procedure and ensure that electrical isolation or grounding is not compromised.

4. Dispose of all opened ENDOPATH Electrosurgery Probe Plus devices, whether used or unused. DO NOT RESTERILIZE. Resterilization may compromise the integrity of the instrument, which may result in unintended injury.

5. In general, monopolar cautery is not intended for contraceptive coagulation of fallopian tissue, but may be used to achieve hemostasis following transection of the fallopian tube.

6. Do not activate the ENDOPATH Electrosurgery Probe Plus device when the electrode tip is in contact with, or in close proximity to, a metal trocar cannula or other conductive instruments. Arcing to a metal trocar cannula may cause a patient burn.

7. To maintain gasket integrity, the barrel sheath should be extended past the electrode tip prior to removing from the trocar.

8. Irrigation pressure limits should not exceed 30 PSIG (61in. Hg, 1600mm Hg).

9. Simultaneous activation of a laser and the electrode is not recommended. The laser fiber should be withdrawn from the operative site prior to electrode use to prevent possible energy transmission to the fiber.

10. Read all instructions carefully. Failure to properly follow the instructions may lead to serious surgical consequences.

INSTRUCTIONS FOR USE:

IMPORTANT: This information is designed to provide instructions for use of the ENDOPATH Electrosurgery Probe Plus

PROBE, ELECTROCAUTERIZATION, SINGLE-USE (cont'd)

device. It is not a reference to electrosurgery techniques.

1. Verify compatibility of all endoscopic instruments and accessories prior to using the ENDOPATH Electrosurgery Probe Plus device. (Refer to paragraphs 2 and 3 under Warnings).

2. Refer to electrosurgical system users manual for use indications and instructions. Ensure that all safety precautions are followed.

3. A patient grounding pad (return electrode) must be firmly affixed to the patient according to proper grounding techniques.

4. Pull the shipping tab, connected to the electrosurgical cord, from the handle to release the suction and irrigation levers. A vacuum line (not provided) and an irrigation supply line (not provided) push into the fluid line fittings located on the butt of the handle. A universal electrosurgical banana jack plugs into the universal adapter, generally supplied with an electrosurgical unit (ESU), or directly into the ESU.

5. Introduce the device through a 5mm diameter ENDOPATH Disposable Surgical Trocar (or larger trocar with 5mm diameter ENDOPATH Trocar Reducer) into the operative site. Expose the electrode tip by retracting the barrel sheath via the slide switch located on the top of the handle. To operate irrigation, push the IRR lever. To operate the suction function, push the VAC lever. Energize the electrode tip to the appropriate power level (cut or coagulate), using the ESU foot pedal.

6. If it is desired to use an electrically non-conductive fiber, a laser, or other implement, pierce the rubber entry port. Push the instrument (not greater than 0.080in. [2mm] diameter) through the port and down the barrel sheath, leaving the surgical end of the instrument at least 5mm beyond the electrosurgical tip. In order to prevent possible energy transmission to the fiber or other implement, withdraw it prior to electrode use.

7. Once the cut, coagulation, or suction/irrigation functions have beencompleted, inspect the area to ensure proper result.

STERILIZATION GUIDELINES: Sterility is guaranteed unless the package is opened or damaged. DO NOT RESTERILIZE.

SPECIFICATIONS/HOW SUPPLIED: The ENDOPATH Electrosurgery Probe Plus device with left hook opening, right hook opening, right angle, and spatula electrode tips are for single-patient use only. Discard after use.

CAUTION: Federal (USA) law restricts this device to sale by or on the order of a physician.

Apple Medical Corp.
93 Nashaway Rd.
Bolton, MA 01740
508-779-2926

Birtcher Medical Systems, Inc.
50 Technology Dr.
Irvine, CA 92718-2301
714-753-9400

Conmed Corp.
310 Broad Street
Utica, NY 13501
315-797-8375

Erbe USA, Inc.
2225 NW Parkway, Ste. 105
Marietta, GA 30067
404-955-4400

Instrument Makar, Inc.
2950 E. Mt. Hope
Okemos, MI 48864-1910
517-332-3593

Laserscope
3052 Orchard Dr.
San Jose, CA 95134-2011
408-943-0636

Leisegang Medical, Inc.
6401 Congress Ave.
Boca Raton, FL 33487-2883
407-994-0202

Marlow Surgical Technologies, Inc.
1810 Joseph Lloyd Pkwy.
Willoughby, OH 44094-8030
216-946-2453

Smith & Nephew Dyonics, Inc.
160 Dascomb Rd.
Andover, MA 01810-5893
508-470-2800

Synectic Engineering, Inc.
4 Oxford Rd.
Milford, CT 06460-7007
203-877-8488

Valleylab, Inc.
5920 Longbow Dr.
Boulder, CO 80301-3202
303-530-2300

W.J. Medical Instruments, Inc.
3537 Old Conejo Rd.
Newbury Park, CA 91320
805-499-8676

Ximed Medical Systems
2195 Trade Zone Blvd.
San Jose, CA 95131
408-945-4040

PROBE, ELECTROSURGERY, ENDOSCOPY

Ethicon Endo-Surgery
4545 Creek Rd.
Cincinnati, OH 45242
513-786-7000

ENDOPATH PROBE PLUS II

DESCRIPTION: The ENDOPATH* Electrosurgery Probe Plus II system offers a choice of four handles and thirteen shafts to allow a handle and shaft configuration to best meet the surgeon's needs. The handles and shafts are completely interchangeable, allowing any shaft to fit any handle. The available handles and shafts are outlined below:

Handles:

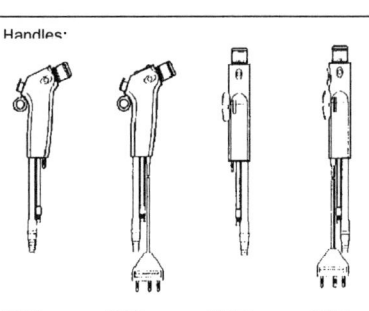

EPH01
Pistol Grip Handle,
Foot Control Electrosurgery

EPH02
Pistol Grip Handle,
Hand Control Electrosurgery

EPH03
Pistol Grip Handle,
Foot Control Electrosurgery

EPH04
Pistol Grip Handle,
Hand Control Electrosurgery

Shaft:

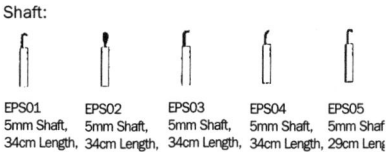

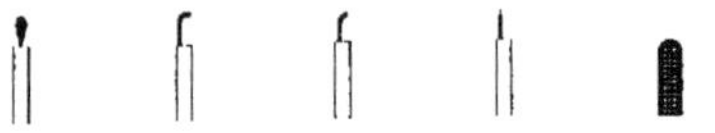

EPS01
5mm Shaft, 34cm Length,
Hook Electrode

EPS02
5mm Shaft, 34cm Length,
Spatula Electrode

EPS03
5mm Shaft, 34cm Length,
Right Angle Electrode

EPS04
5mm Shaft, 34cm Length,
Curved Disector Electrode

EPS05
5mm Shaft, 29cm Length,
Hook Electrode

EPS06
5mm Shaft, 29cm Length,
Spatula Electrode

EPS07
5mm Shaft, 29cm Length,
Right Angle Electrode

EPS08
5mm Shaft, 29cm Length,
Curved Disector Electrode

EPS09
5mm Shaft, 29cm Length,
Needle Electrode

EPS010
5mm Shaft, 34cm Length,
Pool/Sump Suction and Irrigation

ELECTROCAUTERY/65

EPS11
10mm Shaft
34cm Length,
Suction and
Irrigation

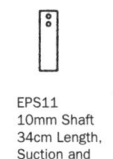

EPS12
10mm Shaft
34cm Length,
Stone
Retrieval

EPS13
5mm Shaft
29cm Length,
Accessory
Port

Shafts EPS01 through EPS09 and EPS13 are for use through a 5mm diameter ENDOPATH Surgical Trocar or a larger trocar with a 5mm reducer. Shafts EPS10 through EPS12 are for use through a 10mm diameter ENDOPATH Surgical Trocar.

The ENDOPATH Electrosurgery Probe Plus II system is compatible with commonly used irrigation and suction devices and monopolar electrosurgery units (ESU).

Illustration and Nomenclature:

ILLUSTRATION AND NOMENCLATURE:

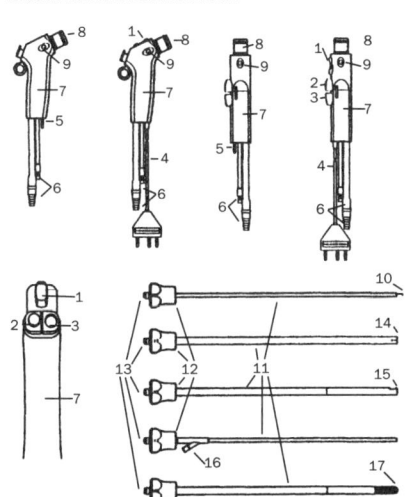

1. ELECTROSURGERY HAND CONTROL
2. IRRIGATION CONTROL
3. SUCTION CONTROL
4. ESU CABLE
5. ESU CONNECTOR
6. FLUID LINE FITTINGS
7. HANDLE
8. SHAFT CONNECTOR
9. RED SHAFT RELEASE BUTTON
10. ELECTRODE TIP
11. SHAFT
12. ELECTRODE ROTATION AND TIP EXPOSURE CONTROL
13. HANDLE CONNECTOR
14. OPEN END SUCTION/ IRRIGATION TIP
15. STONE RETRIEVAL PORT
16. FLEXIBLE DEVICE PORT
17. SUMP/SUCTION

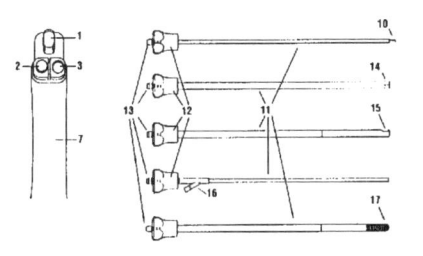

INDICATIONS: The ENDOPATH Electrosurgery Probe Plus II system has application in endoscopic procedures to facilitate tissue dissection, coagulation, irrigation, and fluid evacuation through a common trocar sleeve.

CONTRAINDICATIONS:

1. This device is not intended for contraceptive coagulation of fallopian tissue but may be used to achieve hemostasis following transection of the fallopian tissue.
2. This device is not intended for use when endoscopic techniques are contraindicated.

WARNINGS:

1. Endoscopic procedures should be performed only by persons having adequate training and familiarity with endoscopic techniques. Consult medical literature relative to techniques, complications, and hazards prior to performance of any endoscopic procedure.
2. A thorough understanding of principles and techniques involved in laparoscopic laser and electrosurgical procedures is essential to avoid shock and burn hazards to both patient and medical personnel and damage to the device or other medical instruments. Refer to the appropriate electrosurgical system user manual for indications and instructions to ensure that all safety precautions are followed.
3. Endoscopic instruments may vary in diameter from manufacturer to manufacturer. When endoscopic instruments and accessories from different manufacturers are employed together in a procedure, verify compatibility prior to initiation of procedure and ensure that electrical isolation or grounding is not compromised.
4. Do not activate the ENDOPATH Probe Plus II when the electrode tip is in contact with, or in close proximity to, a metal trocar cannula. Arcing to a metal trocar sleeve may burn the patient.
5. The sheath should cover the electrode tip prior to removal through the trocar sleeve to ensure safety and trocar gasket integrity.
6. Dispose of all opened ENDOPATH Electrosurgery Probe Plus II Shafts and Handles, whether used or unused. DO NOT RESTERILIZE. Resterilization may compromise the integrity of the instrument which may result in unintended injury.

INSTRUCTIONS FOR USE: Read all instructions carefully. Failure to properly follow the instructions may lead to serious surgical consequences.

1. Verify compatibility of all endoscopic instruments and accessories prior to using the ENDOPATH Electrosurgery Probe Plus II System. (Refer to paragraphs 2 and 3 under Warnings.)
2. Refer to electrosurgical system user manual for indications and instructions for use. Ensure that all safety precautions are followed.

3. Firmly affix a patient grounding pad ("return electrode") to the patient according to proper grounding techniques.

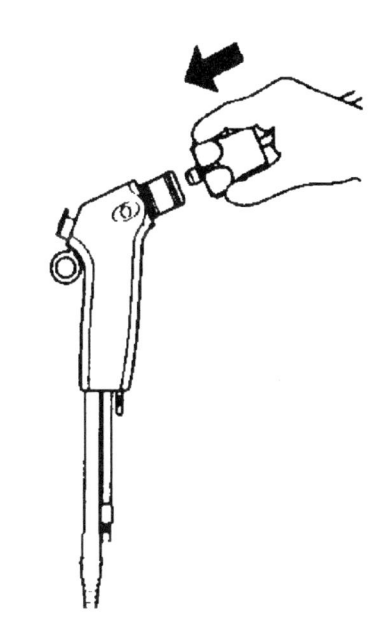

4. Using sterile technique, remove the handle and desired shaft from the package. To avoid damage, do not flip the instrument into the sterile field.

5. Grasping the rotation knob, insert the shaft into the handle until an audible "click" is heard.

CAUTION: The shaft must be properly seated in the handle before use.

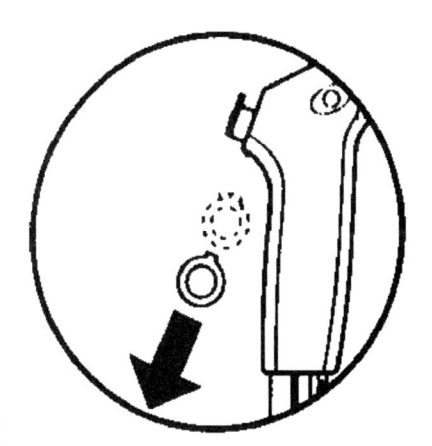

6. Pull out the red shipping tab from the handle to release the suction/irrigation buttons and discard.

7. Connect a suction line (not included) and an irrigation line (not included) to the fluid line fittings located on the tubing extending from the base of the handle.

8. Connect the handle to the electrosurgical generator as follows:

For the handcontrol handle (EPH02, EPH04):

Connect the three-pronged connector at the end of the attached ESU cable to the hand control output of the electrosurgical generator.

PROBE, ELECTROSURGERY, ENDOSCOPY (cont'd)

For the footcontrol handle (EPH01, EPH03):

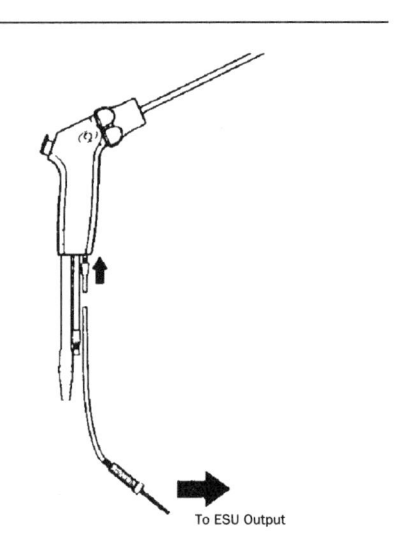

Connect a footcontrol cable to the ESU cable connector located at the base of the handle. Connect the other end of the cable to the footcontrol output of the electrosurgical generator.

9. Introduce the Probe Plus II through the appropriate size ENDOPATH Surgical Trocar (or larger trocar with ENDOPATH 5mm Diameter Trocar Reducer) according to the size of the Probe Plus II Shaft.

10. Use the device in the desired modes as follows:

Electrode tip exposure:
To control exposure of the electrode tip, advance or retract the sheath (product codes EPS01 - EPS09) by sliding the rotation knob forward or backward. (In either position, the knob snaps into place.)

Electrode tip rotation:
Turn the rotation knob to rotate the electrode tip.

Suction/irrigation control:
a. To irrigate, press the convex irrigation button.
b. To suction, press the concave suction button.

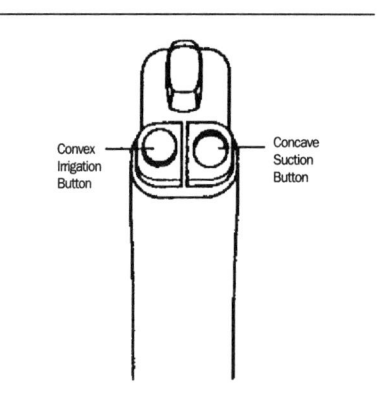

Use of Electrosurgery:
a. Handcontrol handle (EPH02, EPH04): To energize the electrode tip, press the electrosurgery controls on the handle: yellow for CUT and blue for COAG.
b. Footcontrol handle (EPH01, EPH03): To energize the electrode tip, use the Electrosurgical Unit (ESU) footcontrol for CUT or COAG.

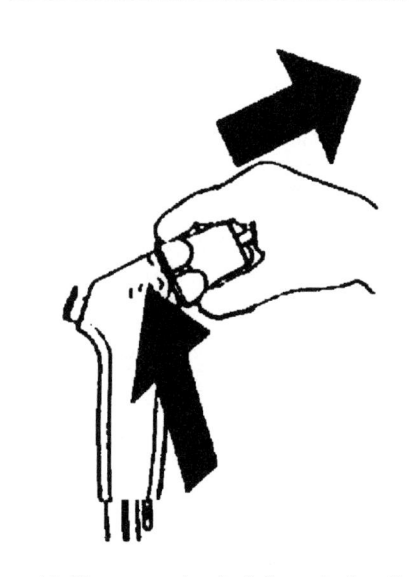

11. To remove the shaft from the handle: Grasp the rotation knob. Press the red shaft release button located on the handle assembly. Pull the shaft away from the handle. Other shafts can be inserted into the handle during the surgical procedure for different surgical needs as follows:

Shafts EPS01 through EPS09: allow monopolar electrosurgery with suction and irrigation in two different shaft lengths and a variety of electrode tips.

Shaft EPS10 and EPS11: allow increased capacity of suction (10mm) with irrigation without electrosurgery.

Shaft EPS12: enables the removal of small stones and blood clots. With suction engaged, the stones or clots are maneuvered into the side port at the distal end of the shaft. The shaft is withdrawn from the trocar with the suction still engaged. The stones or clots can be expelled from the shaft with irrigation.

Shaft EPS13: allows the introduction of a nonconductive flexible device, such as a laser, through the side port of the shaft. The maximum diameter of the flexible device must not exceed 2.5mm. This shaft allows the use of suction and irrigation either with or without the flexible device inserted.

12. Once the cut, coagulation, or suction/irrigation functions have been completed, inspect the area to ensure proper results.

STERILIZATION GUIDELINES: Sterility is guaranteed unless the package is opened or damaged. DO NOT RESTERILIZE.

SPECIFICATIONS/HOW SUPPLIED: The ENDOPATH Electrosurgery Probe Plus II is supplied as a system of interchangeable handles and shafts. The handles and shafts are for single-patient use. Discard after use.

CAUTION: Federal (USA) law restricts this device to sale by or on the order of a physician.

SCALPEL, ULTRASONIC

Ultracision Inc.
25 Thurber Blvd., Unit 3
Smithfield, RI 02917
401-232-7660

ULTRACISION HARMONIC SCALPEL

DESCRIPTION: Unlike lasers and electrosurgery, which use heat to cause hemostasis, the Ultracision Harmonic Scalpel® converts electrical energy to mechanical motion for controlled, cool-blade cutting. Risk of damaging adjacent tissues by stray laser light or arcing electrical current is eliminated. There is no char, smoke or odor to contaminate or obstruct the surgical field.

The blade's exclusive ultrasonic motion causes a tissue's collagen molecules to vibrate and denature, forming a coagulum that seals off the severed vessel.

The Harmonic Scalpel delivers the same tactile feedback provided by conventional scalpels allowing for increased accuracy as well as ease of control compared to other cutting/coagulating systems. The ultrasonic movement prevents accumulation of debris on the blade for continuous unimpaired sharpness.

INDICATIONS: The UltraCision Harmonic Scalpel System is indicated for soft tissue incisions when bleeding control and minimal thermal injury are desired. The Harmonic Scalpel can be used as an adjunct to or substitute for electrosurgery, lasers and steel scalpels.

WARNINGS: The Harmonic Scalpel is not indicated for incising bone.

PRECAUTIONS: Handle hand piece carefully, as damage may shift resonant frequency. Do not bang or drop.

Do not attempt to bend, sharpen or otherwise alter the shape of the blade. Doing so may cause blade failure. The following manner is meant as an overview of the Harmonic Scalpel technology. Refer to complete operating instructions prior to operating the Harmonic Scalpel on any of it's components.

INSTRUCTIONS FOR USE:
Principles of Operation:
The ultrasonic acoustic system, which is housed in the hand piece, is diagrammed in Figure 1 above. The acoustic system or acoustic drive train consists of three components:

Acoustic Transducer: converts the electrical energy to mechanical motion. The acoustic transducer consists of a stack of piezoelectric elements (or ceramics) that are sandwiched under pressure between two metal cylinders.

Acoustic Mount: holds the acoustic system in the hand piece. It amplifies the motion produced by the transducer to increase motion of the blade.

Laparosonic Blade: adds length to the Harmonic Scalpel for laparoscopic use and contains the second amplifier in the system to further amplify the motion.

The system is designed to efficiently transfer the energy from the transducer to the blade. There is no vibration in the Harmonic Scalpel Hand Piece when the acoustic system is activated. All of the components of the drive train are acoustically tuned to integral half wavelengths, so that the entire system resonates at 55.5 kHz when the system is activated.

The ceramic elements in the transducer expand and contract (a positive and negative excursion) when they are electrically activated. By activating the ceramic elements at the resonant frequency of the acoustic system, the longitudinal motion generated at the transducer generates maximum motion at the blade tip. The mount and blade are designed to deliver maximal harmonic motion at the blade tip.

Coagulating Mechanism:
The basic mechanism for coagulating bleeding vessels ultrasonically is similar to that of electrosurgery or lasers. Vessels are sealed by tamponading and coapting with a denatured protein coagulum. The manner in which protein is denatured, however, is different for each of these modalities. Electrosurgery and lasers form the coagulum by heating tissues to denature protein. The former uses electric current whereas the latter uses light.

The ultrasonically activated scalpel denatures protein by the transfer of mechanical energy to the tissues which is sufficient to break tertiary hydrogen bonds, and by the generation of heat from internal tissue friction that results from the high frequency vibration of the tissue.

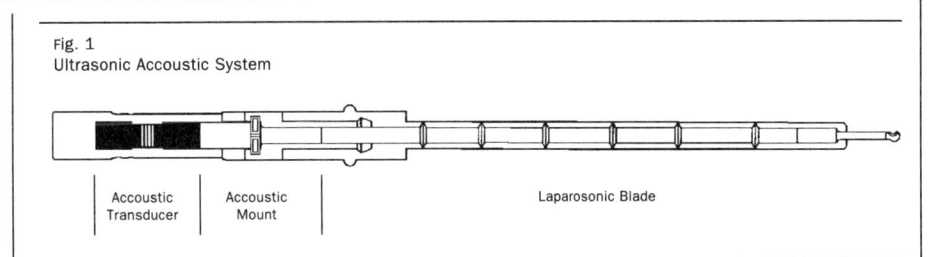

Fig. 1
Ultrasonic Accoustic System

Accoustic Transducer | Accoustic Mount | Laparosonic Blade

As a result, tissue charring and desiccation from the loss of moisture are minimized. The limited heat generation also minimizes the zone of thermal injury. Animal studies at the University of Pittsburgh found the skin incisions made with the ultrasonically activated scalpel or cold steel scalpel healed almost identically and were significantly superior to electrosurgical incisions. Animal studies comparing seromyotomies performed in pigs with either electrosurgery or the ultrasonically activated scalpel noted four times less lateral thermal damage with the ultrasonically activated scalpel (unpublished data). This minimal thermal damage may explain the marked reduction in postoperative adhesions to the liver bed following laparoscopic cholecystectomy with the ultrasonically activated scalpel (22%) when compared to electrosurgery (66%) or laser surgery (77%) in experiments performed in pigs.

The mechanisms of coagulation offer an advantage for the ultrasonically activated scalpel over electrosurgery when coagulating the side wall of a blood vessel. In electrosurgery, the blood vessel is usually not coapted significantly because of the concomitant reduction in power density as the surface area of contact increases with coaptation. The blood within the vessels has a high heat capacity and acts as a heat sink. This allows one side to coagulate prior to the other with resultant bleeding from a hole in the wall of the vessel that was in contact with electrosurgery. In contrast, the ultrasonically activated scalpel relies on pressure and coaptation of the vessel walls for maximum energy transfer to the tissue. Thus, the vessel is sealed together without bleeding from the surface closest to the blade.

Pressure and coaptation are of paramount importance to the coagulative ability of the ultrasonic scalpel. In fact, unsupported tissue such as a transected bleeding blood vessel in a mesentery that can not be compressed against a firm surface, such as the liver, can not be coagulated effectively with the hook-spatula blade. To obviate this problem, the LCS grasping device (Laparosonic Coagulating Shears) has been developed to include a vibrating blade with sharp and blunt edges, as well as a passive (not ultrasonically activated) tissue pad with which tissue is pressed against the active, vibrating blade. This device allows unsupported tissue to be grasped and coagulated without difficulty, or cut and coagulated like scissors. Animal work has shown this device to reproducibly coagulate vessels up to 5mm in diameter (unpublished data).

Cutting Mechanism:
The cutting mechanism for the ultrasonically activated scalpel is also different from the observed with electrosurgery or laser surgery. At least two mechanisms exist. The first is the cavitational fragmentation noted with the ultrasonic cavitational aspirator. However, the cavitational effect for the ultrasonically activated scalpel is not nearly as pronounced as that seen with the ultrasonic cavitational aspirator. Nonetheless, tissue planes separate ahead of the blade of the ultrasonically activated scalpel, which aids in dissection by better visualization of the tissue plane.

The second mechanism for cutting by the ultrasonically activated scalpel, and the most important, is the actual "power cutting" offered by a relatively sharp blade vibrating 55,500 times per second over a distance of 80μm. This is best seen in high protein density areas such as collagen or muscle-rich tissues. In contrast, cutting with electrosurgery or lasers occurs when the temperature of cells increases to such a point that the concomitant increase in gas pressure explodes the cells.

Animal studies have demonstrated the ultrasonically activated scalpel similar in efficacy to an electrosurgical unit with no difference in operative time, complications or bleeding. The ultrasonically activated scalpel is superior with respect to avoidance of inadvertent gallbladder perforation, a finding replicated in humans. In addition, it eliminates many of the disadvantages of monopolar electrosurgery. The ultrasonically activated scalpel is able to cut and coagulate tissue without the generation of smoke. Thus, there is minimal disruption of visualization during the procedure and no need to evacuate the pneumoperitoneum to clear accumulated smoke. Although there is atomization of fluid which creates a transient mist, this does not accumulate, and does not significantly impair the visual field as the droplets rapidly settle out. Furthermore, the ultrasonically activated scalpel eliminates the risks of electrical injury to the patient and surgeon, since there is no current flow through the patient.

SCALPEL, ULTRASONIC *(cont'd)*

Finally, because there is little or no cutting ability with the blade in an inactivated situation, the blunt side of the ultrasonically activated scalpel can be used as a blunt dissector.

Operation of the Harmonic Scalpel Blade Systems:

The blade is ultrasonically energized when either foot switch pedal is depressed.

Pressing the left foot switch pedal (VAR) activates the selected variable level. Pressing the right pedal (FULL) activates full power.

Cutting Rate:
The cutting rate affects the degree of coagulation achieved.

Slower cutting increases coagulation, as more energy couples with the tissue. Strive for a smooth stroke which allows the motion of the blade to do the cutting. A "dragging" feel indicates that cutting speed is too fast for the selected power level.

Tension and Pressure:
Tension and pressure must be applied to the tissue for optimal cutting.

Coaptive Coagulation:
Coaptive coagulation is used to seal large bleeders that are not coagulated during incisions. This is accomplished as follows:

Severed Vessel: If the vessel has already been severed, place the flat surface of the blade proximal to the cut end and not against the opening. Hold the blade in position and apply power until hemostasis occurs.

Unsevered Vessel: When approaching from above, press the blunt edge of the blade against the vessel to flatten it. Move the blade laterally along the length of the vessel until coagulation occurs, as indicated by blanching.

Another strategy is to position the blade underneath the vessel. The blunt edge or flat surface of the blade is moved back and forth while exerting light pressure. The vessel flattens, then blanches, indicating hemostasis. Rotate the blade and sever the vessel.

LCS Operation Guidelines:
Shear Mode:
The shear mode refers to the tissue pad closing against the sharp blade edge. This mode is used to provide rapid hemostatic scissors cutting.

The shear mode provides excellent cutting and hemostasis in relatively avascular tissues. However, hemostasis may not be adequate when cutting speed is too fast.

Unnecessary bleeding can occur when the tissue is under tension (traction/countertraction), or when tissue is grasped too firmly during activation especially when high power is used. Reduced tissue tension and grasper pressure will slow the cutting speed and improve hemostasis.

Coaptive Coagulation Mode:
The coaptive coagulation mode refers to the tissue pad closing against the blunt blade edge. This mode is used to coagulate and bisect vascular tissues and vessels as well as to grasp bleeders and coagulate them.

The LCS can be used to effectively grasp and coagulate bleeders and to coagulate and sever vascular tissues or vessels. When necessary, persistent bleeding is controlled by regrasping the bleeding tissue with the LCS and activating. Coagulation of larger vessels or more vascular tissues can be optimized when the LCS is used first with low power and gradually increasing pressure, then going to higher power and more pressure to bisect the tissue or vessel.

Care should be taken not to apply pressure between LCS blade and tissue pad without having tissue between them. This can result in damping or possible damage of the LCS blade system. Both conditions may cause a system failure signaled by continuous beep when either of the foot pedals is depressed.

Knife Mode:
The knife mode refers to the use of the sharp edge as a scalpel without closure of the tissue pad.

The sharp edge of the LCS blade can be used like a knife or scalpel with the tissue pad in an open position. Reduce cutting speed where increased hemostasis is necessary with the cutting action.

Coagulator Mode:
The coagulator mode refers to the use of the blade tip, back or sides, as a coagulator.

The blade side, back and tip, can be used in a manner similar to the ball coagulator or hook blades for coaptive coagulation. It is recommended that when the LCS is used as a coagulator, the sharp blade edge should be guarded by the tissue pad.

Grasper Mode:
The grasper mode refers to the use of the clamp pad and blade to grasp and hold tissues.

Tissue may be held and manipulated when grasped between the unactivated blunt blade edge and the tissue pad.

Blunt Mode:
The blunt dissector mode refers to the use of the clamp and non-activated blade to separate tissue planes by pushing with the closed clamp and spreading.

REQUIRED ANCILLARY PRODUCTS:
Blade Selection:
Selection of the blade type is a matter of surgeon preference based on the procedure or application. In general, sharper ultrasonically activated edges cut faster with less hemostasis, while more blunt edges and surfaces coagulate more and cut less rapidly. When selecting the appropriate blade, keep in mind that coagulation is a function of the power setting, the extent of blade and tissue coupling, and the duration of the contact between the blade and tissue.

UltraCision makes several blade systems for various applications. Please refer to the following information when selecting the appropriate blade type. Contact UltraCision's Customer Service Department at 1-800-333-9181 for additional information.

Sharp Pointed Hook:
The outer circumference is dull while the inside edge has a 40° angle. The blade surface is flat.

SHARP POINTED HOOK

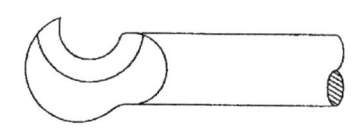

Dissecting Hook:
The outer circumference is dull while the inside edge has a 60° angle. The blade surface is flat.

DISSECTING HOOK

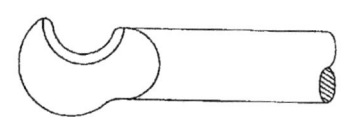

Ball Coagulator:
The tip is spherical, with no edges.

BALL COAGULATOR

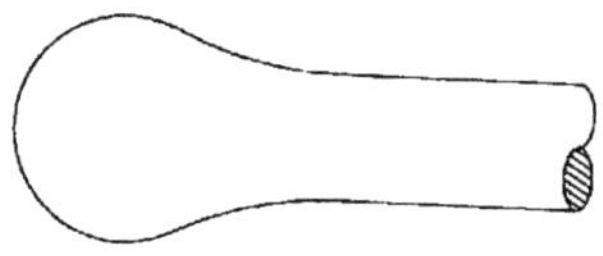

LCS Blade:
The blade is straight with both a sharp edge and a rounded or blunt edge.

LCS BLADE

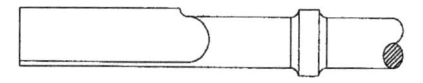

STERILIZATION GUIDELINES:
Hand Piece Decontamination:
Do not immerse the hand piece in liquid.

Wipe the hand piece with a soft cloth moistened with mild soap or hemolyzing detergent. Remove any soap residue with a cloth moistened with plain water. Exposure to liquid sterilizing agents may shorten product life and is therefore not recommended.

10mm Laparosonic Blade System Decontamination Procedure:

Decontaminate the blade and sheath. Remove all surface adherent soil using a cloth moistened with mild soap or hemolyzing detergent. Take special care to decontaminate the inside of the blade sheath with a brush or swab. Remove any soap residue using a cloth moistened with water, and dry. Exposure to liquid sterilizing agent may shorten product life and is therefore not recommended.

Sterilization Procedure:

Bioburden levels can vary significantly and the effectiveness of your cleaning procedure will ultimately determine the bioburden on the product prior to sterilization.

After following the Decontamination and Cleaning steps above, sterilize according to hospital protocol. For additional guidance, please refer to the Association of Operating Room Nurses Recommended Practices for Care of Instruments, Scopes, and Powered Surgical Instruments (AORN Journal, August, 1991) and the AORN Recommended Practices for Steam and Ethylene Oxide Sterilization (AORN Journal, October 1992, Vol. 56, No. 4). Additionally, refer to the Association for the Advancement of Medical Instrumentation (AAMI) recommendations in "Good Hospital Practice: Steam Sterilization and Sterility Assurance" (Approved March 1st, 1988). As a reference, UltraCision offers the following. Reusable Harmonic Scalpel Products have passed sterilization validation tests with a Sterility Assurance Level of 10 -6 using the following sterilization procedures:

	STEAM	FLASH
Sterilizer Type:	Gravity Displacement	Prevacuum
Method:	Wrapped	Unwrapped
Time:	40 Minutes	10 Minutes
Temperature:	250° F	270° F
Pressure:	15 PSIG	30 PSIG
Exhaust:	Slow	Slow

SPECIFICATIONS/HOW SUPPLIED: Federal (USA) law restricts this device to sale by or on the order of a physician.

	ETO
Packaging:	Sterilization pouch with Tyvek® or paper backing
ETO Concentration:	600mg/liter minimum
Preconditioning Time:	Sufficient to allow temperature and relative humidity to rise to specified targets
Sterilization Set Temperature:	130° F
ETO Dwell Period:	2 Hours
Relative Humidity:	50%
Aeration:	12 Hours Minimum
ETO Residuals Dissipation:	24 Hours Minimum

SYSTEM COMPONENTS:

FIGURE 2 HARMONIC SCALPEL GENERATOR

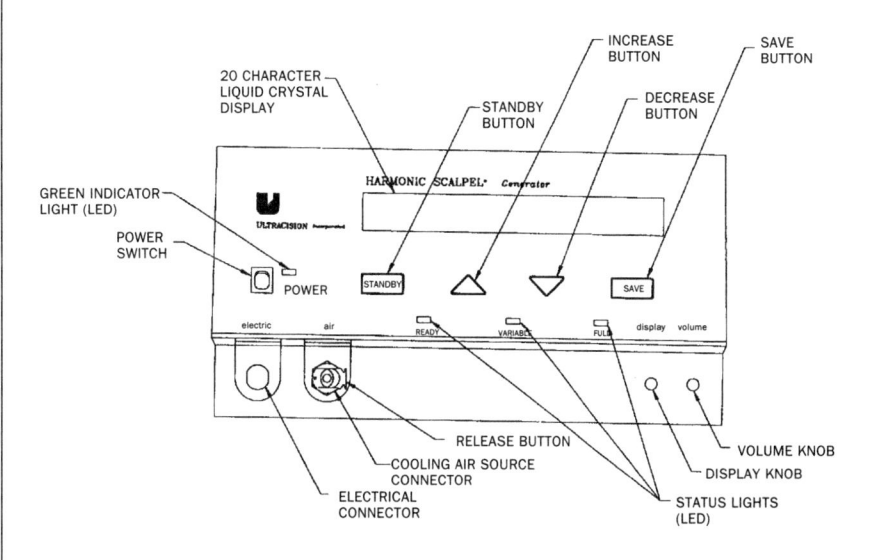

* IN TUV APPROVED UNITS, THE POSITIONS OF THE AIR AND ELECTRICAL CONNECTORS ARE REVERSED.

The Harmonic Scalpel Generator sends an electric signal through a shielded coaxial cable to the transducer in the Harmonic Scalpel Hand Piece. The transducer then converts the electrical energy to mechanical motion. The result is vibration of 55,500 cycles per second at the blade tip.

The electrical signal the generator produces must be identical to the mechanical resonant frequency of the acoustic train (transducer - mount - blade). The Harmonic Scalpel Generator senses changes in the resonant frequency of the acoustic train during use and adjusts the drive frequency to maximize the acoustic efficiency. Also, the generator senses changes in the acoustic train that relate to impending blade fracture or improper use. When this occurs, the generator alerts the user with a continuous beep.

HARMONIC SCALPEL HAND PIECE:

FIGURE 3 HAND PIECE

BLADE WRENCH

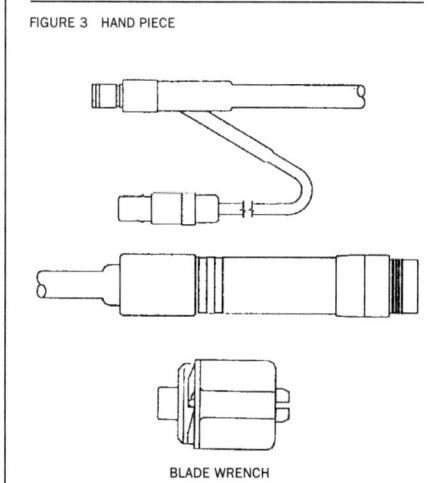

The limited-life reusable Harmonic Scalpel Hand Piece houses the ultrasonic acoustic system. The acoustic system converts electrical energy to mechanical energy resulting in longitudinal motion of the blade edge at ultrasonic frequencies.

SCALPEL HAND PIECE CONFIGURATION:

The ergonomically designed hand piece is compact and lightweight, and is activated by a foot switch.

The hand piece is permanently attached to a 10 foot long silicone cord, which connects to the front of the generator. The cord has two clips to secure the cord to the drapes.

The hand piece is packaged with a blade wrench, which is used to secure the blade to the hand piece. Additional blade wrenches can also be purchased separately. The hand piece and blade wrenches are packaged non-sterile and must be sterilized according to the instructions in the manual prior to use.

FIGURE 4 10mm BLADE AND SHEATH

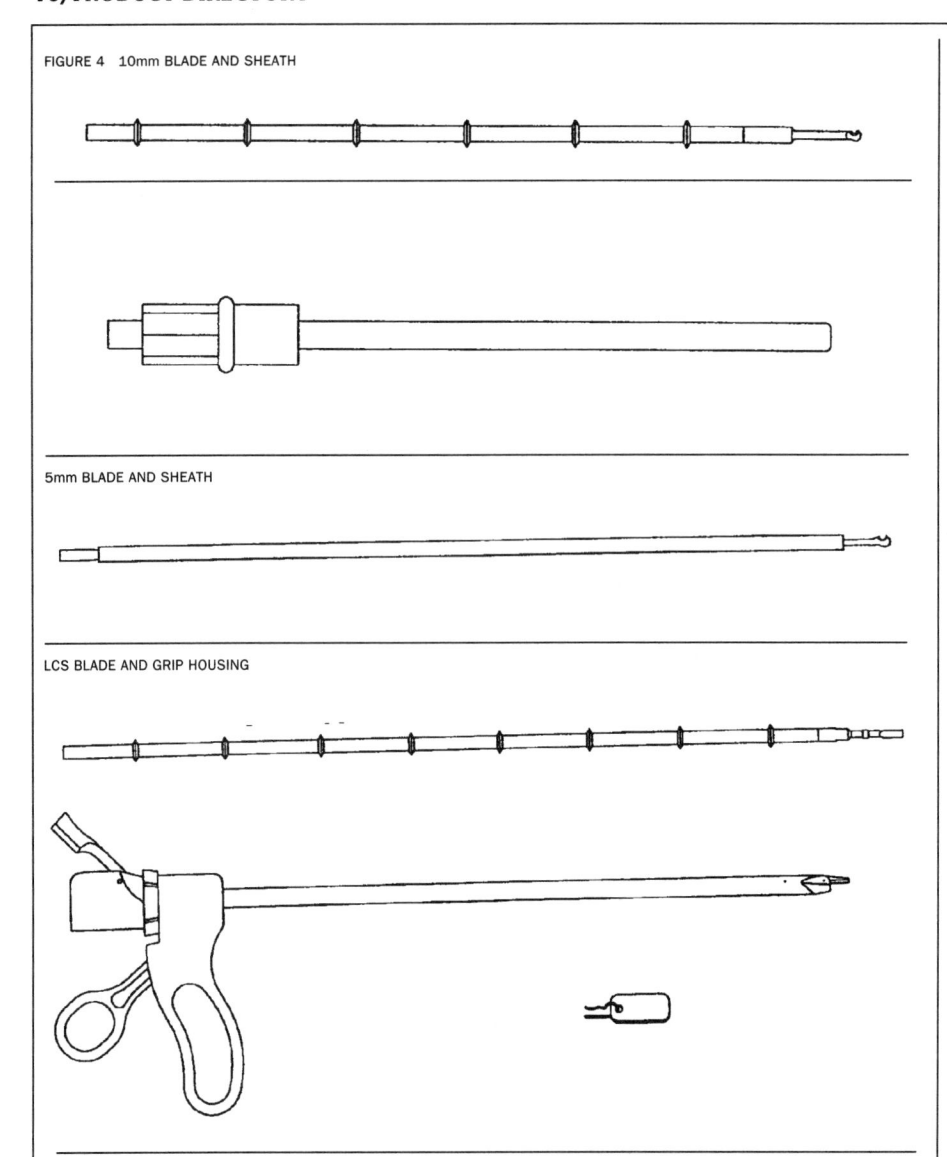

5mm BLADE AND SHEATH

LCS BLADE AND GRIP HOUSING

LAPAROSONIC BLADE SYSTEM:
The Laparosonic 10mm Blades, 5mm Blades, and Coagulating Shears (LCS) are packaged sterile. The shape and precise dimensions of the blade system provide maximal ultrasonic energy at the tip.

10mm Laparosonic Blade Systems are packaged for easy storing and recycling. The 10mm Laparosonic Blade System consists of a titanium blade and a removable stainless steel protective sheath.

The 5mm Laparosonic Blade System consists of a titanium blade with a non-removable PTFE sheath.

The LCS Blade System consists of a titanium blade and grip housing assembly.

HARMONIC SCALPEL SPECIFICATIONS:
Harmonic Generator:
Frequency: 55.5 kHz
Dimensions: 14in. (W) x 8in. (H) x 12in. (D)
Weight: Approximately 20 pounds
UL Flame Rating: V-O
Power Required:
  U.S.: 115 Vac, 60 Hz, 2 Amps, 230 Watts Max
  International: 230 Vac, 50 Hz, 1 Amp, 230 Watts Max

Fuse:
  U.S.: 3AG Slow Blow 1/4in. x 1-1/4in., 2 Amps, 2 required, user changeable
  International: Internal Fused; No user changeable fuses
Air Pressure: 6 PSI Max
Air Flow: Approximately 20 liters per minute

Hand Piece:
Length:
  Hand Piece: 7in.
  Cable: 10 feet without Hand Piece
Weight: 6 oz.
Connectors:
  Electric: 7 pin
  Air: 1/4in. CPC

Foot Switch:
Voltage: 12 Volts maximum at 0.10 Amp

Power Cord:
  U.S.: 15 Foot, 3 Conductor, 16 AWG, Grounded Hospital Grade Power Cord, terminated with IEC 320 Connector
  International: 2 Meter, 3 Conductor, 10A/250 Vac, Grounded Hospital Grade Shielded Power Cord, terminated with an IEC 320 Connector. (Not included).

Endoscope

Endoscopes give the surgeon or gastroenterologist an intraluminal view of the gastrointestinal organs. Although some endoscopists still cling to the older fiber-optic scopes, videoendoscopy is now the standard.

Videoendoscopes are equipped with a camera chip within the tip of the scope. The image transmitted to the video screen has more dimension and better color resolution than that attained by standard fiber optics. Furthermore, the magnified image seen on the screen permits better identification of anatomy; and the operator can view the image comfortably, without the necessity of squinting through an eyepiece. The only drawback of such an integrated scope is that when one part fails, the whole system goes down.

There is one situation in which a fiber-optic scope may still prove superior. For endoscopic retrograde cholangiopancreatography (ERCP), a side-viewing duodenoscope may be called for, because the operator may find it difficult to intubate the papilla of Vater with a videoendoscope.

Endoscopes have become smaller as optical technology has improved. The new smaller scopes are usually better tolerated by patients and are easier to pass, particularly through strictured areas. However, they are also more fragile, and demand more delicate care.

The flexible sigmoidoscope has lost popularity as endoscopists have gained more skill with the longer colonoscope. Inability to render a complete colonic exam has relegated the sigmoidoscope primarily to office use, where it takes the place of the rigid proctoscope.

AMNIOSCOPE, TRANSABDOMINAL (FETOSCOPE)

Origin Medsystems, Inc.
135 Constitution Dr.
Menlo Park, CA 94025
415-617-5000

Rose GmbH
Gottbillstr. 27-30
D-54294 Trier
Germany
0651/89051

Storz GmbH & Co., Karl
Mittelstr. 8
Postfach 230
D-78532 Tuttlingen
Germany
07461/7080

Wolf Medical Instruments Corp., Richard
353 Corporate Woods Pkwy.
Vernon Hills, IL 60061-3110
708-913-1113

ANOSCOPE, NON-POWERED

Abco Dealers, Inc.
6601 W. Mill Rd.
P.O. Box 23090
Milwaukee, WI 53218-0090
414-358-5420

Baxter Healthcare Corp., Hospital Supply
1450 Waukegan Road
McGaw Park, IL 60085-8205
708-473-0400

Baxter Healthcare Corp.
Operating Room Div.
1500 Waukegan Rd.
McGaw Park, IL 60085-8210
708-473-1500

Cabot Medical Corp.
2021 Cabot Blvd. West
Langhorne, PA 19047-1875
215-752-8300

Cameron-Miller, Inc.
3949 S. Racine Ave.
Chicago, IL 60609-2523
312-523-6360

Codman & Shurtleff, Inc.
41 Pacella Park Dr.
Randolph, MA 02368-1755
617-961-2300

Dittmar, Inc.
101 E. Laurel Ave.
P.O. Box 66
Cheltenham, PA 19012-2125
215-379-5533

Grieshaber Manufacturing Co., Inc.
7020 W. Cullom Ave.
Norridge, IL 60634-1325
708-457-1551

Heine Optotechnik GmbH & Co. KG
Kientalstr. 7
D-82211 Herrsching
Germany
08152/380

Himalaya Trading Co., Ltd.
Wazirabad Rd.
P.O. Box No. 59
Sialkot
Pakistan
(0432) 552249

Lawton USA Surgical Instruments
6341 S. Troy Cir.
Englewood, CO 80111-6415
303-790-9416

Link GmbH & Co., Waldemar
Barkhausenweg 10
Postfach 630 565
D-22339 Hamburg 63
Germany
040/5381021

Mader Instrument Corp.
25 Lamington Dr.
Succasunna, NJ 07876-2048
201-584-0816

Martin, Gebr. GmbH & Co. KG
Ludwigstaler Str. 132
Postf. 60
D-78532 Tuttlingen
Germany
07461/7060

Medicon Eg
15 Gansacker
Postfach 4455
D-78532 Tuttlingen
Germany
07462/20090

Medicon Instruments, Inc.
4405 International Blvd.
Norcross, GA 30093-3013
404-381-2858

Miltex Instrument Co., Inc.
6 Ohio Dr.
CB 5006
Lake Success, NY 11042-0006
516-775-7100

Pilling-Rusch
420 Delaware Dr.
Fort Washington, PA 19034-2711
215-643-2600

Sharplan Lasers (Europe) Ltd.
141-155 Brent St.
London NW4 4DJ
United Kingdom
081/203-0006

Sklar Instrument Company
889 South Matlack St.
West Chester, PA 19380
215-430-3200

Storz Endoscopy-America Inc., Karl
10111 W. Jefferson Blvd.
Culver City, CA 90232-3509
310-558-1500

Storz GmbH & Co., Karl
Mittelstr. 8
Postfach 230
D-78532 Tuttlingen
Germany
07461/7080

Surgical Instrument Co. of America
1185 Edgewater Ave.
Ridgefield, NJ 07657-2102
201-941-6500

Ueth & Haug GmbH
Stockacher Str. 41/45
D-78532 Tuttlingen
Germany

Weck & Co. Inc., Edward
1 Weck Dr.
P.O. Box 12600
Research Triangle Park, NC 27709
919-544-8000

Welch Allyn, Inc.
4341 State Street Rd.
P.O. Box 220
Skaneateles Falls, NY 13153-0220
315-685-4100

ANOSCOPE, NON-POWERED (cont'd)

Wolf Medical Instruments Corp., Richard
353 Corporate Woods Pkwy.
Vernon Hills, IL 60061-3110
708-913-1113

Xomed-Treace, Div. of Zimmer of Canada Ltd.
2323 Argentina Rd.
Missisauga, ONT L5N 5N3
Canada
905-858-8588

BRONCHOSCOPE, FLEXIBLE

ACM Endoskopie GmbH
Taunusstr. 38
D-80807 Muenchen 40
Germany
089/352355

Asahi Optical Co., Ltd.
2-36-9, Maeno-Cho, Itabashi-Ku
Tokyo 174
Japan
03/3960-5155

Carsen Group Inc.
151 Telson Rd.
Markham, ONT L3R 1E7
Canada
416-479-4100

Circon Acmi
300 Stillwater Ave.
Stamford, CT 06902-3640
203-328-8689

Daiichi Medical Co. Ltd.
2-27-16, Hongo, Bunkyo-Ku
Tokyo 113
Japan
03/8140111

Fuji Photo Optical Co. Ltd.
1-324, Uetake-Machi, Omiya
Saitama 330
Japan
048/668-2153

Fujinon (Europe) GmbH
Heerdter Lohweg 89
D-40549 Duesseldorf 11
Germany
0211/52050

Fujinon, Inc.
10 High Point Dr.
Wayne, NJ 07470-7434
201-633-5600

Life Medical Technologies, Inc.
3649 W. 1987 S.
Salt Lake City, UT 84104
801-972-1900

Olympus America, Inc.
4 Nevada Drive
Lake Success, NY 11042-1179
516-488-3880

Olympus Optical Co. Ltd.
San-Ei Bldg.
1-22-2, Nishi-Shinjuku
Shinjuku-Ku, Tokyo 163-91
Japan
03/3402111

Ovamed Corporation
111 W. Evelyn Ave. Ste. #214
Sunnyvale, CA 94086-6129
408-720-9876

Pentax Precision Instrument Corp.
30 Ramland Rd.
Orangeburg, NY 10962-2699
914-365-0700

Wolf Medical Instruments Corp., Richard
353 Corporate Woods Pkwy.
Vernon Hills, IL 60061-3110
708-913-1113

BRONCHOSCOPE, FLEXIBLE, ANESTHESIOLOGY

Ulrich KG
Postfach 4060
D-89077 Ulm
Germany
0731/60001

BRONCHOSCOPE, RIGID

ACM Endoskopie GmbH
Taunusstr. 38
D-80807 Muenchen 40
Germany
089/352355

Allgaier Instrumente GmbH
Teuchelgrube 6-10
D-78665 Frittlingen 78665
Germany
07426/1056

Baxter Healthcare Corp.
Operating Room Div.
1500 Waukegan Rd.
McGaw Park, IL 60085-8210
708-473-1500

Boehm Surgical Instrument Corp.
966 Chili Avenue
Rochester, NY 14611-2831
716-436-6584

Bryan Corp.
4 Plympton St.
Woburn, MA 01801-2908
617-935-0004

Kelleher Medical, Inc.
9710 Farrar Court, Suite N
Richmond, VA 23236
804-323-4040

Medicon Eg
15 Gansacker
Postfach 4455
D-78532 Tuttlingen
Germany
07462/20090

Medicon Instruments, Inc.
4405 International Blvd.
Norcross, GA 30093-3013
404-381-2858

Olympus Optical Co. Ltd.
San-Ei Bldg.
1-22-2, Nishi-Shinjuku
Shinjuku-Ku, Tokyo 163-91
Japan
03/3402111

Olympus Winter & Ibe GmbH
Kuehnstrasse 61, Postf. 701709
D-22045 Hamburg 70
Germany
040/66966-0

Pilling-Rusch
420 Delaware Dr.
Fort Washington, PA 19034-2711
215-643-2600

Sharplan Lasers (Europe) Ltd.
141-155 Brent St.
London NW4 4DJ
United Kingdom
081/203-0006

Storz Endoscopy-America Inc., Karl
10111 W. Jefferson Blvd.
Culver City, CA 90232-3509
310-558-1500

Storz GmbH & Co., Karl
Mittelstr. 8
Postfach 230
D-78532 Tuttlingen
Germany
07461/7080

Surgical Instrument Co. of America
1185 Edgewater Ave.
Ridgefield, NJ 07657-2102
201-941-6500

Wolf GmbH, Richard
Pforzheimer Str. 24
Postfach 40
D-75438 Knittlingen
Germany
07043/350

Wolf Medical Instruments Corp., Richard
353 Corporate Woods Pkwy.
Vernon Hills, IL 60061-3110
708-913-1113

BRONCHOSCOPE, RIGID, NON-VENTILATING

Bryan Corp.
4 Plympton St.
Woburn, MA 01801-2908
617-935-0004

Treier Endoscopie AG
Sonnrain
CH-6215 Beromunster
Switzerland
045/512323

Wolf Medical Instruments Corp., Richard
353 Corporate Woods Pkwy.
Vernon Hills, IL 60061-3110
708-913-1113

BRONCHOSCOPE, RIGID, VENTILATING

Bryan Corp.
4 Plympton St.
Woburn, MA 01801-2908
617-935-0004

Pilling-Rusch
420 Delaware Dr.
Fort Washington, PA 19034-2711
215-643-2600

Storz Endoscopy-America Inc., Karl
10111 W. Jefferson Blvd.
Culver City, CA 90232-3509
310-558-1500

Storz GmbH & Co., Karl
Mittelstr. 8
Postfach 230
D-78532 Tuttlingen
Germany
07461/7080

Wolf Medical Instruments Corp., Richard
353 Corporate Woods Pkwy.
Vernon Hills, IL 60061-3110
708-913-1113

COLONOSCOPE, GASTRO-UROLOGY

Circon Acmi
300 Stillwater Ave.
Stamford, CT 06902-3640
203-328-8689

Fuji Photo Optical Co. Ltd.
1-324, Uetake-Machi, Omiya
Saitama 330
Japan
048/668-2153

Fujinon (Europe) GmbH
Heerdter Lohweg 89
D-40549 Duesseldorf 11
Germany
0211/52050

Fujinon, Inc.
10 High Point Dr.
Wayne, NJ 07470-7434
201-633-5600

Olympus America, Inc.
4 Nevada Drive
Lake Success, NY 11042-1179
516-488-3880

Olympus Optical Co. Ltd.
San-Ei Bldg.
1-22-2, Nishi-Shinjuku
Shinjuku-Ku, Tokyo 163-91
Japan
03/3402111

Pentax HgmbH
Julius Vosseler Str. 104
Postf. 540 169
D-22527 Hamburg 54
Germany
040/5617-114

Pentax Precision Instrument Corp.
30 Ramland Rd.
Orangeburg, NY 10962-2699
914-365-0700

Thermotec, Inc.
575 Broad St.
Bridgeport, CT 06604-5122
203-579-4300

COLONOSCOPE, GENERAL & PLASTIC SURGERY

Asahi Optical Co., Ltd.
2-36-9, Maeno-Cho, Itabashi-Ku
Tokyo 174
Japan
03/3960-5155

Carsen Group Inc.
151 Telson Rd.
Markham, ONT L3R 1E7
Canada
416-479-4100

Knight Instrument Co., J. Hugh
226 S. Villere St.
New Orleans, LA 70112-2816
504-524-2797

Thermotec, Inc.
575 Broad St.
Bridgeport, CT 06604-5122
203-579-4300

COLPOSCOPE

Albert-Wetzlar GmbH
Kreisstrasse 120
D-35583 Wetzlar
Germany
06441/45688

Applied Fiberoptics, Inc.
E. Main St.
Southbridge, MA 01550
508-765-9121

Beroflex AG
Haendelstr. 25
D-97688 Bad Kissingen
Germany
0971/1313

Bio Quantum Technologies, Inc.
10270 S. Progress Way
P.O. Box 646
Parker, CO 80134
303-840-9981

Cabot Medical Corp.
2021 Cabot Blvd. West
Langhorne, PA 19047-1875
215-752-8300

Carsen Group Inc.
151 Telson Rd.
Markham, ONT L3R 1E7
Canada
416-479-4100

Codman & Shurtleff, Inc.
41 Pacella Park Dr.
Randolph, MA 02368-1755
617-961-2300

Coopersurgical, Inc.
15 Forest Pkwy.
Shelton, CT 06484-5458
203-929-6321

COLPOSCOPE (cont'd)

Elmed, Inc.
60 W. Fay Ave.
Addison, IL 60101-5198
708-543-2792

Green Medix Corp.
Sun-Family Hongo
4-5-10, Hongo
Bunkyo-Ku, Tokyo 113
Japan
03/8122387

Gyne-Tech Instrument Corp.
1111 Chestnut Street
Burbank, CA 91506-1624
213-849-1512

Kaps GmbH & Co. KG, Karl
Europastrasse - Postfach 1225
D-35614 Asslar
Germany
06441/8404

Leisegang GmbH & Co. KG
Leibnitzstr. 32
D-10625 Berlin
Germany
030-31-9009-0

Leisegang Medical, Inc.
6401 Congress Ave.
Boca Raton, FL 33487-2883
407-994-0202

Medgyn Products, Inc.
328 Eisenhower Ln. #B
Lombard, IL 60148-5405
708-627-4105

Olympus America, Inc.
4 Nevada Drive
Lake Success, NY 11042-1179
516-488-3880

Olympus Optical Co. Ltd.
San-Ei Bldg.
1-22-2, Nishi-Shinjuku
Shinjuku-Ku, Tokyo 163-91
Japan
03/3402111

Sharplan Lasers, Inc.
1 Pearl Ct.
Allendale, NJ 07401-1675
201-327-1666

Smith & Nephew Richards Inc.
1450 Brooks Road
Memphis, TN 38116
901-396-2121

Storz Endoscopy-America Inc., Karl
10111 W. Jefferson Blvd.
Culver City, CA 90232-3509
310-558-1500

Storz GmbH & Co., Karl
Mittelstr. 8
Postfach 230
D-78532 Tuttlingen
Germany
07461/7080

Takizawa Medical Instruments Mfg. Co., Ltd.
38-18 Hongo 2-Chome, Bunkyo-Ku
Tokyo 113
Japan
03/811-9181-2

Technical Enterprises
10023 S.W. 77th Court
Gainesville, FL 32608
904-495-9961

Treier Endoscopie AG
Sonnrain
CH-6215 Beromunster
Switzerland
045/512323

Wallach Surgical Devices, Inc.
P.O. Box 3287
291 Pepe's Farm Road
Milford, CT 06460-3671
203-783-1818

Westco Medical Corp.
7079 Mission Gorge Rd., Bldg. J
San Diego, CA 92120-2455
619-286-1600

Wolf Medical Instruments Corp., Richard
353 Corporate Woods Pkwy.
Vernon Hills, IL 60061-3110
708-913-1113

Zeiss Inc., Carl
One Zeiss Dr.
Thornwood, NY 10594-1939
914-747-1800

Zeiss, Carl Jena GmbH
Tatzendpromenade 1a
D-07745 Jena
Germany
03641/588-0

CULDOSCOPE

Carsen Group Inc.
151 Telson Rd.
Markham, ONT L3R 1E7
Canada
416-479-4100

Rema Medizintechnik GmbH
In Breiten 10
D-78589 Duerbheim-Tuttlingen
Germany
07424-4064

Storz Endoscopy-America Inc., Karl
10111 W. Jefferson Blvd.
Culver City, CA 90232-3509
310-558-1500

Storz GmbH & Co., Karl
Mittelstr. 8
Postfach 230
D-78532 Tuttlingen
Germany
07461/7080

Surgical Instrument Co. of America
1185 Edgewater Ave.
Ridgefield, NJ 07657-2102
201-941-6500

Treier Endoscopie AG
Sonnrain
CH-6215 Beromunster
Switzerland
045/512323

Wolf Medical Instruments Corp., Richard
353 Corporate Woods Pkwy.
Vernon Hills, IL 60061-3110
708-913-1113

CYSTOSCOPE

Asahi Optical Co., Ltd.
2-36-9, Maeno-Cho, Itabashi-Ku
Tokyo 174
Japan
03/3960-5155

Baxter Healthcare Corp.
Operating Room Div.
1500 Waukegan Rd.
McGaw Park, IL 60085-8210
708-473-1500

Boehm Surgical Instrument Corp.
966 Chili Avenue
Rochester, NY 14611-2831
716-436-6584

Cabot Medical Corp.
2021 Cabot Blvd. West
Langhorne, PA 19047-1875
215-752-8300

Carsen Group Inc.
151 Telson Rd.
Markham, ONT L3R 1E7
Canada
416-479-4100

Circon Acmi
300 Stillwater Ave.
Stamford, CT 06902-3640
203-328-8689

Comeg GmbH
Dornierstr. 55
D-78532 Tuttlingen 14
Germany
07461/8036

Depuy, Inc.
700 Orthopaedic Dr.
P.O. Box 988
Warsaw, IN 46581-0988
219-267-8143

Downs Surgical Ltd.
Parkway Industrial Estate
Parkway Close
Sheffield, S9 4WJ
United Kingdom
0742/730346

Electro Fiberoptics Corporation
56 Hudson St.
Northborough, MA 01532-1922
508-393-3753

Encompas Unlimited, Inc.
1110 Pinellas Bayway, Ste. 104
Tierra Verde, FL 33715-8281
813-867-7701

Expanded Optics, Inc.
7382 Bolsa Ave.
Westminster, CA 92683-5212
714-891-3996

Keymed Medical & Industrial Equipment Ltd.
Keymed House, Stock Rd., Southend-on-Sea
Essex SS2 5QH
United Kingdom
0702/616333

Myriadlase, Inc.
4800 S.E. Loop 820
Forest Hill, TX 76140
817-483-9237

Olympus America, Inc.
4 Nevada Drive
Lake Success, NY 11042-1179
516-488-3880

Olympus Optical Co. Ltd.
San-Ei Bldg.
1-22-2, Nishi-Shinjuku
Shinjuku-Ku, Tokyo 163-91
Japan
03/3402111

Olympus Winter & Ibe GmbH
Kuehnstrasse 61, Postf. 701709
D-22045 Hamburg 70
Germany
040/66966-0

Pentax Precision Instrument Corp.
30 Ramland Rd.
Orangeburg, NY 10962-2699
914-365-0700

Schott Fiber Optics, Inc.
122 Charlton St.
Southbridge, MA 01550-1960
508-765-9744

Shinko Optical Co. Ltd.
3-13-4, Hongo, Bunkyo-Ku
Tokyo 113
Japan
03/8114194

Storz Endoscopy-America Inc., Karl
10111 W. Jefferson Blvd.
Culver City, CA 90232-3509
310-558-1500

Storz GmbH & Co., Karl
Mittelstr. 8
Postfach 230
D-78532 Tuttlingen
Germany
07461/7080

Surgitek
3037 Mt. Pleasant St.
Racine, WI 53404-1509
414-639-7205

Wolf Medical Instruments Corp., Richard
353 Corporate Woods Pkwy.
Vernon Hills, IL 60061-3110
708-913-1113

CYSTOURETHROSCOPE

Baxter Healthcare Corp.
Operating Room Div.
1500 Waukegan Rd.
McGaw Park, IL 60085-8210
708-473-1500

Carsen Group Inc.
151 Telson Rd.
Markham, ONT L3R 1E7
Canada
416-479-4100

Circon Acmi
300 Stillwater Ave.
Stamford, CT 06902-3640
203-328-8689

Keymed Medical & Industrial Equipment Ltd.
Keymed House, Stock Rd., Southend-on-Sea
Essex SS2 5QH
United Kingdom
0702/616333

Olympus America, Inc.
4 Nevada Drive
Lake Success, NY 11042-1179
516-488-3880

Olympus Winter & Ibe GmbH
Kuehnstrasse 61, Postf. 701709
D-22045 Hamburg 70
Germany
040/66966-0

Storz Endoscopy-America Inc., Karl
10111 W. Jefferson Blvd.
Culver City, CA 90232-3509
310-558-1500

Storz GmbH & Co., Karl
Mittelstr. 8
Postfach 230
D-78532 Tuttlingen
Germany
07461/7080

Wolf Medical Instruments Corp., Richard
353 Corporate Woods Pkwy.
Vernon Hills, IL 60061-3110
708-913-1113

DUODENOSCOPE, ESOPHAGO/GASTRO

Asahi Optical Co., Ltd.
2-36-9, Maeno-Cho, Itabashi-Ku
Tokyo 174
Japan
03/3960-5155

Carsen Group Inc.
151 Telson Rd.
Markham, ONT L3R 1E7
Canada
416-479-4100

Fujinon, Inc.
10 High Point Dr.
Wayne, NJ 07470-7434
201-633-5600

Olympus America, Inc.
4 Nevada Drive
Lake Success, NY 11042-1179
516-488-3880

Olympus Optical Co. Ltd.
San-Ei Bldg.
1-22-2, Nishi-Shinjuku
Shinjuku-Ku, Tokyo 163-91
Japan
03/3402111

Pentax Precision Instrument Corp.
30 Ramland Rd.
Orangeburg, NY 10962-2699
914-365-0700

ENDOSCOPE

ACM Endoskopie GmbH
Taunusstr. 38
D-80807 Muenchen 40
Germany
089/352355

Bryan Corp.
4 Plympton St.
Woburn, MA 01801-2908
617-935-0004

C.R. Bard Inc., Interventional Products Div.
6091 Heisley Rd.
Mentor, OH 44060-1835
216-352-2935

Cabot Medical Corp.
2021 Cabot Blvd. West
Langhorne, PA 19047-1875
215-752-8300

Chakoff Endoscopy
15405 SW 72 Ct.
Miami, FL 33157
305-253-0321

Circon Acmi
300 Stillwater Ave.
Stamford, CT 06902-3640
203-328-8689

Circon Corporation
460 Ward Drive
Santa Barbara, CA 93111-2310
805-967-0404

Clarus Medical Systems, Inc.
2605 Fernbrook Lane
Minneapolis, MN 55447-4736
612-559-8640

Cogent Light Technologies
26145 W. Technology Dr.
Santa Clarita, CA 91355-1137
805-294-2900

Coopersurgical, Inc.
15 Forest Pkwy.
Shelton, CT 06484-5458
203-929-6321

Cuda Products Corporation
6000 Powers Ave.
Jacksonville, FL 32217-2212
904-737-7611

Dolley/EMC Industries
14 Rue de Saisset
F-92120 Montrouge
France
1/46571205

Endo Image Corporation
1370 Blair Dr.
Odenton, MD 21113
410-551-9700

Endo Optics Inc.
39 Sycamore Ave.
Little Silver, NJ 07739
908-530-6762

Endomedix Corp.
2162 Michelson Drive
Irvine, CA 92715
714-253-1000

ESM Industries
4183 Grove Ave.
Gurnee, IL 60031
708-249-3633

Expanded Optics, Inc.
7382 Bolsa Ave.
Westminster, CA 92683-5212
714-891-3996

Fibertronics, Inc.
100 Foster St.
Southbridge, MA 01550
508-764-3213

Fujinon, Inc.
10 High Point Dr.
Wayne, NJ 07470-7434
201-633-5600

Gabris Surgical Corp.
547 Susan Constant Dr.
Virginia Beach, VA 23451
804-491-6487

Henke-Sass GmbH, Wolf
Kronenstrasse 16
D-78532 Tuttlingen
Germany
07461/189-0

I.S.I. Manufacturing, Inc.
1947 Ivanhoe Dr.
Irwin, PA 15642-4454
412-863-4911

Instrument Technology, Inc.
33 Airport Rd.
P.O. Box 381
Westfield, MA 01086-1357
413-562-3606

Linvatec Corporation
11311 Concept Blvd.
Largo, FL 34643-4908
813-399-5344

Machida Endoscope Co. Ltd.
6-13-8, Honkomagome, Bunkyo-Ku
Tokyo 113
Japan
03/946-2151

Mclean Medical Scientific, Inc.
328 State St.
St. Paul, MN 55107
612-225-9295

Medical Dynamics, Inc.
99 Inverness Dr. E.
Englewood, CO 80112-5115
303-790-2990

Medizintechnik
Wurttemberger Str. 26
D-78567 Fridingen
Germany
07/463-8076

Mizuno Ika Kikai K.k.
7-18 Ajihara-cho, Tennoji-ku
Osaka 543
Japan
06/768-1454

New Life Systems, Inc.
1870 N. State Road 7
Margate, FL 33063-5708
305-972-4600

Olympus America, Inc.
4 Nevada Drive
Lake Success, NY 11042-1179
516-488-3880

Pan Servico Surgical Ltd.
436 Streatham High Rd.
London, SW16 1DA
United Kingdom
081-764-1806

Precision Optics Corp.
22 E. Broadway
Gardner, MA 01440-3338
508-630-1800

Reznik Instrument, Inc.
7337 North Lawndale
Skokie, IL 60076
708-673-3444

RFQ Medizintechnik GmbH & Co. KG
Bruderhofstr. 10-12
Postfach 4652
D-78532 Tuttlingen
Germany
07461/4066

Rudolf GmbH
Tuttlinger Str. 4
Postfach 28
D-78567 Fridingen
Germany
07463/1094

Schott Fiber Optics, Inc.
122 Charlton St.
Southbridge, MA 01550-1960
508-765-9744

Shinko Optical Co. Ltd.
3-13-4, Hongo, Bunkyo-Ku
Tokyo 113
Japan
03/8114194

Storz Endoscopy-America Inc., Karl
10111 W. Jefferson Blvd.
Culver City, CA 90232-3509
310-558-1500

Synectic Engineering, Inc.
4 Oxford Rd.
Milford, CT 06460-7007
203-877-8488

Telmak Pty. Ltd.
131 Sailors Bay Rd., Ste 1, 2nd Floor
Northbridge, NSW 2063
Australia
02/9581077

Tri-Med Specialties, Inc.
P.O. Box 23306
Overland Park, KS 66223
913-888-4440

UMC Incorporated
22510 Highway 55 West
Hamel, MN 55340
612-478-6609

Uresil Corporation
5418 W. Touhy Ave.
Skokie, IL 60077-3232
708-982-0200

Vermont Medical, Inc.
Industrial Park
P.O. Box 556
Bellows Falls, VT 05101-0556
802-463-9976

Weck & Co. Inc., Edward
1 Weck Dr.
P.O. Box 12600
Research Triangle Park, NC 27709
919-544-8000

Wells Johnson Co.
8075 E. Research Ct., Ste. 101
Tucson, AZ 85710-6714
602-298-6069

WM Instrumente GmbH
Panoramastr. 6
D-78604 Rietheim 1
Germany
07424/501310

Wolf GmbH, Richard
Pforzheimer Str. 24
Postfach 40
D-75438 Knittlingen
Germany
07043/350

Zeiss Inc., Carl
One Zeiss Dr.
Thornwood, NY 10594-1939
914-747-1800

Zibra Corp.
105 Ward Hill Ave.
Ward Hill, MA 01835-6928
508-374-9764

Zinnanti Surgical Instruments
21540 B Prairie St.
Chatsworth, CA 91311-5886
818-700-0090

ENDOSCOPE AND ACCESSORIES, AC-POWERED

American International Medicine, Inc.
1917 Glendon Ave., Ste. 201
Los Angeles, CA 90025
310-470-4844

Birtcher Medical Systems, Inc.
50 Technology Dr.
Irvine, CA 92718-2301
714-753-9400

Codman & Shurtleff, Inc.
41 Pacella Park Dr.
Randolph, MA 02368-1755
617-961-2300

Computer Motion, Inc.
250 Storke Rd., Ste. A
Goleta, CA 93117
805-685-3729

Conmed Corp.
310 Broad Street
Utica, NY 13501
315-797-8375

Core Dynamics, Inc.
11222-4 St. Johns Indust. Pkwy.
Jacksonville, FL 32216
904-641-6611

Electroscope, Inc.
4890 Sterling Dr.
Boulder, CO 80301
303-444-2600

Endo Image Corporation
1370 Blair Dr.
Odenton, MD 21113
410-551-9700

Eximed, Inc.
198-03 Hillside Ave.
Hollis, NY 11423-2128
718-479-0020

Heraeus Surgical, Inc.
575 Cottonwood Dr.
Milpitas, CA 95035-7402
408-954-4000

Keymed, Inc.
400 Airport Executive Park
Spring Valley, NY 10977-7404
914-425-3100

Leisegang Medical, Inc.
6401 Congress Ave.
Boca Raton, FL 33487-2883
407-994-0202

Luxtec Corp.
326 Clark St.
Worcester, MA 01606
508-856-9454

Medchem Products, Inc.
232 W. Cummings Pk.
Woburn, MA 01801-6333
617-938-9328

Medicare AG
Mutschellenstr. 115
Ch-8038 Zuerich
Switzerland
01/4824826

Micromedics, Inc.
1285 Corporate Center Dr., Ste. #150
Eagan, MN 55121-1236
612-452-1977

Microsurge, Inc.
150 A St.
Needham, MA 02194
617-444-2300

Microvasive/Boston Scientific Corp.
Urology Div.
480 Pleasant St.
Watertown, MA 02172
617-923-1720

Minorax Corp.
7015 147th St. SW
Edmonds, WA 98026
206-743-0178

NDM Corporation
3040 E. River Rd.
Dayton, OH 45439-1436
513-294-1767

North American Sterilization & Packaging
15 White Lake Rd.
P.O. Box 923
Sparta, NJ 07871-3206
201-579-1397

Redfield Corporation
210 Summit Ave.
Montvale, NJ 07645-1526
201-391-0494

ENDOSCOPE AND ACCESSORIES, AC-POWERED (cont'd)

Reznik Instrument, Inc.
7337 North Lawndale
Skokie, IL 60076
708-673-3444

Sherwood Intrascopic Div.
1915 Olive St.
St. Louis, MO 63103
314-241-5700

Smith & Nephew Richards Inc.
1450 Brooks Road
Memphis, TN 38116
901-396-2121

Snowden-Pencer
5175 S. Royal Atlanta Dr.
Tucker, GA 30084-3053
404-496-0952

Sony Corporation of America
Medical Systems Div.
3 Paragon Drive (S-200)
Montvale, NJ 07645
201-930-7098

Stackhouse Inc.
2059 Atlanta Ave.
Riverside, CA 92507-2439
909-276-4600

Vermont Medical, Inc.
Industrial Park
P.O. Box 556
Bellows Falls, VT 05101-0556
802-463-9976

Wilson-Cook Medical, Inc.
4900 Bethania Station Rd.
Winston-Salem, NC 27105-1203
919-744-0157

ENDOSCOPE AND ACCESSORIES, BATTERY-POWERED

Bag
B.P. 68
M. Rue de Fieuzal
F-33523 Bruges Cedex
France
57/810464

Storz Endoscopy-America Inc., Karl
10111 W. Jefferson Blvd.
Culver City, CA 90232-3509
310-558-1500

Storz GmbH & Co., Karl
Mittelstr. 8
Postfach 230
D-78532 Tuttlingen
Germany
07461/7080

ENDOSCOPE, DIRECT VISION

Aesculap
1000 Gateway Blvd.
South San Francisco, CA 94080-7030
415-876-7000

Bag
B.P. 68
M. Rue de Fieuzal
F-33523 Bruges Cedex
France
57/810464

Bryan Corp.
4 Plympton St.
Woburn, MA 01801-2908
617-935-0004

Coopersurgical, Inc.
15 Forest Pkwy.
Shelton, CT 06484-5458
203-929-6321

Cuda Products Corporation
6000 Powers Ave.
Jacksonville, FL 32217-2212
904-737-7611

Davis & Geck Div.
American Cyanamid Company
One Cyanamid Plaza
Wayne, NJ 07470-2012
201-831-2000

Depuy, Inc.
700 Orthopaedic Dr.
P.O. Box 988
Warsaw, IN 46581-0988
219-267-8143

Electro Surgical Instrument Co.
37 Centennial St.
Rochester, NY 14611-1732
716-235-1430

Instrument Technology, Inc.
33 Airport Rd.
P.O. Box 381
Westfield, MA 01086-1357
413-562-3606

Smith & Nephew Dyonics, Inc.
160 Dascomb Rd.
Andover, MA 01810-5893
508-470-2800

Storz Endoscopy-America Inc., Karl
10111 W. Jefferson Blvd.
Culver City, CA 90232-3509
310-558-1500

Storz GmbH & Co., Karl
Mittelstr. 8
Postfach 230
D-78532 Tuttlingen
Germany
07461/7080

Wolf Medical Instruments Corp., Richard
353 Corporate Woods Pkwy.
Vernon Hills, IL 60061-3110
708-913-1113

ENDOSCOPE, ELECTRONIC (VIDEOENDOSCOPE)

Abinee Assoc.
Av Paulista, 1313-7
01311 Sao Paulo SP
Brazil
11/2511577

Asahi Optical Co., Ltd.
2-36-9, Maeno-Cho, Itabashi-Ku
Tokyo 174
Japan
03/3960-5155

Clarus Medical Systems, Inc.
2605 Fernbrook Lane
Minneapolis, MN 55447-4736
612-559-8640

Endomed Ind.
R. Francisco Leitao 653
05414 Sao Paulo SP
Brazil
11/2110936

Fujinon (Europe) GmbH
Heerdter Lohweg 89
D-40549 Duesseldorf 11
Germany
0211/52050

Fujinon, Inc.
10 High Point Dr.
Wayne, NJ 07470-7434
201-633-5600

Instrument Technology, Inc.
33 Airport Rd.
P.O. Box 381
Westfield, MA 01086-1357
413-562-3606

Karindo Alkestron P.T.
17 Tomang Raya
Jakarta 11440
Indonesia
021/5600896

Welch Allyn, Inc.
4341 State Street Rd.
P.O. Box 220
Skaneateles Falls, NY 13153-0220
315-685-4100

Wolf Medical Instruments Corp., Richard
353 Corporate Woods Pkwy.
Vernon Hills, IL 60061-3110
708-913-1113

ENDOSCOPE, FETAL BLOOD SAMPLING

Bag
B.P. 68
M. Rue de Fieuzal
F-33523 Bruges Cedex
France
57/810464

Nikomed Aps
Glerupvej 20
DK-2610 Rdovre
Denmark
42848000

Rema Medizintechnik GmbH
In Breiten 10
D-78589 Duerbheim-Tuttlingen
Germany
07424-4064

ENDOSCOPE, FLEXIBLE

Clarus Medical Systems, Inc.
2605 Fernbrook Lane
Minneapolis, MN 55447-4736
612-559-8640

Electro Fiberoptics Corporation
56 Hudson St.
Northborough, MA 01532-1922
508-393-3753

Fiber-Tech Medical, Inc.
5020 Campbell Blvd., Ste. K.
Baltimore, MD 21236
410-931-4411

Instrument Technology, Inc.
33 Airport Rd.
P.O. Box 381
Westfield, MA 01086-1357
413-562-3606

Keymed Medical & Industrial Equipment Ltd.
Keymed House, Stock Rd., Southend-on-Sea
Essex SS2 5QH
United Kingdom
0702/616333

Leisegang Medical, Inc.
6401 Congress Ave.
Boca Raton, FL 33487-2883
407-994-0202

Life Medical Technologies, Inc.
3649 W. 1987 S.
Salt Lake City, UT 84104
801-972-1900

Machida Endoscope Co. Ltd.
6-13-8, Honkomagome, Bunkyo-Ku
Tokyo 113
Japan
03/946-2151

Medi-Globe Corp.
6202 South Maple Ave. #131
Tempe, AZ 85283
602-897-2772

Medical Surgical Specialties Ltd.
5148 Lovers Lane
Kalamazoo, MI 49002
616-385-5000

Mitsubishi Cable America, Inc.
520 Madison Ave., 17th Fl.
New York, NY 10022
212-888-2270

Phillips Medical Group
562 East Chatham St.
Cary, NC 27511
919-469-4641

Surgitek
3037 Mt. Pleasant St.
Racine, WI 53404-1509
414-639-7205

Telmak Pty. Ltd.
131 Sailors Bay Rd., Ste 1, 2nd Floor
Northbridge, NSW 2063
Australia
02/9581077

Welch Allyn, Inc.
4341 State Street Rd.
P.O. Box 220
Skaneateles Falls, NY 13153-0220
315-685-4100

Wolf Medical Instruments Corp., Richard
353 Corporate Woods Pkwy.
Vernon Hills, IL 60061-3110
708-913-1113

ENDOSCOPE, NEUROLOGICAL

Electro Fiberoptics Corporation
56 Hudson St.
Northborough, MA 01532-1922
508-393-3753

ENDOSCOPE, RIGID

Davis & Geck Endosurgery
1 Casper St.
Danbury, CT 06810
203-743-4451

PROFESSIONAL LINE 8389 SERIES

DESCRIPTION:

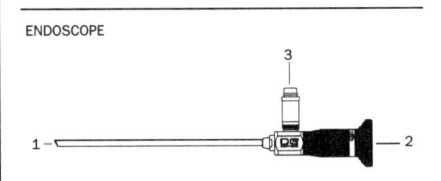

ENDOSCOPE

The DAVIS & GECK endoscopes which are suitable for autoclaving are identified by this symbol on the labeling ring:

ENDOSCOPE AUTOCLAVE SYMBOL

CARE & MAINTENANCE: Cleaning by insertion in cleaning and disinfectant solutions.

Swabs must be used preferably for auxiliary mechanical cleaning.

After chemical cleaning and/or disinfection, rinse sufficiently (i.e., free of residue) under clear, running water.

Use fully-desalinated water in order to avoid water stains.

Remove dirt on window and glass surface [(1) = distal window, (2) = proximal window, (3) = entry surface of the fiber-optic light guide] by gently rubbing with a cotton wool swab moistened with alcohol.

A neutral cleaning agent (washing-up liquid) can also be used in the case of tenacious dirt.

Dry the endoscopes with a soft cloth after treatment.

This is followed by sterilization by autoclaving.

STERILIZATION GUIDELINES: Only endoscopes which are marked as described above must be autoclaved. Place the endoscope in a suitable container or wrap in a towel, whereby no additional instruments must be placed on top. Autoclave up to 273°F (134°C), 29 psig (2 bars) - do not perform flash autoclaving. Hot endoscopes are very sensitive to shocks. For this reason, avoid shocks and vibrations. Do not suddenly expose hot endoscopes to cold after autoclaving.

Autoclaving reduces the service life of endoscopes. For this reason, DAVIS & GECK endoscopes can also be gas sterilized or chemically disinfected (immersion).

In the case of ethylene oxide gas sterilization, please observe the corresponding airing times.

ENDOSCOPE, RIGID (cont'd)

In case of disinfection, observe the instructions of the disinfectant manufacturer. Endoscopes should not be immersed in disinfectant solution for longer than the time recommended by the manufacturer. Equally, avoid long storage times in sterile water. Otherwise, changes may occur on the instrument surface in both cases.

Please use the original packaging when sending in endoscopes for repair in order to avoid transport damage.

SPECIFICATIONS/HOW SUPPLIED:

ACMI/STORZ MALE ATTACHMENT

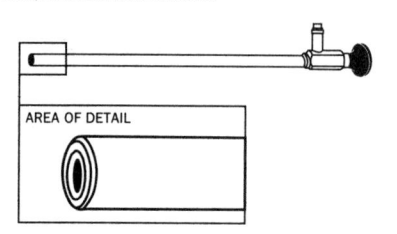

AREA OF DETAIL

ACME/STORZ MALE ATTACHMENT

PRODUCT CODE	DIAMETER	LENGTH	VIEWING ANGLE
8389-01	6.5 mm	27.5 cm	0°
8389-02	10.0 mm	30.0 cm	0°
8389-03	6.5 mm	27.5 cm	30°
8389-04	10.0 mm	30.0 cm	30°

American International Medicine, Inc.
1917 Glendon Ave., Ste. 201
Los Angeles, CA 90025
310-470-4844

Birtcher Medical Systems, Inc.
50 Technology Dr.
Irvine, CA 92718-2301
714-753-9400

Bryan Corp.
4 Plympton St.
Woburn, MA 01801-2908
617-935-0004

Clarus Medical Systems, Inc.
2605 Fernbrook Lane
Minneapolis, MN 55447-4736
612-559-8640

Coopersurgical, Inc.
15 Forest Pkwy.
Shelton, CT 06484-5458
203-929-6321

Cuda Products Corporation
6000 Powers Ave.
Jacksonville, FL 32217-2212
904-737-7611

Davis & Geck Div.
American Cyanamid Company
One Cyanamid Plaza
Wayne, NJ 07470-2012
201-831-2000

Depuy, Inc.
700 Orthopaedic Dr.
P.O. Box 988
Warsaw, IN 46581-0988
219-267-8143

Diener, Christian
Rudolf Diesel Str. 18
D-78532 Tuttlingen
Germany
7461/71067

Electro Fiberoptics Corporation
56 Hudson St.
Northborough, MA 01532-1922
508-393-3753

Electro Surgical Instrument Co.
37 Centennial St.
Rochester, NY 14611-1732
716-235-1430

Elmed, Inc.
60 W. Fay Ave.
Addison, IL 60101-5198
708-543-2792

Heraeus Surgical, Inc.
575 Cottonwood Dr.
Milpitas, CA 95035-7402
408-954-4000

I.S.I. Manufacturing, Inc.
1947 Ivanhoe Dr.
Irwin, PA 15642-4454
412-863-4911

Instrument Technology, Inc.
33 Airport Rd.
P.O. Box 381
Westfield, MA 01086-1357
413-562-3606

Karlheinz Hinze
Endo-engineering
Elbgaustr. 112
D-22532 Hamburg
Germany
40/842510

Key Surgical, Inc.
7101 York Ave. S.
Edina, MN 55435-4450
612-831-7331

Leisegang Medical, Inc.
6401 Congress Ave.
Boca Raton, FL 33487-2883
407-994-0202

Machida Endoscope Co. Ltd.
6-13-8, Honkomagome, Bunkyo-Ku
Tokyo 113
Japan
03/946-2151

Marlow Surgical Technologies, Inc.
1810 Joseph Lloyd Pkwy.
Willoughby, OH 44094-8030
216-946-2453

Medical Surgical Specialties Ltd.
5148 Lovers Lane
Kalamazoo, MI 49002
616-385-5000

Myriadlase, Inc.
4800 S.E. Loop 820
Forest Hill, TX 76140
817-483-9237

Origin Medsystems, Inc.
135 Constitution Dr.
Menlo Park, CA 94025
415-617-5000

Phillips Medical Group
562 East Chatham St.
Cary, NC 27511
919-469-4641

Pioneer Medical, Inc.
34 Laurelcrest Rd.
Madison, CT 06443
203-245-9337

Rema Medizintechnik GmbH
In Breiten 10
D-78589 Duerbheim-Tuttlingen
Germany
07424-4064

Rudolf GmbH
Tuttlinger Str. 4
Postfach 28
D-78567 Fridingen
Germany
07463/1094

Smith & Nephew Dyonics, Inc.
160 Dascomb Rd.
Andover, MA 01810-5893
508-470-2800

Smith & Nephew Richards Inc.
1450 Brooks Road
Memphis, TN 38116
901-396-2121

Storz Endoscopy-America Inc., Karl
10111 W. Jefferson Blvd.
Culver City, CA 90232-3509
310-558-1500

Storz GmbH & Co., Karl
Mittelstr. 8
Postfach 230
D-78532 Tuttlingen
Germany
07461/7080

Telmak Pty. Ltd.
131 Sailors Bay Rd., Ste 1, 2nd Floor
Northbridge, NSW 2063
Australia
02/9581077

Welch Allyn, Inc.
4341 State Street Rd.
P.O. Box 220
Skaneateles Falls, NY 13153-0220
315-685-4100

Wolf Medical Instruments Corp., Richard
353 Corporate Woods Pkwy.
Vernon Hills, IL 60061-3110
708-913-1113

Xomed-Treace
6743 Southpoint Drive N.
Jacksonville, FL 32216-6218
904-296-9600

ENDOSCOPE, TRANSCERVICAL (AMNIOSCOPE)

Bryan Corp.
4 Plympton St.
Woburn, MA 01801-2908
617-935-0004

Caminer Brothers
53-55 Flinders St.
P.O. Box 245
Darlinghurst, NSW 3020
Australia
02/312918

Heine Optotechnik GmbH & Co. KG
Kientalstr. 7
D-82211 Herrsching
Germany
08152/380

Rema Medizintechnik GmbH
In Breiten 10
D-78589 Duerbheim-Tuttlingen
Germany
07424-4064

Storz GmbH & Co., Karl
Mittelstr. 8
Postfach 230
D-78532 Tuttlingen
Germany
07461/7080

Treier Endoscopie AG
Sonnrain
CH-6215 Beromunster
Switzerland
045/512323

Wolf Medical Instruments Corp., Richard
353 Corporate Woods Pkwy.
Vernon Hills, IL 60061-3110
708-913-1113

ENTEROSCOPE

Pentax Precision Instrument Corp.
30 Ramland Rd.
Orangeburg, NY 10962-2699
914-365-0700

GASTRODUODENOSCOPE

Carsen Group Inc.
151 Telson Rd.
Markham, ONT L3R 1E7
Canada
416-479-4100

Fujinon (Europe) GmbH
Heerdter Lohweg 89
D-40549 Duesseldorf 11
Germany
0211/52050

Fujinon, Inc.
10 High Point Dr.
Wayne, NJ 07470-7434
201-633-5600

Olympus America, Inc.
4 Nevada Drive
Lake Success, NY 11042-1179
516-488-3880

Olympus Optical Co. Ltd.
San-Ei Bldg.
1-22-2, Nishi-Shinjuku
Shinjuku-Ku, Tokyo 163-91
Japan
03/3402111

HYSTEROSCOPE

Berkeley Medevices, Inc.
907 Camelia St.
Berkeley, CA 94710-1419
510-526-4046

Bryan Corp.
4 Plympton St.
Woburn, MA 01801-2908
617-935-0004

Cabot Medical Corp.
2021 Cabot Blvd. West
Langhorne, PA 19047-1875
215-752-8300

Carsen Group Inc.
151 Telson Rd.
Markham, ONT L3R 1E7
Canada
416-479-4100

Chakoff Endoscopy
15405 SW 72 Ct.
Miami, FL 33157
305-253-0321

Chirurgische Instrumente
Hauptstrasse 18
D-78582 Balgheim
Germany
7424/501319

Comeg GmbH
Dornierstr. 55
D-78532 Tuttlingen 14
Germany
07461/8036

Conceptus, Inc.
47201 Lakeview Blvd.
Fremont, CA 94538
510-440-7879

Coopersurgical, Inc.
15 Forest Pkwy.
Shelton, CT 06484-5458
203-929-6321

Leisegang GmbH & Co. KG
Leibnitzstr. 32
D-10625 Berlin
Germany
030-31-9009-0

Leisegang Medical, Inc.
6401 Congress Ave.
Boca Raton, FL 33487-2883
407-994-0202

Linvatec, Div. of Zimmer of Canada Ltd.
2323 Argentia Rd.
Mississauga, ONT L5N 5N3
Canada
905-858-8588

Olympus America, Inc.
4 Nevada Drive
Lake Success, NY 11042-1179
516-488-3880

Olympus Optical Co. Ltd.
San-Ei Bldg.
1-22-2, Nishi-Shinjuku
Shinjuku-Ku, Tokyo 163-91
Japan
03/3402111

Rema Medizintechnik GmbH
In Breiten 10
D-78589 Duerbheim-Tuttlingen
Germany
07424-4064

Schoelly Fiberoptic GmbH
Robert Bosch Str. 1-3
Postfach 1280
D-79211 Denzlingen
Germany
07666/1018/1019

Schott Fiber Optics, Inc.
122 Charlton St.
Southbridge, MA 01550-1960
508-765-9744

HYSTEROSCOPE (cont'd)

Smith & Nephew Dyonics, Inc.
160 Dascomb Rd.
Andover, MA 01810-5893
508-470-2800

Storz Endoscopy-America Inc., Karl
10111 W. Jefferson Blvd.
Culver City, CA 90232-3509
310-558-1500

Storz GmbH & Co., Karl
Mittelstr. 8
Postfach 230
D-78532 Tuttlingen
Germany
07461/7080

Treier Endoscopie AG
Sonnrain
CH-6215 Beromunster
Switzerland
045/512323

Weck & Co. Inc., Edward
1 Weck Dr.
P.O. Box 12600
Research Triangle Park, NC 27709
919-544-8000

Wect Instrument Company, Inc.
5645 N. Ravenswood
Chicago, IL 60660-3922
312-769-1944

Wisap Gesellschaft
Rudolf Diesel Ring 20
D-82054 Sauerlach
Germany
08104/1067

Wisap USA
P.O. Box 324
Tomball, TX 77377-0324
713-351-2629

Wolf Medical Instruments Corp., Richard
353 Corporate Woods Pkwy.
Vernon Hills, IL 60061-3110
708-913-1113

LARYNGOSCOPE

Amtec Med. Prod., Inc.
13007 E. Park Ave.
Santa Fe Springs, CA 90670-4005
310-946-8505

Anesthesia Associates, Inc.
460 Enterprise St.
San Marcos, CA 92069-4363
619-744-6561

Anesthesia Medical Specialties, Inc.
13007 E. Park Ave.
Santa Fe Springs, CA 90670-4005
310-946-8303

Bauer & Haselbarth GmbH
Sauerbruchstr. 7 - Postfach
D-25479 Ellerau Bei Hamburg
Germany
04106/72091

Blue Ridge Anesthesia & Critical Care
1201-1207 Jefferson St.
Lynchburg, VA 24504-1813
804-846-2637

Buck GmbH, Rudolf
Obere Hauptstr. 40/1
D-78573 Wurmlingen-Tuttlingen
Germany
07/461-3535

Burton Medical Products, Inc.
7922 Haskell Avenue
Van Nuys, CA 91406-1923
818-989-4700

Caminer Brothers
53-55 Flinders St.
P.O. Box 245
Darlinghurst, NSW 3020
Australia
02/312918

Carley Lamps
1502 West 228th St.
Torrance, CA 90501-5105
310-325-8474

Carsen Group Inc.
151 Telson Rd.
Markham, ONT L3R 1E7
Canada
416-479-4100

Dahlhausen & Co. GmbH, P.J.
Oberbuschweg 76
Postfach 501269
D-5000 Koeln 50
Germany
02236/39130

Dixie USA, Inc.
7800 Amelia, P.O. Box 55549
Houston, TX 77255-5549
713-688-4993

Effner Biomet GmbH
Alt-Lankwitz 102
D-12247 Berlin 46
Germany
49/30-7700920

Frontline Medical Supplies
1601 S.W. 37th St.
Ocala, FL 34474
904-237-1122

Heine Optotechnik GmbH & Co. KG
Kientalstr. 7
D-82211 Herrsching
Germany
08152/380

Intertech Resources, Inc.
300 Tri-State Int'l, Ste. 150
Lincolnshire, IL 60069-4446
708-940-7789

Izumo Rubber Manufacturing Co. Ltd.
7-13, Kitashinagawa 5 Chome
Shinagawa-ku
Tokyo 141
Japan
03/3441-3105

Kay Enterprise Ltd.
Kawada Bldg., 3-21-12, Yushima
Bunkyo-Ku, Tokyo 113
Japan
03/8361316

Kelleher Medical, Inc.
9710 Farrar Court, Suite N
Richmond, VA 23236
804-323-4040

Mabis Healthcare
28401 N. Ballard Dr., Unit H
Lake Forest, IL 60045
708-680-6811

Martin, Gebr. GmbH & Co. KG
Ludwigstaler Str. 132
Postf. 60
D-78532 Tuttlingen
Germany
07461/7060

Medicon Eg
15 Gansacker
Postfach 4455
D-78532 Tuttlingen
Germany
07462/20090

Medicon Instruments, Inc.
4405 International Blvd.
Norcross, GA 30093-3013
404-381-2858

Mercury Medical
11300 49th St. N #A
Clearwater, FL 34622-4800
813-573-0088

Morot-Chopelin
18 Rue Des Cottages
F-92340 Bourg La Reine,
France
1/7028932

Nagashima Medical Instrument Co., Ltd.
24-1 Hongo 5-Chome, Bunkyo-Ku
Tokyo 113
Japan
03/3812-1271

Neutech Corporation
79 Fitzrandolph Road
West Orange, NJ 07052-3527
201-731-2707

Nopa Instruments Medizintechnik GmbH
Gansacker 9 - Postfach 4554
D-78532 Tuttlingen
Germany
07462/7801

North American Medical Products, Inc.
Rotterdam Ind. Pk. Bldg.
901 Vischer Ave.
Schenectady, NY 12306
518-347-1646

Olympus America, Inc.
4 Nevada Drive
Lake Success, NY 11042-1179
516-488-3880

Olympus Optical Co. Ltd.
San-Ei Bldg.
1-22-2, Nishi-Shinjuku
Shinjuku-Ku, Tokyo 163-91
Japan
03/3402111

Opsm Instruments Pty. Ltd.
4 Rothwell Ave.
Concord West, NSW 2138
Australia
02/7361033

Pilling-Rusch
420 Delaware Dr.
Fort Washington, PA 19034-2711
215-643-2600

Professional Surgical Instrument Co.
102 Old Stage Rd.
East Brunswick, NJ 08816
908-390-1133

Riester GmbH & Co. KG., Rudolf
Bruckstrasse 35
D-72417 Jungingen
Germany
07477/2251484

Schott Fiber Optics, Inc.
122 Charlton St.
Southbridge, MA 01550-1960
508-765-9744

Select-Sutter GmbH
Tullastr. 87
D-79108 Freiburg/Breisgau
Germany
0761/515510

Storz Endoscopy-America Inc., Karl
10111 W. Jefferson Blvd.
Culver City, CA 90232-3509
310-558-1500

Storz GmbH & Co., Karl
Mittelstr. 8
Postfach 230
D-78532 Tuttlingen
Germany
07461/7080

Stuemer GmbH & Co.
Sieboldstrasse 2
D-97072 Wuerzburg 1
Germany
0931/885350

Sun-Med, Inc.
5401 Tech Data Dr.
Clearwater, FL 34620-3106
813-530-7099

Surgical Service of London, The
Darenth Mill, Darenth Road
Dartford, Kent
United Kingdom
0322/79772

Tekno-Medical Optik Chirur. GmbH & Co. KG
Sattlerstr. 11
D-78532 Tuttlingen 16
Germany
07461/6067

Timesco of London
176 Pentonville Rd.
London N1 9JP
United Kingdom
071/278-0712-3

Truphatek International Ltd.
Park Poleg, Industrial Area
P.O. Box 8051
Netanya
Israel
09-851155

Vital Signs, Inc.
20 Campus Rd.
Totowa, NJ 07512-1200
201-790-1330

Welch Allyn, Inc.
4341 State Street Rd.
P.O. Box 220
Skaneateles Falls, NY 13153-0220
315-685-4100

NASOPHARYNGOSCOPE (FLEXIBLE OR RIGID)

Asahi Optical Co., Ltd.
2-36-9, Maeno-Cho, Itabashi-Ku
Tokyo 174
Japan
03/3960-5155

Kelleher Medical, Inc.
9710 Farrar Court, Suite N
Richmond, VA 23236
804-323-4040

Machida, Inc.
40 Ramland Rd. South
Orangeburg, NY 10962-2617
914-365-0600

Olympus America, Inc.
4 Nevada Drive
Lake Success, NY 11042-1179
516-488-3880

Olympus Optical Co. Ltd.
San-Ei Bldg.
1-22-2, Nishi-Shinjuku
Shinjuku-Ku, Tokyo 163-91
Japan
03/3402111

Pentax Precision Instrument Corp.
30 Ramland Rd.
Orangeburg, NY 10962-2699
914-365-0700

Schoelly Fiberoptic GmbH
Robert Bosch Str. 1-3
Postfach 1280
D-79211 Denzlingen
Germany
07666/1018/1019

Schott Fiber Optics, Inc.
122 Charlton St.
Southbridge, MA 01550-1960
508-765-9744

Storz Endoscopy-America Inc., Karl
10111 W. Jefferson Blvd.
Culver City, CA 90232-3509
310-558-1500

Storz GmbH & Co., Karl
Mittelstr. 8
Postfach 230
D-78532 Tuttlingen
Germany
07461/7080

Welch Allyn, Inc.
4341 State Street Rd.
P.O. Box 220
Skaneateles Falls, NY 13153-0220
315-685-4100

Wolf Medical Instruments Corp., Richard
353 Corporate Woods Pkwy.
Vernon Hills, IL 60061-3110
708-913-1113

NEPHROSCOPE, FLEXIBLE

Carsen Group Inc.
151 Telson Rd.
Markham, ONT L3R 1E7
Canada
416-479-4100

Circon Acmi
300 Stillwater Ave.
Stamford, CT 06902-3640
203-328-8689

NEPHROSCOPE, FLEXIBLE (cont'd)

Life Medical Technologies, Inc.
3649 W. 1987 S.
Salt Lake City, UT 84104
801-972-1900

Olympus America, Inc.
4 Nevada Drive
Lake Success, NY 11042-1179
516-488-3880

Olympus Optical Co. Ltd.
San-Ei Bldg.
1-22-2, Nishi-Shinjuku
Shinjuku-Ku, Tokyo 163-91
Japan
03/3402111

Pentax Precision Instrument Corp.
30 Ramland Rd.
Orangeburg, NY 10962-2699
914-365-0700

Surgitek
3037 Mt. Pleasant St.
Racine, WI 53404-1509
414-639-7205

Wolf Medical Instruments Corp., Richard
353 Corporate Woods Pkwy.
Vernon Hills, IL 60061-3110
708-913-1113

NEPHROSCOPE, RIGID

Carsen Group Inc.
151 Telson Rd.
Markham, ONT L3R 1E7
Canada
416-479-4100

Circon Acmi
300 Stillwater Ave.
Stamford, CT 06902-3640
203-328-8689

Storz Endoscopy-America Inc., Karl
10111 W. Jefferson Blvd.
Culver City, CA 90232-3509
310-558-1500

Storz GmbH & Co., Karl
Mittelstr. 8
Postfach 230
D-78532 Tuttlingen
Germany
07461/7080

Wolf Medical Instruments Corp., Richard
353 Corporate Woods Pkwy.
Vernon Hills, IL 60061-3110
708-913-1113

OBSERVERSCOPE

Pentax Precision Instrument Corp.
30 Ramland Rd.
Orangeburg, NY 10962-2699
914-365-0700

Storz Endoscopy-America Inc., Karl
10111 W. Jefferson Blvd.
Culver City, CA 90232-3509
310-558-1500

Storz GmbH & Co., Karl
Mittelstr. 8
Postfach 230
D-78532 Tuttlingen
Germany
07461/7080

PANENDOSCOPE

Fuji Photo Optical Co. Ltd.
1-324, Uetake-Machi, Omiya
Saitama 330
Japan
048/668-2153

Fujinon, Inc.
10 High Point Dr.
Wayne, NJ 07470-7434
201-633-5600

PERITONEOSCOPE

Access Surgical International, Inc.
15 Caswell Ln.
Boat Yard Square
Plymouth, MA 02360
508-747-6006

Advanced Surgical, Inc.
305 College Rd. East
Princeton, NJ 08540
609-987-2340

Aesculap
1000 Gateway Blvd.
South San Francisco, CA 94080-7030
415-876-7000

American Hydro-Surgical Instruments, Inc.
430 Commerce Dr., Ste. 50E
Delray Beach, FL 33445
407-278-5664

Automated Medical Products Corp.
2315 Broadway, Ste. 410
New York, NY 10024-4332
212-874-0236

BioEnterics Corporation
1035A Cindy Lane
Carpinteria, CA 93013
805-684-3045

Cabot Medical Corp.
2021 Cabot Blvd. West
Langhorne, PA 19047-1875
215-752-8300

Circon Acmi
300 Stillwater Ave.
Stamford, CT 06902-3640
203-328-8689

Computer Motion, Inc.
250 Storke Rd., Ste. A
Goleta, CA 93117
805-685-3729

Coopersurgical, Inc.
15 Forest Pkwy.
Shelton, CT 06484-5458
203-929-6321

Electroscope, Inc.
4890 Sterling Dr.
Boulder, CO 80301
303-444-2600

Endomedix Corp.
2162 Michelson Drive
Irvine, CA 92715
714-253-1000

Ethicon Endo-Surgery
4545 Creek Road
Cincinnati, OH 45242
513-786-7000

Gabris Surgical Corp.
547 Susan Constant Dr.
Virginia Beach, VA 23451
804-491-6487

Hemostatix Corp.
190 S. Whisman Rd., Bldg. G
Mountain View, CA 94041
415-691-0882

Innovasive Devices, Inc.
100B South St.
Hopkinton, MA 01748
508-435-6000

Koros Surgical Instruments
610 Flinn Ave.
Moorpark, CA 93021-2008
818-889-5077

Laparomed Corp.
9272 Jeronimo Rd., Unit 109
Irvine, CA 92718-1914
714-768-1155

Leonard Medical Inc.
1464 Holcomb Rd.
Huntingdon Valley, PA 19006
215-938-1499

Li Medical Technologies, Inc.
7 Cambridge Dr.
Trumbull, CT 06611
203-371-2227

Linvatec Corporation
11311 Concept Blvd.
Largo, FL 34643-4908
813-399-5344

Marlow Surgical Technologies, Inc.
1810 Joseph Lloyd Pkwy.
Willoughby, OH 44094-8030
216-946-2453

Medchem Products, Inc.
232 W. Cummings Pk.
Woburn, MA 01801-6333
617-938-9328

Mediflex Surgical Products
250 Gibbs Rd.
Islandia, NY 11722-2697
516-582-8440

Megatech Medical, Inc.
1720 Belmont Ave., Bldg. E
Baltimore, MD 21244
410-944-8500

Microsurge, Inc.
150 A St.
Needham, MA 02194
617-444-2300

Microvasive/Boston Scientific Corp.
Urology Div.
480 Pleasant St.
Watertown, MA 02172
617-923-1720

Minorax Corp.
7015 147th St. SW
Edmonds, WA 98026
206-743-0178

Mist, Inc.
6307 E. Angus Dr.
Raleigh, NC 27613
919-787-8377

Multigon Industries, Inc.
559 Gramatan Ave.
Mt. Vernon, NY 10552-2155
914-664-7300

O.R. Concepts, Inc.
12250 Nicollet Ave. South
Burnsville, MN 55337
612-894-7523

Performance Surgical Instruments
40 Norfolk Ave.
Easton, MA 023334
508-230-0010

Quantum Instruments Corp.
17304 Preston Rd., Ste. 800
Dallas, TX 75252
214-733-6566

Redfield Corporation
210 Summit Ave.
Montvale, NJ 07645-1526
201-391-0494

Reznik Instrument, Inc.
7337 North Lawndale
Skokie, IL 60076
708-673-3444

Richard-Allan Medical Industries, Inc.
8850 M-89
P.O. Box 351
Richland, MI 49083-0351
616-629-5811

Rx Honing Machine Corporation
1301 East Fifth St.
Mishawaka, IN 46544-2827
219-259-1606

Sharpe Endosurgical Corp.
3750 Annapolis Lane, Ste. 135
Minneapolis, MN 55447
612-784-0460

Sherwood Intrascopic Div.
1915 Olive St.
St. Louis, MO 63103
314-241-5700

Storz Endoscopy-America Inc., Karl
10111 W. Jefferson Blvd.
Culver City, CA 90232-3509
310-558-1500

Storz GmbH & Co., Karl
Mittelstr. 8
Postfach 230
D-78532 Tuttlingen
Germany
07461/7080

Surgimark, Inc.
4706 West Nob Hill Blvd.
Yakima, WA 98908
509-965-1911

U.S. Endoscopy Group
7123 Industrial Park Blvd.
Mentor, OH 44060
216-269-8226

Unisurge, Inc.
10231 Bubb Rd.
Cupertino, CA 95014
408-996-4700

United States Surgical Corp.
150 Glover Ave.
Norwalk, CT 06856-5080
203-845-1000

Valleylab, Inc.
5920 Longbow Dr.
Boulder, CO 80301-3202
303-530-2300

Wolf Medical Instruments Corp., Richard
353 Corporate Woods Pkwy.
Vernon Hills, IL 60061-3110
708-913-1113

Ximed Medical Systems
2195 Trade Zone Blvd.
San Jose, CA 95131
408-945-4040

PHARYNGOSCOPE

Carsen Group Inc.
151 Telson Rd.
Markham, ONT L3R 1E7
Canada
416-479-4100

Fuji Photo Optical Co. Ltd.
1-324, Uetake-Machi, Omiya
Saitama 330
Japan
048/668-2153

Storz Endoscopy-America Inc., Karl
10111 W. Jefferson Blvd.
Culver City, CA 90232-3509
310-558-1500

Storz GmbH & Co., Karl
Mittelstr. 8
Postfach 230
D-78532 Tuttlingen
Germany
07461/7080

Treier Endoscopie AG
Sonnrain
CH-6215 Beromunster
Switzerland
045/512323

PROCTOSCOPE

ACM Endoskopie GmbH
Taunusstr. 38
D-80807 Muenchen 40
Germany
089/352355

Bashir, Jamil & Bros. Pvt. Ltd.
Khadim Ali Rd.
P.O. Box 7
Sialkot
Pakistan
0432-553862

Baxter Healthcare Corp.
Operating Room Div.
1500 Waukegan Rd.
McGaw Park, IL 60085-8210
708-473-1500

PROCTOSCOPE (cont'd)

Boehm Surgical Instrument Corp.
966 Chili Avenue
Rochester, NY 14611-2831
716-436-6584

Cameron-Miller, Inc.
3949 S. Racine Ave.
Chicago, IL 60609-2523
312-523-6360

Codman & Shurtleff, Inc.
41 Pacella Park Dr.
Randolph, MA 02368-1755
617-961-2300

Dittmar, Inc.
101 E. Laurel Ave.
P.O. Box 66
Cheltenham, PA 19012-2125
215-379-5533

Effner Biomet GmbH
Alt-Lankwitz 102
D-12247 Berlin 46
Germany
49/30-7700920

Electro Surgical Instrument Co.
37 Centennial St.
Rochester, NY 14611-1732
716-235-1430

Himalaya Trading Co., Ltd.
Wazirabad Rd.
P.O. Box No. 59
Sialkot
Pakistan
(0432) 552249

Link GmbH & Co., Waldemar
Barkhausenweg 10
Postfach 630 565
D-22339 Hamburg 63
Germany
040/5381021

Mader Instrument Corp.
25 Lamington Dr.
Succasunna, NJ 07876-2048
201-584-0816

Martin, Gebr. GmbH & Co. KG
Ludwigstaler Str. 132
Postf. 60
D-78532 Tuttlingen
Germany
07461/7060

Medicon Eg
15 Gansacker
Postfach 4455
D-78532 Tuttlingen
Germany
07462/20090

Medicon Instruments, Inc.
4405 International Blvd.
Norcross, GA 30093-3013
404-381-2858

Miltex Instrument Co., Inc.
6 Ohio Dr.
CB 5006
Lake Success, NY 11042-0006
516-775-7100

Rema Medizintechnik GmbH
In Breiten 10
D-78589 Duerbheim-Tuttlingen
Germany
07424-4064

Rose GmbH
Gottbillstr. 27-30
D-54294 Trier
Germany
0651/89051

Sharplan Lasers (Europe) Ltd.
141-155 Brent St.
London NW4 4DJ
United Kingdom
081/203-0006

Sklar Instrument Company
889 South Matlack St.
West Chester, PA 19380
215-430-3200

Storz Endoscopy-America Inc., Karl
10111 W. Jefferson Blvd.
Culver City, CA 90232-3509
310-558-1500

Storz GmbH & Co., Karl
Mittelstr. 8
Postfach 230
D-78532 Tuttlingen
Germany
07461/7080

Surgical Instrument Co. of America
1185 Edgewater Ave.
Ridgefield, NJ 07657-2102
201-941-6500

Ueth & Haug GmbH
Stockacher Str. 41/45
D-78532 Tuttlingen
Germany

Welch Allyn, Inc.
4341 State Street Rd.
P.O. Box 220
Skaneateles Falls, NY 13153-0220
315-685-4100

Wolf Medical Instruments Corp., Richard
353 Corporate Woods Pkwy.
Vernon Hills, IL 60061-3110
708-913-1113

PROCTOSIGMOIDOSCOPE

Abco Dealers, Inc.
6601 W. Mill Rd.
P.O. Box 23090
Milwaukee, WI 53218-0090
414-358-5420

Boehm Surgical Instrument Corp.
966 Chili Avenue
Rochester, NY 14611-2831
716-436-6584

Cameron-Miller, Inc.
3949 S. Racine Ave.
Chicago, IL 60609-2523
312-523-6360

Carsen Group Inc.
151 Telson Rd.
Markham, ONT L3R 1E7
Canada
416-479-4100

Electro Surgical Instrument Co.
37 Centennial St.
Rochester, NY 14611-1732
716-235-1430

Medicon Eg
15 Gansacker
Postfach 4455
D-78532 Tuttlingen
Germany
07462/20090

Medicon Instruments, Inc.
4405 International Blvd.
Norcross, GA 30093-3013
404-381-2858

Sharplan Lasers (Europe) Ltd.
141-155 Brent St.
London NW4 4DJ
United Kingdom
081/203-0006

Surgical Instrument Co. of America
1185 Edgewater Ave.
Ridgefield, NJ 07657-2102
201-941-6500

Welch Allyn, Inc.
4341 State Street Rd.
P.O. Box 220
Skaneateles Falls, NY 13153-0220
315-685-4100

PYELOSCOPE

Wolf Medical Instruments Corp., Richard
353 Corporate Woods Pkwy.
Vernon Hills, IL 60061-3110
708-913-1113

RESECTOSCOPE

Baxter Healthcare Corp.
Operating Room Div.
1500 Waukegan Rd.
McGaw Park, IL 60085-8210
708-473-1500

Cabot Medical Corp.
2021 Cabot Blvd. West
Langhorne, PA 19047-1875
215-752-8300

Carsen Group Inc.
151 Telson Rd.
Markham, ONT L3R 1E7
Canada
416-479-4100

Circon Acmi
300 Stillwater Ave.
Stamford, CT 06902-3640
203-328-8689

Coopersurgical, Inc.
15 Forest Pkwy.
Shelton, CT 06484-5458
203-929-6321

Keymed Medical & Industrial Equipment Ltd.
Keymed House, Stock Rd., Southend-on-Sea
Essex SS2 5QH
United Kingdom
0702/616333

Leisegang Medical, Inc.
6401 Congress Ave.
Boca Raton, FL 33487-2883
407-994-0202

Olympus America, Inc.
4 Nevada Drive
Lake Success, NY 11042-1179
516-488-3880

Olympus Optical Co. Ltd.
San-Ei Bldg.
1-22-2, Nishi-Shinjuku
Shinjuku-Ku, Tokyo 163-91
Japan
03/3402111

Storz Endoscopy-America Inc., Karl
10111 W. Jefferson Blvd.
Culver City, CA 90232-3509
310-558-1500

Storz GmbH & Co., Karl
Mittelstr. 8
Postfach 230
D-78532 Tuttlingen
Germany
07461/7080

Treier Endoscopie AG
Sonnrain
CH-6215 Beromunster
Switzerland
045/512323

Wid-Med, Inc.
111 N. Wabash Ave.
Chicago, IL 60602-1903
312 236-8586

Wolf Medical Instruments Corp., Richard
353 Corporate Woods Pkwy.
Vernon Hills, IL 60061-3110
708-913-1113

SIGMOIDOSCOPE, FLEXIBLE

Asahi Optical Co., Ltd.
2-36-9, Maeno-Cho, Itabashi-Ku
Tokyo 174
Japan
03/3960-5155

Carsen Group Inc.
151 Telson Rd.
Markham, ONT L3R 1E7
Canada
416-479-4100

Circon Acmi
300 Stillwater Ave.
Stamford, CT 06902-3640
203-328-8689

Fuji Photo Optical Co. Ltd.
1-324, Uetake-Machi, Omiya
Saitama 330
Japan
048/668-2153

Fujinon (Europe) GmbH
Heerdter Lohweg 89
D-40549 Duesseldorf 11
Germany
0211/52050

Fujinon, Inc.
10 High Point Dr.
Wayne, NJ 07470-7434
201-633-5600

Olympus America, Inc.
4 Nevada Drive
Lake Success, NY 11042-1179
516-488-3880

Olympus Optical Co. Ltd.
San-Ei Bldg.
1-22-2, Nishi-Shinjuku
Shinjuku-Ku, Tokyo 163-91
Japan
03/3402111

Pentax Precision Instrument Corp.
30 Ramland Rd.
Orangeburg, NY 10962-2699
914-365-0700

Schott Fiber Optics, Inc.
122 Charlton St.
Southbridge, MA 01550-1960
508-765-9744

Timesco of London
176 Pentonville Rd.
London N1 9JP
United Kingdom
071/278-0712-3

Welch Allyn, Inc.
4341 State Street Rd.
P.O. Box 220
Skaneateles Falls, NY 13153-0220
315-685-4100

SIGMOIDOSCOPE, RIGID, ELECTRICAL

Himalaya Trading Co., Ltd.
Wazirabad Rd.
P.O. Box No. 59
Sialkot
Pakistan
(0432) 552249

Martin, Gebr. GmbH & Co. KG
Ludwigstaler Str. 132
Postf. 60
D-78532 Tuttlingen
Germany
07461/7060

Welch Allyn, Inc.
4341 State Street Rd.
P.O. Box 220
Skaneateles Falls, NY 13153-0220
315-685-4100

SIGMOIDOSCOPE, RIGID, NON-ELECTRICAL

Abco Dealers, Inc.
6601 W. Mill Rd.
P.O. Box 23090
Milwaukee, WI 53218-0090
414-358-5420

Baxter Healthcare Corp.
Operating Room Div.
1500 Waukegan Rd.
McGaw Park, IL 60085-8210
708-473-1500

Boehm Surgical Instrument Corp.
966 Chili Avenue
Rochester, NY 14611-2831
716-436-6584

Cameron-Miller, Inc.
3949 S. Racine Ave.
Chicago, IL 60609-2523
312-523-6360

SIGMOIDOSCOPE, RIGID, NON-ELECTRICAL (cont'd)

Himalaya Trading Co., Ltd.
Wazirabad Rd.
P.O. Box No. 59
Sialkot
Pakistan
(0432) 552249

Leibinger GmbH
Botzinger Strasse 41
D-70437 Freiburg
Germany
0761/49058-0

Martin, Gebr. GmbH & Co. KG
Ludwigstaler Str. 132
Postf. 60
D-78532 Tuttlingen
Germany
07461/7060

Medicon Instruments, Inc.
4405 International Blvd.
Norcross, GA 30093-3013
404-381-2858

Sharplan Lasers (Europe) Ltd.
141-155 Brent St.
London NW4 4DJ
United Kingdom
081/203-0006

Storz Endoscopy-America Inc., Karl
10111 W. Jefferson Blvd.
Culver City, CA 90232-3509
310-558-1500

Storz GmbH & Co., Karl
Mittelstr. 8
Postfach 230
D-78532 Tuttlingen
Germany
07461/7080

Surgical Instrument Co. of America
1185 Edgewater Ave.
Ridgefield, NJ 07657-2102
201-941-6500

Ueth & Haug GmbH
Stockacher Str. 41/45
D-78532 Tuttlingen
Germany

Welch Allyn, Inc.
4341 State Street Rd.
P.O. Box 220
Skaneateles Falls, NY 13153-0220
315-685-4100

Wolf Medical Instruments Corp., Richard
353 Corporate Woods Pkwy.
Vernon Hills, IL 60061-3110
708-913-1113

SPHINCTEROSCOPE

Himalaya Trading Co., Ltd.
Wazirabad Rd.
P.O. Box No. 59
Sialkot
Pakistan
(0432) 552249

Sklar Instrument Company
889 South Matlack St.
West Chester, PA 19380
215-430-3200

Ueth & Haug GmbH
Stockacher Str. 41/45
D-78532 Tuttlingen
Germany

THORACOSCOPE

Access Surgical International, Inc.
15 Caswell Ln.
Boat Yard Square
Plymouth, MA 02360
508-747-6006

Advanced Surgical, Inc.
305 College Rd. East
Princeton, NJ 08540
609-987-2340

Aesculap
1000 Gateway Blvd.
South San Francisco, CA 94080-7030
415-876-7000

Bei Medical Systems
83 Hobart St.
Hackensack, NJ 07601
201-489-4222

BioEnterics Corporation
1035A Cindy Lane
Carpinteria, CA 93013
805-684-3045

Birtcher Medical Systems, Inc.
50 Technology Dr.
Irvine, CA 92718-2301
714-753-9400

Bryan Corp.
4 Plympton St.
Woburn, MA 01801-2908
617-935-0004

Cabot Medical Corp.
2021 Cabot Blvd. West
Langhorne, PA 19047-1875
215-752-8300

Circon Acmi
300 Stillwater Ave.
Stamford, CT 06902-3640
203-328-8689

Depuy, Inc.
700 Orthopaedic Dr.
P.O. Box 988
Warsaw, IN 46581-0988
219-267-8143

Fujinon, Inc.
10 High Point Dr.
Wayne, NJ 07470-7434
201-633-5600

Gabris Surgical Corp.
547 Susan Constant Dr.
Virginia Beach, VA 23451
804-491-6487

K+A Medical
413 Oak Pl., Bldg. 6J
Port Orange, FL 32127-4352
904-767-0229

Leonard Medical Inc.
1464 Holcomb Rd.
Huntingdon Valley, PA 19006
215-938-1499

Linvatec Corporation
11311 Concept Blvd.
Largo, FL 34643-4908
813-399-5344

Microsurge, Inc.
150 A St.
Needham, MA 02194
617-444-2300

Olympus America, Inc.
4 Nevada Drive
Lake Success, NY 11042-1179
516-488-3880

Pilling-Rusch
420 Delaware Dr.
Fort Washington, PA 19034-2711
215-643-2600

Precision Optics Corp.
22 E. Broadway
Gardner, MA 01440-3338
508-630-1800

Sherwood Intrascopic Div.
1915 Olive St.
St. Louis, MO 63103
314-241-5700

Smith & Nephew Dyonics, Inc.
160 Dascomb Rd.
Andover, MA 01810-5893
508-470-2800

Snowden-Pencer
5175 S. Royal Atlanta Dr.
Tucker, GA 30084-3053
404-496-0952

Storz Endoscopy-America Inc., Karl
10111 W. Jefferson Blvd.
Culver City, CA 90232-3509
310-558-1500

Storz GmbH & Co., Karl
Mittelstr. 8
Postfach 230
D-78532 Tuttlingen
Germany
07461/7080

Surgical Technologies International, Inc.
4715 NW 157th St., #212
Miami, FL 33014
305-623-0363

Welch Allyn, Inc.
4341 State Street Rd.
P.O. Box 220
Skaneateles Falls, NY 13153-0220
315-685-4100

Wolf Medical Instruments Corp., Richard
353 Corporate Woods Pkwy.
Vernon Hills, IL 60061-3110
708-913-1113

Ximed Medical Systems
2195 Trade Zone Blvd.
San Jose, CA 95131
408-945-4040

TRANSFORMER, ENDOSCOPE

Berchtold KG, Gebr.
Weimarstr. 13-15
D-78532 Tuttlingen
Germany
07461/2345

Buck GmbH, Rudolf
Obere Hauptstr. 40/1
Wurmlingen-Tuttlingen D-78573
Germany
07/461-3535

Martin, Gebr. GmbH & Co. KG
Ludwigstaler Str. 132
Postf. 60
D-78532 Tuttlingen
Germany
07461/7060

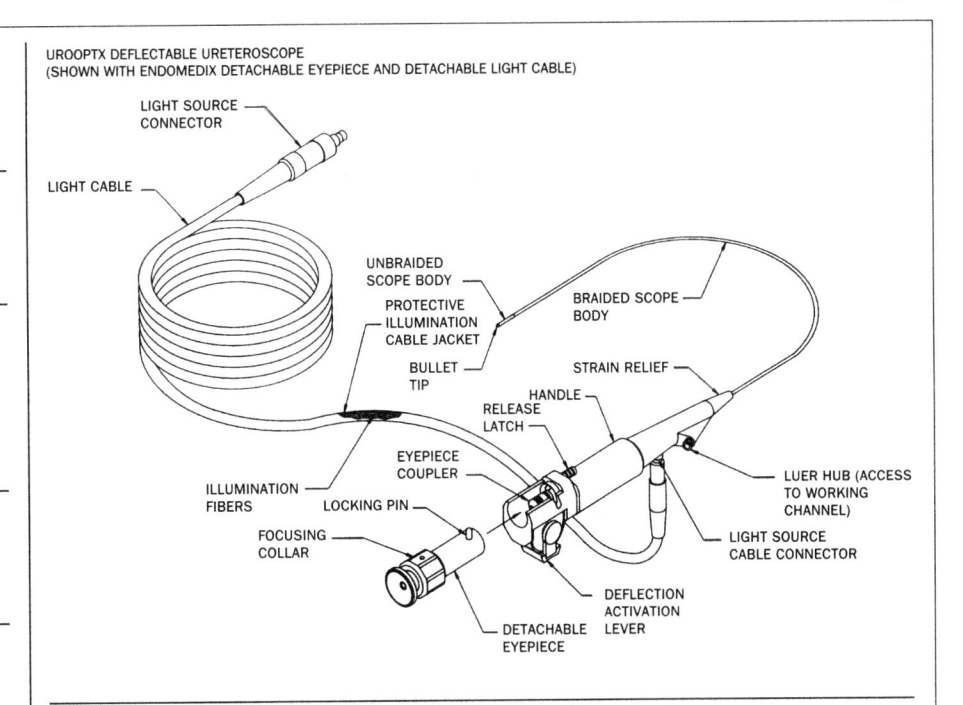

UROOPTX DEFLECTABLE URETEROSCOPE
(SHOWN WITH ENDOMEDIX DETACHABLE EYEPIECE AND DETACHABLE LIGHT CABLE)

URETEROSCOPE

Endomedix Corp.
2162 Michelson Dr.
Irvine, CA 92715
714-253-1000

UROOPTX

DESCRIPTION: The UroOptx™ Deflectable Ureteroscope is a device intended for diagnostic and therapeutic procedures within the urinary system. This Ureteroscope is a flexible, actively deflectable, fiberoptic endoscope which can be introduced into the ureter directly or through an instrument from natural or created orifices. The UroOptx Ureteroscope is nonrepairable; however, it may be reused following appropriate inspection, cleaning, and sterilization or disinfection. The small size, bi-directional deflectable tip and high level of torque make this Ureteroscope suitable for use in routine and specialized urologic procedures. Use of the UroOptx Ureteroscope is limited to physicians who have been trained in the use of flexible ureteroscopes and in generally accepted techniques for performing ureteroscopy.

WARNINGS: Do not force the UroOptx Ureteroscope if it will not pass easily, this may cause trauma to the tissue or damage the device. Potential complications from use of the UroOptx Ureteroscope are the same as those generally associated with catheterization or endoscopy of the ureter. They include ureteral avulsion, ureteral perforation, infection, hemorrhage, extravasation, stenosis and stricture.

INSTRUCTIONS FOR USE: Using standard operative procedures, insert the Deflectable Tip of the UroOptx Ureteroscope in an undeflected position directly or through a cystoscope or introducer into a natural or created orifice into the ureter. Infuse sterile saline through the working channel as necessary to maintain a clear field of view. Continue advancing the UroOptx Ureteroscope, as appropriate, using the deflection mechanism to maintain the lumen within the field of view until the desired endpoint is reached. At the conclusion of the procedure, withdraw the UroOptx Ureteroscope with the tip in the undeflected position using standard techniques.

Accessory instruments measuring 3 Fr, or smaller, are optimal for use with the UroOptx Ureteroscope and may be passed through the working channel. Instrument sizes should be selected to allow for sufficient irrigation. Simultaneous irrigation while using an instrument in the working channel can be achieved by connecting a Y-Adaptor such as the EndoMedix Y-Adaptor (Model S160) to the Luer Hub on the Scope Handle.

CARE & MAINTENANCE: The UroOptx Ureteroscope must be sterilized by an ethylene oxide (EtO) gas sterilization process. If the UroOptx Ureteroscope is disinfected after previous sterilization (such as between consecutive cases), it may be totally immersed in a high level chemical disinfectant such as 2% alkaline glutaraldehyde. Keep the Ureteroscope and Eyepiece joined together during cleaning and disinfecting between consecutive cases, until preparation for the next sterilization cycle, at which time they should be separated for cleaning and EtO sterilizing. Do not autoclave.

The number of times the UroOptx Ureteroscope may be used depends upon the amount of care exerted when handling, using, cleaning, sterilizing or disinfecting, and storing this device.

URETEROSCOPE (cont'd)

SPECIFICATIONS/HOW SUPPLIED: The UroOptx Ureteroscope is supplied as a single nonsterile unit with the UroOptx Scope Sheath attached. The EndoMedix Detachable Eyepiece is required for use with the UroOptx Ureteroscope, but it must be procured separately. The UroOptx Ureteroscope (Model S760UR) has a 7.6 Fr body size, 3.6 Fr working channel diameter, usable length of 70 cm and a tip deflecting range of -60° to +60°.

Bard Urological
8195 Industrial Blvd.
Covington, GA 30209-2656
404-784-6113

Circon Acmi
300 Stillwater Ave.
Stamford, CT 06902-3640
203-328-8689

Electro Fiberoptics Corporation
56 Hudson St.
Northborough, MA 01532-1922
508-393-3753

Intramed Labs
11100 Roselle Street
San Diego, CA 92121-1210
619-455-5000

Life Medical Technologies, Inc.
3649 W. 1987 S.
Salt Lake City, UT 84104
801-972-1900

Olympus America, Inc.
4 Nevada Drive
Lake Success, NY 11042-1179
516-488-3880

Olympus Optical Co. Ltd.
San-Ei Bldg.
1-22-2, Nishi-Shinjuku
Shinjuku-Ku, Tokyo 163-91
Japan
03/3402111

Omega Universal Technologies Ltd.
Omega House, 211 New North Rd.
London, N1 6UT
United Kingdom
71/490-1318

Ovamed Corporation
111 W. Evelyn Ave. Ste. #214
Sunnyvale, CA 94086-6129
408-720-9876

Pentax Precision Instrument Corp.
30 Ramland Rd.
Orangeburg, NY 10962-2699
914-365-0700

Schott Fiber Optics, Inc.
122 Charlton St.
Southbridge, MA 01550-1960
508-765-9744

Storz Endoscopy-America Inc., Karl
10111 W. Jefferson Blvd.
Culver City, CA 90232-3509
310-558-1500

Storz GmbH & Co., Karl
Mittelstr. 8
Postfach 230
D-78532 Tuttlingen
Germany
07461/7080

Surgitek
3037 Mt. Pleasant St.
Racine, WI 53404-1509
414-639-7205

Wolf Medical Instruments Corp., Richard
353 Corporate Woods Pkwy.
Vernon Hills, IL 60061-3110
708-913-1113

URETHROSCOPE

Bauer & Haselbarth GmbH
Sauerbruchstr. 7 - Postfach
D-25479 Ellerau Bei Hamburg
Germany
04106/72091

Baxter Healthcare Corp.
Operating Room Div.
1500 Waukegan Rd.
McGaw Park, IL 60085-8210
708-473-1500

Carsen Group Inc.
151 Telson Rd.
Markham, ONT L3R 1E7
Canada
416-479-4100

Keymed Medical & Industrial Equipment Ltd.
Keymed House, Stock Rd., Southend-on-Sea
Essex SS2 5QH
United Kingdom
0702/616333

Storz Endoscopy-America Inc., Karl
10111 W. Jefferson Blvd.
Culver City, CA 90232-3509
310-558-1500

Storz GmbH & Co., Karl
Mittelstr. 8
Postfach 230
D-78532 Tuttlingen
Germany
07461/7080

Wolf Medical Instruments Corp., Richard
353 Corporate Woods Pkwy.
Vernon Hills, IL 60061-3110
708-913-1113

VAGINOSCOPE

Rema Medizintechnik GmbH
In Breiten 10
D-78589 Duerbheim-Tuttlingen
Germany
07424-4064

Storz Endoscopy-America Inc., Karl
10111 W. Jefferson Blvd.
Culver City, CA 90232-3509
310-558-1500

Storz GmbH & Co., Karl
Mittelstr. 8
Postfach 230
D-78532 Tuttlingen
Germany
07461/7080

Wisap USA
P.O. Box 324
Tomball, TX 77377-0324
713-351-2629

Wolf Medical Instruments Corp., Richard
353 Corporate Woods Pkwy.
Vernon Hills, IL 60061-3110
708-913-1113

Esophagoscope

ESOPHAGOSCOPE (FLEXIBLE OR RIGID)

Asahi Optical Co., Ltd.
2-36-9, Maeno-Cho, Itabashi-Ku
Tokyo 174
Japan
03/3960-5155

Baxter Healthcare Corp.
Operating Room Div.
1500 Waukegan Rd.
McGaw Park, IL 60085-8210
708-473-1500

Boehm Surgical Instrument Corp.
966 Chili Avenue
Rochester, NY 14611-2831
716-436-6584

Carsen Group Inc.
151 Telson Rd.
Markham, ONT L3R 1E7
Canada
416-479-4100

Fuji Photo Optical Co. Ltd.
1-324, Uetake-Machi, Omiya
Saitama 330
Japan
048/668-2153

Life Medical Technologies, Inc.
3649 W. 1987 S.
Salt Lake City, UT 84104
801-972-1900

Medicon Eg
15 Gansacker
Postfach 4455
D-78532 Tuttlingen
Germany
07462/20090

Olympus America, Inc.
4 Nevada Drive
Lake Success, NY 11042-1179
516-488-3880

Olympus Optical Co. Ltd.
San-Ei Bldg.
1-22-2, Nishi-Shinjuku
Shinjuku-Ku, Tokyo 163-91
Japan
03/3402111

Pilling-Rusch
420 Delaware Dr.
Fort Washington, PA 19034-2711
215-643-2600

Storz Endoscopy-America Inc., Karl
10111 W. Jefferson Blvd.
Culver City, CA 90232-3509
310-558-1500

Storz GmbH & Co., Karl
Mittelstr. 8
Postfach 230
D-78532 Tuttlingen
Germany
07461/7080

Wolf Medical Instruments Corp., Richard
353 Corporate Woods Pkwy.
Vernon Hills, IL 60061-3110
708-913-1113

ESOPHAGOSCOPE, RIGID, GASTRO-UROLOGY

Kelleher Medical, Inc.
9710 Farrar Court, Suite N
Richmond, VA 23236
804-323-4040

Medicon Instruments, Inc.
4405 International Blvd.
Norcross, GA 30093-3013
404-381-2858

Forceps

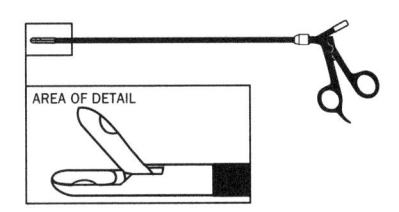

FORCEPS, BIOPSY

Davis & Geck Endosurgery
1 Casper St.
Danbury, CT 06810
203-743-4451

PROFESSIONAL LINE 8377 SERIES

DESCRIPTION:
Spoon Cup Biopsy Forceps (order number 8377-01):
 Locking spring incorporated in the instrument shaft, 10mm diameter, insulated, monopolar connection, working length 33cm. For gallstone retrieval in the abdomen and tissue biopsy:

SPOON CUP BIOPSY FORCEPS

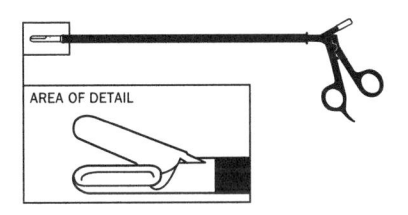

AREA OF DETAIL

Excision Biopsy Forceps (order number 8377-02):
 Locking spring incorporated in the instrument shaft, 5mm diameter, insulated, monopolar connection, working length 33cm, color coded yellow. For removing tissue samples:

EXCISION BIOPSY FORCEPS

AREA OF DETAIL

FORCEPS, BIOPSY *(cont'd)*

Cutting Biopsy Forceps (order number 8377-03):

Serrated, locking spring incorporated in the instrument shaft, 5mm diameter, insulated, monopolar connection, working length 33cm, color coded yellow. For removing tissue samples:

CUTTING BIOPSY FORCEPS

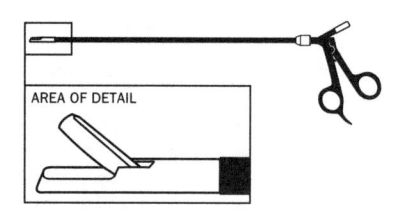

AREA OF DETAIL

Baxter Healthcare Corp., V. Mueller Div.
6600 W. Touhy
Niles, IL 60714
708-647-9383

Chirurgische Instrumente
Hauptstrasse 18
D-78582 Balgheim
Germany
7424/501319

Davis & Geck Div.
American Cyanamid Company
One Cyanamid Plaza
Wayne, NJ 07470-2012
201-831-2000

Leisegang Medical, Inc.
6401 Congress Ave.
Boca Raton, FL 33487-2883
407-994-0202

U.S. Endoscopy Group
7123 Industrial Park Blvd.
Mentor, OH 44060
216-269-8226

FORCEPS, ELECTROSURGICAL

Accurate Surgical & Scientific Instrument Corp.
300 Shames Dr.
Westbury, NY 11590-1736
516-333-2570

Aspen Laboratories, Inc.
P.O. Box 3936
Englewood, CO 80155-3936
303-798-5800

Birtcher Medical Systems, Inc.
50 Technology Dr.
Irvine, CA 92718-2301
714-753-9400

Cabot Medical Corp.
2021 Cabot Blvd. West
Langhorne, PA 19047-1875
215-752-8300

Cameron-Miller, Inc.
3949 S. Racine Ave.
Chicago, IL 60609-2523
312-523-6360

Codman & Shurtleff, Inc.
41 Pacella Park Dr.
Randolph, MA 02368-1755
617-961-2300

Elmed, Inc.
60 W. Fay Ave.
Addison, IL 60101-5198
708-543-2792

Erbe Elektromedizin GmbH
Waldhoernle Str. 17
D-72072 Tuebingen
Germany
07071/70010

Everest Medical Corp.
13755 First Avenue. N.
Minneapolis, MN 55441-5454
612-473-6262

Geister Medizintechnik GmbH
Foehrenstr. 2
Postfach 4228
D-78532 Tuttlingen
Germany
7461-8084

Jedmed Instruments Co.
6096 Lemay Ferry Rd.
St. Louis, MO 63129-2217
314-845-3770

Kirwan Surgical Products, Inc.
83 East Water St.
P.O. Box 545
Rockland, MA 02370-1837
617-878-2706

L&M Instruments, Inc.
P.O.Box 2070
Sunnyvale, CA 94087-0070
408-733-5858

Nopa Instruments Medizintechnik GmbH
Gansacker 9 - Postfach 4554
D-78532 Tuttlingen
Germany
07462/7801

Olsen Electrosurgical Inc.
2100 Meridian Park Blvd.
Concord, CA 94520-5709
510-825-8151

Pilling-Rusch
420 Delaware Dr.
Fort Washington, PA 19034-2711
215-643-2600

Storz Endoscopy-America Inc., Karl
10111 W. Jefferson Blvd.
Culver City, CA 90232-3509
310-558-1500

Storz GmbH & Co., Karl
Mittelstr. 8
Postfach 230
D-78532 Tuttlingen
Germany
07461/7080

Surgical Instrument Co. of America
1185 Edgewater Ave.
Ridgefield, NJ 07657-2102
201-941-6500

Valleylab, Inc.
5920 Longbow Dr.
Boulder, CO 80301-3202
303-530-2300

Weck & Co. Inc., Edward
1 Weck Dr.
P.O. Box 12600
Research Triangle Park, NC 27709
919-544-8000

Wect Instrument Company, Inc.
5645 N. Ravenswood
Chicago, IL 60660-3922
312-769-1944

Westco Medical Corp.
7079 Mission Gorge Rd., Bldg. J
San Diego, CA 92120-2455
619-286-1600

Wolf Medical Instruments Corp., Richard
353 Corporate Woods Pkwy.
Vernon Hills, IL 60061-3110
708-913-1113

Yole Company
51 Boulevard
Greenlawn, NY 11740-1401
516-757-9336

FORCEPS, ENDOSCOPIC

A&A Medical, Inc.
11485 Mountain Laurel Dr.
Roswell, GA 30075
800-424-1234

Access Surgical International, Inc.
15 Caswell Ln.
Boat Yard Square
Plymouth, MA 02360
508-747-6006

Aesculap
1000 Gateway Blvd.
South San Francisco, CA 94080-7030
415-876-7000

Aesculap AG
Moehringerstr. 125
Postfach 40
D-78532 Tuttlingen
Germany
00149/0746951

Bard Ventures
1200 Technology Park Dr.
Billerica, MA 01821
508-667-1300

Baxter Healthcare Corp.
Operating Room Div.
1500 Waukegan Rd.
McGaw Park, IL 60085-8210
708-473-1500

Birtcher Medical Systems, Inc.
50 Technology Dr.
Irvine, CA 92718-2301
714-753-9400

Bryan Corp.
4 Plympton St.
Woburn, MA 01801-2908
617-935-0004

Cabot Medical Corp.
2021 Cabot Blvd. West
Langhorne, PA 19047-1875
215-752-8300

Cameron-Miller, Inc.
3949 S. Racine Ave.
Chicago, IL 60609-2523
312-523-6360

Circon Acmi
300 Stillwater Ave.
Stamford, CT 06902-3640
203-328-8689

Collin - Gentile Drapier
69 71 Ave. La Place
Boite Postal 31
F-94114 Arcueil
France
1/46571235

Coopersurgical, Inc.
15 Forest Pkwy.
Shelton, CT 06484-5458
203-929-6321

Core Dynamics, Inc.
11222-4 St. Johns Indust. Pkwy.
Jacksonville, FL 32216
904-641-6611

Davis & Geck Div.
American Cyanamid Company
One Cyanamid Plaza
Wayne, NJ 07470-2012
201-831-2000

Davol, Inc.
100 Sockanossett
P.O. Box 8500
Cranston, RI 02920-0500
401-463-7000

Depuy, Inc.
700 Orthopaedic Dr.
P.O. Box 988
Warsaw, IN 46581-0988
219-267-8143

Diener, Christian
Rudolf Diesel Str. 18
D-78532 Tuttlingen
Germany
7461/71067

Elekta Instruments, Inc.
8 Executive Park West, Ste. 809
Atlanta, GA 30329
404-315-1225

Elmed, Inc.
60 W. Fay Ave.
Addison, IL 60101-5198
708-543-2792

Ethicon Endo-Surgery
4545 Creek Road
Cincinnati, OH 45242
513-786-7000

Everest Medical Corp.
13755 First Avenue. N.
Minneapolis, MN 55441-5454
612-473-6262

Frantz Medical Development Ltd.
7740 Metric Drive
Mentor, OH 44060-4862
216-255-1155

Geister Medizintechnik GmbH
Foehrenstr. 2
Postfach 4228
D-78532 Tuttlingen
Germany
7461-8084

Globe Medical, Inc. (Endo Scientific)
9291 130th Ave. N., Ste. 410
Largo, FL 34643
813-585-9700

Heraeus Surgical, Inc.
575 Cottonwood Dr.
Milpitas, CA 95035-7402
408-954-4000

Innovative Surgical, Inc.
3071 Continental Dr., Ste. 102
West Palm Beach, FL 33407
407-697-5051

Instrument Makar, Inc.
2950 E. Mt. Hope
Okemos, MI 48864-1910
517-332-3593

Jarit Instruments
9 Skyline Dr.
Hawthorne, NY 10532-2119
914-592-9050

Kensey Nash Corporation
55 E. Uwchlan Ave., Ste. 204
Exton, PA 19341-1247
215-524-0188

Kirwan Surgical Products, Inc.
83 East Water St.
P.O. Box 545
Rockland, MA 02370-1837
617-878-2706

L&M Instruments, Inc.
P.O.Box 2070
Sunnyvale, CA 94087-0070
408-733-5858

Leisegang Medical, Inc.
6401 Congress Ave.
Boca Raton, FL 33487-2883
407-994-0202

Life Medical Technologies, Inc.
3649 W. 1987 S.
Salt Lake City, UT 84104
801-972-1900

FORCEPS, ENDOSCOPIC
(cont'd)

Marlow Surgical Technologies, Inc.
1810 Joseph Lloyd Pkwy.
Willoughby, OH 44094-8030
216-946-2453

Medicon Eg
15 Gansacker
Postfach 4455
D-78532 Tuttlingen
Germany
07462/20090

Medicon Instruments, Inc.
4405 International Blvd.
Norcross, GA 30093-3013
404-381-2858

Mill-Rose Laboratories
7310 Corporate Blvd.
Mentor, OH 44060-4856
216-255-7995

Mist, Inc.
6307 E. Angus Dr.
Raleigh, NC 27613
919-787-8377

Nopa Instruments Medizintechnik GmbH
Gansacker 9 - Postfach 4554
D-78532 Tuttlingen
Germany
07462/7801

Olympus America, Inc.
4 Nevada Drive
Lake Success, NY 11042-1179
516-488-3880

Olympus Optical Co. Ltd.
San-Ei Bldg.
1-22-2, Nishi-Shinjuku
Shinjuku-Ku, Tokyo 163-91
Japan
03/3402111

Olympus Winter & Ibe GmbH
Kuehnstrasse 61, Postf. 701709
D-22045 Hamburg 70
Germany
040/66966-0

Origin Medsystems, Inc.
135 Constitution Dr.
Menlo Park, CA 94025
415-617-5000

Performance Surgical Instruments
40 Norfolk Ave.
Easton, MA 023334
508-230-0010

Phillips Medical Group
562 East Chatham St.
Cary, NC 27511
919-469-4641

Pilling-Rusch
420 Delaware Dr.
Fort Washington, PA 19034-2711
215-643-2600

Portlyn Medical Products
Route 25
Moultonboro, NH 03254
603-476-5538

Smith & Nephew Dyonics, Inc.
160 Dascomb Rd.
Andover, MA 01810-5893
508-470-2800

Smith & Nephew Richards Inc.
1450 Brooks Road
Memphis, TN 38116
901-396-2121

Snowden-Pencer
5175 S. Royal Atlanta Dr.
Tucker, GA 30084-3053
404-496-0952

Storz Endoscopy-America Inc., Karl
10111 W. Jefferson Blvd.
Culver City, CA 90232-3509
310-558-1500

Storz GmbH & Co., Karl
Mittelstr. 8
Postfach 230
D-78532 Tuttlingen
Germany
07461/7080

Surgical Instrument Co. of America
1185 Edgewater Ave.
Ridgefield, NJ 07657-2102
201-941-6500

Synectic Engineering, Inc.
4 Oxford Rd.
Milford, CT 06460-7007
203-877-8488

Unisurge, Inc.
10231 Bubb Rd.
Cupertino, CA 95014
408-996-4700

United States Surgical Corp.
150 Glover Ave.
Norwalk, CT 06856-5080
203-845-1000

Weck & Co. Inc., Edward
1 Weck Dr.
P.O. Box 12600
Research Triangle Park, NC 27709
919-544-8000

Wect Instrument Company, Inc.
5645 N. Ravenswood
Chicago, IL 60660-3922
312-769-1944

WM Instrumente GmbH
Panoramastr. 6
D-78604 Rietheim 1
Germany
07424/501310

Wolf Medical Instruments Corp., Richard
353 Corporate Woods Pkwy.
Vernon Hills, IL 60061-3110
708-913-1113

FORCEPS, GRASPING, ATRAUMATIC

Davis & Geck Endosurgery
1 Casper St.
Danbury, CT 06810
203-743-4451

PROFESSIONAL LINE 8375 SERIES

DESCRIPTION:

Tubal Grasping Forceps:
Smooth, insulated monopolar connection, color coded green. For fixing and holding the fallopian tube. May also be used for blunt dissecting:

TUBAL GRASPING FORCEPS

TUBAL GRASPING FORCEPS

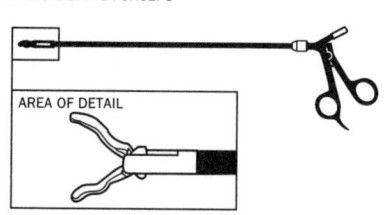

PRODUCT CODE	DIAMETER MM	SHAFT LENGTH CM	FLUSH PORT
8375-08	5	33	No
8375-14	10	33	No
8375-15	5	45	Yes

Davis & Geck Endosurgery
1 Casper St.
Danbury, CT 06810
203-743-4451

PROFESSIONAL LINE
8376 - 8450-14 SERIES
DESCRIPTION:
Babcock Tissue Grasping Forceps:
Atraumatic forceps with single-action jaw pattern and ratchet lock for fixation, holding and manipulation of organs:

BABCOCK TISSUE GRASPING FORCEPS

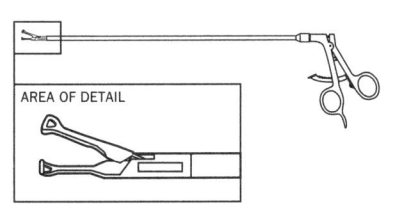

AREA OF DETAIL

Intestinal Grasping Forceps (Dorsey) (order number 8376-21):
For fixation, holding and manipulation of intestinal tissue, with ratchet handle. The long branches and fenestration in the branches allow safe and careful grasping of tissue:

INTESTINAL GRASPING FORCEPS

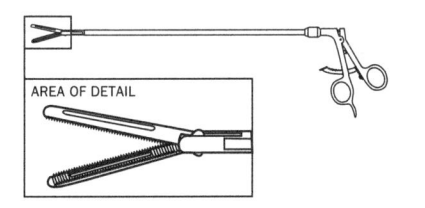

AREA OF DETAIL

Davis & Geck Endosurgery
1 Casper St.
Danbury, CT 06810
203-743-4451

PROFESSIONAL LINE
8376 - 8450-15 SERIES
DESCRIPTION:
Tissue and Swab Forceps (Heywood-Smith):
Insulated, monopolar connection with ratchet lock, without closing spring, color coded green. For blunt dissection by sponge: also for fixation, holding and manipulation of organs and tissue:

TISSUE AND SWAB FORCEPS

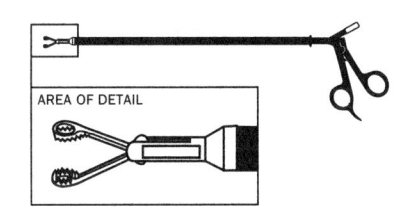

AREA OF DETAIL

BABCOCK TISSUE GRASPING FORCEPS

PRODUCT CODE	DIAMETER MM	SHAFT LENGTH CM	360° ROTATION	INSULATED MONOPOLAR	CURVED SHAFT	D-TACH
8376-19	5	33	No	No	No	No
8376-20	10	40	No	No	No	No
8390-25	5	35	Yes	Yes	No	Yes
8390-32	10	42	Yes	Yes	No	Yes
8450-14	5	33	Yes	No	Yes	No

INTESTINAL GRASPING FORCEPS

PRODUCT CODE	DIAMETER MM	SHAFT LENGTH CM	360° ROTATION	INSULATED MONOPOLAR	RATCHET LOCK	D-TACH
8376-21	5	40	No	No	Yes	No
8390-34	5	42	Yes	Yes	Yes	Yes

TISSUE AND SWAB FORCEPS

PRODUCT CODE	DIAMETER MM	SHAFT LENGTH CM	360° ROTATION	INSULATED MONOPOLAR	RATCHET LOCK	CURVED SHAFT	D-TACH
8376-22	10	33	No	Yes	Yes	No	No
8376-23	10	40	No	Yes	Yes	No	No
8390-33	10	35	Yes	Yes	Yes	No	Yes
8450-15	10	33	Yes	Yes	Yes	Yes	No

Access Surgical International, Inc.
15 Caswell Ln.
Boat Yard Square
Plymouth, MA 02360
508-747-6006

Aesculap
1000 Gateway Blvd.
South San Francisco, CA 94080-7030
415-876-7000

Birtcher Medical Systems, Inc.
50 Technology Dr.
Irvine, CA 92718-2301
714-753-9400

Boss Instruments, Ltd.
1310 Central Ct.
Hermitage, TN 37076
615-885-2231

Bryan Corp.
4 Plympton St.
Woburn, MA 01801-2908
617-935-0004

Cabot Medical Corp.
2021 Cabot Blvd. West
Langhorne, PA 19047-1875
215-752-8300

Chirurgische Instrumente
Hauptstrasse 18
D-78582 Balgheim
Germany
7424/501319

Coopersurgical, Inc.
15 Forest Pkwy.
Shelton, CT 06484-5458
203-929-6321

Core Dynamics, Inc.
11222-4 St. Johns Indust. Pkwy.
Jacksonville, FL 32216
904-641-6611

DaVinci Medical, Inc.
13700 First Ave. North
Minneapolis, MN 55441
612-473-4245

Davis & Geck Div.
American Cyanamid Company
One Cyanamid Plaza
Wayne, NJ 07470-2012
201-831-2000

Davol, Inc.
100 Sockanossett
P.O. Box 8500
Cranston, RI 02920-0500
401-463-7000

Elekta Instruments, Inc.
8 Executive Park West, Ste. 809
Atlanta, GA 30329
404-315-1225

FORCEPS, GRASPING, ATRAUMATIC (cont'd)

Elmed, Inc.
60 W. Fay Ave.
Addison, IL 60101-5198
708-543-2792

Ethicon Endo-Surgery
4545 Creek Road
Cincinnati, OH 45242
513-786-7000

Heraeus Surgical, Inc.
575 Cottonwood Dr.
Milpitas, CA 95035-7402
408-954-4000

Innovative Surgical, Inc..
3071 Continental Dr., Ste. 102
West Palm Beach, FL 33407
407-697-5051

Instrument Makar, Inc.
2950 E. Mt. Hope
Okemos, MI 48864-1910
517-332-3593

Kensey Nash Corporation
55 E. Uwchlan Ave., Ste. 204
Exton, PA 19341-1247
215-524-0188

Leisegang Medical, Inc.
6401 Congress Ave.
Boca Raton, FL 33487-2883
407-994-0202

Marlow Surgical Technologies, Inc.
1810 Joseph Lloyd Pkwy.
Willoughby, OH 44094-8030
216-946-2453

Medicon Instruments, Inc.
4405 International Blvd.
Norcross, GA 30093-3013
404-381-2858

Mist, Inc.
6307 E. Angus Dr.
Raleigh, NC 27613
919-787-8377

Origin Medsystems, Inc.
135 Constitution Dr.
Menlo Park, CA 94025
415-617-5000

Performance Surgical Instruments
40 Norfolk Ave.
Easton, MA 023334
508-230-0010

Sharpe Endosurgical Corp.
3750 Annapolis Lane, Ste. 135
Minneapolis, MN 55447
612-784-0460

Smith & Nephew Dyonics, Inc.
160 Dascomb Rd.
Andover, MA 01810-5893
508-470-2800

Synectic Engineering, Inc.
4 Oxford Rd.
Milford, CT 06460-7007
203-877-8488

T.A.G. Medical Products
Kibbutz Gaaton 25130
Israel
4-859810

Unisurge, Inc.
10231 Bubb Rd.
Cupertino, CA 95014
408-996-4700

United States Surgical Corp.
150 Glover Ave.
Norwalk, CT 06856-5080
203-845-1000

Wolf Medical Instruments Corp., Richard
353 Corporate Woods Pkwy.
Vernon Hills, IL 60061-3110
708-913-1113

FORCEPS, GRASPING, FLEXIBLE ENDOSCOPIC

Aesculap AG
Moehringerstr. 125
Postfach 40
D-78532 Tuttlingen
Germany
00149/0746951

Aspen Laboratories, Inc.
P.O. Box 3936
Englewood, CO 80155-3936
303-798-5800

Cabot Medical Corp.
2021 Cabot Blvd. West
Langhorne, PA 19047-1875
215-752-8300

Circon Acmi
300 Stillwater Ave.
Stamford, CT 06902-3640
203-328-8689

Cook Urological, Inc.
1100 West Morgan St.
P.O. Box 227
Spencer, IN 47460-9426
812-829-4891

Coopersurgical, Inc.
15 Forest Pkwy.
Shelton, CT 06484-5458
203-929-6321

Corpak, Inc.
100 Chaddick Dr.
Wheeling, IL 60090-6006
708-537-4601

Davis & Geck Endosurgery
1 Casper Street
Danbury, CT 06810
203-743-4451

Design Standards Corp.
643 North Ave.
Bridgeport, CT 06606-5745
203-366-7046

Diener, Christian
Rudolf Diesel Str. 18
D-78532 Tuttlingen
Germany
7461/71067

Elmed, Inc.
60 W. Fay Ave.
Addison, IL 60101-5198
708-543-2792

Ethicon Endo-Surgery
4545 Creek Road
Cincinnati, OH 45242
513-786-7000

Hobbs Medical, Inc.
P.O. Box 46
Stafford Springs, CT 06076-0046
203-684-5875

Instrument Makar, Inc.
2950 E. Mt. Hope
Okemos, MI 48864-1910
517-332-3593

Leisegang Medical, Inc.
6401 Congress Ave.
Boca Raton, FL 33487-2883
407-994-0202

Life Medical Technologies, Inc.
3649 W. 1987 S.
Salt Lake City, UT 84104
801-972-1900

Medi-Tech/Boston Scientific Corp.
480 Pleasant St.
Watertown, MA 02172-2414
617-923-1720

Medicon Eg
15 Gansacker
Postfach 4455
D-78532 Tuttlingen
Germany
07462/20090

Medicon Instruments, Inc.
4405 International Blvd.
Norcross, GA 30093-3013
404-381-2858

Mill-Rose Laboratories
7310 Corporate Blvd.
Mentor, OH 44060-4856
216-255-7995

Nopa Instruments Medizintechnik GmbH
Gansacker 9 - Postfach 4554
D-78532 Tuttlingen
Germany
07462/7801

Portlyn Medical Products
Route 25
Moultonboro, NH 03254
603-476-5538

Questus Corp.
Lime St.
P.O. Box 9
Marblehead, MA 01945-0009
617-639-1900

Snowden-Pencer
5175 S. Royal Atlanta Dr.
Tucker, GA 30084-3053
404-496-0952

Storz Endoscopy-America Inc., Karl
10111 W. Jefferson Blvd.
Culver City, CA 90232-3509
310-558-1500

Storz GmbH & Co., Karl
Mittelstr. 8
Postfach 230
D-78532 Tuttlingen
Germany
07461/7080

Surgitek
3037 Mt. Pleasant St.
Racine, WI 53404-1509
414-639-7205

Synectic Engineering, Inc.
4 Oxford Rd.
Milford, CT 06460-7007
203-877-8488

United Instrument Corp.
P.O. Box 20924
Philadelphia, PA 19141-0924
215-635-4000

United States Surgical Corp.
150 Glover Ave.
Norwalk, CT 06856-5080
203-845-1000

Weck & Co. Inc., Edward
1 Weck Dr.
P.O. Box 12600
Research Triangle Park, NC 27709
919-544-8000

Wolf Medical Instruments Corp., Richard
353 Corporate Woods Pkwy.
Vernon Hills, IL 60061-3110
708-913-1113

FORCEPS, GRASPING, TRAUMATIC

Davis & Geck Endosurgery
1 Casper St.
Danbury, CT 06810
203-743-4451

PRESTIGE 10MM SERIES

INDICATIONS: DAVIS & GECK PRESTIGE endoscopic instruments are designed to grasp, cut, and/or dissect tissue during endoscopic surgical procedures. DAVIS & GECK PRESTIGE endoscopic instruments are designed to be used through a cannula or port commonly referred to as a trocar.

DAVIS & GECK PRESTIGE endoscopic instruments are designed for the purpose of manipulating soft tissue structures. DAVIS & GECK PRESTIGE endoscopic instruments are delicate surgical instruments. Any use of the instrument for tasks other than for which it is intended will usually result in a damaged or broken instrument.

CONTRAINDICATIONS: The use of DAVIS & GECK PRESTIGE endoscopic instruments is contraindicated when, in the judgment of the physician, their use would be contrary to the best interests of the patient.

PRECAUTIONS: Instruments must be handled carefully during surgery to avoid misusing the instrument. Misuse will usually result in damage or breakage. Instruments are designed to be held with one finger and the thumb in the ring handles. Do not hold handles in a whole hand grip (fingers outside ring handles). This grip applies excessive force to the linkage mechanism and results in damage to the instrument.

Use extreme care when inserting or removing endoscopic instruments through a cannula. Upon insertion, ensure that the cannula "trap-door" or trumpet valve has been fully opened to allow passage of the instrument. During removal, pull the instrument straight out until completely clear of the cannula, as any lateral pressure on the instrument may damage the working tip. Instrument jaws should be closed completely so that they do not catch on the cannula's internal valve assembly. Care must be taken to avoid tissue being inadvertently trapped in the jaws of the instrument on removal; therefore, visualize instrument prior to and during removal.

Any type of misuse or abuse of the instrument will render the warranty void. DAVIS & GECK assumes no liability if the instrument is misused or otherwise abused.

CARE & MAINTENANCE: Before using the instrument for the first time, and after each surgical procedure, clean all instruments thoroughly as follows:

1. Open all portions of the instrument by disassembling the 10mm shaft from the handle. With one hand, grip the 10mm shaft near the instrument handle. While holding the handle with the other hand, disengage the shaft from the handle. Applying a slight turning motion while pulling will make this easier. The instrument's flush ports are now exposed for cleaning and sterilization (see Figure 1).

2. Open the jaws by spreading the ring handles. Rinse the instrument thoroughly with deionized water to remove any accumulated debris. Hand wash instruments using a neutral pH instrument detergent or enzymatic instrument cleaner, being sure to thoroughly flush all lumen channels of the instrument with the solution (Figures 1 and 2). Be sure to clean the lumen between the 10mm non-rotating shaft and the 5mm rotating shaft.

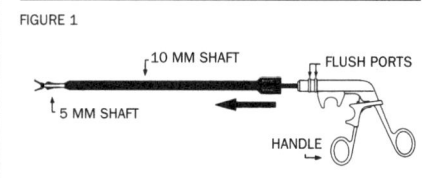

FIGURE 1

3. Hand wash each surface and "O" rings of the instrument with an instrument cleaning brush to remove visible residual debris. Using the flushing syringe supplied, thoroughly flush the instrument with enzymatic instrument cleaner, then with water through each flush port to remove all blood and debris that may obstruct the shaft lumen and handle (Figure 2). The distal flush port flushes the inner shaft and linkage while the proximal flush port flushes the inner handle mechanism. Continue flushing at each port until the flushing water is clear and no residue of cleaning solution remains.

4. DAVIS & GECK PRESTIGE endoscopic instruments should be handled with care. Avoid the use of steel wool, wire brushes, and highly abrasive detergents. Use of anything other than high quality brushes designed for instrument cleaning may result in damage to the instrument. Care should be taken not to scratch the surface of the instrument.

FORCEPS, GRASPING, TRAUMATIC (cont'd)

FIGURE 2

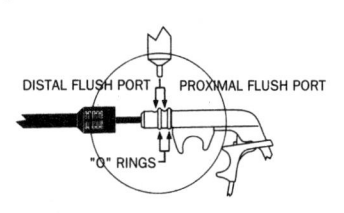

5. Thoroughly rinse the instrument again with deionized water and visually inspect the instrument after washing, making sure the internal lumens and channels are thoroughly rinsed and free of any cleaning solutions.

6. All instrument surfaces and individual parts should be visually inspected for burrs, nicks, misalignment, or bent tips.

7. Thoroughly dry all components using a towel or pressurized air to ensure removal of residual moisture. Moisture which is not removed may cause corrosion of the instrument.

8. Prior to sterilizing, lubricate with a non-silicone, antimicrobial, water-soluble surgical instrument lubricant solution. Do not rinse or towel dry. Do not use mineral oil, petroleum jelly, or silicone sprays which can inhibit sterilization and cause build-up in the crevices of the instrument.

9. Return instrument to its designated storage container. DAVIS & GECK PRESTIGE endoscopic instruments should be stored in a tray with silicone holders designed to protect them. Proceed with sterilization.

Storage: DAVIS & GECK PRESTIGE endoscopic instruments must be completely dry before storing and must be handled with care to prevent damage. Instruments should be stored in areas which provide protection from extremes of temperature and humidity.

STERILIZATION GUIDELINES: Ensure that the 10mm shaft is disconnected before sterilization (Figure 3). With one hand, grip the 10mm shaft near the instrument handle. While holding the handle with the other hand, disengage the shaft from the handle. Applying a slight turning motion while pulling will make this easier.

FIGURE 3

Clean and sterilize product before each use. Steam sterilize at a minimum of 250°F (121°C).

1. Sterilizing in ethylene oxide is not recommended.

2. Sterilizing in liquid solutions is not recommended.

3. Do not sterilize at temperatures greater than 275°F (135°C).

NOTE: Time and temperature parameters required for steam sterilization vary according to type of sterilizer, cycle design, and packaging material.

Minimum exposure times for steam sterilizers are as follows:

Gravity Displacement: 250° to 254°F, wrapped 30 minutes

Prevacuum: 270° to 274°F, wrapped 4 minutes

The use of "flash" sterilization should be avoided whenever possible, as it may result in shortening the life of the instrument.

Prior to use, using aseptic techniques, lubricate the white "O" rings on the handle with sterile water and reassemble the 10mm shaft to the handle, so that the 10mm shaft snaps over both "O" rings (Figure 4).

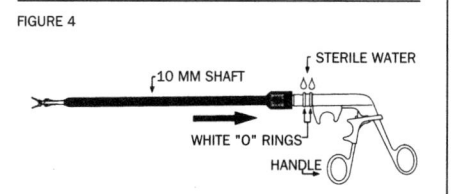

FIGURE 4

SPECIFICATIONS/HOW SUPPLIED: DAVIS & GECK PRESTIGE endoscopic instruments are provided non-sterile and must be sterilized before using, according to the procedures in the Sterilization section.

Contact your local DAVIS & GECK Endosurgery Representative to place an order, or call or write to the following:

DAVIS & GECK
American Cyanamid Company
ATTN: Customer Service Department
One Casper Street
Danbury, CT 06810
1-800-225-5341: Select the option to place an order
Fax Number: (203) 796-9534

SERVICE REQUIREMENTS & CONTACTS: DAVIS & GECK warrants its instruments against breakage or failure to function in normal use in surgery. If a DAVIS & GECK instrument breaks or fails to function in normal use due to defects in materials or workmanship, DAVIS & GECK will repair or replace such instrument at no cost to the customer after an evaluation has been made by DAVIS & GECK.

Any disassembly, alterations, re-sharpening or repair performed by persons not specifically authorized by DAVIS & GECK will void the above warranties.

The above warranties exclude: instrument coating, scissor edge sharpening, refurbishment due to normal wear and tear and apply only to the original buyer and are in lieu of all other warranties, either expressed or implied.

REPAIRS:
DAVIS & GECK provides repair services for all DAVIS & GECK instruments, as well as for instruments from other manufacturers. Repaired instruments will be sent back to the customer within 10 business days of receipt by DAVIS & GECK.

When an instrument needs repair please use the following procedure:

1. Clean instruments thoroughly, then sterilize before shipping them to DAVIS & GECK.

2. To ship instruments, use a sturdy shipping box with soft packaging material to protect your instruments.

3. Use tip protectors and individually wrap micro and delicate instruments.

Return instruments for repair to:
DAVIS & GECK
American Cyanamid Company
INSTRUMENT REPAIR SERVICE
Commerce Park, Commerce Drive
Danbury, CT 06810
1-800-225-5341: Select the option to inquire about repairs.

Davis & Geck Endosurgery
1 Casper St.
Danbury, CT 06810
203-743-4451

PROFESSIONAL LINE
8375 - 8450-17 SERIES

DESCRIPTION:

Pike-Mouth Forceps:
For fixing and holding tissue and for tissue extraction, with reservoir in jaws, color coded green:

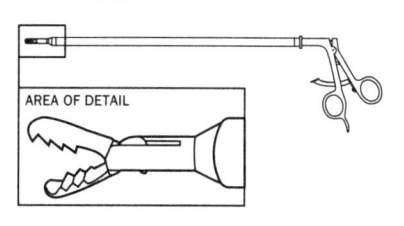

Large Pike-Mouth Forceps:
For extracting organs and tissue masses, with extra-wide jaws and ratchet lock:

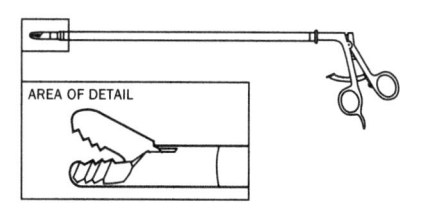

Grasping Forceps, 2x3 Teeth:
For extracting organs and tissue masses, with single action jaws and ratchet lock:

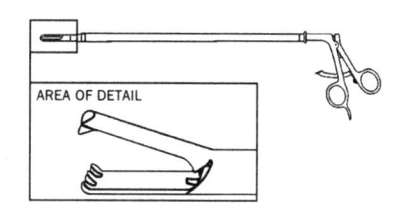

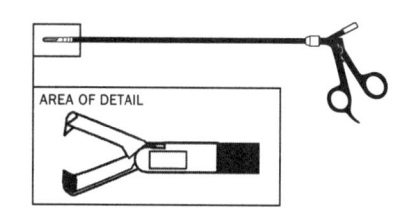

PIKE-MOUTH FORCEPS

PRODUCT CODE	DIAMETER MM	SHAFT LENGTH CM	360° ROTATION	INSULATED MONOPOLAR	RATCHET LOCK	CLOSING SPRING	CURVED SHAFT	D-TACH
8375-02	10	33	No	No	Yes	No	No	No
8376-01	5	33	No	Yes	No	Yes	No	No
8376-10	5	33	Yes	Yes	Yes	No	No	No
8376-11	10	33	Yes	Yes	Yes	No	No	No
8376-12	10	40	Yes	Yes	Yes	No	No	No
8376-25	10	40	No	Yes	No	Yes	No	No
8390-22	5	35	Yes	Yes	Yes	No	No	Yes
8390-28	10	35	Yes	Yes	Yes	No	No	Yes
8390-40	5	26	Yes	Yes	Yes	No	No	Yes
8450-16	5	33	Yes	Yes	No	No	Yes	No
8450-17	5	26	Yes	Yes	Yes	No	No	No

LARGE PIKE-MOUTH FORCEPS

PRODUCT CODE	DIAMETER MM	SHAFT LENGTH CM	360° ROTATION	INSULATED MONOPOLAR	D-TACH
8375-04	10	33	No	No	No
8375-10	10	40	No	No	No
8390-29	10	35	Yes	Yes	Yes

GRASPING FORCEPS

PRODUCT CODE	DIAMETER MM	SHAFT LENGTH CM	360° ROTATION	INSULATED MONOPOLAR	D-TACH
8375-05	10	33	No	No	No
8375-11	10	40	No	No	No
8390-30	10	35	Yes	Yes	Yes

SHARP GRASPING FORCEPS (NELSON)

PRODUCT CODE	DIAMETER MM	SHAFT LENGTH CM	360° ROTATION	INSULATED MONOPOLAR	RATCHET LOCK	CLOSING SPRING	CURVED SHAFT	D-TACH
8376-24	5	33	No	Yes	No	Yes	No	No
8390-27	5	35	Yes	Yes	Yes	No	No	Yes
8450-11	5	33	Yes	Yes	No	Yes	Yes	No

Davis & Geck Endosurgery
1 Casper St.
Danbury, CT 06810
203-743-4451

PROFESSIONAL LINE
8375-09 - 8450-11 SERIES

DESCRIPTION:

Grasping Forceps:
1x2 teeth, locking spring incorporated in the instrument shaft, insulated, monopolar connection, working length 33cm, color coded green.

For holding the peritoneum. May be used in the case of hernias, myomas, and polyps:

GRASPING FORCEPS

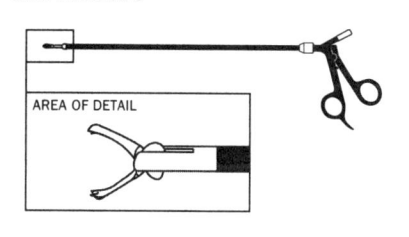

PRODUCT CODE	DIAMETER MM	SHAFT LENGTH CM	INSULATED MONOPOLAR
8375-09	5	33	Yes
8375-15	10	33	Yes

Sharp Grasping Forceps (Nelson):
5x6 teeth, closing spring, insulated, monopolar connection, working length 33cm, color coded green:

PRODUCT DIRECTORY

FORCEPS, GRASPING, TRAUMATIC (cont'd)

Davis & Geck Endosurgery
1 Casper St.
Danbury, CT 06810
203-743-4451

PROFESSIONAL LINE 8376 & 8390 SERIES

DESCRIPTION:
Pike-Mouth Forceps:
Reservoir in jaws, insulated, monopolar connection, color coded green. For fixing and holding organs and tissue:

PIKE-MOUTH FORCEPS

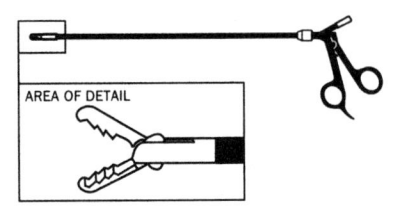

AREA OF DETAIL

INSTRUMENT KNOB

360° ROTATION

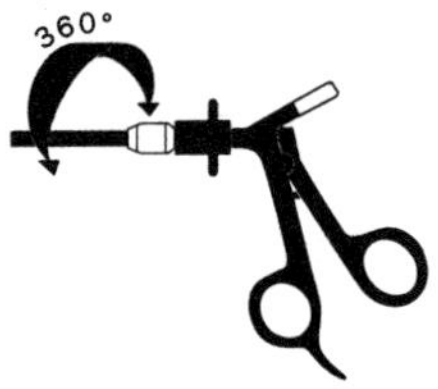

Pike-Mouth Forceps:

PRODUCT CODE	DIAMETER	WORKING LENGTH	ROTATABLE	RATCHET LOCK	CLOSING SPRING	D-TACH
8376-10	5 mm	33 cm	Yes	Yes	No	No
8376-11	10 mm	33 cm	Yes	Yes	No	No
8376-12	10 mm	40 cm	Yes	Yes	No	No
8376-01	5 mm	33 cm	No	No	Yes	No
8376-25	10 mm	40 cm	No	No	Yes	No
8390-23	5 mm	35 cm	Yes	No	No	Yes
8390-36	10 mm	35 cm	Yes	No	No	Yes

Crocodile Forceps:
Extra-long jaws, locking spring incorporated in the instrument shaft (except for products 8390-23 and 8390-36), without ratchet lock, insulated, monopolar connection, color coded green. For fixing and holding organs and tissue:

CROCODILE FORCEPS

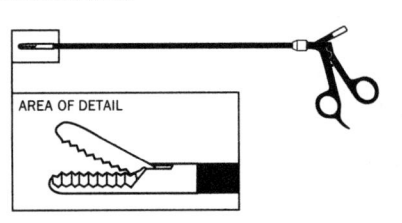

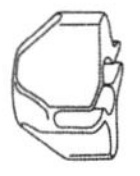

AREA OF DETAIL

Crocodile Forceps:

PRODUCT CODE	DIAMETER	WORKING LENGTH	ROTATABLE
8376-13	5 mm	33 cm	Yes
8376-14	10 mm	33 cm	Yes
8376-15	10 mm	40 cm	Yes
8376-02	5 mm	33 cm	No
8376-27	10 mm	33 cm	No
8376-28	10 mm	40 cm	No

Access Surgical International, Inc.
15 Caswell Ln.
Boat Yard Square
Plymouth, MA 02360
508-747-6006

Aesculap
1000 Gateway Blvd.
South San Francisco, CA 94080-7030
415-876-7000

Birtcher Medical Systems, Inc.
50 Technology Dr.
Irvine, CA 92718-2301
714-753-9400

Bryan Corp.
4 Plympton St.
Woburn, MA 01801-2908
617-935-0004

Chirurgische Instrumente
Hauptstrasse 18
D-78582 Balgheim
Germany
7424/501319

Circon Acmi
300 Stillwater Ave.
Stamford, CT 06902-3640
203-328-8689

Coopersurgical, Inc.
15 Forest Pkwy.
Shelton, CT 06484-5458
203-929-6321

Core Dynamics, Inc.
11222-4 St. Johns Indust. Pkwy.
Jacksonville, FL 32216
904-641-6611

DaVinci Medical, Inc.
13700 First Ave. North
Minneapolis, MN 55441
612-473-4245

Davis & Geck Div.
American Cyanamid Company
One Cyanamid Plaza
Wayne, NJ 07470-2012
201-831-2000

Davol, Inc.
100 Sockanossett
P.O. Box 8500
Cranston, RI 02920-0500
401-463-7000

Elekta Instruments, Inc.
8 Executive Park West, Ste. 809
Atlanta, GA 30329
404-315-1225

Elmed, Inc.
60 W. Fay Ave.
Addison, IL 60101-5198
708-543-2792

Heraeus Surgical, Inc.
575 Cottonwood Dr.
Milpitas, CA 95035-7402
408-954-4000

Kensey Nash Corporation
55 E. Uwchlan Ave., Ste. 204
Exton, PA 19341-1247
215-524-0188

Leisegang Medical, Inc.
6401 Congress Ave.
Boca Raton, FL 33487-2883
407-994-0202

Marlow Surgical Technologies, Inc.
1810 Joseph Lloyd Pkwy.
Willoughby, OH 44094-8030
216-946-2453

Mist, Inc.
6307 E. Angus Dr.
Raleigh, NC 27613
919-787-8377

Origin Medsystems, Inc.
135 Constitution Dr.
Menlo Park, CA 94025
415-617-5000

Performance Surgical Instruments
40 Norfolk Ave.
Easton, MA 023334
508-230-0010

Portlyn Medical Products
Route 25
Moultonboro, NH 03254
603-476-5538

Schwarz Medical
Kirchstrasse 24
D-86935 Rott
Germany
8869/1881

Smith & Nephew Dyonics, Inc.
160 Dascomb Rd.
Andover, MA 01810-5893
508-470-2800

Synectic Engineering, Inc.
4 Oxford Rd.
Milford, CT 06460-7007
203-877-8488

United States Surgical Corp.
150 Glover Ave.
Norwalk, CT 06856-5080
203-845-1000

Wolf Medical Instruments Corp., Richard
353 Corporate Woods Pkwy.
Vernon Hills, IL 60061-3110
708-913-1113

FORCEPS, LAPAROSCOPY, ELECTROSURGICAL

Davis & Geck Endosurgery
1 Casper St.
Danbury, CT 06810
203-743-4451

PRESTIGE 8364 SERIES
DESCRIPTION:

Fine Tip Dissecting Forceps (Electrosurgical):
Cone shaped dual action jaws, insulated handle, monopolar electrosurgical connection, 360° rotating shaft with integral flush port (cleaning syringe included). Also includes one 8370-03 PRESTIGE Monopolar Cord Adaptor. For precise dissection, i.e., to expose cystic artery or cystic duct. Also for fixing and holding fine structures:

FINE TIP DISSECTING FORCEPS

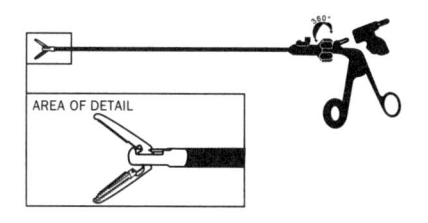

AREA OF DETAIL

FINE TIP DISSECTING FORCEPS		
PRODUCT CODE	DIAMETER MM	SHAFT LENGTH CM
8364-24	5	33
8364-34	5	22
8364-44	5	44

SPECIFICATIONS/HOW SUPPLIED: Dual action jaws. 5mm diameter, working length 33cm. Insulated handle, monopolar electrosurgical connection, rotating shaft with integral flush port (cleaning syringe included, order number 8364-24). Also includes one 8370-03 PRESTIGE Monopolar Cord Adaptor.

Davis & Geck Endosurgery
1 Casper St.
Danbury, CT 06810
203-743-4451

PROFESSIONAL LINE 8382 SERIES
DESCRIPTION:

Bipolar Fixation Forceps (order number 8382-01):
5mm diameter, working length 33cm. For hemostasis during a variety of surgical procedures:

BIPOLAR FIXATION FORCEPS

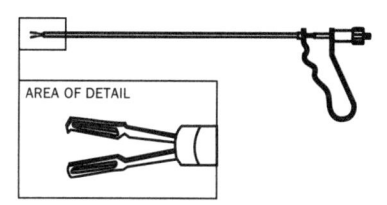

AREA OF DETAIL

Bipolar Micro Coagulation Forceps (order number 8382-02):
For hemostasis using micro-fine tips. 5mm diameter, width of jaw parts 1mm:

BIPOLAR MICRO COAGULATION FORCEPS

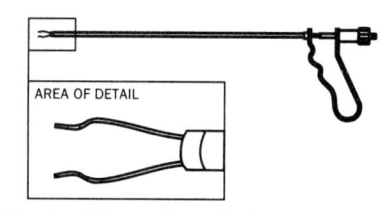

AREA OF DETAIL

Bipolar Micro Coagulation Forceps with Olive Tip (order number 8382-03) for fine hemostasis. Olive space to accomodate tissue.

Reusable Bipolar Cable (order number 8370-06); dual banana pin connects DAVIS & GECK bipolar forceps to any bipolar unit.

INDICATIONS: DAVIS & GECK's bipolar fixation forceps or micro-forceps are used for coagulating tissue in laparoscopic operating techniques.

IMPORTANT: Bipolar autocoagulation, which some coagulation instruments offer, cannot be used with these instruments. Here coagulation is only possible in conjunction with the foot switch.

ASSEMBLY GUIDELINES: To disassemble the instrument, remove the union nut and contact jack from the housing and pull out the forceps forwards. Next, remove the clamping element from the housing. To assemble the instrument, insert clamping element and contact jack into the housing and slightly screw on the union nut (pin of the contact jack must lie in the groove of the housing). Insert forceps into the housing at the front while carefully closing the mouthparts of the forceps with your thumb and index finger. Gently push the forceps as far as they will go and tighten the union nut.

CARE & MAINTENANCE: It is best to clean the instrument immediately after use. To do this, the instrument should be disassembled and its component parts cleaned with a soft sponge or cloth under running water. The inside of the tube of the housing should be cleaned with a soft cylindrical brush. Dry well with a soft cloth or compressed air.

STERILIZATION GUIDELINES: The instrument must be reassembled dry before sterilization and sprayed with oil spray. It is preferable to sterilize the instrument with steam at max. 3 bar (143°C).

Everest Medical Corp.
13755 First Ave. N.
Minneapolis, MN 55441-5454
612-473-6262

BICOAG FORCEPS
DESCRIPTION: BiCOAG™ bipolar coagulating forceps from Everest Medical provide a new level of safety and precision in minimally invasive surgery. The BiCOAG Forceps use bipolar current to localize current flow, minimize lateral tissue damage, and reduce the

risk of alternate site burns and other monopolar complications.

Both Macro Jaw and Micro Jaw forcep designs allow effective use of the BiCOAG Forceps in a variety of applications. The proprietary handle design of BiCOAG Forceps incorporates smooth and stable action with fingertip rotation for accurate orientation of the jaws. BiCOAG Forceps are compatible with the bipolar output of common electrosurgical generators.

SPECIFICATIONS/HOW SUPPLIED: Technical specifications: working length 33cm, shaft diameter 4.8mm, single use/sterile package/5 per box; compatible with the bipolar output of most electrosurgical generators.

Ordering information: BiCOAG macro jaw forceps (model 3600), BiCOAG micro jaw forceps (model 3601), extension cord: BiCOAG forceps to Wolf bipolar units (model 3998), adapter cord: BiCOAG forceps to dual male banana jack (model 3999); other adapter cords available upon request.

Apple Medical Corp.
93 Nashaway Rd.
Bolton, MA 01740
508-779-2926

Berchtold Corp.
2050 Mabeline Rd., Ste. C
North Charlestown, SC 29418-4643
803-569-6100

Marlow Surgical Technologies, Inc.
1810 Joseph Lloyd Pkwy.
Willoughby, OH 44094-8030
216-946-2453

Medicon Instruments, Inc.
4405 International Blvd.
Norcross, GA 30093-3013
404-381-2858

Mediflex Surgical Products
250 Gibbs Rd.
Islandia, NY 11722-2697
516-582-8440

Microsurge, Inc.
150 A St.
Needham, MA 02194
617-444-2300

Performance Surgical Instruments
40 Norfolk Ave.
Easton, MA 023334
508-230-0010

Reznik Instrument, Inc.
7337 North Lawndale
Skokie, IL 60076
708-673-3444

Gastroscope

GASTROSCOPE, FLEXIBLE

ACM Endoskopie GmbH
Taunusstr. 38
D-80807 Muenchen 40
Germany
089/352355

Asahi Optical Co., Ltd.
2-36-9, Maeno-Cho, Itabashi-Ku
Tokyo 174
Japan
03/3960-5155

Carsen Group Inc.
151 Telson Rd.
Markham, ONT L3R 1E7
Canada
416-479-4100

Effner Biomet GmbH
Alt-Lankwitz 102
D-12247 Berlin 46
Germany
49/30-7700920

Fuji Photo Optical Co. Ltd.
1-324, Uetake-Machi, Omiya
Saitama 330
Japan
048/668-2153

Fujinon (Europe) GmbH
Heerdter Lohweg 89
D-40549 Duesseldorf 11
Germany
0211/52050

Fujinon, Inc.
10 High Point Dr.
Wayne, NJ 07470-7434
201-633-5600

Life Medical Technologies, Inc.
3649 W. 1987 S.
Salt Lake City, UT 84104
801-972-1900

Olympus America, Inc.
4 Nevada Drive
Lake Success, NY 11042-1179
516-488-3880

Olympus Optical Co. Ltd.
San-Ei Bldg.
1-22-2, Nishi-Shinjuku
Shinjuku-Ku, Tokyo 163-91
Japan
03/3402111

Pentax HgmbH
Julius Vosseler Str. 104
Postf. 540 169
D-22527 Hamburg 54
Germany
040/5617-114

Pentax Precision Instrument Corp.
30 Ramland Rd.
Orangeburg, NY 10962-2699
914-365-0700

Treier Endoscopie AG
Sonnrain
CH-6215 Beromunster
Switzerland
045/512323

GASTROSCOPE, GASTRO-UROLOGY

Circon Acmi
300 Stillwater Ave.
Stamford, CT 06902-3640
203-328-8689

Effner Biomet GmbH
Alt-Lankwitz 102
D-12247 Berlin 46
Germany
49/30-7700920

Fujinon, Inc.
10 High Point Dr.
Wayne, NJ 07470-7434
201-633-5600

Olympus Optical Co. Ltd.
San-Ei Bldg.
1-22-2, Nishi-Shinjuku
Shinjuku-Ku, Tokyo 163-91
Japan
03/3402111

Pentax HgmbH
Julius Vosseler Str. 104
Postf. 540 169
D-22527 Hamburg 54
Germany
040/5617-114

GASTROSCOPE, GENERAL & PLASTIC SURGERY

Effner Biomet GmbH
Alt-Lankwitz 102
D-12247 Berlin 46
Germany
49/30-7700920

Pentax HgmbH
Julius Vosseler Str. 104
Postf. 540 169
D-22527 Hamburg 54
Germany
040/5617-114

Wolf Medical Instruments Corp., Richard
353 Corporate Woods Pkwy.
Vernon Hills, IL 60061-3110
708-913-1113

GASTROSCOPE, RIGID

ACM Endoskopie GmbH
Taunusstr. 38
D-80807 Muenchen 40
Germany
089/352355

Effner Biomet GmbH
Alt-Lankwitz 102
D-12247 Berlin 46
Germany
49/30-7700920

Treier Endoscopie AG
Sonnrain
CH-6215 Beromunster
Switzerland
045/512323

Wolf Medical Instruments Corp., Richard
353 Corporate Woods Pkwy.
Vernon Hills, IL 60061-3110
708-913-1113

Holder

HOLDER, INSTRUMENT, LAPAROSCOPIC

Access Surgical International, Inc.
15 Caswell Ln.
Boat Yard Square
Plymouth, MA 02360
508-747-6006

Aesculap
1000 Gateway Blvd.
South San Francisco, CA 94080-7030
415-876-7000

Apple Medical Corp.
93 Nashaway Rd.
Bolton, MA 01740
508-779-2926

Computer Motion, Inc.
250 Storke Rd., Ste. A
Goleta, CA 93117
805-685-3729

Coopersurgical, Inc.
15 Forest Pkwy.
Shelton, CT 06484-5458
203-929-6321

Ideas For Medicine, Inc.
12167 49th St. N
Clearwater, FL 34622-4304
813-576-2747

Koros Surgical Instruments
610 Flinn Ave.
Moorpark, CA 93021-2008
818-889-5077

Leisegang Medical, Inc.
6401 Congress Ave.
Boca Raton, FL 33487-2883
407-994-0202

Origin Medsystems, Inc.
135 Constitution Dr.
Menlo Park, CA 94025
415-617-5000

Resorba Surgical Sutures
Schonerstr. 7
D-90443 Nurnberg
Germany
0911/442344

Thompson Surgical Instruments, Inc.
10170 E. Cherry Bend Rd.
P.O. Box 1051
Traverse City, MI 49685
616-922-0177

HOLDER, LAPAROSCOPE

Access Surgical International, Inc.
15 Caswell Ln.
Boat Yard Square
Plymouth, MA 02360
508-747-6006

Automated Medical Products Corp.
2315 Broadway, Ste. 410
New York, NY 10024-4332
212-874-0236

Elmed, Inc.
60 W. Fay Ave.
Addison, IL 60101-5198
708-543-2792

Leisegang Medical, Inc.
6401 Congress Ave.
Boca Raton, FL 33487-2883
407-994-0202

Leonard Medical Inc.
1464 Holcomb Rd.
Huntingdon Valley, PA 19006
215-938-1499

Mediflex Surgical Products
250 Gibbs Rd.
Islandia, NY 11722-2697
516-582-8440

Omni-Tract Surgical Div.
Minnesota Scientific Co.
403 County Rd. E2 West
St. Paul, MN 55112-6858
612-633-8448

Surgical Technologies International, Inc.
4715 NW 157th St., #212
Miami, FL 33014
305-623-0363

HOLDER, LAPAROSCOPE (cont'd)

Thompson Surgical Instruments, Inc.
10170 E. Cherry Bend Rd.
P.O. Box 1051
Traverse City, MI 49685
616-922-0177

W.J. Medical Instruments, Inc.
3537 Old Conejo Rd.
Newbury Park, CA 91320
805-499-8676

Wolf Medical Instruments Corp., Richard
353 Corporate Woods Pkwy.
Vernon Hills, IL 60061-3110
708-913-1113

HOLDER, LEG, ARTHROSCOPY

Abco Dealers, Inc.
6601 W. Mill Rd.
P.O. Box 23090
Milwaukee, WI 53218-0090
414-358-5420

Allen Medical Systems, Inc.
5198 Richmond Rd.
Bedford Heights, OH 44146-1331
216-765-0990

Arthrex Arthroscopy Instrument
3050 North Horseshoe Dr., Ste. 168
Naples, FL 33942-7909
813-643-5553

Arthrex Medical Instrument GmbH
Von Kahr Str. 2
D-80997 Muenchen 50
Germany
89/142257

Arthro-Medic, Inc.
4203 Belfort Rd., Ste. 150
Jacksonville, FL 32216-5896
904-296-1188

Chamco
10 Rue de L'Armee D'Orient
P.O. Box 162
F-06300 Nice, CEDEX
France
93/891145

Contec Medical Ltd.
11 Haroshet Street
P.O. Box 1400
Ramat Hasharon 47113
Israel
03/5491153

Faro Technologies, Inc.
125 Technology Park
Lake Mary, FL 32746-6204
407-333-9911

Instrument Makar, Inc.
2950 E. Mt. Hope
Okemos, MI 48864-1910
517-332-3593

Maramed Orthopedic Systems
2480 W. 82nd St.
Hialeah, FL 33016-2753
305-823-8300

Medin Corporation
111 Lester St.
Wallington, NJ 07057-1012
201-779-2400

Meditek
120 East Hudson
Royal Oak, MI 48067
313-544-2230

Medrecon, Inc.
257 South Ave.
Garwood, NJ 07027-1341
908-789-2050

Orthopedic Systems, Inc.
1897 National Ave.
Hayward, CA 94545-1794
510-785-1020

Performance Orthopedics
3971 Deep Rock Rd.
Richmond, VA 23233-1433
804-270-0140

Smith & Nephew Dyonics, Inc.
160 Dascomb Rd.
Andover, MA 01810-5893
508-470-2800

Sodem Systems
110, Chemin du Pont du Centenaire
Pont-du-Centenaire
CH-1228 Plan-les-Quates/Geneva
Switzerland
22/794-9696

Tecnol, Inc.
7201 Industrial Park Blvd.
Fort Worth, TX 76180-6153
817-581-6424

Wolf Medical Instruments Corp., Richard
353 Corporate Woods Pkwy.
Vernon Hills, IL 60061-3110
708-913-1113

HOLDER, NEEDLE, CURVED, LAPAROSCOPIC

Access Surgical International, Inc.
15 Caswell Ln.
Boat Yard Square
Plymouth, MA 02360
508-747-6006

Birtcher Medical Systems, Inc.
50 Technology Dr.
Irvine, CA 92718-2301
714-753-9400

Cabot Medical Corp.
2021 Cabot Blvd. West
Langhorne, PA 19047-1875
215-752-8300

Coopersurgical, Inc.
15 Forest Pkwy.
Shelton, CT 06484-5458
203-929-6321

Elmed, Inc.
60 W. Fay Ave.
Addison, IL 60101-5198
708-543-2792

Leisegang Medical, Inc.
6401 Congress Ave.
Boca Raton, FL 33487-2883
407-994-0202

Marlow Surgical Technologies, Inc.
1810 Joseph Lloyd Pkwy.
Willoughby, OH 44094-8030
216-946-2453

Medicon Instruments, Inc.
4405 International Blvd.
Norcross, GA 30093-3013
404-381-2858

Performance Surgical Instruments
40 Norfolk Ave.
Easton, MA 023334
508-230-0010

Sharpe Endosurgical Corp.
3750 Annapolis Lane, Ste. 135
Minneapolis, MN 55447
612-784-0460

Smith & Nephew Dyonics, Inc.
160 Dascomb Rd.
Andover, MA 01810-5893
508-470-2800

HOLDER, NEEDLE, LAPAROSCOPIC

Davis & Geck Endosurgery
1 Casper St.
Danbury, CT 06810
203-743-4451

PROFESSIONAL LINE 8377 SERIES

DESCRIPTION:

Tungsten Carbide Needle Holder (order number 8377-04):

Ratchet handle, 5mm diameter, non-insulated, working length 33cm, color coded gray. For guiding the needle and suture and for placing ligatures:

TUNGSTEN CARBIDE NEEDLE HOLDER

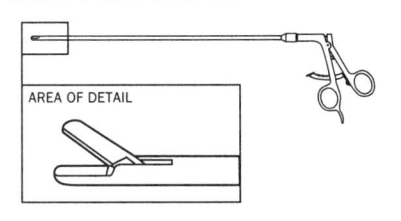

AREA OF DETAIL

Micro-Needle Holder with Tungsten Carbide Inserts (order number 8377-05):

Ratchet handle, 3mm diameter, non-insulated, working length 33cm, color coded gray. To control fine needles and introduce small curved needles through cannulas:

MICRO-NEEDLE HOLDER WITH TUNGSTEN CARBIDE INSERTS

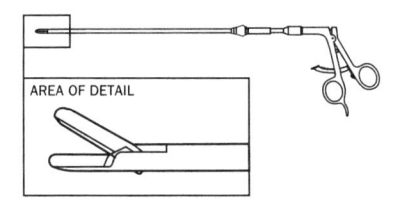

AREA OF DETAIL

Nu Surg Medical, Inc.
4440 Glen Este-Withamsville Rd., Ste.780
Cincinnati, OH 45245
513-753-3633

ENDOVISE

DESCRIPTION:

ENDOVISE™
CLEANING PORT
MOVABLE JAW
"IN-LINE" HANDLE

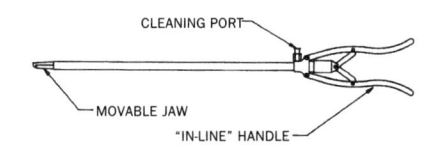

The Nu Surg Endovise Needle Holder is available in 5mm or 10mm sizes of stainless steel construction. The Endovise is available in 3 jaw configurations: 30° Right Angle Jaw, 30° Left Angle Jaw, and 90° Universal Angle Jaw. The crosshatched tungsten carbide jaw inserts permit a secure hold on the needle. The spring-tensioned "in-line" handle is designed to lessen frustration and hand fatigue in suturing procedures.

INDICATIONS: The Endovise is suited for endoscopic suturing with large needles. It has applications in laparoscopic general surgery procedures, gynecology, urology, and thoracic surgery fields where large structures are to be sutured. Some uses for Endovise suturing are: Nissen Fundoplication, Hiatal hernia repair, Inguinal hernia repair, Bladder suspensions, Closure of enterotomies, suture ligation of uterine vessel. The Right or Left 30° Endovise Needle Holder allows the surgeon to insert the needle through a trocar sleeve while the needle is held firmly in jaws.

WARNINGS: Gas sterilization can be used only if the instrument is thoroughly dry prior to sterilization.

PRECAUTIONS: Care should be taken when using this device to ensure direct visualization of the jaw and needle. Avoid any inadvertent needle injuries to viscera.

INSTRUCTIONS FOR USE: To deliver a SH, CT2 (or smaller) needle on the Endovise Needle Holder through a trocar sleeve (possible only with right and left 30° angle jaw configurations) proceed as follows: Position the needle in the jaw with the needle point oriented toward the tip of the instrument. Carefully insert needle and needle holder into a 10mm trocar sleeve. Under visualization, use a grasper to rotate the needle 90° to the instrument shaft. The needle holder and suture is now ready for suturing.

The universal or 90° Endovise Needle Holder requires the use of an assisting forceps to grasp the suture and push the needle into the peritoneal cavity. Then the needle is aligned on the Endovise for suturing.

Inspection: A routine check should be completed before each case. This check should include the following:
1. Ensure free movement of the jaws when actuated by the handle (no sticking).
2. Ensure the luer lock cap is in position.
3. Return for repair if wear is noted.

CARE & MAINTENANCE:

Lubrication: It is extremely important that movable parts be properly lubricated to maintain instrument function. It is recommended that the Endovise be completely immersed in a water-soluble lubricant and dried completely prior to sterilization. Use Lubriteck™ (Proprietary name of Baxter International) or equivalent product.

Cleaning: Rinse and softly brush instrument with water to remove blood and debris. Flush instrument through cleaning port. Wash instrument with a neutral pH detergent and brush. Mechanical washer sterilizers may be utilized following manufacturer's recommendations. It is also recommended that the instrument be ultrasonically cleaned. Rinse instrument thoroughly and flush cleaning port. Dry instrument completely.

STERILIZATION GUIDELINES: The instrument may be autoclaved or gas sterilized. Refer to sterilizer manufacturer's instructions for correct time, temperature and pressure settings.

SERVICE REQUIREMENTS & CONTACTS: Send all instruments for service or repair to:

Nu Surg Medical, Inc.
4440 Glen Este-Withamsville Road
Suite 780
Cincinnati, OH 45245
800-225-2922

Always include the purchase order number and a written description of the problem.

Warranty: This device is warranted for one full year from date of purchase. Devices are guaranteed to be free from defects in both materials and workmanship. Disassembly, alteration or repair performed by any person not specifically authorized by Nu Surg Medical Inc., will invalidate the warranty. Devices under warranty should be returned to Nu Surg Medical Inc. and will be repaired without charge to the purchaser, assuming they were used for their intended purpose. The above warranties are in lieu of all other warranties either expressed or implied. Suitability for use of this device for any surgical procedure shall be determined by the user. Nu Surg Medical Inc., shall not be liable for incidental or consequential damages of any kind.

Access Surgical International, Inc.
15 Caswell Ln.
Boat Yard Square
Plymouth, MA 02360
508-747-6006

Birtcher Medical Systems, Inc.
50 Technology Dr.
Irvine, CA 92718-2301
714-753-9400

Boss Instruments, Ltd.
1310 Central Ct.
Hermitage, TN 37076
615-885-2231

Bryan Corp.
4 Plympton St.
Woburn, MA 01801-2908
617-935-0004

Chirurgische Instrumente
Hauptstrasse 18
D-78582 Balgheim
Germany
7424/501319

Coopersurgical, Inc.
15 Forest Pkwy.
Shelton, CT 06484-5458
203-929-6321

HOLDER, NEEDLE, LAPROSCOPIC (cont'd)

Elekta Instruments, Inc.
8 Executive Park West, Ste. 809
Atlanta, GA 30329
404-315-1225

Elmed, Inc.
60 W. Fay Ave.
Addison, IL 60101-5198
708-543-2792

Ethicon Endo-Surgery
4545 Creek Road
Cincinnati, OH 45242
513-786-7000

Koros Surgical Instruments
610 Flinn Ave.
Moorpark, CA 93021-2008
818-889-5077

Leisegang Medical, Inc.
6401 Congress Ave.
Boca Raton, FL 33487-2883
407-994-0202

Medicon Instruments, Inc.
4405 International Blvd.
Norcross, GA 30093-3013
404-381-2858

Origin Medsystems, Inc.
135 Constitution Dr.
Menlo Park, CA 94025
415-617-5000

Performance Surgical Instruments
40 Norfolk Ave.
Easton, MA 023334
508-230-0010

Smith & Nephew Dyonics, Inc.
160 Dascomb Rd.
Andover, MA 01810-5893
508-470-2800

Smith & Nephew Richards Inc.
1450 Brooks Road
Memphis, TN 38116
901-396-2121

Synectic Engineering, Inc.
4 Oxford Rd.
Milford, CT 06460-7007
203-877-8488

W.J. Medical Instruments, Inc.
3537 Old Conejo Rd.
Newbury Park, CA 91320
805-499-8676

Ximed Medical Systems
2195 Trade Zone Blvd.
San Jose, CA 95131
408-945-4040

HOLDER, RING, ANASTOMOSIS

Davis & Geck Endosurgery
1 Casper Street
Danbury, CT 06810
203-743-4451

HOLDER, SHOULDER, ARTHROSCOPY

All Orthopedic Appliances
9690 Deereco Road, Suite 600
Timonium, MD 21093
410-560-3333

Allen Medical Systems, Inc.
5198 Richmond Rd.
Bedford Heights, OH 44146-1331
216-765-0990

Arthrex Arthroscopy Instrument
3050 North Horseshoe Dr., Ste. 168
Naples, FL 33942-7909
813-643-5553

Bauerfeind USA, Inc.
Suite 114
1590 North Roberts Rd.
Kennesaw, GA 30144-3679
404-429-8330

Biodynamic Technologies, Inc.
1425 E. Newport Center Dr.
Deerfield Beach, FL 33442
305-421-3166

Instrument Makar, Inc.
2950 E. Mt. Hope
Okemos, MI 48864-1910
517-332-3593

Medin Corporation
111 Lester St.
Wallington, NJ 07057-1012
201-779-2400

Smith & Nephew Donjoy, Inc.
2777 Loker West
Carlsbad, CA 92008-6601
619-438-9091

Smith & Nephew Dyonics, Inc.
160 Dascomb Rd.
Andover, MA 01810-5893
508-470-2800

Sodem Systems
110, Chemin du Pont du Centenaire
Pont-du-Centenaire
CH-1228 Plan-les-Quates/Geneva
Switzerland
22/794-9696

HOLDER/SCISSORS, NEEDLE, LAPAROSCOPIC

Access Surgical International, Inc.
15 Caswell Ln.
Boat Yard Square
Plymouth, MA 02360
508-747-6006

Elekta Instruments, Inc.
8 Executive Park West, Ste. 809
Atlanta, GA 30329
404-315-1225

Elmed, Inc.
60 W. Fay Ave.
Addison, IL 60101-5198
708-543-2792

Leisegang Medical, Inc.
6401 Congress Ave.
Boca Raton, FL 33487-2883
407-994-0202

Origin Medsystems, Inc.
135 Constitution Dr.
Menlo Park, CA 94025
415-617-5000

Smith & Nephew Dyonics, Inc.
160 Dascomb Rd.
Andover, MA 01810-5893
508-470-2800

Smith & Nephew Richards, Inc.
1450 Brooks Road
Memphis, TN 38116
901-396-2121

Synectic Engineering, Inc.
4 Oxford Rd.
Milford, CT 06460-7007
203-877-8488

Wolf Medical Instruments Corp., Richard
353 Corporate Woods Pkwy.
Vernon Hills, IL 60061-3110
708-913-1113

Ximed Medical Systems
2195 Trade Zone Blvd.
San Jose, CA 95131
408-945-4040

Imaging

COMPUTER, IMAGE, ENDOSCOPIC

Machida, Inc.
40 Ramland Rd. South
Orangeburg, NY 10962-2617
914-365-0600

Pentax Precision Instrument Corp.
30 Ramland Rd.
Orangeburg, NY 10962-2699
914-365-0700

Vicom Systems
46107 Landing Parkway
Fremont, CA 94538-6407
415-498-3200

PROBE, DETECTOR, FLOW, BLOOD, LAPAROSCOPY, ULTRASONIC

Aloka (US Headquarters)
10 Fairfield Blvd.
P.O. Box 5002
Wallingford, CT 06492-7502
203-269-5088

Endomedix Corp.
2162 Michelson Drive
Irvine, CA 92715
714-253-1000

SYSTEM, IMAGING, LAPAROSCOPY, ULTRASONIC

Endomedix Corp.
2162 Michelson Dr.
Irvine, CA 92715
714-253-1000

LAPAROSCAN

DESCRIPTION: Laparoscopic ultrasonography is employed to visualize the structure and orientation of intra-abdominal tissues to assist in procedure planning and identification of target tissues. The LaparoScan™ System is designed to offer surgeons the opportunity to perform real-time intraoperative ultrasonography during laparoscopic surgery using a handheld probe which can be inserted through standard 10-11mm laparoscopic portals.

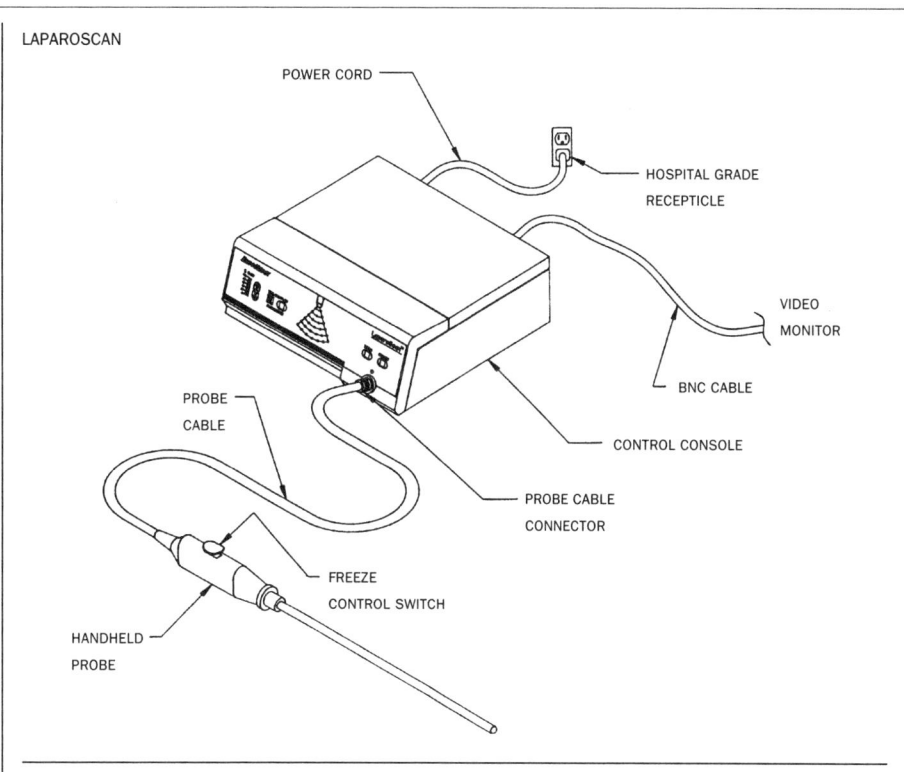

The LaparoScan System is a unique ultrasound unit designed specifically for laparoscopic use. It is a B-mode scanner/real-time imager operating at a frame rate of 15 fps with a gray shade capability of up to 128 levels. The modular unit is compact enough to fit on a typical laparoscopic cart, and is incorporated into the laparoscopic video system via a video mixer, which presents the ultrasound and the camera image in a picture-in-picture format on the monitor. This is a suitable format for laparoscopic use, since all the visual information is on one monitor and thus facilitates the use of the ultrasound while maintaining the orientation of the viewer. The console has four functions for image control: gain, TGC, zoom, and freeze. The gain and TGC affect the signal strength and thus the brightness of the image. The zoom and freeze are used to control the dynamics of the image on the monitor. The system comes complete with two 7.5MHz mechanical sector probes, which can be inserted through 10mm trocars. The probes provide a wide 90° sector field of view on the monitor with a scan depth of up to 6cm, and are available in two configurations. The first is a front viewing/end-fire probe which has a viewing angle of 0° (straight forward) from the transducer tip. This type of probe can be useful in providing multiple planes of view from a single port by simple rotation of the probe handle. The second is a side viewing probe which has a viewing angle of 45° off axis from the transducer tip. This angled view facilitates imaging tissue and organs when a side approach is used. This system is user friendly and facilitates diagnostic procedures during laparoscopy.

INDICATIONS: The LaparoScan System is intended to visualize abdominal anatomy through existing portals during laparoscopic surgery. The device is intended for use by physicians who have been trained in generally accepted techniques of laparoscopic surgery and specifically trained on use of the LaparoScan System.

WARNINGS: Contraindicated for fetal use.

STERILIZATION GUIDELINES: For sterilization of the handheld probes, the STERIS PROCESS™ can be used. Do not steam sterilize. The metal probe shield should always be used during the disinfection or sterilization process. Hospitals may elect to use high level disinfection with 2% glutaraldehyde solution. Disinfection is acceptable only when the LaparoScan handheld probe is used with a sterile probe sheath. Use only high level disinfectants such as Cidex® or Omnicide®.

SPECIFICATIONS/HOW SUPPLIED: A complete LaparoScan System (Model U4000) consists of: LaparoScan control console and power cord, forward viewing handheld probe, side viewing handheld probe, probe shield (one per probe), and a BNC cable (6 feet). A picture-in-picture video mixer (Model U460) and other accessories are also available.

SERVICE REQUIREMENTS & CONTACTS: For information or service contact: EndoMedix Customer Service at 1-800-553-6361.

Cooper-Endoscopy
951 Calle Amanecer
San Clemente, CA 92673
714-361-5390

Instrument

BRUSH, CYTOLOGY, ENDOSCOPIC

Annex Medical, Inc.
7098 Shady Oak Rd.
Eden Prairie, MN 55344-3505
612-942-7576

Bard Ventures
1200 Technology Park Dr.
Billerica, MA 01821
508-667-1300

Carsen Group Inc.
151 Telson Rd.
Markham, ONT L3R 1E7
Canada
416-479-4100

Circon Acmi
300 Stillwater Ave.
Stamford, CT 06902-3640
203-328-8689

Cook Urological, Inc.
1100 West Morgan St.
P.O. Box 227
Spencer, IN 47460-9426
812-829-4891

Coopersurgical, Inc.
15 Forest Pkwy.
Shelton, CT 06484-5458
203-929-6321

Endovations, Inc.
Hill & George Avenues
Reading, PA 19610
215-378-1606

Fujinon (Europe) GmbH
Heerdter Lohweg 89
D-40549 Duesseldorf 11
Germany
0211/52050

Fujinon, Inc.
10 High Point Dr.
Wayne, NJ 07470-7434
201-633-5600

Hobbs Medical, Inc.
P.O. Box 46
Stafford Springs, CT 06076-0046
203-684-5875

Inben Brothers Company
5250 N. Leamington Ave.
Chicago, IL 60630-1622
312-286-7241

Mill-Rose Laboratories
7310 Corporate Blvd.
Mentor, OH 44060-4856
216-255-7995

Olympus America, Inc.
4 Nevada Drive
Lake Success, NY 11042-1179
516-488-3880

Olympus Optical Co. Ltd.
San-Ei Bldg.
1-22-2, Nishi-Shinjuku
Shinjuku-Ku, Tokyo 163-91
Japan
03/3402111

Pentax Precision Instrument Corp.
30 Ramland Rd.
Orangeburg, NY 10962-2699
914-365-0700

R-Group International
2321 N.W. 66th Court, Ste. W4
Gainesville, FL 32606
904-378-3633

Sanderson-Macleod, Inc.
199 S. Main St.
P.O. Box 50
Palmer, MA 01069-1899
413-283-3481

U.S. Endoscopy Group
7123 Industrial Park Blvd.
Mentor, OH 44060
216-269-8226

Wilson-Cook Medical, Inc.
4900 Bethania Station Rd.
Winston-Salem, NC 27105-1203
919-744-0157

Wolf Medical Instruments Corp., Richard
353 Corporate Woods Pkwy.
Vernon Hills, IL 60061-3110
708-913-1113

CARRIER, SPONGE, ENDOSCOPIC

Aesculap
1000 Gateway Blvd.
South San Francisco, CA 94080-7030
415-876-7000

Encompas Unlimited, Inc.
1110 Pinellas Bayway, Ste. 104
Tierra Verde, FL 33715-8281
813-867-7701

Marlow Surgical Technologies, Inc.
1810 Joseph Lloyd Pkwy.
Willoughby, OH 44094-8030
216-946-2453

Pilling-Rusch
420 Delaware Dr.
Fort Washington, PA 19034-2711
215-643-2600

Plastofilm Industries, Inc.
P.O. Box 531
Wheaton, IL 60189-0531
708-668-2838

Wolf Medical Instruments Corp., Richard
353 Corporate Woods Pkwy.
Vernon Hills, IL 60061-3110
708-913-1113

EXTRACTOR, GALL BLADDER

Davis & Geck Endosurgery
1 Casper St.
Danbury, CT 06810
203-743-4451

PROFESSIONAL LINE 8381-05
Description:
Gall Bladder Extractor (order number 8381-05):

GALL BLADDER EXTRACTOR

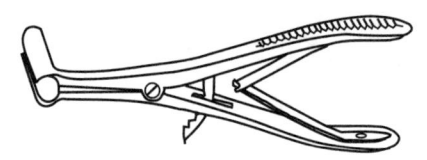

Used as an auxiliary instrument for extracting small organs like a gallbladder or appendix.

Apple Medical Corp.
93 Nashaway Rd.
Bolton, MA 01740
508-779-2926

Davis & Geck Div.
American Cyanamid Company
One Cyanamid Plaza
Wayne, NJ 07470-2012
201-831-2000

Schwarz Medical
Kirchstrasse 24
D-86935 Rott
Germany
8869/1881

GAUGE, THICKNESS, TISSUE

Beta Instrument, Inc.
125 John Hancock Rd.
Taunton, MA 02780
508-880-0771

United States Surgical Corp.
150 Glover Ave.
Norwalk, CT 06856-5080
203-845-1000

INSTRUMENT, DISSECTING, LAPAROSCOPIC

Davis & Geck Endosurgery
1 Casper St.
Danbury, CT 06810
203-743-4451

PRESTIGE 8364-21

DESCRIPTION:

Maryland Dissecting Forceps (Electrosurgical):
Dual action jaws curved 30°, 5mm diameter. Insulated handle, monopolar electrosurgical connection, 360° rotating shaft with integral flush port (cleaning syringe included). Also includes one 8370-03 PRESTIGE Monopolar Cord Adaptor. For precise dissection of mesentery tissue. Also for fixing and holding fine structures:

MARYLAND DISSECTING FORCEPS

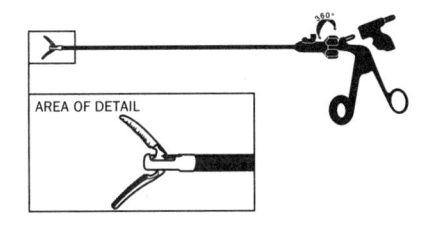

PRODUCT CODE	DIAMETER MM	SHAFT LENGTH CM
8364-21	5	33
8364-31	5	22
8364-41	5	44

Davis & Geck Endosurgery
1 Casper St.
Danbury, CT 06810
203-743-4451

PRESTIGE 8364-22

DESCRIPTION:

Olive Tip Dissecting Forceps (Electrosurgical):
Delicate dual action jaws, 5mm diameter, insulated handle, monopolar electrosurgical connection, 360° rotating shaft with integral flush port (cleaning syringe included). Also includes one 8370-03 PRESTIGE Monopolar Cord Adaptor. For precise, delicate dissection of tubular structures, i.e., to expose cystic artery or cystic duct. Also for fixing and holding fine structures:

OLIVE TIP DISSECTING FORCEPS

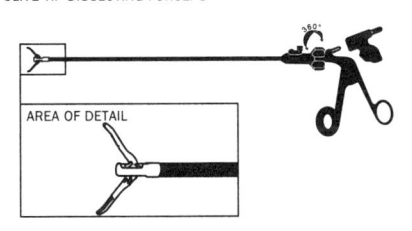

PRODUCT CODE	DIAMETER MM	SHAFT LENGTH CM
8364-22	5	33
8364-32	5	22
8364-42	5	44

Davis & Geck Endosurgery
1 Casper St.
Danbury, CT 06810
203-743-4451

PRESTIGE 8364-23

DESCRIPTION:

Dolphin Nose Dissecting Forceps (Electrosurgical):
Delicate dual action jaws with very fine tapered tips, insulated handle, monopolar electrosurgical connection, 360° rotating shaft with integral flush port (cleaning syringe included). Also includes one 8370-03 PRESTIGE Monopolar Cord Adaptor. For fine dissection. Also for fixing and holding fine structures:

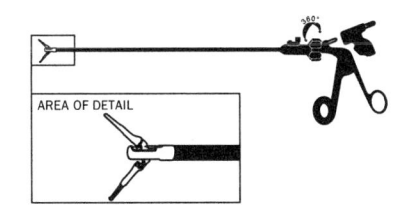

DOLPHIN NOSE DISSECTING FORCEPS

PRODUCT CODE	DIAMETER MM	SHAFT LENGTH CM
8364-23	5	33
8364-33	5	22
8364-43	5	44

Davis & Geck Endosurgery
1 Casper St.
Danbury, CT 06810
203-743-4451

PROFESSIONAL LINE 8375 & 8376 SERIES

DESCRIPTION:

Micro Dissecting Forceps:
5mm diameter (order number 8375-06) or 10mm diameter (order number 8375-12), insulated, monopolar connection, working length 33cm, color coded green. For fixing and holding fine structures. May also be used for dissecting:

MICRO DISSECTING FORCEPS

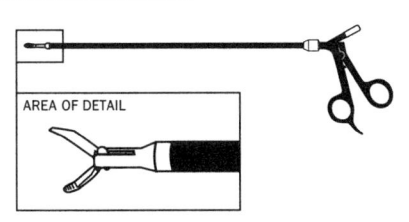

Atraumatic Dissecting Forceps:
Insulated, monopolar connection, color coded green. For fixing and holding organs and tissue. May be used for dissecting:

ATRAUMATIC DISSECTING FORCEPS

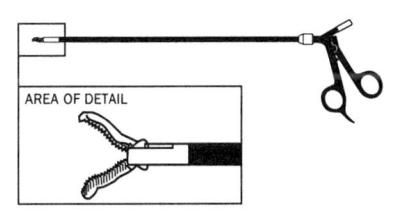

INSTRUMENT, DISSECTING, LAPAROSCOPIC *(cont'd)*

INSTRUMENT KNOB

360° ROTATION

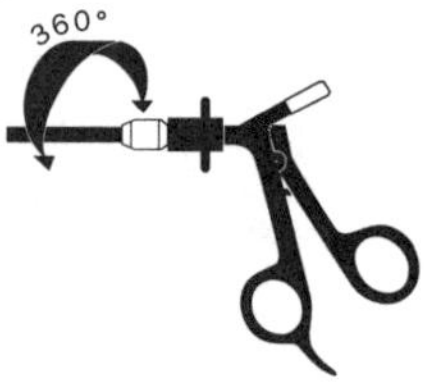

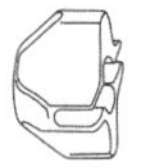

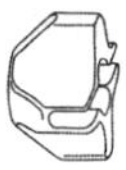

ATRAUMATIC DISSECTING FORCEPS

PRODUCT CODE	DIAMETER	WORKING LENGTH	ROTATABLE
8376-07	5 mm	33 cm	Yes
8376-08	10 mm	33 cm	Yes
8376-09	10 mm	40 cm	Yes
8375-07	5 mm	33 cm	No
8375-13	10 mm	33 cm	No

Davis & Geck Endosurgery
1 Casper St.
Danbury, CT 06810
203-743-4451

PROFESSIONAL LINE 8376 & 8390 SERIES

DESCRIPTION:

Fine Dissecting Forceps:
Flat nose tip, insulated, monopolar connection, color coded green. For dissecting near vessels:

FINE DISSECTING FORCEPS

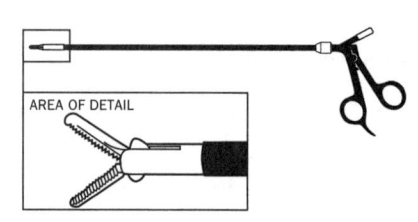

AREA OF DETAIL

FINE DISSECTING FORCEPS

PRODUCT CODE	DIAMETER	WORKING LENGTH
8376-03	5 mm	33 cm
8376-29	10 mm	33 cm
8376-30	10 mm	40 cm

Micro-Dissecting Forceps:
5mm diameter (order number 8376-04) or 10mm diameter single action (order number 8376-26), insulated, monopolar connection, working length 33cm, color coded green. For dissecting very fine structures:

MICRO-DISSECTING FORCEPS

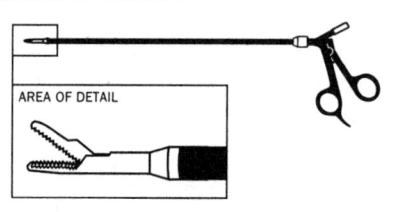

AREA OF DETAIL

Maryland Dissecting Forceps:
Jaws angled 30°, insulated, monopolar connection, color coded green. For precise dissection, i.e. to expose cystic artery or cystic duct:

INSTRUMENT KNOB

360° ROTATION

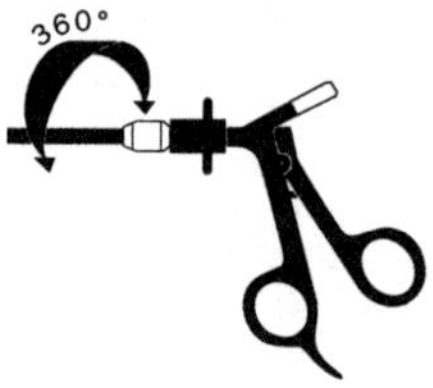

MARYLAND DISSECTING FORCEPS

AREA OF DETAIL

MARYLAND DISSECTING FORCEPS

PRODUCT CODE	DIAMETER	WORKING LENGTH	ROTATABLE	D-TACH
8376-16	5 mm	33 cm	Yes	No
8376-17	10 mm	33 cm	Yes	No
8376-18	10 mm	40 cm	Yes	No
8376-05	5 mm	33 cm	No	No
8376-06	10 mm	33 cm	No	No
8376-31	10 mm	40 cm	No	No
8390-24	5 mm	35 cm	Yes	Yes
8390-38	5 mm	26 cm	Yes	Yes

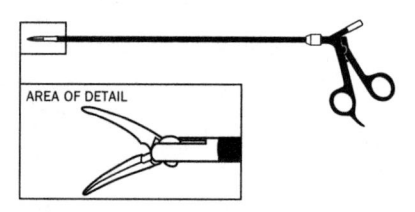

Access Surgical International, Inc.
15 Caswell Ln.
Boat Yard Square
Plymouth, MA 02360
508-747-6006

Aesculap
1000 Gateway Blvd.
South San Francisco, CA 94080-7030
415-876-7000

Birtcher Medical Systems, Inc.
50 Technology Dr.
Irvine, CA 92718-2301
714-753-9400

Boss Instruments, Ltd.
1310 Central Ct.
Hermitage, TN 37076
615-885-2231

Bryan Corp.
4 Plympton St.
Woburn, MA 01801-2908
617-935-0004

Cabot Medical Corp.
2021 Cabot Blvd. West
Langhorne, PA 19047-1875
215-752-8300

Circon Acmi
300 Stillwater Ave.
Stamford, CT 06902-3640
203-328-8689

Core Dynamics, Inc.
11222-4 St. Johns Indust. Pkwy.
Jacksonville, FL 32216
904-641-6611

Davinci Medical, Inc.
13700 First Ave. North
Minneapolis, MN 55441
612-473-4245

Davis & Geck Div.
American Cyanamid Company
One Cyanamid Plaza
Wayne, NJ 07470-2012
201-831-2000

Davol, Inc.
100 Sockanossett
P.O. Box 8500
Cranston, RI 02920-0500
401-463-7000

Elekta Instruments, Inc.
8 Executive Park West, Ste. 809
Atlanta, GA 30329
404-315-1225

Elmed, Inc.
60 W. Fay Ave.
Addison, IL 60101-5198
708-543-2792

Ethicon Endo-Surgery
4545 Creek Road
Cincinnati, OH 45242
513-786-7000

Heraeus Surgical, Inc.
575 Cottonwood Dr.
Milpitas, CA 95035-7402
408-954-4000

Innovative Surgical, Inc.
3071 Continental Dr., Ste. 102
West Palm Beach, FL 33407
407-697-5051

Kensey Nash Corporation
55 E. Uwchlan Ave., Ste. 204
Exton, PA 19341-1247
215-524-0188

Leisegang Medical, Inc.
6401 Congress Ave.
Boca Raton, FL 33487-2883
407-994-0202

Marlow Surgical Technologies, Inc.
1810 Joseph Lloyd Pkwy.
Willoughby, OH 44094-8030
216-946-2453

Microsurge, Inc.
150 A St.
Needham, MA 02194
617-444-2300

Mist, Inc.
6307 E. Angus Dr.
Raleigh, NC 27613
919-787-8377

Origin Medsystems, Inc.
135 Constitution Dr.
Menlo Park, CA 94025
415-617-5000

P.A.K. Orthopaedics, Inc.
3 De Camp Ct.
West Long Branch, NJ 07764-1165
201-939-6906

Performance Surgical Instruments
40 Norfolk Ave.
Easton, MA 023334
508-230-0010

Smith & Nephew Dyonics, Inc.
160 Dascomb Rd.
Andover, MA 01810-5893
508-470-2800

Synectic Engineering, Inc.
4 Oxford Rd.
Milford, CT 06460-7007
203-877-8488

Unisurge, Inc.
10231 Bubb Rd.
Cupertino, CA 95014
408-996-4700

United States Surgical Corp.
150 Glover Ave.
Norwalk, CT 06856-5080
203-845-1000

Wolf Medical Instruments Corp., Richard
353 Corporate Woods Pkwy.
Vernon Hills, IL 60061-3110
708-913-1113

INSTRUMENT, DISSECTING, MYOMA, LAPAROSCOPIC

Davis & Geck Div.
American Cyanamid Company
One Cyanamid Plaza
Wayne, NJ 07470-2012
201-831-2000

Davol, Inc.
100 Sockanossett
P.O. Box 8500
Cranston, RI 02920-0500
401-463-7000

Elmed, Inc.
60 W. Fay Ave.
Addison, IL 60101-5198
708-543-2792

Leisegang Medical, Inc.
6401 Congress Ave.
Boca Raton, FL 33487-2883
407-994-0202

Marlow Surgical Technologies, Inc.
1810 Joseph Lloyd Pkwy.
Willoughby, OH 44094-8030
216-946-2453

Wolf Medical Instruments Corp., Richard
353 Corporate Woods Pkwy.
Vernon Hills, IL 60061-3110
708-913-1113

INSTRUMENT, ELECTROSURGERY, LAPAROSCOPIC

Davis & Geck Endosurgery
1 Casper St.
Danbury, CT 06810
203-743-4451

PRESTIGE 5MM SERIES

INDICATIONS: DAVIS & GECK Prestige endoscopic instruments are designed to grasp, cut, and/or dissect tissue during endoscopic surgical procedures. DAVIS & GECK Prestige endoscopic instruments are designed to be used through a cannula or port, commonly referred to as a trocar.

DAVIS & GECK Prestige endoscopic instruments are designed for the purpose of manipulating soft tissue structures. DAVIS & GECK Prestige endoscopic instruments are delicate surgical instruments. Any use of an instrument for tasks other than for which it is intended will usually result in a damaged or broken instrument.

CONTRAINDICATIONS: The use of DAVIS & GECK Prestige endoscopic instruments is contraindicated when, in the judgment of the physician, their use would be contrary to the best interests of the patient.

PRECAUTIONS: Instruments must be handled carefully during surgery to avoid misusing the instrument. Misuse will usually result in damage or breakage. Instruments are designed to be held with one finger and the thumb in the ring handles. Do not hold handles in a whole hand grip (fingers outside ring handles). This grip applies excessive force to the linkage mechanism and results in damage to the instrument.

Use extreme care when inserting or removing endoscopic instruments through a cannula. Upon insertion, ensure that the cannula "trap door" or trumpet valve has been

INSTRUMENT, ELECTROSURGERY, LAPAROSCOPIC (cont'd)

fully opened to allow passage of the instrument. During removal, pull the instrument straight out until completely clear of the cannula, as any lateral pressure on the instrument may damage the working tip. Instrument jaws should be closed completely so that they do not catch on the cannula's internal valve assembly. Care must be taken to avoid tissue being inadvertantly trapped in the jaws of the instrument on removal; therefore, visualize instrument prior to and during removal.

Any type of misuse or abuse of the instrument will render the warranty void. DAVIS & GECK assumes no liability if the instrument is misused or otherwise abused.

CARE & MAINTENANCE: Before using the instrument for the first time, and after each surgical procedure, clean all instruments thoroughly as follows:

1. Open the jaws by spreading the ring handles. Rinse the instrument thoroughly with deionized water to remove any accumulated debris. Hand wash instruments using a neutral pH instrument detergent or enzymatic instrument cleaner, being sure to thoroughly flush all lumen channels of the instrument with the solution (Figures 1 and 2).

FIGURE 1

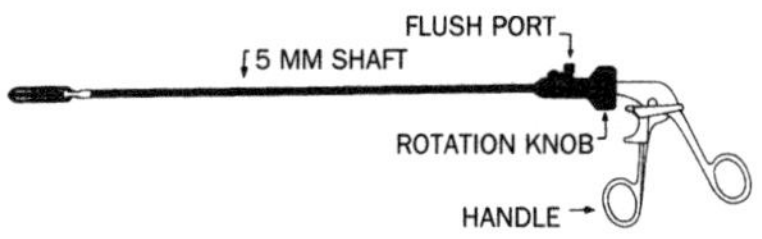

2. Hand wash each surface of the instrument with an instrument cleaning brush to remove visible residual debris. Using the flushing syringe supplied, thoroughly flush the instrument with enzymatic instrument cleaner, then with water through the flush port to remove all blood and debris that may obstruct the shaft lumen (Figures 1 and 2). The flush port flushes the inner shaft and linkage. Continue flushing until the flushing water is clear and no residue of cleaning solution remains.

3. DAVIS & GECK Prestige endoscopic instruments should be handled with care. Avoid the use of steel wool, wire brushes, and highly abrasive detergents. Use of anything other than high quality brushes designed for instrument cleaning may result in damage to the instrument. Care should be taken not to scratch the surface of the instrument.

4. Thoroughly rinse the instrument again with deionized water and visually inspect the instrument after washing, making sure the internal lumens and channels are thoroughly rinsed and free of any cleaning solutions.

5. All instrument surfaces and individual parts should be visually inspected for burrs, nicks, misalignment, or bent tips.

FIGURE 2

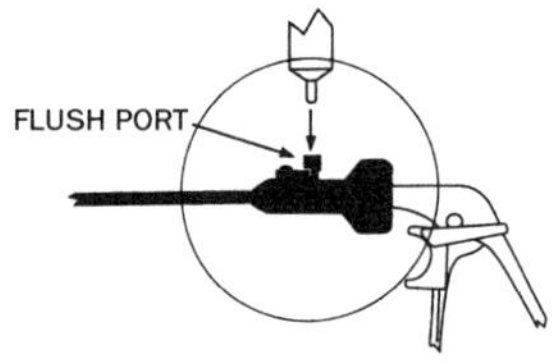

6. Thoroughly dry all components using a towel or pressurized air to ensure removal of residual moisture. Moisture which is not removed may cause corrosion of the instrument.

7. Prior to sterilizing, lubricate with a non-silicone, antimicrobial, water-soluble surgical instrument lubricant solution. Do not rinse or towel dry. Do not use mineral oil, petroleum jelly, or silicone sprays which can inhibit sterilization and cause build-up in the crevices of the instrument.

8. Return item to its designated storage container. DAVIS & GECK Prestige endoscopic instruments should be stored in a tray with silicone holders designed to protect them. Proceed with sterilization.

Storage: DAVIS & GECK Prestige endoscopic instruments must be completely dry before storing and must be handled with care to prevent damage. Instruments should be stored in areas which provide protection from extremes of temperature and humidity.

STERILIZATION GUIDELINES: Clean and sterilize product before each use. Steam sterilize at a minimum of 250°F (121°C).

1. Sterilizing in ethylene oxide is not recommended.
2. Sterilizing in liquid solutions is not recommended.
3. Do not sterilize at temperatures greater than 275°F (135°C).

NOTE: Time and temperature parameters required for steam sterilization vary according to type of sterilizer, cycle design, and packaging material.

Minimum exposure times for steam sterilizers are as follows:

Gravity Displacement: 250° to 254°F, wrapped 30 minutes
Prevacuum: 270° to 274°F, wrapped 4 minutes

The use of "flash" sterilization should be avoided whenever possible, as it may result in shortening the life of the instrument.

SPECIFICATIONS/HOW SUPPLIED: DAVIS & GECK Prestige endoscopic instruments are provided non-sterile and must be sterilized before use according to the procedures in the Sterilization section.

Contact your local DAVIS & GECK Endosurgery Representative to place an order, or call or write to the following:

DAVIS & GECK
American Cyanamid Company
ATTN: Customer Service Department
One Casper Street
Danbury, CT 06810
1-800-225-5341: Select the option to place an order
Fax Number: (203) 796-9534

SERVICE REQUIREMENTS & CONTACTS: DAVIS & GECK warrants its instruments against breakage or failure to function in normal use in surgery. If a DAVIS & GECK instrument breaks or fails to function in normal use due to defects in materials or workmanship, DAVIS & GECK will repair or replace such instrument at no cost to the customer after an evaluation has been made by DAVIS & GECK.

Any disassembly, alterations, re-sharpening or repair performed by persons not specifically authorized by DAVIS & GECK will void the above warranties.

The above warranties exclude: instrument coating, scissor edge sharpening, refurbishment due to normal wear and tear, and apply only to the original buyer and are in lieu of all other warranties, either expressed or implied.

REPAIRS:
DAVIS & GECK provides repair services for all DAVIS & GECK instruments, as well as for instruments from other manufacturers. Repaired instruments will be sent back to the customer within 10 business days of receipt by DAVIS & GECK.

When an instrument needs repair, please use the following procedure:

1. Clean instruments thoroughly, then sterilize before shipping them to DAVIS & GECK.
2. To ship instruments, use a sturdy shipping box with soft packaging material to protect your instruments.
3. Use tip protectors and individually wrap micro and delicate instruments.

Return instruments for repair to:

DAVIS & GECK
American Cyanamid Company
INSTRUMENT REPAIR SERVICE
Commerce Park, Commerce Drive
Danbury, CT 06810
1-800-225-5341: Select the option to inquire about repairs.

Ethicon Endo-Surgery
4545 Creek Road
Cincinnati, OH 45242
513-786-7000

INSTRUMENT, KNOT TYING, SUTURE, LAPAROSCOPIC

Davis & Geck Endosurgery
1 Casper St.
Danbury, CT 06810
203-743-4451

PROFESSIONAL LINE 8378-02

DESCRIPTION:

Insulated Suture Fixation Forceps (order number 8378-02):

SUTURE FIXATION FORCEPS, INSULATED

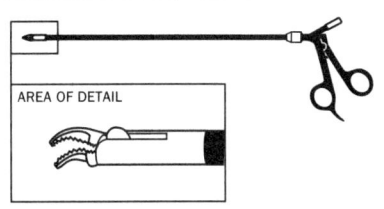

AREA OF DETAIL

U-shaped jaws, incorporated locking spring, 5mm diameter, insulated, monopolar connection, working length 33cm, color coded gray. For simultaneous coagulation while guiding needle and suture.

Davis & Geck Endosurgery
1 Casper St.
Danbury, CT 06810
203-743-4451

PROFESSIONAL LINE 8380 SERIES

DESCRIPTION:

Loop Applicator (order number 8380-01):
For holding prepared (Roeder style) loops and applying ligatures. 3mm diameter (can be used with 5mm trocars):

LOOP APPLICATOR

Knot Tying Instrument (order number 8380-02):
For accurately placing and fixing sutures and knots. 5mm diameter:

KNOT TYING INSTRUMENT

Access Surgical International, Inc.
15 Caswell Ln.
Boat Yard Square
Plymouth, MA 02360
508-747-6006

Advanced Surgical, Inc.
305 College Rd. East
Princeton, NJ 08540
609-987-2340

Aesculap
1000 Gateway Blvd.
South San Francisco, CA 94080-7030
415-876-7000

American Surgical Technologies Corp.
300 Billerica Rd.
Chelmsford, MA 01824
508-250-0150

Boss Instruments, Ltd.
1310 Central Ct.
Hermitage, TN 37076
615-885-2231

Cabot Medical Corp.
2021 Cabot Blvd. West
Langhorne, PA 19047-1875
215-752-8300

Core Dynamics, Inc.
11222-4 St. Johns Indust. Pkwy.
Jacksonville, FL 32216
904-641-6611

Davis & Geck Div.
American Cyanamid Company
One Cyanamid Plaza
Wayne, NJ 07470-2012
201-831-2000

Davol, Inc.
100 Sockanossett
P.O. Box 8500
Cranston, RI 02920-0500
401-463-7000

Elmed, Inc.
60 W. Fay Ave.
Addison, IL 60101-5198
708-543-2792

Instrument Makar, Inc.
2950 E. Mt. Hope
Okemos, MI 48864-1910
517-332-3593

Leisegang Medical, Inc.
6401 Congress Ave.
Boca Raton, FL 33487-2883
407-994-0202

Linvatec Corporation
11311 Concept Blvd.
Largo, FL 34643-4908
813-399-5344

Marlow Surgical Technologies, Inc.
1810 Joseph Lloyd Pkwy.
Willoughby, OH 44094-8030
216-946-2453

Medicon Instruments, Inc.
4405 International Blvd.
Norcross, GA 30093-3013
404-381-2858

Mist, Inc.
6307 E. Angus Dr.
Raleigh, NC 27613
919-787-8377

Performance Surgical Instruments
40 Norfolk Ave.
Easton, MA 023334
508-230-0010

Ranfac Corp.
Avon Indus. Pk./30 Doherty Ave., Box 635
Avon, MA 02322-1125
508-588-4400

Sharpe Endosurgical Corp.
3750 Annapolis Lane, Ste. 135
Minneapolis, MN 55447
612-784-0460

Wolf Medical Instruments Corp., Richard
353 Corporate Woods Pkwy.
Vernon Hills, IL 60061-3110
708-913-1113

INSTRUMENT, NEEDLE HOLDER/KNOT TYING

Access Surgical International, Inc.
15 Caswell Ln.
Boat Yard Square
Plymouth, MA 02360
508-747-6006

Boss Instruments, Ltd.
1310 Central Ct.
Hermitage, TN 37076
615-885-2231

Cabot Medical Corp.
2021 Cabot Blvd. West
Langhorne, PA 19047-1875
215-752-8300

INSTRUMENT, NEEDLE HOLDER/KNOT TYING (cont'd)

Core Dynamics, Inc.
11222-4 St. Johns Indust. Pkwy.
Jacksonville, FL 32216
904-641-6611

Elmed, Inc.
60 W. Fay Ave.
Addison, IL 60101-5198
708-543-2792

Instrument Makar, Inc.
2950 E. Mt. Hope
Okemos, MI 48864-1910
517-332-3593

Leisegang Medical, Inc.
6401 Congress Ave.
Boca Raton, FL 33487-2883
407-994-0202

Marlow Surgical Technologies, Inc.
1810 Joseph Lloyd Pkwy.
Willoughby, OH 44094-8030
216-946-2453

Origin Medsystems, Inc.
135 Constitution Dr.
Menlo Park, CA 94025
415-617-5000

Performance Surgical Instruments
40 Norfolk Ave.
Easton, MA 023334
508-230-0010

Smith & Nephew Dyonics, Inc.
160 Dascomb Rd.
Andover, MA 01810-5893
508-470-2800

Synectic Engineering, Inc.
4 Oxford Rd.
Milford, CT 06460-7007
203-877-8488

W.J. Medical Instruments, Inc.
3537 Old Conejo Rd.
Newbury Park, CA 91320
805-499-8676

Wolf Medical Instruments Corp., Richard
353 Corporate Woods Pkwy.
Vernon Hills, IL 60061-3110
708-913-1113

INSTRUMENT, PASSING, SUTURE, LAPAROSCOPIC

Access Surgical International, Inc.
15 Caswell Ln.
Boat Yard Square
Plymouth, MA 02360
508-747-6006

Boss Instruments, Ltd.
1310 Central Ct.
Hermitage, TN 37076
615-885-2231

Cabot Medical Corp.
2021 Cabot Blvd. West
Langhorne, PA 19047-1875
215-752-8300

Davis & Geck Div.
American Cyanamid Company
One Cyanamid Plaza
Wayne, NJ 07470-2012
201-831-2000

Elmed, Inc.
60 W. Fay Ave.
Addison, IL 60101-5198
708-543-2792

Linvatec Corporation
11311 Concept Blvd.
Largo, FL 34643-4908
813-399-5344

Marlow Surgical Technologies, Inc.
1810 Joseph Lloyd Pkwy.
Willoughby, OH 44094-8030
216-946-2453

Mist, Inc.
6307 E. Angus Dr.
Raleigh, NC 27613
919-787-8377

Performance Surgical Instruments
40 Norfolk Ave.
Easton, MA 023334
508-230-0010

Ranfac Corp.
Avon Indus. Pk./30 Doherty Ave., Box 635
Avon, MA 02322-1125
508-588-4400

Surgical Safety Products, Inc.
434 S. Washington Blvd., Ste. 2
Sarasota, FL 34236
813-953-7889

Wolf Medical Instruments Corp., Richard
353 Corporate Woods Pkwy.
Vernon Hills, IL 60061-3110
708-913-1113

INSTRUMENT, SEPARATING, NERVE

Nu Surg Medical, Inc.
4440 Glen Este-Withamsville Rd., Ste.780
Cincinnati, OH 45245
513-753-3633

NUSURG LAPAROSCOPIC PROBE/NERVE HOOK
DESCRIPTION:

The Nu Surg Laparoscopic Probe/Nerve Hook incorporates a unique tip enabling the surgeon to separate, isolate, and support structures with one instrument. The ball tip minimizes the possibility of puncturing viscera. The Laparoscopic Probe is a 5mm curved shaft placed through 5mm trocar sleeves. The surgeon is able to support and separate structures without grasping which may cause vessel trauma. The Laparoscopic Probe/Nerve Hook is suited for truncal and highly selective vagotomies. It has been useful in isolating cystic ducts and cystic arteries, vas deferens, sympathetic pelvic nerve trunk, ureters, and mesenteric vessels.

WARNINGS: Failure to read and follow instructions furnished in this product insert may result in serious injury.

PRECAUTIONS: Care should be taken when using this device to ensure direct visualization of the hook and tip in order to avoid any inadvertent injuries to viscera.

INSTRUCTIONS FOR USE: Insert Laparoscopic Probe/Nerve Hook into a 5mm trocar sleeve with the ball tip oriented in the 12:00 position. Rotate the instrument 180° in a clockwise manner so that the ball tip is at the 6:00 position, inferior to the structure, (i.e., nerve vessel). Separate beneath the structure until a window in the surrounding tissues is made. Roll the instrument 90° in a counter clockwise direction and capture the structure. Support and separate the structure from the surrounding tissues by moving the instrument longitudinally along the length of the structure.

CARE & MAINTENANCE:
Inspection: A routine check should be completed before each case. This check should include the following:
 1. Check tip for correct configuration.

ENLARGED VIEW

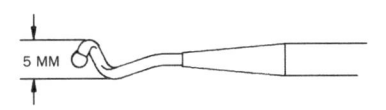

 2. Check to ensure tip is secure to shaft.
 3. Insert instrument through a 5mm (or larger) trocar sleeve ensuring proper instrument shaft configuration.

Cleaning: Use a soft brush and a neutral ph detergent to remove all traces of blood and debris. Rinse thoroughly and dry completely. Mechanical washer/sterilizer may be utilized following the manufacturer's recommendations of that equipment and facility protocol. Ultrasonic cleaning could also be utilized, but instrument is to be rinsed thoroughly and dried completely.

STERILIZATION GUIDELINES: The instrument may be autoclaved or gas sterilized. Refer to the sterilizer manufacturer's instructions for correct time and temperature settings. Warning: Gas sterilization can be used only if the instrument is thoroughly dry after cleaning.

SERVICE REQUIREMENTS & CONTACTS: Send all instruments for service or repair to:

Nu Surg Medical, Inc.
4440 Glen Este-Withamsville Road
Suite 780
Cincinnati, OH 45245
800-225-2922

Always include the purchase order number and a written description of the problem.
 Warranty: This device is warranted for one full year from date of purchase. Devices are guaranteed to be free from defects in both materials and workmanship. Disassembly, alteration or repair performed by any person not specifically authorized by Nu Surg Medical Inc., will invalidate the warranty. Devices under warranty should be returned to Nu Surg Medical Inc. and will be repaired without charge to the purchaser, assuming they were used for their intended purpose. The above warranties are in lieu of all other warranties either expressed or implied. Suitability for use of this device for any surgical procedure shall be determined by the user. Nu Surg Medical Inc., shall not be liable for incidental or consequential damages of any kind.

INTRODUCER, T-TUBE

Access Surgical International, Inc.
15 Caswell Ln.
Boat Yard Square
Plymouth, MA 02360
508-747-6006

Performance Surgical Instruments
40 Norfolk Ave.
Easton, MA 023334
508-230-0010

Smith & Nephew Richards Inc.
1450 Brooks Road
Memphis, TN 38116
901-396-2121

MIRROR, ENDOSCOPIC

Aesculap
1000 Gateway Blvd.
South San Francisco, CA 94080-7030
415-876-7000

Lawton USA Surgical Instruments
6341 S. Troy Cir.
Englewood, CO 80111-6415
303-790-9416

Surgimedics/SLP
2828 N. Crescent Ridge Dr.
The Woodlands, TX 77381
713-363-4949

RACK, INSTRUMENT, LAPAROSCOPY

Davis & Geck Endosurgery
1 Casper St.
Danbury, CT 06810
203-743-4451

PROFESSIONAL LINE 8381-09
DESCRIPTION: The DAVIS & GECK **Professional Line Sterilization and Storage Rack 8381-09** provides secure and clearly arranged instrument storage. In addition, the product is suitable for use during instrument sterilization.

STERILIZATION/STORAGE RACK

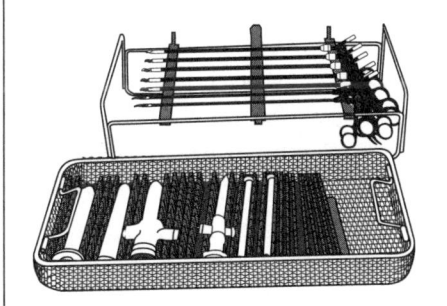

Upper rack securely holds up to ten 5mm and/or 10mm hand-held instruments. Lower rack holds trocars, small parts, etc.

INSTRUCTIONS FOR USE: To prepare the product for use during the sterilization cycle, the product can either be double-wrapped in a woven or non-woven wrapper, or placed within an appropriately sized rigid container system. In either case, the wrapper or container system used must be suitable for the type of sterilization to be utilized according to the manufacturer's directions.

SPECIFICATIONS/HOW SUPPLIED:
Replacement Parts For Storage Rack:
 8381-29 silicone insert, 5mm diameter, 9/pkg.; 8381-30 silicone insert, 10mm diameter, 9/pkg.; 8381-31 silicone insert, 12mm diameter, 9/pkg.; 8381-32 rack only; 8381-33 silicone pad only, 8381-34 basket only.

Davis & Geck Div.
American Cyanamid Company
One Cyanamid Plaza
Wayne, NJ 07470-2012
201-831-2000

SNARE, ENDOSCOPIC

Cameron-Miller, Inc.
3949 S. Racine Ave.
Chicago, IL 60609-2523
312-523-6360

Carsen Group Inc.
151 Telson Rd.
Markham, ONT L3R 1E7
Canada
416-479-4100

Davol, Inc.
100 Sockanossett
P.O. Box 8500
Cranston, RI 02920-0500
401-463-7000

Electro Surgical Instrument Co.
37 Centennial St.
Rochester, NY 14611-1732
716-235-1430

Elmed, Inc.
60 W. Fay Ave.
Addison, IL 60101-5198
708-543-2792

Kensey Nash Corporation
55 E. Uwchlan Ave., Ste. 204
Exton, PA 19341-1247
215-524-0188

SNARE, ENDOSCOPIC (cont'd)

Laparomed Corp.
9272 Jeronimo Rd., Unit 109
Irvine, CA 92718-1914
714-768-1155

Life Medical Technologies, Inc.
3649 W. 1987 S.
Salt Lake City, UT 84104
801-972-1900

Marlow Surgical Technologies, Inc.
1810 Joseph Lloyd Pkwy.
Willoughby, OH 44094-8030
216-946-2453

Meditron Devices, Inc.
83 Hobart St.
Hackensack, NJ 07601-3912
201-489-4222

Mill-Rose Laboratories
7310 Corporate Blvd.
Mentor, OH 44060-4856
216-255-7995

Pentax Precision Instrument Corp.
30 Ramland Rd.
Orangeburg, NY 10962-2699
914-365-0700

Performance Surgical Instruments
40 Norfolk Ave.
Easton, MA 023334
508-230-0010

Storz Endoscopy-America Inc., Karl
10111 W. Jefferson Blvd.
Culver City, CA 90232-3509
310-558-1500

Storz GmbH & Co., Karl
Mittelstr. 8
Postfach 230
D-78532 Tuttlingen
Germany
07461/7080

U.S. Endoscopy Group
7123 Industrial Park Blvd.
Mentor, OH 44060
216-269-8226

Wolf Medical Instruments Corp., Richard
353 Corporate Woods Pkwy.
Vernon Hills, IL 60061-3110
708-913-1113

Insufflator

Insufflators provide the pressurized gas needed to maintain pneumoperitoneum during laparoscopic surgery. All modern insufflators are pressure-regulated. They instill gas at a specified flow rate until a preset pressure is reached, then maintain that pressure by delivering additional gas as needed. Constant, reproducible pressure permits improved fluid and airway management and better maintenance of acid-base balance.

As laparoscopic procedures become ever more complex, higher and higher flow rates are needed to maintain a given pressure. Large trocars at multiple sites, frequent instrument changes, and increased intra-abdominal suctioning all serve to bleed off pressure more rapidly, making low-flow insufflators obsolete. The minimum flow rate necessary for today's surgeries is six liters per minute. Ten is more common; 15 is desirable.

A typical modern insufflator has a solid-state regulator and requires very little maintenance. It should have indicators that permit monitoring and adjustment of flow rate and intra-abdominal pressure; and these readouts should be legible from across the room. Some models also have an indicator that shows when the insufflation needle has entered the peritoneal cavity. This, however, is not only of questionable accuracy, but also promotes an unsafe method of introduction. The needle should never be connected to the insufflator until its presence in the peritoneal cavity has been confirmed by other means.

Some machines now include a filtered recirculation system for removing intra-abdominal smoke. This eliminates the need for other corrective measures. However, the system is bulky and slow to do its work; and many surgeons still prefer to clear the cavity with a standard suction machine.

INSUFFLATOR, CARBON-DIOXIDE, AUTOMATIC (FOR ENDOSCOPE)

Bryan Corp.
4 Plympton St.
Woburn, MA 01801-2908
617-935-0004

Cabot Medical Corp.
2021 Cabot Blvd. West
Langhorne, PA 19047-1875
215-752-8300

CMT, Inc.
648 Bay Road
P.O. Box 297
Hamilton, MA 01936
508-468-5640

Coopersurgical, Inc.
15 Forest Pkwy.
Shelton, CT 06484-5458
203-929-6321

Elmed, Inc.
60 W. Fay Ave.
Addison, IL 60101-5198
708-543-2792

Leisegang Medical, Inc.
6401 Congress Ave.
Boca Raton, FL 33487-2883
407-994-0202

Marlow Surgical Technologies, Inc.
1810 Joseph Lloyd Pkwy.
Willoughby, OH 44094-8030
216-946-2453

Mist, Inc.
6307 E. Angus Dr.
Raleigh, NC 27613
919-787-8377

Smith & Nephew Dyonics, Inc.
160 Dascomb Rd.
Andover, MA 01810-5893
508-470-2800

Spiess Design, Inc.
495 Lindberg Lane
Northbrook, IL 60062-2412
708-564-1098

Storz Endoscopy-America Inc., Karl
10111 W. Jefferson Blvd.
Culver City, CA 90232-3509
310-558-1500

Storz GmbH & Co., Karl
Mittelstr. 8
Postfach 230
D-78532 Tuttlingen
Germany
07461/7080

Wolf Medical Instruments Corp., Richard
353 Corporate Woods Pkwy.
Vernon Hills, IL 60061-3110
708-913-1113

Zinnanti Surgical Instruments
21540 B Prairie St.
Chatsworth, CA 91311-5886
818-700-0090

INSUFFLATOR, CARBON-DIOXIDE, UTEROTUBAL

Haiss KG, K.
Postfach 7
D-72417 Jungingen
Germany
07477/1023

Storz Endoscopy-America Inc., Karl
10111 W. Jefferson Blvd.
Culver City, CA 90232-3509
310-558-1500

Storz GmbH & Co., Karl
Mittelstr. 8
Postfach 230
D-78532 Tuttlingen
Germany
07461/7080

Unimar, Inc.
475 Danbury Rd.
Wilton, CT 06897-2126
203-762-9550

INSUFFLATOR, HYSTEROSCOPIC

Bristol-Myers Squibb Company Australia
556 Princes Highway
P.O. Box 39
Noble Park, VIC 3174
Australia
03/7953722

Bryan Corp.
4 Plympton St.
Woburn, MA 01801-2908
617-935-0004

Cabot Medical Corp.
2021 Cabot Blvd. West
Langhorne, PA 19047-1875
215-752-8300

CMT, Inc.
648 Bay Road
P.O. Box 297
Hamilton, MA 01936
508-468-5640

Coopersurgical, Inc.
15 Forest Pkwy.
Shelton, CT 06484-5458
203-929-6321

Elmed, Inc.
60 W. Fay Ave.
Addison, IL 60101-5198
708-543-2792

F.M. Wiest Mdeizintechnik GmbH
82004 Unterhaching
Postfach 1449
Muenchen 82204
Germany
49-89/6129080

Leisegang Medical, Inc.
6401 Congress Ave.
Boca Raton, FL 33487-2883
407-994-0202

Unimar, Inc.
475 Danbury Rd.
Wilton, CT 06897-2126
203-762-9550

Wiest USA, Inc.
P.O. Box 637
Oradell, NJ 07649
201-262-4662

Wisap Gesellschaft
Rudolf Diesel Ring 20
D-82054 Sauerlach
Germany
08104/1067

Wisap USA
P.O. Box 324
Tomball, TX 77377-0324
713-351-2629

WM Instrumente GmbH
Panoramastr. 6
D-78604 Rietheim 1
Germany
07424/501310

Wolf Medical Instruments Corp., Richard
353 Corporate Woods Pkwy.
Vernon Hills, IL 60061-3110
708-913-1113

Zimmer, Patient Care Div.
200 W. Ohio Ave.
Dover, OH 44622-9642
216-343-8801

INSUFFLATOR, LAPAROSCOPIC

Birtcher Medical Systems, Inc.
50 Technology Dr.
Irvine, CA 92718-2301
714-753-9400

Bryan Corp.
4 Plympton St.
Woburn, MA 01801-2908
617-935-0004

Cabot Medical Corp.
2021 Cabot Blvd. West
Langhorne, PA 19047-1875
215-752-8300

CMT, Inc.
648 Bay Road
P.O. Box 297
Hamilton, MA 01936
508-468-5640

Coopersurgical, Inc.
15 Forest Pkwy.
Shelton, CT 06484-5458
203-929-6321

Elmed, Inc.
60 W. Fay Ave.
Addison, IL 60101-5198
708-543-2792

F.M. Wiest Medizintechnik GmbH
Postfach 1449
D-82204 Muenchen
Germany
49-89/6129080

Geister Medizintechnik GmbH
Foehrenstr. 2
Postfach 4228
D-78532 Tuttlingen
Germany
7461-8084

Leisegang Medical, Inc.
6401 Congress Ave.
Boca Raton, FL 33487-2883
407-994-0202

INSUFFLATOR, LAPAROSCOPIC (cont'd)

Marlow Surgical Technologies, Inc.
1810 Joseph Lloyd Pkwy.
Willoughby, OH 44094-8030
216-946-2453

Meditron Devices, Inc.
83 Hobart St.
Hackensack, NJ 07601-3912
201-489-4222

Mist, Inc.
6307 E. Angus Dr.
Raleigh, NC 27613
919-787-8377

Northgate Technologies, Inc.
3930 Ventura Dr., Ste. 150
Arlington Heights, IL 60004
708-506-9872

Optik, Inc.
1370 Blair Dr.
Odenton, MD 21113
410-551-9700

Progressive Dynamics, Inc.
507 Industrial Rd.
Marshall, MI 49068-1758
616-781-4241

Reznik Instrument, Inc.
7337 North Lawndale
Skokie, IL 60076
708-673-3444

Smith & Nephew Dyonics, Inc.
160 Dascomb Rd.
Andover, MA 01810-5893
508-470-2800

Storz Endoscopy-America Inc., Karl
10111 W. Jefferson Blvd.
Culver City, CA 90232-3509
310-558-1500

Storz GmbH & Co., Karl
Mittelstr. 8
Postfach 230
D-78532 Tuttlingen
Germany
07461/7080

Synectic Engineering, Inc.
4 Oxford Rd.
Milford, CT 06460-7007
203-877-8488

W.J. Medical Instruments, Inc.
3537 Old Conejo Rd.
Newbury Park, CA 91320
805-499-8676

Wiest USA, Inc.
P.O. Box 637
Oradell, NJ 07649
201-262-4662

WM Instrumente GmbH
Panoramastr. 6
D-78604 Rietheim 1
Germany
07424/501310

Wolf Medical Instruments Corp., Richard
353 Corporate Woods Pkwy.
Vernon Hills, IL 60061-3110
708-913-1113

Xylog Corp.
83 Hobart St.
Hackensack, NJ 07601-3948
201-489-4040

INSUFFLATOR, OTHER

Arbor Technologies
3728 Plaza Dr.
Ann Arbor, MI 48108-7354
313-665-3300

Bei Medical Systems
83 Hobart St.
Hackensack, NJ 07601
201-489-4222

Bryan Corp.
4 Plympton St.
Woburn, MA 01801-2908
617-935-0004

Coopersurgical, Inc.
15 Forest Pkwy.
Shelton, CT 06484-5458
203-929-6321

Endovations, Inc.
Hill & George Avenues
Reading, PA 19610
215-378-1606

Escalon Ophthalmics
182 Tamarack Circle
Skillman, NJ 08558-9662
609-497-9141

Hemox, Inc.
P.O. Box 362115
Melbourne, FL 32902-0115
407-777-4772

Linvatec Corporation
11311 Concept Blvd.
Largo, FL 34643-4908
813-399-5344

M.D. Engineering
3464 Depot Rd.
Hayward, CA 94545-2714
510-732-9950

Marlow Surgical Technologies, Inc.
1810 Joseph Lloyd Pkwy.
Willoughby, OH 44094-8030
216-946-2453

Med-Co Hospital Supplies Ltd.
7, Shelf House Ind. Est
New Farm Rd.
Alresford, Hampshire SO24 9QE
United Kingdom
096/273-4629

Meditron Devices, Inc.
83 Hobart St.
Hackensack, NJ 07601-3912
201-489-4222

MP Video, Inc.
63 South St.
Hopkinton, MA 01748-2212
508-435-2131

Optik, Inc.
1370 Blair Dr.
Odenton, MD 21113
410-551-9700

Picker International Inc.
Health Care Products Div.
6700 Beta Dr.
Mayfield Village, OH 44143-2321
216-473-6787

Progressive Dynamics, Inc.
507 Industrial Rd.
Marshall, MI 49068-1758
616-781-4241

Smith & Nephew Dyonics, Inc.
160 Dascomb Rd.
Andover, MA 01810-5893
508-470-2800

Snowden-Pencer
5175 S. Royal Atlanta Dr.
Tucker, GA 30084-3053
404-496-0952

Storz Endoscopy-America Inc., Karl
10111 W. Jefferson Blvd.
Culver City, CA 90232-3509
310-558-1500

Storz GmbH & Co., Karl
Mittelstr. 8
Postfach 230
D-78532 Tuttlingen
Germany
07461/7080

Veriflo Corporation
250 Canal Blvd.
P.O. Box 4034
Richmond, CA 94804-0034
510-235-9590

Visioneering, Inc.
3178 Pullman St.
Costa Mesa, CA 92626-3319
714-549-2557

Wect Instrument Company, Inc.
5645 N. Ravenswood
Chicago, IL 60660-3922
312-769-1944

Wolf Medical Instruments Corp., Richard
353 Corporate Woods Pkwy.
Vernon Hills, IL 60061-3110
708-913-1113

INSUFFLATOR, VAGINAL

CMT, Inc.
648 Bay Road
P.O. Box 297
Hamilton, MA 01936
508-468-5640

Leisegang Medical, Inc.
6401 Congress Ave.
Boca Raton, FL 33487-2883
407-994-0202

Wisap Gesellschaft
Rudolf Diesel Ring 20
D-82054 Sauerlach
Germany
08104/1067

Wisap USA
P.O. Box 324
Tomball, TX 77377-0324
713-351-2629

PUMP, AIR, NON-MANUAL, ENDOSCOPIC

Circon Acmi
300 Stillwater Ave.
Stamford, CT 06902-3640
203-328-8689

Frantz Medical Development Ltd.
7740 Metric Drive
Mentor, OH 44060-4862
216-255-1155

Intramed Labs
11100 Roselle Street
San Diego, CA 92121-1210
619-455-5000

Irrigator

There are laparoscopic irrigators powered by pneumatic bags, gravity, manual syringes, and electric pumps. All work equally well; and all have specific advantages and drawbacks.

The electric models permit fast instillation of large amounts of fluid. However, most of their parts are not disposable; and the cost of cleaning and maintenance is therefore a continuing consideration. These models can also be rather loud, adding to the already high decibel level in the typical laparoscopic operating room. Nevertheless, if aqua-dissection and large-volume irrigation are requirements, an electric model is the superior choice.

Manually activated systems are less expensive. However, they do not generate the high pressure needed for aqua-dissection, and can become quite tiring for the operator if copious or frequent irrigation is needed. They are most cost-effective in situations that require infrequent, low-volume irrigation.

Most irrigators have suction mechanisms, which means that large amounts of contaminated fluid will routinely be traveling through the system. Maintaining clean valves and tubes can therefore be a major problem. Disposable systems completely eliminate this worry; and for that reason, disposables are more common in this application than almost any other.

When selecting an irrigator, make sure that the tubing is flexible enough to permit easy handling and manipulation, yet rigid enough to resist collapse under maximum suction. In some designs, the conduit gradually increases in diameter as it recedes from the abdomen. However, this reduces suctioning power and should be avoided. The tubing should be uniform throughout the apparatus.

Check the valves of the cannula to make certain they are wide enough to allow free flow of fluid; and make sure they are easy to depress. Valves with strong springs tend to tire the surgeon during sustained irrigation or suctioning. Also check the location of the valve buttons. They should be ergonomically placed to allow the surgeon maximum flexibility during use.

CONNECTOR, SUCTION/IRRIGATION

Davis & Geck Endosurgery
1 Casper Street
Danbury, CT 06810
203-743-4451

Schwarz Medical
Kirchstrasse 24
D-86935 Rott
Germany
8869/1881

EQUIPMENT, SUCTION/IRRIGATION, LAPAROSCOPIC

Conmed Corp.
310 Broad St.
Utica, NY 13501
315-797-8375

GLEESON FLOVAC

DESCRIPTION: The Gleeson FloVac™ is a high flow volume (up to 10mm capacity), multi-functional sterile, single-patient use suction/irrigation instrument for laparoscopic,

EQUIPMENT, SUCTION/IRRIGATION, LAPAROSCOPIC *(cont'd)*

pelviscopic and thoracoscopic procedures. The device consists of a handle assembly having two unique flow-through push-button valves for control of suction and irrigation flow, and interchangeable suction/irrigation cannulae of various sizes and tip configurations. All components are furnished sterile.

By pressing the appropriate instrument button, the specific suction or irrigation tube is opened proportionately to the depth to which the button is pressed, allowing the clinician to control the amount of flow.

The suction/irrigation cannulae, most of which can be reused, can be interchanged on the handle via the special locking mechanism. The cannulae are available in various lengths, diameters and tip configurations for endoscopic use.

The Gleeson FloVac should be connected to a pressurized irrigation source, such as an inflatable pressure infusion bag, mechanical pump or other source approved for laparoscopic use.

The manufacturer recommends that the suction tubing of Gleeson FloVac be connected to a high-flow regulated suction source. 10ft. of sterile suction/irrigation tubing is included.

CONTRAINDICATIONS: Gleeson FloVac should only be used by surgeons trained in surgical endoscopy according to established protocols.

See package insert for use directions, cautions, warnings, and detailed product descriptions.

American Hydro-Surgical Instruments, Inc.
430 Commerce Dr., Ste. 50E
Delray Beach, FL 33445
407-278-5664

Apple Medical Corp.
93 Nashaway Rd.
Bolton, MA 01740
508-779-2926

Biosearch Medical Products, Inc.
P.O. Box 1700
35 Industrial Pkwy.
Somerville, NJ 08876-1276
908-722-5000

Birtcher Medical Systems, Inc.
50 Technology Dr.
Irvine, CA 92718-2301
714-753-9400

Boss Instruments, Ltd.
1310 Central Ct.
Hermitage, TN 37076
615-885-2231

Bryan Corp.
4 Plympton St.
Woburn, MA 01801-2908
617-935-0004

Cabot Medical Corp.
2021 Cabot Blvd. West
Langhorne, PA 19047-1875
215-752-8300

Chirurgische Instrumente
Hauptstrasse 18
D-78582 Balgheim
Germany
7424/501319

Clarus Medical Systems, Inc.
2605 Fernbrook Lane
Minneapolis, MN 55447-4736
612-559-8640

Core Dynamics, Inc.
11222-4 St. Johns Indust. Pkwy.
Jacksonville, FL 32216
904-641-6611

Davis & Geck Div.
American Cyanamid Company
One Cyanamid Plaza
Wayne, NJ 07470-2012
201-831-2000

Davol, Inc.
100 Sockanossett
P.O. Box 8500
Cranston, RI 02920-0500
401-463-7000

Dexide, Inc.
7509 Flagstone Dr.
P.O. Box 185789
Fort Worth, TX 76118-6953
817-589-1454

Elmed, Inc.
60 W. Fay Ave.
Addison, IL 60101-5198
708-543-2792

Ethicon Endo-Surgery
4545 Creek Road
Cincinnati, OH 45242
513-786-7000

Inlet Medical, Inc.
9951 Valley View Rd.
Eden Prairie, MN 55344
612-942-5034

Leisegang Medical, Inc.
6401 Congress Ave.
Boca Raton, FL 33487-2883
407-994-0202

Marlow Surgical Technologies, Inc.
1810 Joseph Lloyd Pkwy.
Willoughby, OH 44094-8030
216-946-2453

Megadyne Medical Products, Inc.
11506 S. State St.
Draper, UT 84020
801-576-9669

Microsurge, Inc.
150 A St.
Needham, MA 02194
617-444-2300

Northgate Technologies, Inc.
3930 Ventura Dr., Ste. 150
Arlington Heights, IL 60004
708-506-9872

Origin Medsystems, Inc.
135 Constitution Dr.
Menlo Park, CA 94025
415-617-5000

Sherwood Medical Company
1915 Olive St.
St. Louis, MO 63103-1625
314-621-7788

Surgin, Inc.
14762 Bentley Circle
Tustin, CA 92680
714-832-6300

Synectic Engineering, Inc.
4 Oxford Rd.
Milford, CT 06460-7007
203-877-8488

Unisurge, Inc.
10231 Bubb Rd.
Cupertino, CA 95014
408-996-4700

United States Surgical Corp.
150 Glover Ave.
Norwalk, CT 06856-5080
203-845-1000

Valleylab, Inc.
5920 Longbow Dr.
Boulder, CO 80301-3202
303-530-2300

W.J. Medical Instruments, Inc.
3537 Old Conejo Rd.
Newbury Park, CA 91320
805-499-8676

Wolf Medical Instruments Corp., Richard
353 Corporate Woods Pkwy.
Vernon Hills, IL 60061-3110
708-913-1113

Ximed Medical Systems
2195 Trade Zone Blvd.
San Jose, CA 95131
408-945-4040

HANDLE, INSTRUMENT, LAPAROSCOPIC (IRRIGATION)

Davis & Geck Endosurgery
1 Casper St.
Danbury, CT 06810
203-743-4451

LAPAROSCOPIC ASSIST DEVICE 8575-02

DESCRIPTION: Suction/Irrigation Handpiece (order number 8575-02):

SUCTION/IRRIGATION HANDPIECE

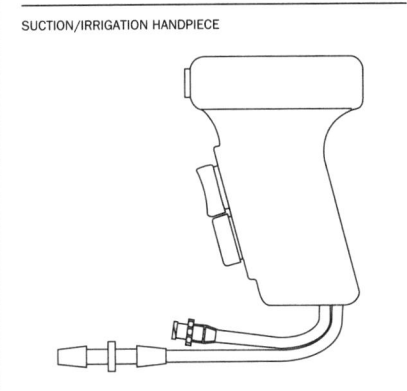

SPECIFICATIONS/HOW SUPPLIED: Supplied sterile, in boxes of 5 units.

Davis & Geck Div.
American Cyanamid Company
One Cyanamid Plaza
Wayne, NJ 07470-2012
201-831-2000

Ethicon Endo-Surgery
4545 Creek Road
Cincinnati, OH 45242
513-786-7000

PROBE, SUCTION, IRRIGATOR/ASPIRATOR, LAPAROSCOPIC

Davis & Geck Endosurgery
1 Casper St.
Danbury, CT 06810
203-743-4451

LAPAROSCOPIC ASSIST DEVICES 8572 SERIES

DESCRIPTION: Dual Trumpet Valve-Probe with Suction/Irrigation (no electrocautery). Luer lock-type fittings for suction and irrigation ports; barb fitting to luer lock adaptor included.

Suction/Irrigation Probe (order number 8572-01):

SUCTION/IRRIGATION PROBE

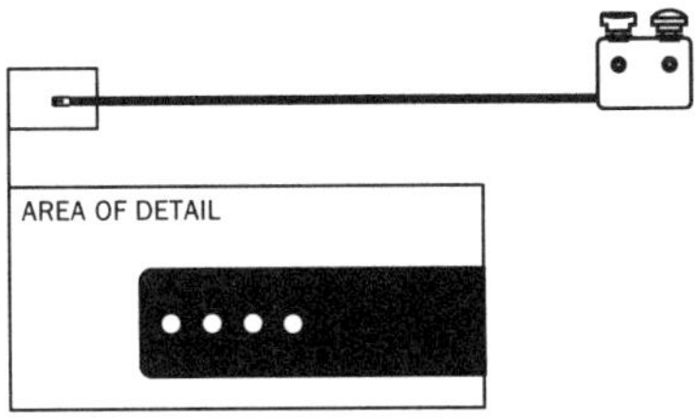

AREA OF DETAIL

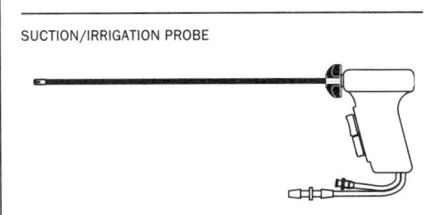

Tapered Tip Probe (order number 8572-02):

TAPERED TIP PROBE

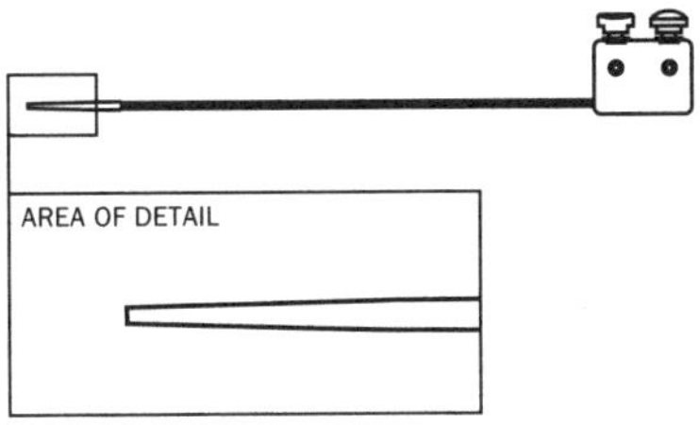

AREA OF DETAIL

WARNINGS: Do not use the probe if the insulation appears cracked, flawed or otherwise damaged.

INSTRUCTIONS FOR USE: Refer to your irrigation system's operator manual for proper setup and use.

Assure that all irrigation/suction manufacturer's safety precautions are followed.

Use accepted aseptic technique when removing the single-use Laparoscopic Probe from the package.

Attach suction system or wall suction to the suction port (1) and the irrigation system to the irrigation port (2) using tubing or luer lock connectors.

Before surgical use, depress each trumpet valve firmly once to prime the valve.

PRODUCT SETUP

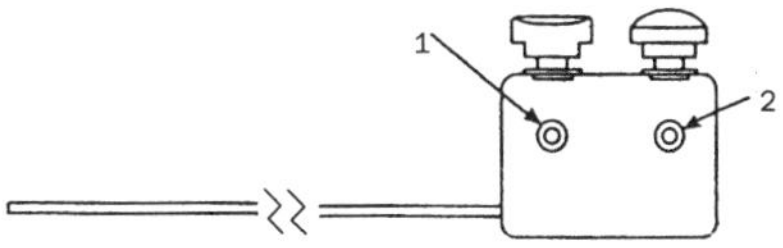

Select the appropriate suction irrigation settings on the respective units to obtain the desired effect.

STERILIZATION GUIDELINES: This product is intended for single use only. Do not attempt to resterilize by any method.

SPECIFICATIONS/HOW SUPPLIED: This product is provided sterile in boxes of 5 units. Do not utilize the product if the package is opened or damaged.

Davis & Geck Endosurgery
1 Casper St.
Danbury, CT 06810
203-743-4451

LAPAROSCOPIC ASSIST DEVICES 8574 SERIES

DESCRIPTION: Multifunction Pistol Grip Device with Modular Interchangeable Probes for suction/irrigation (no electrocautery). Luer lock-type connector for irrigation; barb connector for suction.

Suction/Irrigation Probe (order number 8574-01):

SUCTION/IRRIGATION PROBE

Tapered Tip Probe (order number 8574-02):

TAPERED TIP PROBE

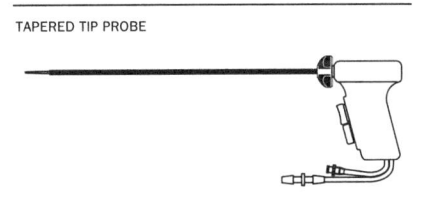

WARNINGS: Do not use the electrode if the insulation appears cracked, flawed or otherwise damaged.

INSTRUCTIONS FOR USE: Refer to your suction/irrigation unit's operator manual for proper setup and use. Assure that all manufacturer's safety precautions are followed.

Follow all precautions normally used with suction/irrigation devices.

Use accepted aseptic technique when removing the single-use Laparoscopic Probe and Multifunction Pistol Grip from the package.

Attach suction system or wall suction to the suction port (1) and the irrigation system to the irrigation port (2) using tube or luer lock connectors.

Before surgical use, depress each trigger valve firmly once to prime the valves.

Davis & Geck Endosurgery

PROBE, SUCTION, IRRIGATOR/ASPIRATOR, LAPAROSCOPIC (cont'd)

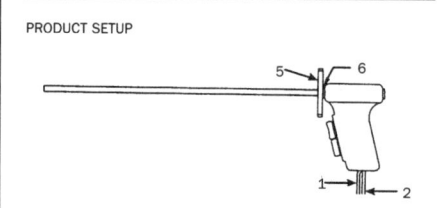

PRODUCT SETUP

To change probes grasp the black knurled knob (5) on the probe shaft and remove it from the pistol grip handpiece by gently separating the two units.

Replace the probe in similar fashion. Grip the black knurled knob on the probe shaft and insert it into the probe recess (6) on the front of the pistol grip handle. Ensure that the probe is securely seated all the way into the probe recess prior to use.

STERILIZATION GUIDELINES: The probe is intended for single use only. Do not attempt to resterilize by any method.

SPECIFICATIONS/HOW SUPPLIED: This product is provided sterile in boxes of 5 units. Do not utilize the product if the package is opened or damaged.

Davis & Geck Endosurgery
1 Casper St.
Danbury, CT 06810
203-743-4451

LAPAROSCOPIC ASSIST DEVICES 8577-01/-02

DESCRIPTION: Single-use Suction/Irrigation Probes for use with Multifunction Pistol Grip Devices 8573, 8574, 8575 (no electrocautery).

Suction/Irrigation Probe (order number 8577-01):

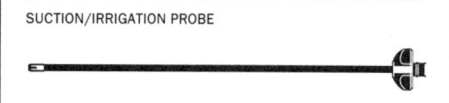

SUCTION/IRRIGATION PROBE

Tapered Tip Probe (order number 8577-02):

TAPERED TIP PROBE

Davis & Geck Endosurgery
1 Casper St.
Danbury, CT 06810
203-743-4451

LAPAROSCOPIC ASSIST DEVICES 8579 SERIES

DESCRIPTION: Reusable Suction/Irrigation Probes for use with Multifunction Pistol Grip Devices 8573, 8574, 8575 (no electrocautery):

Suction/Irrigation Probe (order number 8579-01 for 5mm, 8579-04 for 10mm model):

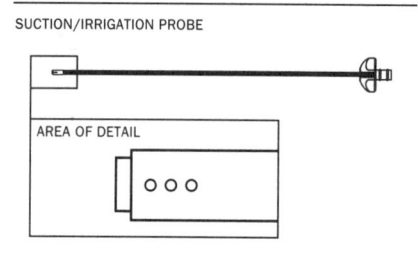

SUCTION/IRRIGATION PROBE

AREA OF DETAIL

Tapered Tip Probe (order number 8579-02):

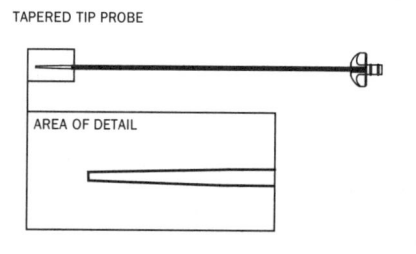

TAPERED TIP PROBE

AREA OF DETAIL

INSTRUCTIONS FOR USE: All surgeons and surgical staff involved in the performance of endoscopic procedures should read these instructions, warnings, and precautions prior to performing endoscopic procedures. The surgical staff and other related hospital personnel should be fully trained in this surgical technique prior to use of all endoscopic devices.

Usage: Refer to your suction/irrigation unit's operator manual for proper setup and use. Assure that all manufacturer's safety precautions are followed.

Follow all precautions normally used with suction and irrigation devices.

Product Setup:
1. Use accepted aseptic technique when removing the single-use Laparoscopic Multi-Function Pistol Grip from the sterile package.
2. Attach suction system or wall suction to the suction port (1) using tubing and the irrigation system to the irrigation port, (2) using tubing and luer lock connectors.
3. Before surgical use, depress each trigger valve firmly once to prime the valve.

PRODUCT SETUP/REMOVAL

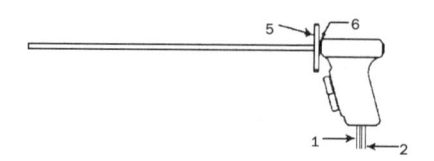

4. Select the irrigation aspiration rate on the suction/irrigation unit to obtain the desired effect.

Probe Removal:
1. To remove probes from the handle, grasp the white finger wheel (5) on the reusable probe shaft and remove it from the pistol grip handpiece by gently rotating and separating the two units.
2. Install the sterile probe in similar fashion by gripping the white finger wheel on the probe shaft and insert it into the probe recess (6) on the front of the pistol grip handle.
3. You may want to lubricate the "O" rings on the finger wheel with sterile water to facilitate assembly.
4. Ensure that the probe is securely seated all the way into the probe recess prior to use.
Sterilize this product before use.

CARE & MAINTENANCE:
1. Do not use any alcohol or acetone based solvents on the instruments.
2. Do not use clamps or forceps when handling the instruments as they may damage the instruments.
3. Do not pile instruments on top of the reusable probes as damage to the instrument may be caused.

STERILIZATION GUIDELINES: Sterilize the device in accordance with approved hospital steam sterilization methods:
1. Do not disinfect or sterilize in EtO/Freon;
2. Do not disinfect or sterilize in liquid solutions;
3. Do not sterilize at temperatures greater than 275°F (135°C).

After removal of the instruments from the autoclave, they should be allowed to cool naturally to room temperature.

Do not cold quench instruments in cold water or any other liquid following sterilization.

SPECIFICATIONS/HOW SUPPLIED: The Reusable Laparoscopic Suction/Irrigation Probe for use with the DAVIS & GECK Multifunction Pistol Grip is supplied non-sterile, one unit per box.

Access Surgical International, Inc.
15 Caswell Ln.
Boat Yard Square
Plymouth, MA 02360
508-747-6006

Apple Medical Corp.
93 Nashaway Rd.
Bolton, MA 01740
508-779-2926

Birtcher Medical Systems, Inc.
50 Technology Dr.
Irvine, CA 92718-2301
714-753-9400

Boss Instruments, Ltd.
1310 Central Ct.
Hermitage, TN 37076
615-885-2231

Bryan Corp.
4 Plympton St.
Woburn, MA 01801-2908
617-935-0004

Cabot Medical Corp.
2021 Cabot Blvd. West
Langhorne, PA 19047-1875
215-752-8300

Conmed Corp.
310 Broad Street
Utica, NY 13501
315-797-8375

Core Dynamics, Inc.
11222-4 St. Johns Indust. Pkwy.
Jacksonville, FL 32216
904-641-6611

Davis & Geck Div.
American Cyanamid Company
One Cyanamid Plaza
Wayne, NJ 07470-2012
201-831-2000

Davol, Inc.
100 Sockanossett
P.O. Box 8500
Cranston, RI 02920-0500
401-463-7000

Elmed, Inc.
60 W. Fay Ave.
Addison, IL 60101-5198
708-543-2792

Ethicon Endo-Surgery
4545 Creek Road
Cincinnati, OH 45242
513-786-7000

Inlet Medical, Inc.
9951 Valley View Rd.
Eden Prairie, MN 55344
612-942-5034

Leisegang Medical, Inc.
6401 Congress Ave.
Boca Raton, FL 33487-2883
407-994-0202

Marlow Surgical Technologies, Inc.
1810 Joseph Lloyd Pkwy.
Willoughby, OH 44094-8030
216-946-2453

Megadyne Medical Products, Inc.
11506 S. State St.
Draper, UT 84020
801-576-9669

Mist, Inc.
6307 E. Angus Dr.
Raleigh, NC 27613
919-787-8377

Origin Medsystems, Inc.
135 Constitution Dr.
Menlo Park, CA 94025
415-617-5000

Sharpe Endosurgical Corp.
3750 Annapolis Lane, Ste. 135
Minneapolis, MN 55447
612-784-0460

Sharplan Lasers, Inc.
1 Pearl Ct.
Allendale, NJ 07401-1675
201-327-1666

Surgin, Inc.
14762 Bentley Circle
Tustin, CA 92680
714-832-6300

Synectic Engineering, Inc.
4 Oxford Rd.
Milford, CT 06460-7007
203-877-8488

Unisurge, Inc.
10231 Bubb Rd.
Cupertino, CA 95014
408-996-4700

Valleylab, Inc.
5920 Longbow Dr.
Boulder, CO 80301-3202
303-530-2300

Wolf Medical Instruments Corp., Richard
353 Corporate Woods Pkwy.
Vernon Hills, IL 60061-3110
708-913-1113

Ximed Medical Systems
2195 Trade Zone Blvd.
San Jose, CA 95131
408-945-4040

TUBING, IRRIGATION

Davis & Geck Endosurgery
1 Casper St.
Danbury, CT 06810
203-743-4451

LAPAROSCOPIC ASSIST DEVICE 8580-03

DESCRIPTION: The Dual Bottle Irrigation Set (order number 8580-03) is designed to allow the attachment of the DAVIS & GECK Trumpet Valve and Multifunction Pistol Grip Devices to Bottle Irrigation Pump Devices.

INSTRUCTIONS FOR USE: Refer to your suction/irrigation unit's manual for proper setup and use. Assure that all manufacturer's safety precautions are followed.

Refer to the instructions for DAVIS & GECK Multifunction Pistol Grip and Dual Trumpet Valve for proper setup and use.

ASSEMBLY GUIDELINES:
Irrigation Tubing Attachment (dual irrigation bottle systems):
1) slide the irrigation bottle attachment tubes over the male barbs on the irrigation bottle caps;
2) ensure that the tubing is pushed all the way down over the male barb fitting and is securely attached to the cap;
3) attach the male luer on the attachment tube to the luer lock on the irrigation device;
4) ensure that the luer locks are engaged completely, to prevent any fluid leakage;
5) select the appropriate pressure flow on the suction/irrigation system to obtain the desired irrigation flow rates.

Irrigation Tubing Attachment (single irrigation bottle systems):
1) using the dual bottle irrigation tubing set with single bottle irrigation systems, follow instructions 1-4 above;
2) apply a clamp to the non-utilized bottle attachment tube to prevent any retrograde fluid leakage;
3) select the appropriate pressure flow on the suction/irrigation system to obtain the desired irrigation flow rates.

Pressure Line Attachment:
1) insert the pressure line fittings into the pressure outlets on the irrigation system;
2) attach the luer lock fittings to the top of the irrigation bottles;
3) ensure that the luer locks are engaged completely, to prevent any pressure loss.

Should the irrigation system's pressure lines utilize male barb attachments rather than those fittings supplied, remove the supplied fittings from the pressure tubes by cutting them off:
1) slide the pressure lines over the male barbs on the irrigation bottle caps;
2) ensure that the tubing is pushed all the way down over the male barb fitting and is securely attached to the cap.

TUBING, IRRIGATION
(cont'd)

STERILIZATION GUIDELINES: This product is intended for single-patient use only. Do not attempt to resterilize by any manner.

SPECIFICATIONS/HOW SUPPLIED:
Package Contains:
- one (1) 10 ft. device attachment tube with bifurcation and two bottle attachment tubes;
- one (1) male luer lock on the device attachment tube;
- two (2) anti-reflux valves on bottle attachment tubes;
- two (2) CO_2 pressure line attachments with luer locks and pump attachments which may be cut off to attach to a 1/4 inch barb fitting.

Contents sterile unless package opened or damaged.

CAUTION: Federal (USA) law restricts this device to sale by or on the order of a physician.

Davis & Geck Endosurgery
1 Casper St.
Danbury, CT 06810
203-743-4451

LAPAROSCOPIC ASSIST DEVICE 8580-04

DESCRIPTION: The Dual Bag Irrigation Tubing Set (order number 8580-04) is designed to allow the attachment of the DAVIS & GECK Trumpet Valve and Multifunction Pistol Grip Devices to Pressure Bag Irrigation Devices.

INSTRUCTIONS FOR USE: Refer to your suction/irrigation unit's manual for proper setup and use. Assure that all manufacturer's safety precautions are followed.

Refer to the instructions for DAVIS & GECK Multifunction Pistol Grip and Dual Trumpet Valve for proper setup and use.

ASSEMBLY GUIDELINES:
Irrigation Tubing Attachment (dual irrigation bag systems):
1) insert the irrigation bag attachment spikes into the fittings on the irrigation bags;
2) ensure that the spikes are pushed all the way into the fittings and are securely attached to the bag;
3) attach the male luer on the attachment tube to the luer lock on the irrigation device;
4) ensure that the luer locks are engaged completely, to prevent any fluid leakage;
5) select the appropriate pressure flow on the suction/irrigation system to obtain the desired irrigation flow rates.

Irrigation Tubing Attachment (single irrigation bag systems):
1) using the dual bag irrigation tubing set with single irrigation bag systems, follow instructions 1-4 above;
2) apply a clamp to the non-utilized bag attachment tube to prevent any retrograde fluid leakage;
3) select the appropriate pressure flow on the suction/irrigation system to obtain the desired irrigation flow rates.

STERILIZATION GUIDELINES: Contents sterile unless package opened or damaged. This product is intended for single-patient use only. Do not attempt to resterilize by any manner.

SPECIFICATIONS/HOW SUPPLIED:
Package Contains:
- one (1) 10 ft. device attachment tube with bifurcation and two saline bag attachment tubes with spikes;
- one (1) male luer lock on the device attachment tube;
- two (2) anti-reflux valves on the bag attachment tubes.

CAUTION: Federal (USA) law restricts this device to sale by or on the order of a physician.

Davis & Geck Div.
American Cyanamid Company
One Cyanamid Plaza
Wayne, NJ 07470-2012
201-831-2000

Inlet Medical, Inc.
9951 Valley View Rd.
Eden Prairie, MN 55344
612-942-5034

Polygon Co.
P.O. Box 176
Walkerton, IN 46574-0176
219-586-3122

Kit

KIT, BOWEL

Ethicon Endo-Surgery
4545 Creek Road
Cincinnati, OH 45242
513-786-7000

Reznik Instrument, Inc.
7337 North Lawndale
Skokie, IL 60076
708-673-3444

KIT, CHOLECYSTECTOMY

Access Surgical International, Inc.
15 Caswell Ln.
Boat Yard Square
Plymouth, MA 02360
508-747-6006

Advanced Surgical, Inc.
305 College Rd. East
Princeton, NJ 08540
609-987-2340

Aesculap
1000 Gateway Blvd.
South San Francisco, CA 94080-7030
415-876-7000

Conmed Corp.
310 Broad Street
Utica, NY 13501
315-797-8375

Coopersurgical, Inc.
15 Forest Pkwy.
Shelton, CT 06484-5458
203-929-6321

Core Dynamics, Inc.
11222-4 St. Johns Indust. Pkwy.
Jacksonville, FL 32216
904-641-6611

Elmed, Inc.
60 W. Fay Ave.
Addison, IL 60101-5198
708-543-2792

Ethicon Endo-Surgery
4545 Creek Road
Cincinnati, OH 45242
513-786-7000

Gabris Surgical Corp.
547 Susan Constant Dr.
Virginia Beach, VA 23451
804-491-6487

Jarit Instruments
9 Skyline Dr.
Hawthorne, NY 10532-2119
914-592-9050

K+A Medical
413 Oak Pl., Bldg. 6J
Port Orange, FL 32127-4352
904-767-0229

Leonard Medical Inc.
1464 Holcomb Rd.
Huntingdon Valley, PA 19006
215-938-1499

Marlow Surgical Technologies, Inc.
1810 Joseph Lloyd Pkwy.
Willoughby, OH 44094-8030
216-946-2453

Medchem Products, Inc.
232 W. Cummings Pk.
Woburn, MA 01801-6333
617-938-9328

Medicon Instruments, Inc.
4405 International Blvd.
Norcross, GA 30093-3013
404-381-2858

Megatech Medical, Inc.
1720 Belmont Ave., Bldg. E
Baltimore, MD 21244
410-944-8500

Microsurge, Inc.
150 A St.
Needham, MA 02194
617-444-2300

Microvasive/Boston Scientific Corp.
Urology Div.
480 Pleasant St.
Watertown, MA 02172
617-923-1720

Mist, Inc.
6307 E. Angus Dr.
Raleigh, NC 27613
919-787-8377

Performance Surgical Instruments
40 Norfolk Ave.
Easton, MA 023334
508-230-0010

Reznik Instrument, Inc.
7337 North Lawndale
Skokie, IL 60076
708-673-3444

Richard-Allan Medical Industries, Inc.
8850 M-89
P.O. Box 351
Richland, MI 49083-0351
616-629-5811

Sharpe Endosurgical Corp.
3750 Annapolis Lane, Ste. 135
Minneapolis, MN 55447
612-784-0460

Storz Endoscopy-America Inc., Karl
10111 W. Jefferson Blvd.
Culver City, CA 90232-3509
310-558-1500

Surgical Technologies International, Inc.
4715 NW 157th St., #212
Miami, FL 33014
305-623-0363

U.S. Endoscopy Group
7123 Industrial Park Blvd.
Mentor, OH 44060
216-269-8226

Unisurge, Inc.
10231 Bubb Rd.
Cupertino, CA 95014
408-996-4700

Ximed Medical Systems
2195 Trade Zone Blvd.
San Jose, CA 95131
408-945-4040

KIT, GASTROSTOMY, ENDOSCOPIC, PERCUTANEOUS

Wilson-Cook Medical, Inc.
4900 Bethania Station Rd.
Winston-Salem, NC 27105-1203
919-744-0157

KIT, LAPAROSCOPY

Access Surgical International, Inc.
15 Caswell Ln.
Boat Yard Square
Plymouth, MA 02360
508-747-6006

Accurate Surgical & Scientific
Instrument Corp.
300 Shames Dr.
Westbury, NY 11590-1736
516-333-2570

American Medical Devices, Inc.
287 S. Stoddard Ave.
San Bernardino, CA 92401-2021
714-381-4364

B.E.C. Medical Products
615 Front St.
Toledo, OH 43605-2105
419-693-5307

Bristol-Myers Squibb Company Australia
556 Princes Highway
P.O. Box 39
Noble Park, VIC 3174
Australia
03/7953722

Bryan Corp.
4 Plympton St.
Woburn, MA 01801-2908
617-935-0004

Circon Acmi
300 Stillwater Ave.
Stamford, CT 06902-3640
203-328-8689

Clinipad Corp.
66 High St.
P.O. Box 387
Guilford, CT 06437
203-453-6543

Coopersurgical, Inc.
15 Forest Pkwy.
Shelton, CT 06484-5458
203-929-6321

Cuda Products Corporation
6000 Powers Ave.
Jacksonville, FL 32217-2212
904-737-7611

Davol, Inc.
100 Sockanosset
P.O. Box 8500
Cranston, RI 02920-0500
401-463-7000

Deroyal Industries, Inc.
200 DeBusk Lane
Powell, TN 37849-4703
615-938-7828

KIT, LAPAROSCOPY (cont'd)

Electroscope, Inc.
4890 Sterling Dr.
Boulder, CO 80301
303-444-2600

Elmed, Inc.
60 W. Fay Ave.
Addison, IL 60101-5198
708-543-2792

Ethicon Endo-Surgery
4545 Creek Road
Cincinnati, OH 45242
513-786-7000

Fujinon, Inc.
10 High Point Dr.
Wayne, NJ 07470-7434
201-633-5600

GM Engineering, Inc.
2549 Sierra Way #B
La Verna, CA 91750-5800
909-596-5065

Hipp GmbH, Anton
Annastr. 25/1
Postfach 80
D-78567 Fridingen
Germany
07463/7776-5088

Lapac, Inc.
130 Overlook Ave.
Hackensack, NJ 07601-2225
201-646-0101

Leisegang Medical, Inc.
6401 Congress Ave.
Boca Raton, FL 33487-2883
407-994-0202

Life Medical Technologies, Inc.
3649 W. 1987 S.
Salt Lake City, UT 84104
801-972-1900

Mader Instrument Corp.
25 Lamington Dr.
Succasunna, NJ 07876-2048
201-584-0816

Marlow Surgical Technologies, Inc.
1810 Joseph Lloyd Pkwy.
Willoughby, OH 44094-8030
216-946-2453

Med-Surg Industries, Inc.
251 Exchange Place
Herndon, VA 22070-4822
703-742-9700

Medizintechnik
Wurttemberger Str. 26
D-78567 Fridingen
Germany
07/463-8076

Minorax Corp.
7015 147th St. SW
Edmonds, WA 98026
206-743-0178

Mist, Inc.
6307 E. Angus Dr.
Raleigh, NC 27613
919-787-8377

Multigon Industries, Inc.
559 Gramatan Ave.
Mt. Vernon, NY 10552-2155
914-664-7300

Needletech Products, Inc.
428 Towne St.
North Attleborough, MA 02760-3407
508-699-4148

O.R. Concepts, Inc.
12250 Nicollet Ave. South
Burnsville, MN 55337
612-894-7523

Omni-Tract Surgical Div.
Minnesota Scientific Co.
403 County Rd. E2 West
St. Paul, MN 55112-6858
612-633-8448

Origin Medsystems, Inc.
135 Constitution Dr.
Menlo Park, CA 94025
415-617-5000

Performance Surgical Instruments
40 Norfolk Ave.
Easton, MA 023334
508-230-0010

Snowden-Pencer
5175 S. Royal Atlanta Dr.
Tucker, GA 30084-3053
404-496-0952

Storz Endoscopy-America Inc., Karl
10111 W. Jefferson Blvd.
Culver City, CA 90232-3509
310-558-1500

Surgical Technologies International, Inc.
4715 NW 157th St., #212
Miami, FL 33014
305-623-0363

Unisurge, Inc.
10231 Bubb Rd.
Cupertino, CA 95014
408-996-4700

United States Surgical Corp.
150 Glover Ave.
Norwalk, CT 06856-5080
203-845-1000

Wolf Medical Instruments Corp., Richard
353 Corporate Woods Pkwy.
Vernon Hills, IL 60061-3110
708-913-1113

KIT, PELVISCOPY

Ethicon Endo-Surgery
4545 Creek Road
Cincinnati, OH 45242
513-786-7000

Laparomed Corp.
9272 Jeronimo Rd., Unit 109
Irvine, CA 92718-1914
714-768-1155

Microsurge, Inc.
150 A St.
Needham, MA 02194
617-444-2300

Minorax Corp.
7015 147th St. SW
Edmonds, WA 98026
206-743-0178

Sherwood Intrascopic Div.
1915 Olive St.
St. Louis, MO 63103
314-241-5700

Wolf Medical Instruments Corp., Richard
353 Corporate Woods Pkwy.
Vernon Hills, IL 60061-3110
708-913-1113

KIT, TROCAR

Ethicon Endo-Surgery
4545 Creek Road
Cincinnati, OH 45242
513-786-7000

Unisurge, Inc.
10231 Bubb Rd.
Cupertino, CA 95014
408-996-4700

Knife

BLADE, KNIFE, LAPAROSCOPIC

Access Surgical International, Inc.
15 Caswell Ln.
Boat Yard Square
Plymouth, MA 02360
508-747-6006

Elmed, Inc.
60 W. Fay Ave.
Addison, IL 60101-5198
708-543-2792

Sharpe Endosurgical Corp.
3750 Annapolis Lane, Ste. 135
Minneapolis, MN 55447
612-784-0460

KNIFE, LAPAROSCOPIC

DaVinci Medical, Inc.
13700 First Ave. North
Minneapolis, MN 55441
612-473-4245

Nu Surg Medical, Inc.
4440 Glen Este-Withamsville Road
Suite 780
Cincinnati, OH 45245
513-753-3633

Laparoscope

COVER, LAPAROSCOPE

Civco Medical Instruments Co., Inc.
Medical Pkwy.
102 Hwy. 1 South
Kalona, IA 52247
319-656-4447

Coopersurgical, Inc.
15 Forest Pkwy.
Shelton, CT 06484-5458
203-929-6321

Depuy, Inc.
700 Orthopaedic Dr.
P.O. Box 988
Warsaw, IN 46581-0988
219-267-8143

Electroscope, Inc.
4890 Sterling Dr.
Boulder, CO 80301
303-444-2600

Elmed, Inc.
60 W. Fay Ave.
Addison, IL 60101-5198
708-543-2792

Leisegang Medical, Inc.
6401 Congress Ave.
Boca Raton, FL 33487-2883
407-994-0202

W.J. Medical Instruments, Inc.
3537 Old Conejo Rd.
Newbury Park, CA 91320
805-499-8676

LAPAROSCOPE, FLEXIBLE

Birtcher Medical Systems, Inc.
50 Technology Dr.
Irvine, CA 92718-2301
714-753-9400

Clarus Medical Systems, Inc.
2605 Fernbrook Lane
Minneapolis, MN 55447-4736
612-559-8640

Contec Medical Ltd.
11 Haroshet Street
P.O. Box 1400
Ramat Hasharon 47113
Israel
03/5491153

Fuji Photo Optical Co. Ltd.
1-324, Uetake-Machi, Omiya
Saitama 330
Japan
048/668-2153

Fujinon (Europe) GmbH
Heerdter Lohweg 89
D-40549 Duesseldorf 11
Germany
0211/52050

Fujinon, Inc.
10 High Point Dr.
Wayne, NJ 07470-7434
201-633-5600

Lican Medical Products Ltd.
5120 Halford Dr., R.R. 1
Windsor, ONT N9A 6J3
Canada
519-737-1142

Olympus Winter & Ibe GmbH
Kuehnstrasse 61, Postf. 701709
D-22045 Hamburg 70
Germany
040/66966-0

PLC Systems, Laser Engineering, Inc. Div.
113 Cedar St.
Milford, MA 01757-1154
508-478-5991

Sklar Instrument Company
889 South Matlack St.
West Chester, PA 19380
215-430-3200

Welch Allyn, Inc.
4341 State Street Rd.
P.O. Box 220
Skaneateles Falls, NY 13153-0220
315-685-4100

LAPAROSCOPE, GENERAL & PLASTIC SURGERY

Aesculap
1000 Gateway Blvd.
South San Francisco, CA 94080-7030
415-876-7000

Baxter Healthcare Corp.
Operating Room Div.
1500 Waukegan Rd.
McGaw Park, IL 60085-8210
708-473-1500

Biocare International, Inc.
3375 Park Ave., Suite 2000A
Wantagh, NY 11793-3712
516-781-5800

Boss Instruments, Ltd.
1310 Central Ct.
Hermitage, TN 37076
615-885-2231

Cabot Medical Corp.
2021 Cabot Blvd. West
Langhorne, PA 19047-1875
215-752-8300

Carsen Group Inc.
151 Telson Rd.
Markham, ONT L3R 1E7
Canada
416-479-4100

Chakoff Endoscopy
15405 SW 72 Ct.
Miami, FL 33157
305-253-0321

Chirurgische Instrumente
Hauptstrasse 18
D-78582 Balgheim
Germany
7424/501319

Comeg GmbH
Dornierstr. 55
D-78532 Tuttlingen 14
Germany
07461/8036

Contec Medical Ltd.
11 Haroshet Street
P.O. Box 1400
Ramat Hasharon 47113
Israel
03/5491153

Coopersurgical, Inc.
15 Forest Pkwy.
Shelton, CT 06484-5458
203-929-6321

Cuda Products Corporation
6000 Powers Ave.
Jacksonville, FL 32217-2212
904-737-7611

Davis & Geck Div.
American Cyanamid Company
One Cyanamid Plaza
Wayne, NJ 07470-2012
201-831-2000

DCG Precision Manufacturing Corp.
9 Trowbridge Dr.
Bethel, CT 06801
203-743-5525

Depuy, Inc.
700 Orthopaedic Dr.
P.O. Box 988
Warsaw, IN 46581-0988
219-267-8143

Electro Fiberoptics Corporation
56 Hudson St.
Northborough, MA 01532-1922
508-393-3753

Elmed, Inc.
60 W. Fay Ave.
Addison, IL 60101-5198
708-543-2792

Endotec, Inc.
2225 Skyland Ct.
Norcross, GA 30071
404-840-1883

Endomedix Corp.
2162 Michelson Drive
Irvine, CA 92715
714-253-1000

Expanded Optics, Inc.
7382 Bolsa Ave.
Westminster, CA 92683-5212
714-891-3996

Fujinon, Inc.
10 High Point Dr.
Wayne, NJ 07470-7434
201-633-5600

Geister Medizintechnik GmbH
Foehrenstr. 2
Postfach 4228
D-78532 Tuttlingen
Germany
7461-8084

Hipp GmbH, Anton
Annastr. 25/1
Postfach 80
D-78567 Fridingen
Germany
07463/7776-5088

Jarit Instruments
9 Skyline Dr.
Hawthorne, NY 10532-2119
914-592-9050

K-Medic, Inc.
117 Fort Lee Rd.
Leonia, NJ 07605-2216
201-944-8731

Leisegang Medical, Inc.
6401 Congress Ave.
Boca Raton, FL 33487-2883
407-994-0202

Li Medical Technologies, Inc.
7 Cambridge Dr.
Trumbull, CT 06611
203-371-2227

Lican Medical Products Ltd.
5120 Halford Dr., R.R. 1
Windsor, ONT N9A 6J3
Canada
519-737-1142

Linvatec, Div. of Zimmer of Canada Ltd.
2323 Argentia Rd.
Mississauga, ONT L5N 5N3
Canada
905-858-8588

Mark Medical Manufacturing, Inc.
484 Douglas Drive
West Chester, PA 19380-1120
215-296-3020

McLean Medical Scientific, Inc.
328 State St.
St. Paul, MN 55107
612-225-9295

Mediflex Surgical Products
250 Gibbs Rd.
Islandia, NY 11722-2697
516-582-8440

Mist, Inc.
6307 E. Angus Dr.
Raleigh, NC 27613
919-787-8377

Nextec Surgical Corp.
2629 South Horseshoe Dr.
Naples, FL 33942-6122
813-643-2553

Olympus America, Inc.
4 Nevada Drive
Lake Success, NY 11042-1179
516-488-3880

Olympus Optical Co. Ltd.
San-Ei Bldg.
1-22-2, Nishi-Shinjuku
Shinjuku-Ku, Tokyo 163-91
Japan
03/3402111

Precision Optics Corp.
22 E. Broadway
Gardner, MA 01440-3338
508-630-1800

Rema Medizintechnik GmbH
In Breiten 10
D-78589 Duerbheim-Tuttlingen
Germany
07424-4064

Schott Fiber Optics, Inc.
122 Charlton St.
Southbridge, MA 01550-1960
508-765-9744

Sharplan Lasers, Inc.
1 Pearl Ct.
Allendale, NJ 07401-1675
201-327-1666

Simal Belgium Instrument Co.
2131 Espey Court, Suite 7
Crofton, MD 21114-2424

Sklar Instrument Company
889 South Matlack St.
West Chester, PA 19380
215-430-3200

Smith & Nephew Dyonics, Inc.
160 Dascomb Rd.
Andover, MA 01810-5893
508-470-2800

Storz Endoscopy-America Inc., Karl
10111 W. Jefferson Blvd.
Culver City, CA 90232-3509
310-558-1500

Storz GmbH & Co., Karl
Mittelstr. 8
Postfach 230
D-78532 Tuttlingen
Germany
07461/7080

Surgical Safety Products, Inc.
434 S. Washington Blvd., Ste. 2
Sarasota, FL 34236
813-953-7889

Wect Instrument Company, Inc.
5645 N. Ravenswood
Chicago, IL 60660-3922
312-769-1944

Welch Allyn, Inc.
4341 State Street Rd.
P.O. Box 220
Skaneateles Falls, NY 13153-0220
315-685-4100

WM Instrumente GmbH
Panoramastr. 6
D-78604 Rietheim 1
Germany
07424/501310

Wolf Medical Instruments Corp., Richard
353 Corporate Woods Pkwy.
Vernon Hills, IL 60061-3110
708-913-1113

LAPAROSCOPE, GYNECOLOGIC

Biocare International, Inc.
3375 Park Ave., Suite 2000A
Wantagh, NY 11793-3712
516-781-5800

Cabot Medical Corp.
2021 Cabot Blvd. West
Langhorne, PA 19047-1875
215-752-8300

Circon Acmi
300 Stillwater Ave.
Stamford, CT 06902-3640
203-328-8689

Comeg GmbH
Dornierstr. 55
D-78532 Tuttlingen 14
Germany
07461/8036

Coopersurgical, Inc.
15 Forest Pkwy.
Shelton, CT 06484-5458
203-929-6321

Cuda Products Corporation
6000 Powers Ave.
Jacksonville, FL 32217-2212
904-737-7611

Elmed, Inc.
60 W. Fay Ave.
Addison, IL 60101-5198
708-543-2792

Ethicon Endo-Surgery
4545 Creek Road
Cincinnati, OH 45242
513-786-7000

Expanded Optics, Inc.
7382 Bolsa Ave.
Westminster, CA 92683-5212
714-891-3996

Geister Medizintechnik GmbH
Foehrenstr. 2
Postfach 4228
D-78532 Tuttlingen
Germany
7461-8084

Heraeus Surgical, Inc.
575 Cottonwood Dr.
Milpitas, CA 95035-7402
408-954-4000

Hipp GmbH, Anton
Annastr. 25/1
Postfach 80
D-78567 Fridingen
Germany
07463/7776-5088

Keymed Medical & Industrial
Equipment Ltd.
Keymed House, Stock Rd., Southend-on-Sea
Essex SS2 5QH
United Kingdom
0702/616333

Leisegang Medical, Inc.
6401 Congress Ave.
Boca Raton, FL 33487-2883
407-994-0202

Lican Medical Products Ltd.
5120 Halford Dr., R.R. 1
Windsor, ONT N9A 6J3
Canada
519-737-1142

Linvatec, Div. of Zimmer of Canada Ltd.
2323 Argentia Rd.
Mississauga, ONT L5N 5N3
Canada
905-858-8588

Marlow Surgical Technologies, Inc.
1810 Joseph Lloyd Pkwy.
Willoughby, OH 44094-8030
216-946-2453

Northgate Technologies, Inc.
3930 Ventura Dr., Ste. 150
Arlington Heights, IL 60004
708-506-9872

Olympus America, Inc.
4 Nevada Drive
Lake Success, NY 11042-1179
516-488-3880

Pioneer Medical, Inc.
34 Laurelcrest Rd.
Madison, CT 06443
203-245-9337

Rema Medizintechnik GmbH
In Breiten 10
D-78589 Duerbheim-Tuttlingen
Germany
07424-4064

LAPAROSCOPE GYNECOLOGIC (cont'd)

Sharplan Lasers (Europe) Ltd.
141-155 Brent St.
London NW4 4DJ
United Kingdom
081/203-0006

Sklar Instrument Company
889 South Matlack St.
West Chester, PA 19380
215-430-3200

Smith & Nephew Dyonics, Inc.
160 Dascomb Rd.
Andover, MA 01810-5893
508-470-2800

Storz Endoscopy-America Inc., Karl
10111 W. Jefferson Blvd.
Culver City, CA 90232-3509
310-558-1500

Storz GmbH & Co., Karl
Mittelstr. 8
Postfach 230
D-78532 Tuttlingen
Germany
07461/7080

Surgical Safety Products, Inc.
434 S. Washington Blvd., Ste. 2
Sarasota, FL 34236
813-953-7889

Valley Forge Scientific, Inc.
P.O. Box 925
Valley Forge, PA 19482-0925
215-666-7500

W.J. Medical Instruments, Inc.
3537 Old Conejo Rd.
Newbury Park, CA 91320
805-499-8676

Wect Instrument Company, Inc.
5645 N. Ravenswood
Chicago, IL 60660-3922
312-769-1944

Welch Allyn, Inc.
4341 State Street Rd.
P.O. Box 220
Skaneateles Falls, NY 13153-0220
315-685-4100

WM Instrumente GmbH
Panoramastr. 6
D-78604 Rietheim 1
Germany
07424/501310

Wolf Medical Instruments Corp., Richard
353 Corporate Woods Pkwy.
Vernon Hills, IL 60061-3110
708-913-1113

Zinnanti Surgical Instruments
21540 B Prairie St.
Chatsworth, CA 91311-5886
818-700-0090

LAPAROSCOPE, SEMI-FLEXIBLE

Clarus Medical Systems, Inc.
2605 Fernbrook Lane
Minneapolis, MN 55447-4736
612-559-8640

Welch Allyn, Inc.
4341 State Street Rd.
P.O. Box 220
Skaneateles Falls, NY 13153-0220
315-685-4100

TELESCOPE, RIGID, ENDOSCOPIC

Olympus America, Inc.
4 Nevada Dr.
Lake Success, NY 11042-1179
516-488-3880

OES TELESCOPE
DESCRIPTION:

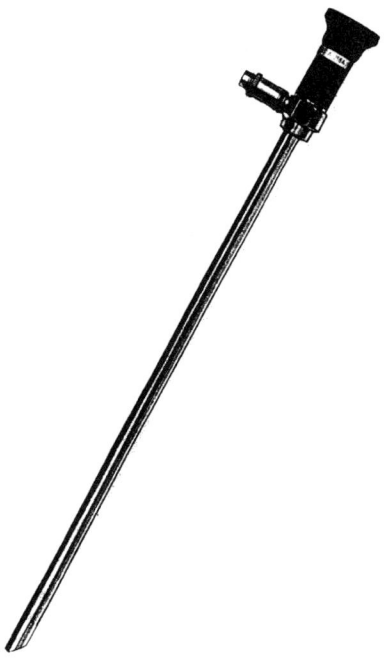

OES Telescopes provide a 100% distortion-free image in rigid endoscopy. The fish-eye effect, previously accepted as inevitable, has disappeared.

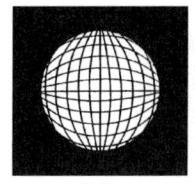

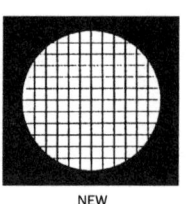

OLD   NEW

The new OES telescopes A5287, A5288, and A5289, specially designed for the use with the new Olympus video camera OTV-S4 and OTV-SX, provide a 37% increase in depth of field to improve image clarity and eliminate the need to refocus.

Birtcher Medical Systems, Inc.
50 Technology Dr.
Irvine, CA 92718-2301
714-753-9400

Bryan Corp.
4 Plympton St.
Woburn, MA 01801-2908
617-935-0004

Cabot Medical Corp.
2021 Cabot Blvd. West
Langhorne, PA 19047-1875
215-752-8300

Circon Acmi
300 Stillwater Ave.
Stamford, CT 06902-3640
203-328-8689

Coopersurgical, Inc.
15 Forest Pkwy.
Shelton, CT 06484-5458
203-929-6321

Cuda Products Corporation
6000 Powers Ave.
Jacksonville, FL 32217-2212
904-737-7611

Davis & Geck Div.
American Cyanamid Company
One Cyanamid Plaza
Wayne, NJ 07470-2012
201-831-2000

Designs For Vision, Inc.
760 Koehler Ave.
Ronkonkoma, NY 11779-7405
516-585-3300

Leisegang Medical, Inc.
6401 Congress Ave.
Boca Raton, FL 33487-2883
407-994-0202

Pilling-Rusch
420 Delaware Dr.
Fort Washington, PA 19034-2711
215-643-2600

Pioneer Medical, Inc.
34 Laurelcrest Rd.
Madison, CT 06443
203-245-9337

Storz Endoscopy-America Inc., Karl
10111 W. Jefferson Blvd.
Culver City, CA 90232-3509
310-558-1500

Storz GmbH & Co., Karl
Mittelstr. 8
Postfach 230
D-78532 Tuttlingen
Germany
07461/7080

Wid-Med, Inc.
111 N. Wabash Ave.
Chicago, IL 60602-1903
312-236-8586

Wolf Medical Instruments Corp., Richard
353 Corporate Woods Pkwy.
Vernon Hills, IL 60061-3110
708-913-1113

Laser

Due to their expense and the expertise they require of the surgeon, lasers have taken a back seat to other forms of energy in recent years. Nevertheless, they remain excellent dissection tools. Indeed, when sufficiently skilled, a surgeon can cut and coagulate with a laser more precisely than with any other instrument.

Most medical lasers employ fiber optics. In these fiber lasers, light energy is carried from its source to the tissue by flexible optical fibers. However, the CO_2 laser is a notable exception to this rule. The long wavelength employed in this laser is difficult to conduct through fibers, so a series of mirrors is usually employed instead. This arrangement yields a highly focused beam suitable for cutting and vaporization. (With a slightly softer focus, the beam is capable of coagulation as well.) The device is used primarily for removing cutaneous raised lesions such as condylomata and keloids, and, in laparoscopy, for cutting, drilling, and vaporizing. Its beam can cause damage several centimeters beyond the focus point, so a backstop should be used to control the forward spread of energy.

When shorter wavelengths are acceptable, a fiber laser is the preferred mode of delivery, since it can easily be passed through a small hole into the abdominal cavity. The shorter wavelengths do not vaporize and cut as well as a CO_2 laser beam, but they are better for coagulation and, because they have less forward penetration, may be safer to use. Most of these wavelengths are color-sensitive, making them excellent for ablation of colored lesions such as endometriomas, port wine stains, and tattoos.

The fibers in fiber lasers come in three types: bare fiber, sapphire-tipped, and sculptured. They are also available in a variety of sizes, with diameters usually ranging from 0.3 to 0.6 microns. The smaller the fiber, the higher the power-density at the tip; so thinner fibers are better for cutting, and thicker fibers better for coagulation.

Among fiber lasers, the Nd:YAG laser gives the deepest penetration and the best coagulation. KTP and Argon lasers provide less penetration and coagulation, but offer superior cutting ability. To boost the YAG laser's cutting power, it can be fitted with a sculptured fiber or disposable synthetic sapphire tip, both of which deliver increased power-density. Another approach to the problem 'the FiberTome laser' uses a built-in feedback mechanism to achieve cutting and coagulation with bare fibers much like those employed in the KTP and Argon lasers.

EQUIPMENT/ACCESSORIES, LASER, LAPAROSCOPY

Davis & Geck Endosurgery
1 Casper St.
Danbury, CT 06810
203-743-4451

LAPAROSCOPIC ASSIST DEVICE 8572-03

DESCRIPTION: Dual Trumpet Valve-Probe with Suction/Irrigation (no electrocautery). Luer lock-type fittings for suction and irrigation ports; barb fitting to luer lock adaptor included.

Laser Port Probe (order number 8572-03):

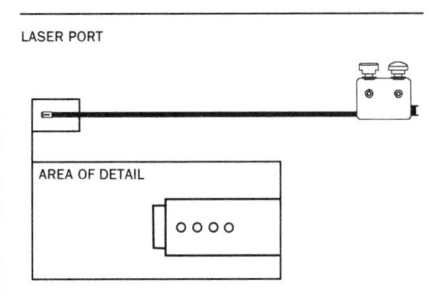

SPECIFICATIONS/HOW SUPPLIED: Supplied in boxes of 5 units.

Davis & Geck Endosurgery
1 Casper St.
Danbury, CT 06810
203-743-4451

LAPAROSCOPIC ASSIST DEVICE 8580-05

DESCRIPTION: Laser Fiber Delivery Sheath (order number 8580-05) for use with Laser Port-equipped Dual Trumpet Valve or Pistol Grip Handpiece:

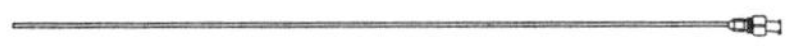

INSTRUCTIONS FOR USE: Refer to your laser unit and suction irrigation unit operator manuals for proper setup and use. Follow all safety precautions normally used with laser cutting and coagulation devices.

Use accepted aseptic technique when removing the single-use Laser Fiber Delivery Sheath from the sterile package.

To utilize the Laser Fiber Delivery Sheath, insert the laser fiber into the rear of the Laser Fiber Delivery Sheath, by slightly unscrewing the rear seal on the fiber sheath to allow fiber passage.

Do not extend the laser fiber beyond the tip of the Laser Fiber Delivery Sheath prior to insertion into the rear port of the Suction/Irrigation Device, as you may damage the laser fiber upon introduction into the device.

Prior to insertion of the Laser Fiber Delivery Sheath into the rear port on the Suction/Irrigation Device, lubricate both the Laser Fiber Delivery Sheath and the rear port of the Suction/Irrigation Device with sterile water.

Insert the Laser Fiber Delivery Sheath into the rear port of the Suction/Irrigation Device and ensure that the sheath is visible beyond the tip of the Suction/Irrigation Probe.

Extend the tip of the laser fiber beyond the Laser Fiber Delivery Sheath by advancing it through the delivery sheath's rear screw seal. The laser fiber must be visible by approximately 5mm beyond the Delivery Sheath. Tighten the rear screw seal on the Laser Fiber Delivery Sheath to ensure that the laser fiber is locked in place and can not accidentally retract within the Laser Fiber Delivery Sheath.

The laser fiber must be visible beyond both the Laser Fiber Delivery Sheath and the suction probe before any activation of the laser unit can be initiated.

To remove the laser fiber from the Suction/Irrigation Device, draw the laser fiber into the fiber sheath by first loosening the rear screw seal and withdrawing the fiber into the sheath. Withdraw the Laser Fiber Delivery Sheath from the Suction/Irrigation Device by pulling straight back on the sheath.

Do not bend the Laser Fiber Delivery Sheath, as it may damage the laser fiber inside.

STERILIZATION GUIDELINES: This product is provided sterile. Do not utilize the product if the package is opened or damaged. This product is intended for single use only. Do not attempt to resterilize by any method.

SPECIFICATIONS/HOW SUPPLIED: Supplied sterile, 5 units per box.

Davis & Geck Endosurgery
1 Casper St.
Danbury, CT 06810
203-743-4451

LAPAROSCOPIC ASSIST DEVICES 8574 & 8575

DESCRIPTION: Multifunction Pistol Grip Device with Modular Interchangeable Probes for suction/irrigation (no electrocautery). Luer lock-type connector for irrigation; barb connector for suction.

Laser Port Probe (order number 8574-03):

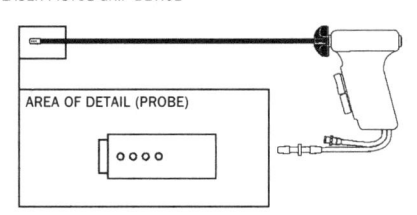

Multifunction Pistol Grip Handpieces for use with products 8576, 8577, 8578, 8579 (probes not included). Luer lock-type connector for irrigation; barb connector for suction.

Laser Port Handpiece (order number 8575-03):

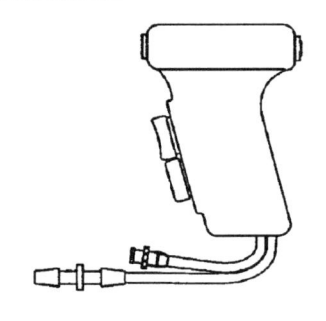

SPECIFICATIONS/HOW SUPPLIED: Supplied in boxes of 5 units.

Aerotech, Inc.
101 Zeta Dr.
Pittsburgh, PA 15238
412-963-7470

Davis & Geck Div.
American Cyanamid Company
One Cyanamid Plaza
Wayne, NJ 07470-2012
201-831-2000

Haraeus Lasersonics, Inc.
575 Cottonwood Dr.
Milpitas, CA 95035-7434
408-954-4000

Ligature

LIGATURE, LAPAROSCOPIC

Davis & Geck Endosurgery
1 Casper St.
Danbury, CT 06810
203-743-4451

LAPRO-LOOP

DESCRIPTION: Chromic or plain gut absorbable surgical ligature:

LAPRO-LOOP LIGATURE

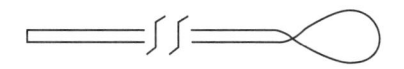

The LAPRO-LOOP* chromic or plain gut ligature consists of a plastic tube that is narrowed on one end and scored on the other. An 18in. gut strand is inserted into the tube, protrudes from the narrowed end, and is formed into a ligature loop with a knot, which becomes secure after the device is activated. The opposite end of the strand is fastened to the scored end of the tube, which acts as the handle.

INDICATIONS: LAPRO-LOOP is indicated to ligate blood vessels and small tubular structures.

CONTRAINDICATIONS: LAPRO-LOOP is not intended for contraceptive tubal occlusion, but may be used to achieve hemostasis following transection of the fallopian tubes.

INSTRUCTIONS FOR USE: Standard endoscopic procedures should be followed up to the point of tissue ligation. The LAPRO-LOOP ligature is then introduced through a cannula. An appropriate surgical instrument is used to grasp and position the tissue. This may involve either pulling the tissue through the loop or encompassing the tissue with the loop. The LAPRO-LOOP ligature tube is then broken at the scored point. This allows the tube to slide over the suture and cinches the loop around the tissue. When the ligature has provided hemostasis, the ligature is cut behind the knot leaving an appropriate length of material. The tube is then removed. Several ligatures may be applied to ensure secure hemostasis.

SPECIFICATIONS/HOW SUPPLIED: Chromic gut ligatures, size 0, length 18in. (45cm), order number 8501-63 (one box contains 12 envelopes).

Heraeus Surgical, Inc.
575 Cottonwood Dr.
Milpitas, CA 95035-7402
408-954-4000

Laserscope
3052 Orchard Dr.
San Jose, CA 95134-2011
408-943-0636

Leisegang Medical, Inc.
6401 Congress Ave.
Boca Raton, FL 33487-2883
407-994-0202

Sharplan Lasers, Inc.
1 Pearl Ct.
Allendale, NJ 07401-1675
201-327-1666

Surgilase, Inc.
33 Plan Way
Warwick, RI 02886
401-732-6440

LASER, ND:YAG, LAPAROSCOPY

Continuum Biomedical Inc.
547 Rhea Way
Livermore, CA 94550
510-606-6118

Dermalase Inc.
3 Main St.
Hopkinton, MA 01748
508-435-0277

Heraeus Surgical, Inc.
575 Cottonwood Dr.
Milpitas, CA 95035-7402
408-954-4000

Kentek Corp., The
4 Depot St.
Pittsfield, NH 03263-1108
603-225-1117

Laserscope
3052 Orchard Dr.
San Jose, CA 95134-2011
408-943-0636

Myriadlase, Inc.
4800 S.E. Loop 820
Forest Hill, TX 76140
817-483-9237

Sharplan Lasers, Inc.
1 Pearl Ct.
Allendale, NJ 07401-1675
201-327-1666

Surgilase, Inc.
33 Plan Way
Warwick, RI 02886
401-732-6440

Davis & Geck Div.
American Cyanamid Company
One Cyanamid Plaza
Wayne, NJ 07470-2012
201-831-2000

Ethicon Endo-Surgery
4545 Creek Road
Cincinnati, OH 45242
513-786-7000

Laparomed Corp.
9272 Jeronimo Rd., Unit 109
Irvine, CA 92718-1914
714-768-1155

Light

ILLUMINATOR, FIBEROPTIC (FOR ENDOSCOPE)

Apple Medical Corp.
93 Nashaway Rd.
Bolton, MA 01740
508-779-2926

Bryan Corp.
4 Plympton St.
Woburn, MA 01801-2908
617-935-0004

Chiu Technical Corp.
252 Indian Head Rd.
Kings Park, NY 11754-4814
516-544-0606

Codman & Shurtleff, Inc.
41 Pacella Park Dr.
Randolph, MA 02368-1755
617-961-2300

Cuda Products Corporation
6000 Powers Ave.
Jacksonville, FL 32217-2212
904-737-7611

Electro Fiberoptics Corporation
56 Hudson St.
Northborough, MA 01532-1922
508-393-3753

Elmed, Inc.
60 W. Fay Ave.
Addison, IL 60101-5198
708-543-2792

Galileo Electro-Optics Corp.
Galileo Park, Rte. 20
P.O. Box 550
Sturbridge, MA 01566
508-347-9191

Heraeus Surgical, Inc.
575 Cottonwood Dr.
Milpitas, CA 95035-7402
408-954-4000

Leisegang Medical, Inc.
6401 Congress Ave.
Boca Raton, FL 33487-2883
407-994-0202

Microlux, Inc.
6000-1 Powers Ave., Medical Bldg.
Jacksonville, FL 32217
904-737-9660

Midwest Dental Products Corp.
901 W. Oakton St.
Des Plaines, IL 60018-1884
708-640-4800

Mist, Inc.
6307 E. Angus Dr.
Raleigh, NC 27613
919-787-8377

Nextec Surgical Corp.
2629 South Horseshoe Dr.
Naples, FL 33942-6122
813-643-2553

Optical Radiation Corp.
1300 Optical Drive
Azusa, CA 91702-3251
818-969-3344

Progressive Dynamics, Inc.
507 Industrial Rd.
Marshall, MI 49068-1758
616-781-4241

Schott Fiber Optics, Inc.
122 Charlton St.
Southbridge, MA 01550-1960
508-765-9744

Smith & Nephew Dyonics, Inc.
160 Dascomb Rd.
Andover, MA 01810-5893
508-470-2800

Storz Endoscopy-America Inc., Karl
10111 W. Jefferson Blvd.
Culver City, CA 90232-3509
310-558-1500

Storz GmbH & Co., Karl
Mittelstr. 8
Postfach 230
D-78532 Tuttlingen
Germany
07461/7080

Thezard
7 Rue Jules Ferry
F-78800 Houilles
France
1/39146509

Wolf Medical Instruments Corp., Richard
353 Corporate Woods Pkwy.
Vernon Hills, IL 60061-3110
708-913-1113

LAMP, ENDOSCOPIC, INCANDESCENT

Applied Fiberoptics, Inc.
E. Main St.
Southbridge, MA 01550
508-765-9121

Bulbtronics
45 Banfi Plaza
P.O. Box 306
Farmingdale, NY 11735-1539
516-249-2272

Cabot Medical Corp.
2021 Cabot Blvd. West
Langhorne, PA 19047-1875
215-752-8300

Carley Lamps
1502 West 228th St.
Torrance, CA 90501-5105
310-325-8474

Cuda Products Corporation
6000 Powers Ave.
Jacksonville, FL 32217-2212
904-737-7611

Effner Biomet GmbH
Alt-Lankwitz 102
D-12247 Berlin 46
Germany
49/30-7700920

Electro Surgical Instrument Co.
37 Centennial St.
Rochester, NY 14611-1732
716-235-1430

Lamp Technology, Inc.
1645 Sycamore Ave.
Bohemia, NY 11716-1729
516-567-1800

Leisegang Medical, Inc.
6401 Congress Ave.
Boca Raton, FL 33487-2883
407-994-0202

Martin, Gebr. GmbH & Co. KG
Ludwigstaler Str. 132
Postf. 60
D-78532 Tuttlingen
Germany
07461/7060

Microlux, Inc.
6000-1 Powers Ave., Medical Bldg.
Jacksonville, FL 32217
904-737-9660

Osram Corp.
110 Bracken Road
Montgomery, NY 12549-2600
914-457-4040

Osram GmbH
Hellabrunner Str. 1
Postfach 900 620
D-81543 Muenchen
Germany
089/62131

Pilling-Rusch
420 Delaware Dr.
Fort Washington, PA 19034-2711
215-643-2600

Schott Fiber Optics, Inc.
122 Charlton St.
Southbridge, MA 01550-1960
508-765-9744

Storz Endoscopy-America Inc., Karl
10111 W. Jefferson Blvd.
Culver City, CA 90232-3509
310-558-1500

Storz GmbH & Co., Karl
Mittelstr. 8
Postfach 230
D-78532 Tuttlingen
Germany
07461/7080

Wolf Medical Instruments Corp., Richard
353 Corporate Woods Pkwy.
Vernon Hills, IL 60061-3110
708-913-1113

LIGHT SOURCE, ENDOSCOPE, XENON ARC

Birtcher Medical Systems Inc.
Endoscopy Div.
41 Brooks Dr.
Braintree, MA 02184
617-356-4830

Birtcher Medical Systems, Inc.
50 Technology Dr.
Irvine, CA 92718-2301
714-753-9400

Bryan Corp.
4 Plympton St.
Woburn, MA 01801-2908
617-935-0004

Bulbtronics
45 Banfi Plaza
P.O. Box 306
Farmingdale, NY 11735-1539
516-249-2272

Cabot Medical Corp.
2021 Cabot Blvd. West
Langhorne, PA 19047-1875
215-752-8300

Chiu Technical Corp.
252 Indian Head Rd.
Kings Park, NY 11754-4814
516-544-0606

Coopersurgical, Inc.
15 Forest Pkwy.
Shelton, CT 06484-5458
203-929-6321

Cuda Products Corporation
6000 Powers Ave.
Jacksonville, FL 32217-2212
904-737-7611

Depuy, Inc.
700 Orthopaedic Dr.
P.O. Box 988
Warsaw, IN 46581-0988
219-267-8143

Elmed, Inc.
60 W. Fay Ave.
Addison, IL 60101-5198
708-543-2792

Fuji Photo Optical Co. Ltd.
1-324, Uetake-Machi, Omiya
Saitama 330
Japan
048/668-2153

Fujinon (Europe) GmbH
Heerdter Lohweg 89
D-40549 Duesseldorf 11
Germany
0211/52050

Fujinon, Inc.
10 High Point Dr.
Wayne, NJ 07470-7434
201-633-5600

Karlheinz Hinze
Endo-Engineering
Elbgaustr. 112
D-22532 Hamburg
Germany
40/842510

Leisegang Medical, Inc.
6401 Congress Ave.
Boca Raton, FL 33487-2883
407-994-0202

Luxtec Corp.
326 Clark St.
Worcester, MA 01606
508-856-9454

Mediflex Surgical Products
250 Gibbs Rd.
Islandia, NY 11722-2697
516-582-8440

Mist, Inc.
6307 E. Angus Dr.
Raleigh, NC 27613
919-787-8377

Origin Medsystems, Inc.
135 Constitution Dr.
Menlo Park, CA 94025
415-617-5000

Pentax Precision Instrument Corp.
30 Ramland Rd.
Orangeburg, NY 10962-2699
914-365-0700

Pioneer Medical, Inc.
34 Laurelcrest Rd.
Madison, CT 06443
203-245-9337

Smith & Nephew Dyonics, Inc.
160 Dascomb Rd.
Andover, MA 01810-5893
508-470-2800

Spiess Design, Inc.
495 Lindberg Lane
Northbrook, IL 60062-2412
708-564-1098

Storz Endoscopy-America Inc., Karl
10111 W. Jefferson Blvd.
Culver City, CA 90232-3509
310-558-1500

Storz GmbH & Co., Karl
Mittelstr. 8
Postfach 230
D-78532 Tuttlingen
Germany
07461/7080

Transamerican Technologies International
7026 Koll Center Pkwy., Ste. 207
Pleasanton, CA 94566-3108
510-484-0700

Wolf Medical Instruments Corp., Richard
353 Corporate Woods Pkwy.
Vernon Hills, IL 60061-3110
708-913-1113

Xenon Corp.
20 Commerce Way
Woburn, MA 01801
617-938-3594

Xylog Corp.
83 Hobart St.
Hackensack, NJ 07601-3948
201-489-4040

LIGHT, SURGICAL, ENDOSCOPIC

Applied Fiberoptics, Inc.
E. Main St.
Southbridge, MA 01550
508-765-9121

Birtcher Medical Systems, Inc.
50 Technology Dr.
Irvine, CA 92718-2301
714-753-9400

Contec Medical Ltd.
11 Haroshet Street
P.O. Box 1400
Ramat Hasharon 47113
Israel
03/5491153

Coopersurgical, Inc.
15 Forest Pkwy.
Shelton, CT 06484-5458
203-929-6321

Cory Brothers Co.
4 Dollis Pk.
London, N3 1HG
United Kingdom
081/349/1081

Cuda Products Corporation
6000 Powers Ave.
Jacksonville, FL 32217-2212
904-737-7611

Depuy, Inc.
700 Orthopaedic Dr.
P.O. Box 988
Warsaw, IN 46581-0988
219-267-8143

Electro Surgical Instrument Co.
37 Centennial St.
Rochester, NY 14611-1732
716-235-1430

Expanded Optics, Inc.
7382 Bolsa Ave.
Westminster, CA 92683-5212
714-891-3996

Leisegang Medical, Inc.
6401 Congress Ave.
Boca Raton, FL 33487-2883
407-994-0202

Link GmbH & Co., Waldemar
Barkhausenweg 10
Postfach 630 565
D-22339 Hamburg 63
Germany
040/5381021

Microlux, Inc.
6000-1 Powers Ave., Medical Bldg.
Jacksonville, FL 32217
904-737-9660

Redfield Corporation
210 Summit Ave.
Montvale, NJ 07645-1526
201-391-0494

Welch Allyn, Inc.
4341 State Street Rd.
P.O. Box 220
Skaneateles Falls, NY 13153-0220
315-685-4100

Wolf Medical Instruments Corp., Richard
353 Corporate Woods Pkwy.
Vernon Hills, IL 60061-3110
708-913-1113

Miscellaneous

ARTHROGRAM SET

Baxter Healthcare Corp.
Pharmaseal Division
27200 North Tourney Rd.
Valencia, CA 91355-1895
805-253-1300

Becton Dickinson And Co.
Becton Dickinson Div.
One Becton Dr.
Franklin Lakes, NJ 07417-1815
201-847-6800

International General Medical Systems Ltd.
Picker Div.
P.O. Box 2, East Lane
GB-Wembley, Middlesex HA9 7PR
United Kingdom
01/904-1288

Med-Surg Industries, Inc.
251 Exchange Place
Herndon, VA 22070-4822
703-742-9700

Picker International GmbH
Barmannstrasse 38
D-80689 Muenchen 60
Germany
089/839-42-0

Picker International, Inc.
595 Miner Rd.
Cleveland, OH 44143-2131
216-473-3000

Radiographics
3013 Regina Dr. Ste. B
Silver Spring, MD 20906-5364
301-460-1736

BOUGIE, ESOPHAGEAL, AND GASTROINTESTINAL, GASTRO-UROLOGY

Bioenterics Corporation
1035A Cindy Lane
Carpinteria, CA 93013
805-684-3045

ENDOLUMINA

DESCRIPTION: The BioEnterics EndoLumina® Illuminated Bougies are designed to aid in the identification of the esophagus, rectum and other structures by transillumination during laparoscopy, thoracoscopy, or open procedures. The EndoLumina Bougie is a silicone elastomer tube filled with a glass fiberoptic bundle which transmits light into a clear, soft flexible silicone tip. The adapter end of the bougie is designed to be attached via a longer fiberoptic cable to a high intensity (300 Watt) light source usually available in the well-equipped laparoscopic facility. The fiberoptic bundle transmits the intense light to the bougie tip without dangerous heat generation. The light transilluminates the esophagus, rectosigmoid, and other organs.

The EndoLumina Bougie is available in multiple tip shapes and diameters. The clear tips are either tapered or rounded in shape and vary in length. A stainless steel connector and silicone adhesive permanently bond the tip to the silicone-sheathed fiberoptic cable. Adapters are provided with the EndoLumina Bougie for light source extension cables from Storz, Olympus, Wolf, Dyonics, ACMI and other companies with compatible connections.

INDICATIONS: The EndoLumina Bougie is intended for use:

To transilluminate the esophagus to assist in the identification and location of the esophagus and its surrounding tissues during laparoscopic, thoracoscopic and open procedures.

To transilluminate the rectum and rectosigmoid to assist in the identification and location of these and the surrounding tissues during gynecological and colorectal laparoscopic and open procedures.

To transilluminate other organs or provide illumination to other natural or surgically-produced cavities.

CONTRAINDICATIONS: Use of the EndoLumina Bougie is contraindicated in any situation where the size or presence of the bougie could cause injury or contamination. The bougie is contraindicated if the patient has a severe stricture which would not allow any size of the bougie to be inserted.

WARNINGS: Care must be taken to ensure that the metal adapter portion of the bougie at its distal end does not come in contact with the patient. When in use, the metal adapter can produce thermal injury.

A damaged bougie should not be used. Care must be taken in handling and inserting the bougie to prevent nicks, cuts or tears in the bougie.

Use of a damaged bougie could result in detachment of some portion of the tip or exposure of the glass fiber cable, and injury to the patient.

PRECAUTIONS:

CAUTION: The bougie must be completely cooled after autoclaving prior to use to avoid possible tissue damage from residual heat. Our testing indicates that a minimum cooling time of 20 minutes at room temperature (25°C) is required.

The bougie should be checked for integrity prior to use. A bougie which has been damaged, or on which repairs have been attempted, should not be used. A standby bougie should be available at the time of use.

The tip of the bougie may be easily penetrated or cut by needles, scalpels or surgical instruments.

Care should be taken to prevent scratching or biting of the bougie. Breakage of individual glass fibers, or nicks, cuts or gouges in the silicone tip will affect light transmission.

Do not kink, stretch, pull or tightly coil the light cable as this can damage the glass fibers.

Care should be taken to prevent any scratching on the face of the adapter end, which could result in a loss of light transmission.

Care must be taken when disconnecting the bougie from the light source cable. Grasp the bougie within 2cm of the attachment point when pulling to disconnect.

The bougie may last longer or wear out sooner, depending on the care, cleaning and the amount of use of the bougie. Cracking, discoloration, and broken fibers will be the most obvious indications of aging and will affect the safety and effectiveness of the device. An opaque or damaged bougie must be replaced.

ADVERSE REACTIONS: Inability to place the bougie may occur. It is possible that severe strictures or other conditions may prevent insertion of a bougie, in which case a smaller EndoLumina Bougie may be used.

If not inserted with care and lubrication, bougies may perforate the walls of the esophagus or other cavities.

Active severe inflammation may interfere with the passage of the larger bougies and may require the use of a smaller diameter bougie.

Active bleeding may interfere with the transillumination of the esophagus.

INSTRUCTIONS FOR USE:
Prior to each surgery:

1. Ensure that a functional 300 Watt light source with a high quality fiberoptic extension cable (5, 5.5 or 7mm) and the appropriate bougie adapter are available for the time of surgery. A low power light source, damaged extension cable, or incorrect adapter will result in inadequate transillumination.

2. Inspect the EndoLumina Bougie for defects by the following steps:

   a. Examine the cable and tip for cracks, splits, gouges and rents;

   b. Examine the junction between the tip and the cable for cracks, peeling, gaps or general deterioration and loosening and;

   c. Hold the tip to light and examine the adapter end of the fiberoptic bundle for broken fibers. Replace bougie if too many fibers are broken (see Figure 3 Bougie Replacement Chart).

Damage to the tip or to the fibers will reduce the amount of light transmission and the bougie may not provide adequate illumination. If light transmission is decreased, replace the bougie.

Esophageal Transillumination:

The patient is prepared for surgery and the surgical procedure initiated. The tipped end of the bougie is passed by the standard technique through the mouth and into the esophagus. The bougie must be lubricated for passage down the esophagus. Water, sterile saline or a clear lubricant can be used to lubricate the bougie.

FIGURE 1 ADAPTERS FOR 40 FRENCH AND SMALLER SIZES

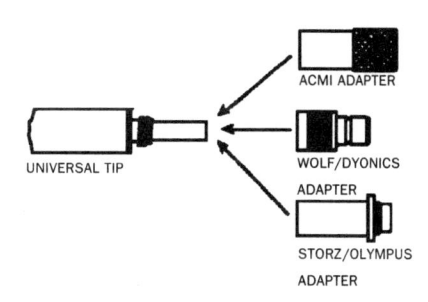

FIGURE 2 ADAPTERS FOR 50 FRENCH AND LARGER SIZES

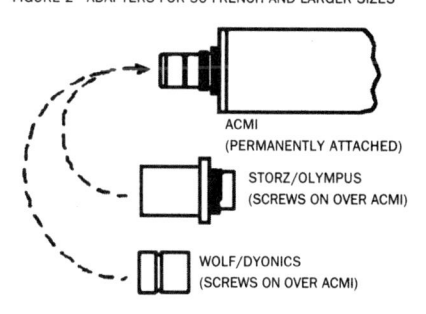

At the appropriate time during surgery, the end of the bougie is attached to a longer fiberoptic cable connected to a high intensity (300 Watt) light source, using one of the supplied adapters (see Figures 1 and 2).

The light source is then turned on. Care must be taken to ensure that the metal adapter portion of the bougie does not come in contact with the patient. When the surgical procedure is completed, the bougie is disconnected from the light source cable, removed from the esophagus, cleaned and sterilized for future use.

Other Transillumination:

The same principles apply for rectosigmoid or other uses. It is customary to have separate bougies for esophageal and rectal uses.

CARE & MAINTENANCE:

General Instrument Cleaning Guidelines:

1. Clean instruments thoroughly immediately after use with a soft-bristled brush in lukewarm soapy water to remove contaminants. Use a non-oily cleaner or mild non-abrasive soap. Do not use synthetic detergents or oil-based soaps as these may be absorbed and may subsequently leach out and cause tissue reaction.

2. Rinse thoroughly in lukewarm water. Follow with a thorough rinse in distilled water and sterilize.

3. Sterilize with gas sterilization, steam autoclave, or the Steris™ process.

CAUTION: Do not soak the BioEnterics EndoLumina Bougie in a disinfectant because the silicone elastomer may absorb some of the solution which may subsequently leach out and cause tissue reaction.

General Guidelines for Care and Maintenance:

1. Meticulous care must be taken to avoid bougie contact with any sharp edges or pointed objects. Any cut or puncture will possibly expose the optical fibers and render the bougie unusable.

2. Do not use any solvent, except alcohol on the bougie.

3. Do not allow the bougie to soak in any solution, including disinfectants.

4. Do not use germicides such as bichloride of mercury or other corrosive solutions.

5. Do not use clamps or forceps on the bougie.

BOUGIE, ESOPHAGEAL, AND GASTROINTESTINAL, GASTRO-UROLOGY (cont'd)

6. Do not twist, stretch, kink or shake the bougie. The glass fibers in the bougie can be irreversibly damaged by careless handling, which could result in a loss of light transmission.

7. Do not clean the bougie in an ultrasonic cleaning device.

8. Do not use a prevacuum high temperature sterilizer as this type will cause the silicone tubing to bubble excessively.

9. Make certain that the autoclave is properly operating regarding maximum temperature. The bougie should be cooled down slowly. To avoid breakage of the glass fibers, do not immerse or rinse in cold liquid. Extensive fiber breakage will result in loss of light intensity.

10. Fiberoptic breakage can result in light and function loss. Hold the tip to light and examine the adapter end of the bougie for broken fibers. Small black dots within the fiberoptic bundle indicate broken fibers.

FIGURE 3   BOUGIE REPLACEMENT CHART

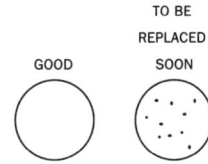

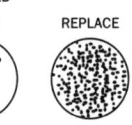

GOOD | TO BE REPLACED SOON | REPLACE

STERILIZATION GUIDELINES:

Gas Sterilization Guidelines:
Ethylene oxide (EtO) gas is recommended. Do not gas sterilize the bougie in a plastic bag or plastic container. The temperature should not exceed 60°C (140°F). The pressure should not exceed 8 psi. Temperature and pressure must be stabilized throughout the cycle.

Recommended aeration time following gas sterilization is noted:
Ambient room air, without aeration chamber: 7 days.
Elevated temperature in an aeration cabinet at 50°C: 12 hours.
Elevated temperature in an aeration cabinet at 60°C: 8 hours.

Other parameters, such as cycle time, temperature, humidification, vacuum, gas concentration and aeration, are all determined by many factors and are established by the sterilizer manufacturer.

Steam (Autoclave) Sterilization Guidelines:

1. Standard gravity sterilization: For a standard gravity sterilizer, conventional double-wrap packaging is recommended. Sterilize for 60 minutes at 250°F and 15 psi or at 121°C and 1 kg/cm2.

2. High Speed Instrument (Flash) Sterilizer: Flash sterilization is not recommended because it reduces the useful life of the product. Flash sterilization accelerates discoloration, which reduces light transmission. If flash sterilization is necessary, wrap the bougie in a surgical towel and place in a clean open tray. Sterilize for 10 minutes at 270°F and 30 psi or at 132°C and 2 kg/cm2.

Do not use autoclaves that incorporate a fast vacuum system to initiate faster heating and/or cooling as this could damage the fiberoptic bundles. Allow the bougie to cool naturally to room temperature. Do not immerse in cool liquids.

Pressure differential during steam autoclaving may cause small bubbles in the silicone tubing. The bubbles will not affect the fiber cables and will dissipate with time.

While the bougie is hot, avoid contact of the adapter metal tip with plastics.

Liquid Sterilant Guidelines:
CAUTION: Do not soak the BioEnterics EndoLumina Bougie in a disinfectant because the silicone elastomer may absorb some of the solution which may subsequently leach out and cause tissue reaction.

The bougie may be sterilized using a Steris System 1™ Processor and Steris 20™ Sterilant. The general processing instructions in the System 1 Operator Manual should be followed.

SPECIFICATIONS/HOW SUPPLIED: The BioEnterics EndoLumina Bougie will be provided clean and non-sterile.

Special Order Devices:
If this Product Insert Data Sheet accompanies a Special Order Device, please note that because of the specifications set out by the physician for this special order device, there will be slight differences between the physical characteristics of the product enclosed and the product description as specified in this brochure. These differences will not affect the safety of this product.

Limited Warranty, Limitation of Liability and Disclaimer of Other Warranties:
BioEnterics Corporation warrants that reasonable care was used in the manufacture and production of this product. Because BioEnterics Corporation has no control over the conditions of use, patient selections, surgical procedure, post-surgical stresses, or handling of the device after it leaves our possession, BioEnterics Corporation does not warrant either a good effect, or against an ill effect following its use. BioEnterics Corporation's sole responsibility in the event that BioEnterics Corporation determines the product was defective when shipped by BioEnterics Corporation, shall be replacement of the product. This warranty is in lieu of and excludes all other warranties not expressly set forth herein, whether expressed or implied by operation of law or otherwise, including, but not limited to, any implied warranties of merchantability or fitness for use.

Returned Goods Policy:
Authorization for return of merchandise should be obtained from your respective dealer. Merchandise returned must have all manufacturer's seals intact and be received within 60 days of invoice to be eligible for credit or replacement. Returned products may be subject to restocking charges.

Product Ordering Information:
For additional product and ordering information, please contact your local dealer or:

BioEnterics Corporation
1035 A Cindy Lane
Carpinteria, CA 93013
Tel: 800 435-4353
805 684-3045
Fax: 805 684-0812

The EndoLumina Illuminated Bougie is manufactured by:

BioEnterics Corporation
1035 A Cindy Lane
Carpinteria, CA 93013, USA
Tel: 805 684-3045
Fax: 805 684-0812

CAUTION: This device is restricted to sale by or on the order of a physician.

EndoLumina is a registered trademark of BioEnterics Corporation.

Steris 1 and Steris 20 are trademarks of Steris Corporation.

U.S. and international patents pending.

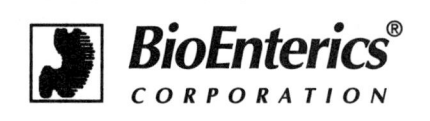

BioEnterics® CORPORATION

Baxter Healthcare Corp.
Operating Room Div.
1500 Waukegan Rd.
McGaw Park, IL 60085-8210
708-473-1500

Berchtold KG, Gebr.
Weimarstr. 13-15
D-78532 Tuttlingen
Germany
07461/2345

Martin, Gebr. GmbH & Co. KG
Ludwigstaler Str. 132
Postf. 60
D-78532 Tuttlingen
Germany
07461/7060

Pilling-Rusch
420 Delaware Dr.
Fort Washington, PA 19034-2711
215-643-2600

Rusch, Inc.
2450 Meadowbrook Pkwy.
Duluth, GA 30136-4635
404-623-0816

Wilson-Cook Medical, Inc.
4900 Bethania Station Rd.
Winston-Salem, NC 27105-1203
919-744-0157

BOUGIE, ESOPHAGEAL, ENT

Baxter Healthcare Corp.
Operating Room Div.
1500 Waukegan Rd.
McGaw Park, IL 60085-8210
708-473-1500

BioEnterics Corporation
1035A Cindy Lane
Carpinteria, CA 93013
805-684-3045

Carsen Group Inc.
151 Telson Rd.
Markham, ONT L3R 1E7
Canada
416-479-4100

Medovations, Inc.
102 East Keefe Ave.
Milwaukee, WI 53212-1535
414-265-7620

Pilling-Rusch
420 Delaware Dr.
Fort Washington, PA 19034-2711
215-643-2600

Rusch, Inc.
2450 Meadowbrook Pkwy.
Duluth, GA 30136-4635
404-623-0816

Sklar Instrument Company
889 South Matlack St.
West Chester, PA 19380
215-430-3200

Wect Instrument Company, Inc.
5645 N. Ravenswood
Chicago, IL 60660-3922
312-769-1944

CABINET, STORAGE, ENDOSCOPE

Chris Lutz Medical, Inc.
23011 Houlton Pkwy. B-3
Laguna Hills, CA 92653
714-830-2472

Custom Ultrasonics, Inc.
P.O. Box 850
Buckingham, PA 18912-0850
215-364-1477

Elmed, Inc.
60 W. Fay Ave.
Addison, IL 60101-5198
708-543-2792

Encompas Unlimited, Inc.
1110 Pinellas Bayway, Ste. 104
Tierra Verde, FL 33715-8281
813-867-7701

Harloff Company
650 Ford St.
Colorado Springs, CO 80915-3712
719-637-0300

Keymed, Inc.
400 Airport Executive Park
Spring Valley, NY 10977-7404
914-425-3100

Medivators, Inc.
6352 320 St. Way
P.O. Box 487
Cannon Falls, MN 55009
507-263-4721

CART, EQUIPMENT, VIDEO

Anthro Corporation
3221 N.W. Yeon St.
Portland, OR 97210
503-241-7113

Armstrong Medical Industries, Inc.
575 Knightsbridge Pkwy.
P.O. Box 700
Lincolnshire, IL 60069-3616
708-913-0101

ATD-American Co.
115-149 Greenwood Ave.
Wyncote, PA 19095-1325
215-576-1000

Berchtold Corp.
2050 Mabeline Rd., Ste. C
North Charlestown, SC 29418-4643
803-569-6100

Blickman Health Industries
39 Robinson Rd. (at Rt. 17S)
Lodi, NJ 07644
201-909-0807

Blue Bell Bio-Medical
P.O. Box 455
Blue Bell, PA 19422
215-699-2266

Cabot Medical Corp.
2021 Cabot Blvd. West
Langhorne, PA 19047-1875
215-752-8300

Cine Graphics Inc.
933 Egyptian Way
Grand Prairie, TX 75050
214-264-5212

Clarus Medical Systems, Inc.
2605 Fernbrook Lane
Minneapolis, MN 55447-4736
612-559-8640

Contec Medical Ltd.
11 Haroshet Street
P.O. Box 1400
Ramat Hasharon 47113
Israel
03/5491153

Coopersurgical, Inc.
15 Forest Pkwy.
Shelton, CT 06484-5458
203-929-6321

Datel Medical Storage Systems, Inc.
2748 Courier Ct. NW
P.O. Box 3740 ZIP 49501-3740
Grand Rapids, MI 49504
616-791-7675

Elmed, Inc.
60 W. Fay Ave.
Addison, IL 60101-5198
708-543-2792

Encompas Unlimited, Inc.
1110 Pinellas Bayway, Ste. 104
Tierra Verde, FL 33715-8281
813-867-7701

Endotec, Inc.
2225 Skyland Ct.
Norcross, GA 30071
404-840-1883

CART, EQUIPMENT, VIDEO

(cont'd)

Envirosurgical, Inc.
7195 E. Kemper Rd.
Cincinnati, OH 45249-1030
513-489-6074

Harloff Company
650 Ford St.
Colorado Springs, CO 80915-3712
719-637-0300

Heraeus Surgical, Inc.
575 Cottonwood Dr.
Milpitas, CA 95035-7402
408-954-4000

Leisegang Medical, Inc.
6401 Congress Ave.
Boca Raton, FL 33487-2883
407-994-0202

Linvatec, Div. of Zimmer of Canada Ltd.
2323 Argentia Rd.
Mississauga, ONT L5N 5N3
Canada
905-858-8588

Northgate Technologies, Inc.
3930 Ventura Dr., Ste. 150
Arlington Heights, IL 60004
708-506-9872

Pentax Precision Instrument Corp.
30 Ramland Rd.
Orangeburg, NY 10962-2699
914-365-0700

Practical Design, Inc.
4711 126th Ave. North, Ste. J
Clearwater, FL 34622
813-572-4820

Promedica, Inc.
5501 D Airport Blvd.
Tampa, FL 33634-5171
813-889-9250

Sharn, Inc.
4801 George Rd., Ste. 180
Tampa, FL 33634-6236
813-889-9614

Smith & Nephew Dyonics, Inc.
160 Dascomb Rd.
Andover, MA 01810-5893
508-470-2800

Smith & Nephew Richards, Inc.
1450 Brooks Road
Memphis, TN 38116
901-396-2121

Snowden-Pencer
5175 S. Royal Atlanta Dr.
Tucker, GA 30084-3053
404-496-0952

Storz Endoscopy-America Inc., Karl
10111 W. Jefferson Blvd.
Culver City, CA 90232-3509
310-558-1500

Waterloo Industries, Inc.
300 Ansborough Ave.
P.O. Box 2095
Waterloo, IA 50704-2095
319-235-7131

Wolf Medical Instruments Corp., Richard
353 Corporate Woods Pkwy.
Vernon Hills, IL 60061-3110
708-913-1113

CART, INSTRUMENT/EQUIPMENT, LAPAROSCOPY

Clarus Medical Systems, Inc.
2605 Fernbrook Lane
Minneapolis, MN 55447-4736
612-559-8640

Elmed, Inc.
60 W. Fay Ave.
Addison, IL 60101-5198
708-543-2792

Leisegang Medical, Inc.
6401 Congress Ave.
Boca Raton, FL 33487-2883
407-994-0202

CONTAINER, SPECIMEN, LAPAROSCOPIC

Cabot Medical Corp.
2021 Cabot Blvd. West
Langhorne, PA 19047-1875
215-752-8300

Dexide, Inc.
7509 Flagstone Dr.
P.O. Box 185789
Fort Worth, TX 76118-6953
817-589-1454

Encompas Unlimited, Inc.
1110 Pinellas Bayway, Ste. 104
Tierra Verde, FL 33715-8281
813-867-7701

DEVICE, ANASTOMOSIS, BIOFRAGMENTABLE

Davis & Geck
Endosurgery
Casper St.
Danbury, CT 06810
203-743-4451

KNOB, INSTRUMENT, ROTATING

Davis & Geck Div.
American Cyanamid Company
One Cyanamid Plaza
Wayne, NJ 07470-2012
201-831-2000

LITHOTRIPTOR, LAPAROSCOPIC

Endomedix Corp.
2162 Michelson Dr.
Irvine, CA 92715
714-253-1000

LAPAROLITH

DESCRIPTION: The LaparoLith™ System allows for removal of a gallstone-laden gallbladder during laparoscopic cholecystectomy without enlarging the laparoscopic incision beyond 10mm. The LaparoLith System spins a rotor inside a protective basket, creating a fluid vortex which draws the stones into contact with the rotor where they are rapidly fragmented into sand. The sand is then aspirated which allows for easier extraction of the gallbladder through the small laparoscopic incision, thus preserving all the advantages of laparoscopic cholecystectomy. The LaparoLith System is intended for use by physicians who have been specifically trained

LAPAROLITH

- HANDPLACE CABLE
- TO MOTOR CONTROLLER
- ACTIVATION SWITCH
- HANDPLACE ASSEMBLY
- SYRINGE
- SLIDE (OPEN)
- INTRODUCER
- SKIN
- GALLBLADDER CLAMP
- PERITONEAL CAVITY
- CAGE (DEPLOYED)
- GALLBLADDER WALL

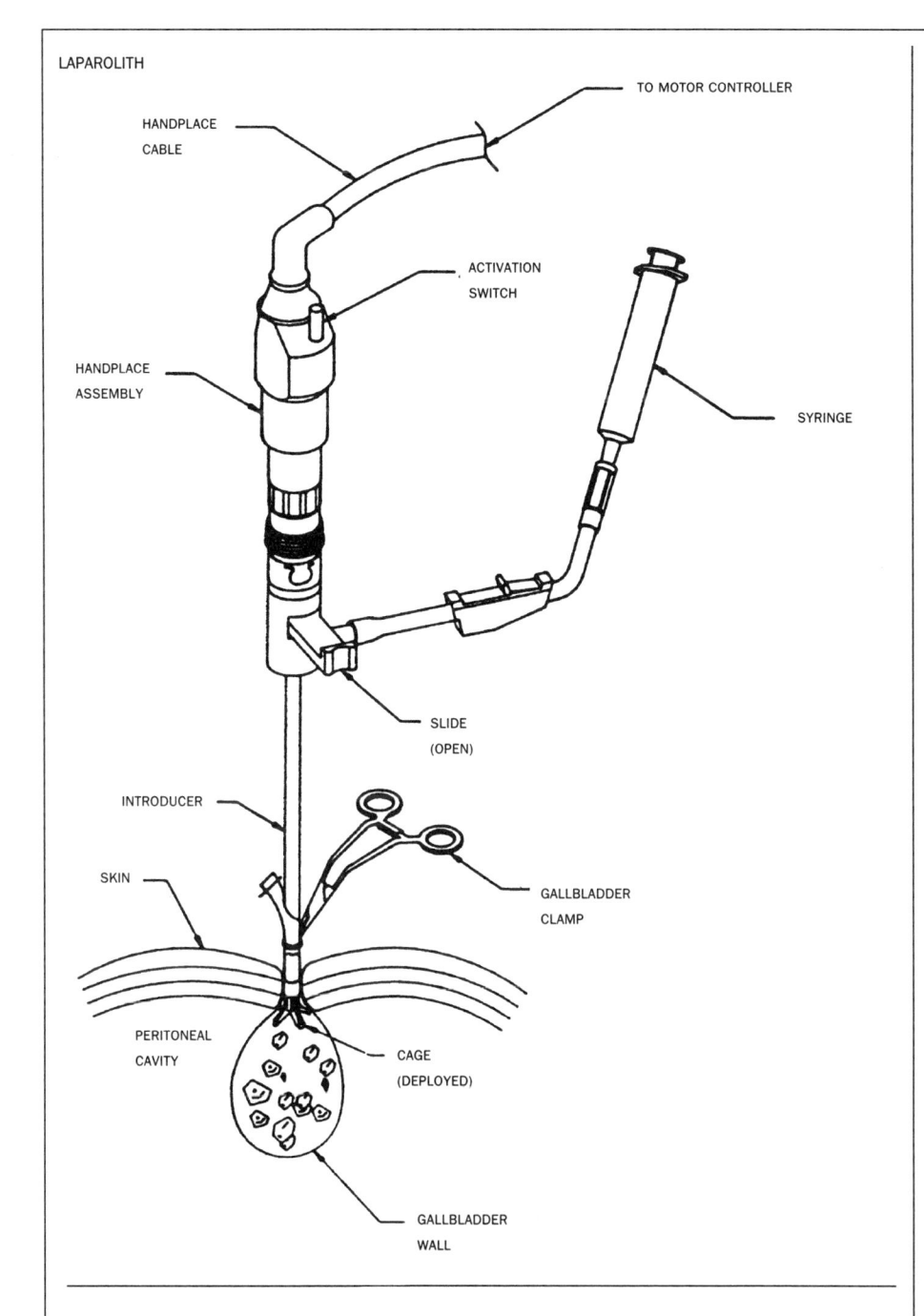

in the use of this device along with generally accepted techniques for performing laparoscopic cholecystectomy.

WARNINGS: Gallstones that are impacted within the gallbladder or adherent to the gallbladder wall may not be capable of entering the fluid vortex. Therefore, the fragmentation that can occur with these types of stones may be limited.

Sufficient void space within the gallbladder is necessary to allow the cage to open and allow for free movement of gallstones.

Do not touch the Spindle or Rotor while they are rotating.

Activation of the Rotor outside of the Introducer could cause serious injury.

INSTRUCTIONS FOR USE: After the gallbladder has been detached from its ductal, vascular and hepatic attachments, and the neck of the gallbladder has been pulled through the laparoscopic incision and exposed on the anterior abdominal wall, cut a small incision high on the gallbladder neck and decompress the gallbladder by aspirating the bile. If gentle traction on the gallbladder does not deliver the gallbladder through the laparoscopic incision, continue the LaparoLith procedure by performing the following steps: Insert the Introducer; distend the gallbladder with saline; pass the Handpiece Assembly into the Introducer until it snaps into place (this will open the protective basket on the Introducer within the gallbladder lumen); aspirate air from the gallbladder; then, activate the device. Activation should not exceed a total of three minutes with an intermittent opera-

tion mode of 15 sec. on/5 sec. off. The device should be run until it reaches a state of "smooth operation" (as detected both audibly and by touch) following an appropriate period of palpable grinding. When aspiration is complete, gently retract the Gallbladder Clamp (still tightly clamped) and Introducer simultaneously, thereby pulling the gallbladder through the laparoscopic incision.

STERILIZATION GUIDELINES: The LaparoLith System Tray may be autoclaved. Under no circumstances should the temperature exceed 275°F (135°C) or 30 minutes of autoclave exposure time. Do not soak, disinfect or immerse in liquid to cool.

SPECIFICATIONS/HOW SUPPLIED: The LaparoLith System consists of two packaged sets. The LaparoLith Drive System (Model L3000) consists of the reusables and includes the Motor Controller and System Tray (Handpiece, Drive Train, Gallbladder Clamp, Obturator and Spindle in an Autoclave Tray). The LaparoLith Kit (Model L300S) is a sterile disposable kit that includes the Introducer, Rotor (with Rotor Cap), Clamp Sleeves and Syringe. Sterile physiological saline (0.9%) is used during the procedure and must be supplied by the hospital.

SERVICE REQUIREMENTS & CONTACTS: For information or service contact: EndoMedix Customer Service at 1-800-553-6361.

PROSTHESIS, ESOPHAGEAL

Carsen Group, Inc.
151 Telson Rd.
Markham, ONT L3R 1E7
Canada
416-479-4100

Keymed Medical & Industrial
Equipment Ltd.
Keymed House, Stock Rd., Southend-on-Sea
Essex SS2 5QH
United Kingdom
0702/616333

Keymed, Inc.
400 Airport Executive Park
Spring Valley, NY 10977-7404
914-425-3100

Rusch, Inc.
2450 Meadowbrook Pkwy.
Duluth, GA 30136-4635
404-623-0816

Wilson-Cook Medical, Inc.
4900 Bethania Station Rd.
Winston-Salem, NC 27105-1203
919-744-0157

SHEATH, ENDOSCOPIC

Bryan Corp.
4 Plympton St.
Woburn, MA 01801-2908
617-935-0004

Circon Acmi
300 Stillwater Ave.
Stamford, CT 06902-3640
203-328-8689

Clarus Medical Systems, Inc.
2605 Fernbrook Lane
Minneapolis, MN 55447-4736
612-559-8640

Coopersurgical, Inc.
15 Forest Pkwy.
Shelton, CT 06484-5458
203-929-6321

Electroscope, Inc.
4890 Sterling Dr.
Boulder, CO 80301
303-444-2600

Endovations, Inc.
Hill & George Avenues
Reading, PA 19610
215-378-1606

Greenwald Surgical Co., Inc.
2688 Dekalb Street
Lake Station, IN 46405-1519
219-962-1604

Instrument Makar, Inc.
2950 E. Mt. Hope
Okemos, MI 48864-1910
517-332-3593

Keymed Medical & Industrial
Equipment Ltd.
Keymed House, Stock Rd., Southend-on-Sea
Essex SS2 5QH
United Kingdom
0702/616333

Keymed, Inc.
400 Airport Executive Park
Spring Valley, NY 10977-7404
914-425-3100

Leisegang Medical, Inc.
6401 Congress Ave.
Boca Raton, FL 33487-2883
407-994-0202

Martin, Gebr. Gmbh & Co. Kg
Ludwigstaler Str. 132
Postf. 60
D-78532 Tuttlingen
Germany
07461/7060

Mist, Inc.
6307 E. Angus Dr.
Raleigh, NC 27613
919-787-8377

Myriadlase, Inc.
4800 S.E. Loop 820
Forest Hill, TX 76140
817-483-9237

Storz Endoscopy-america Inc., Karl
10111 W. Jefferson Blvd.
Culver City, CA 90232-3509
310-558-1500

Storz Gmbh & Co., Karl
Mittelstr. 8
Postfach 230
D-78532 Tuttlingen
Germany
07461/7080

Wect Instrument Company, Inc.
5645 N. Ravenswood
Chicago, IL 60660-3922
312-769-1944

Wells Johnson Co.
8075 E. Research Ct., Ste. 101
Tucson, AZ 85710-6714
602-298-6069

Wid-med, Inc.
111 N. Wabash Ave.
Chicago, IL 60602-1903
312-236-8586

Wolf Medical Instruments Corp., Richard
353 Corporate Woods Pkwy.
Vernon Hills, IL 60061-3110
708-913-1113

SIZER, DEVICE, ANASTOMOSIS

Davis & Geck Endosurgery
1 Casper Street
Danbury, CT 06810
203-743-4451

Davis & Geck Div.
American Cyanamid Company
One Cyanamid Plaza
Wayne, NJ 07470-2012
201-831-2000

STERILIZER/WASHER, ENDOSCOPE

American Medical Concepts, Inc.
1544 Sawdust Rd., Ste. 120
The Woodlands, TX 77380
713-364-8700

Amsco
2424 West 23rd Street
P.O. Box 620
Erie, PA 16506
814-452-3100

Amsco Healthcare
2 Chatham Ctr., Ste. 1100
112 Washington Plaza
Pittsburgh, PA 15219
412-338-6565

Avenatech, Inc.
5001 SW 74th Ct., Ste. 104
Miami, FL 33155
305-667-4117

Bard Ventures
1200 Technology Park Dr.
Billerica, MA 01821
508-667-1300

Bilmar Enterprises, Inc.
1211 W. La Palma Ave. #707
Anaheim, CA 92801-2855
714-991-9170

C.r. Bard Inc., Interventional Products Div.
6091 Heisley Rd.
Mentor, OH 44060-1835
216-352-2935

Custom Ultrasonics, Inc.
P.O. Box 850
Buckingham, PA 18912-0850
215-364-1477

Encompas Unlimited, Inc.
1110 Pinellas Bayway, Ste. 104
Tierra Verde, FL 33715-8281
813-867-7701

Keymed, Inc.
400 Airport Executive Park
Spring Valley, NY 10977-7404
914-425-3100

Medivators, Inc.
6352 320 St. Way
P.O. Box 487
Cannon Falls, MN 55009
507-263-4721

Miele Professional Products Group
22D Worlds Fair Dr.
Somerset, NJ 08873
908-560-0899

Mutoh Co. Ltd.
1-19-2,iriya, Taito-Ku
Tokyo 110
Japan
03/8747141

Sparco, Inc.
2141-A Industrial Court
Vista, CA 92083-7960
619-727-8309

SYSTEM, TRACTION, ARTHROSCOPY

Allen Medical Systems, Inc.
5198 Richmond Rd.
Bedford Heights, OH 44146-1331
216-765-0990

Depuy, Inc.
700 Orthopaedic Dr.
P.O. Box 988
Warsaw, IN 46581-0988
219-267-8143

Promedica, Inc.
5501 D Airport Blvd.
Tampa, FL 33634-5171
813-889-9250

Simal Belgium Instrument Co.
2131 Espey Court, Suite 7
Crofton, MD 21114-2424

TRAY, STERILIZATION, INSTRUMENT

Davis & Geck Endosurgery
1 Casper St.
Danbury, CT 06810
203-743-4451

PRESTIGE 8482-00

DESCRIPTION: Instrument Tray (order number 8482-00):

INSTRUMENT TRAY

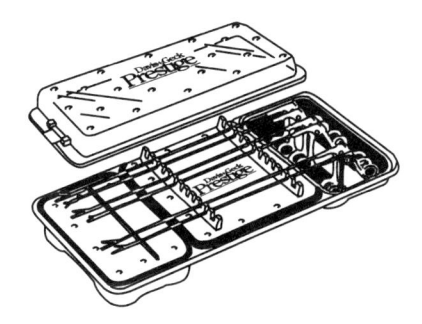

For instrument storage and sterilization. Holds up to 12 instruments (10 5mm and 2 10mm).

SPECIFICATIONS/HOW SUPPLIED:
Standard Instrument Tray:
Order number 8482-10: Replacement Lid
Order number 8482-11: Replacement Base

Large Instrument Tray:
Holds 16 instruments (5mm, or 10mm), up to 52cm in length, 13in. x 25in. x 6in., extra strength polymer, order number 8482-01.
Order number 8482-02: Replacement Lid
Order number 8482-03: Replacement Base

Davis & Geck Div.
American Cyanamid Company
One Cyanamid Plaza
Wayne, NJ 07470-2012
201-831-2000

Ethicon Endo-Surgery
4545 Creek Road
Cincinnati, OH 45242
513-786-7000

Medical Device Technologies, Inc.
4445-310 SW 35th Terrace
Gainesville, FL 32608
904-338-0440

Micromedics, Inc.
1285 Corporate Center Dr., Ste. #150
Eagan, MN 55121-1236
612-452-1977

Needle

NEEDLE, ASPIRATION, CYST, LAPAROSCOPIC

Cabot Medical Corp.
2021 Cabot Blvd. West
Langhorne, PA 19047-1875
215-752-8300

Ranfac Corp.
Avon Indus. Pk./30 Doherty Ave., Box 635
Avon, MA 02322-1125
508-588-4400

Surgin, Inc.
14762 Bentley Circle
Tustin, CA 92680
714-832-6300

Wolf Medical Instruments Corp., Richard
353 Corporate Woods Pkwy.
Vernon Hills, IL 60061-3110
708-913-1113

NEEDLE, BIOPSY, MAMMARY

Pan Servico Surgical Ltd.
436 Streatham High Rd.
London, SW16 1DA
United Kingdom
081-764-1806

Ranfac Corp.
Avon Indus. Pk./30 Doherty Ave., Box 635
Avon, MA 02322-1125
508-588-4400

NEEDLE, ENDOSCOPIC

Bryan Corp.
4 Plympton St.
Woburn, MA 01801-2908
617-935-0004

Cook Urological, Inc.
1100 West Morgan St.
P.O. Box 227
Spencer, IN 47460-9426
812-829-4891

Endovations, Inc.
Hill & George Avenues
Reading, PA 19610
215-378-1606

NEEDLE ENDOSCOPIC (cont'd)

Erbe USA, Inc.
2225 NW Parkway, Ste. 105
Marietta, GA 30067
404-955-4400

Greenwald Surgical Co., Inc.
2688 Dekalb Street
Lake Station, IN 46405-1519
219-962-1604

Hobbs Medical, Inc.
P.O. Box 46
Stafford Springs, CT 06076-0046
203-684-5875

Mill-Rose Laboratories
7310 Corporate Blvd.
Mentor, OH 44060-4856
216-255-7995

Nopa Instruments Medizintechnik GmbH
Gansacker 9 - Postfach 4554
D-78532 Tuttlingen
Germany
07462/7801

Origin Medsystems, Inc.
135 Constitution Dr.
Menlo Park, CA 94025
415-617-5000

Pentax Precision Instrument Corp.
30 Ramland Rd.
Orangeburg, NY 10962-2699
914-365-0700

Pilling-Rusch
420 Delaware Dr.
Fort Washington, PA 19034-2711
215-643-2600

Ranfac Corp.
Avon Indus. Pk./30 Doherty Ave., Box 635
Avon, MA 02322-1125
508-588-4400

Storz Endoscopy-America Inc., Karl
10111 W. Jefferson Blvd.
Culver City, CA 90232-3509
310-558-1500

Storz GmbH & Co., Karl
Mittelstr. 8
Postfach 230
D-78532 Tuttlingen
Germany
07461/7080

U.S. Endoscopy Group
7123 Industrial Park Blvd.
Mentor, OH 44060
216-269-8226

United States Surgical Corp.
150 Glover Ave.
Norwalk, CT 06856-5080
203-845-1000

Wilson-Cook Medical, Inc.
4900 Bethania Station Rd.
Winston-Salem, NC 27105-1203
919-744-0157

Wolf Medical Instruments Corp., Richard
353 Corporate Woods Pkwy.
Vernon Hills, IL 60061-3110
708-913-1113

NEEDLE, INSUFFLATION, LAPAROSCOPIC

Davis & Geck Endosurgery
1 Casper St.
Danbury, CT 06810
203-743-4451

PROFESSIONAL LINE 8381-07
DESCRIPTION: Verres Needle (order number 8381-07):

VERRES NEEDLE
AREA OF DETAIL

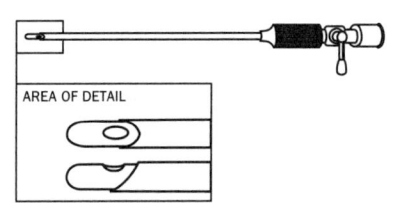

For insufflation of the abdomen (10cm long).

Access Surgical International, Inc.
15 Caswell Ln.
Boat Yard Square
Plymouth, MA 02360
508-747-6006

Advanced Surgical, Inc.
305 College Rd. East
Princeton, NJ 08540
609-987-2340

Aesculap
1000 Gateway Blvd.
South San Francisco, CA 94080-7030
415-876-7000

Apple Medical Corp.
93 Nashaway Rd.
Bolton, MA 01740
508-779-2926

Boss Instruments, Ltd.
1310 Central Ct.
Hermitage, TN 37076
615-885-2231

Bryan Corp.
4 Plympton St.
Woburn, MA 01801-2908
617-935-0004

Cabot Medical Corp.
2021 Cabot Blvd. West
Langhorne, PA 19047-1875
215-752-8300

Chirurgische Instrumente
Hauptstrasse 18
D-78582 Balgheim
Germany
7424/501319

Conmed Corp.
310 Broad Street
Utica, NY 13501
315-797-8375

Coopersurgical, Inc.
15 Forest Pkwy.
Shelton, CT 06484-5458
203-929-6321

Core Dynamics, Inc.
11222-4 St. Johns Indust. Pkwy.
Jacksonville, FL 32216
904-641-6611

Davis & Geck Div.
American Cyanamid Company
One Cyanamid Plaza
Wayne, NJ 07470-2012
201-831-2000

Dexide, Inc.
7509 Flagstone Dr.
P.O. Box 185789
Fort Worth, TX 76118-6953
817-589-1454

Elmed, Inc.
60 W. Fay Ave.
Addison, IL 60101-5198
708-543-2792

Ethicon Endo-Surgery
4545 Creek Road
Cincinnati, OH 45242
513-786-7000

Heraeus Surgical, Inc.
575 Cottonwood Dr.
Milpitas, CA 95035-7402
408-954-4000

Leisegang Medical, Inc.
6401 Congress Ave.
Boca Raton, FL 33487-2883
407-994-0202

Linvatec, Div. of Zimmer of Canada Ltd.
2323 Argentia Rd.
Mississauga, ONT L5N 5N3
Canada
905-858-8588

Marlow Surgical Technologies, Inc.
1810 Joseph Lloyd Pkwy.
Willoughby, OH 44094-8030
216-946-2453

Medicon Instruments, Inc.
4405 International Blvd.
Norcross, GA 30093-3013
404-381-2858

Origin Medsystems, Inc.
135 Constitution Dr.
Menlo Park, CA 94025
415-617-5000

Ranfac Corp.
Avon Indus. Pk./30 Doherty Ave., Box 635
Avon, MA 02322-1125
508-588-4400

Smith & Nephew Dyonics, Inc.
160 Dascomb Rd.
Andover, MA 01810-5893
508-470-2800

Synectic Engineering, Inc.
4 Oxford Rd.
Milford, CT 06460-7007
203-877-8488

United States Surgical Corp.
150 Glover Ave.
Norwalk, CT 06856-5080
203-845-1000

Wolf Medical Instruments Corp., Richard
353 Corporate Woods Pkwy.
Vernon Hills, IL 60061-3110
708-913-1113

NEEDLE, PUNCTURE

Davis & Geck Endosurgery
1 Casper St.
Danbury, CT 06810
203-743-4451

PROFESSIONAL LINE 8381-02
DESCRIPTION: Puncture Needle (order number 8381-02):

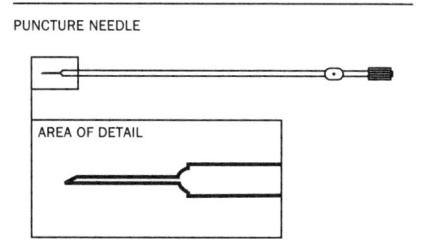

PUNCTURE NEEDLE

AREA OF DETAIL

With luer lock connection and finger valve, 5mm diameter, working length 33cm. Can be used with Y-Connector (8381-06).

Chirurgische Instrumente
Hauptstrasse 18
D-78582 Balgheim
Germany
7424/501319

Davis & Geck Div.
American Cyanamid Company
One Cyanamid Plaza
Wayne, NJ 07470-2012
201-831-2000

Schwarz Medical
Kirchstrasse 24
D-86935 Rott
Germany
8869/1881

NEEDLE, SUTURE, ARTHROSCOPY

Flexmedics Corp.
12400 Whitewater Dr. #2040
Minnetonka, MN 55343
612-939-0900

Instrument Makar, Inc.
2950 E. Mt. Hope
Okemos, MI 48864-1910
517-332-3593

JSB-Medizintechnik
Hauptstr. 24
D-78549 Spaichingen
Germany
07424/4303

Power Supply

BOX, BATTERY, POCKET (ENDOSCOPIC)

Alexander Batteries, New Product/OEM Div.
P.O. Box 1508
Mason City, IA 50402
515-423-8955

Martin, Gebr. GmbH & Co. KG
Ludwigstaler Str. 132
Postf. 60
D-78532 Tuttlingen
Germany
07461/7060

Zarges Leichtbau GmbH
Zargesstr. 7
D-82362 Weilheim
Germany
0881/687-0

BOX, BATTERY, RECHARGEABLE (ENDOSCOPIC)

Access/God Loves You
651 Topeka Way
P.O. Box 1630
Castle Rock, CO 80104-1630
303-688-1808

Alexander Batteries, New Product/OEM Div.
P.O. Box 1508
Mason City, IA 50402
515-423-8955

Johnson Controls Inc., Specialty Battery Div.
900 E. Keefe Ave.
Milwaukee, WI 53212-1709
414-961-6500

Nesa Corp.
12 Silvermine Road
Brookfield Center, CT 06804-3316
203-775-0578

Zarges Leichtbau GmbH
Zargesstr. 7
D-82362 Weilheim
Germany
0881/687-0

CORD, ELECTRIC, ENDOSCOPE

Apple Medical Corp.
93 Nashaway Rd.
Bolton, MA 01740
508-779-2926

Bard Ventures
1200 Technology Park Dr.
Billerica, MA 01821
508-667-1300

Bryan Corp.
4 Plympton St.
Woburn, MA 01801-2908
617-935-0004

Circon Acmi
300 Stillwater Ave.
Stamford, CT 06902-3640
203-328-8689

Electro Surgical Instrument Co.
37 Centennial St.
Rochester, NY 14611-1732
716-235-1430

Elmed, Inc.
60 W. Fay Ave.
Addison, IL 60101-5198
708-543-2792

Erbe USA, Inc.
2225 NW Parkway, Ste. 105
Marietta, GA 30067
404-955-4400

Kirwan Surgical Products, Inc.
83 East Water St.
P.O. Box 545
Rockland, MA 02370-1837
617-878-2706

Leisegang Medical, Inc.
6401 Congress Ave.
Boca Raton, FL 33487-2883
407-994-0202

Martin, Gebr. GmbH & Co. KG
Ludwigstaler Str. 132
Postf. 60
D-78532 Tuttlingen
Germany
07461/7060

Wolf Medical Instruments Corp., Richard
353 Corporate Woods Pkwy.
Vernon Hills, IL 60061-3110
708-913-1113

Yole Company
51 Boulevard
Greenlawn, NY 11740-1401
516-757-9336

GENERATOR, POWER, ELECTROSURGICAL

Access Surgical International, Inc.
15 Caswell Ln.
Boat Yard Square
Plymouth, MA 02360
508-747-6006

Birtcher Medical Systems, Inc.
50 Technology Dr.
Irvine, CA 92718-2301
714-753-9400

Hemostatix Corp.
190 S. Whisman Rd., Bldg. G
Mountain View, CA 94041
415-691-0882

Leisegang Medical, Inc.
6401 Congress Ave.
Boca Raton, FL 33487-2883
407-994-0202

Quantum Instruments Corp.
17304 Preston Rd., Ste. 800
Dallas, TX 75252
214-733-6566

Valley Forge Scientific, Inc.
P.O. Box 925
Valley Forge, PA 19482-0925
215-666-7500

Valleylab, Inc.
5920 Longbow Dr.
Boulder, CO 80301-3202
303-530-2300

Wolf Medical Instruments Corp., Richard
353 Corporate Woods Pkwy.
Vernon Hills, IL 60061-3110
708-913-1113

POWER SUPPLY, ENDOSCOPIC, BATTERY OPERATED

Aaron Medical Industries, Inc.
7100 30th Ave. North
St. Petersburg, FL 33710-2902
813-384-2323

Chiu Technical Corp.
252 Indian Head Rd.
Kings Park, NY 11754-4814
516-544-0606

Ethnor
192 Ave. Charles De Gaulle
F-92523 Neuilly S/Seine Cedex
France
1/47382233

Frankignoul & Cie. S.A.
Zoning Industriel
B-4330 Grace-Hollogne
Belgium
41/633920

Storz Endoscopy-America Inc., Karl
10111 W. Jefferson Blvd.
Culver City, CA 90232-3509
310-558-1500

Storz GmbH & Co., Karl
Mittelstr. 8
Postfach 230
D-78532 Tuttlingen
Germany
07461/7080

Welch Allyn, Inc.
4341 State Street Rd.
P.O. Box 220
Skaneateles Falls, NY 13153-0220
315-685-4100

POWER SUPPLY, ENDOSCOPIC, LINE OPERATED

Cameron-Miller, Inc.
3949 S. Racine Ave.
Chicago, IL 60609-2523
312-523-6360

Carsen Group Inc.
151 Telson Rd.
Markham, ONT L3R 1E7
Canada
416-479-4100

Condor D.C. Power Supplies, Inc.
2311 Statham Pkwy.
Oxnard, CA 93033-3911
805-486-4565

Remover

REMOVER, CLIP

Davis & Geck Endosurgery
1 Casper St.
Danbury, CT 06810
203-743-4451

LAPRO-CLIP 8487-99

DESCRIPTION: Lapro-Clip* Ligating Clip Remover is stainless steel and designed to fit through a 10mm cannula.

LIGATING CLIP REMOVER

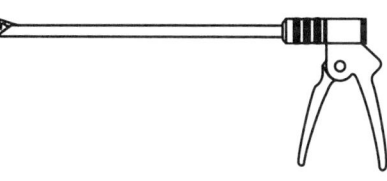

INDICATIONS: Lapro-Clip Ligating Clip Remover is used during those surgical applications where, in the opinion of the surgeon, removal of the Lapro-Clip Ligating Clip is indicated.

WARNINGS: The clip remover must be properly positioned on the Lapro-Clip Ligating Clip as illustrated in the instructions for use.

INSTRUCTIONS FOR USE:
1. Position the grasping hook in front of the trunnion post, seating the Lapro-Clip ligating clip onto the lower platform of the remover.

LIGATING CLIP REMOVER

Detail of Ligating Clip Remover

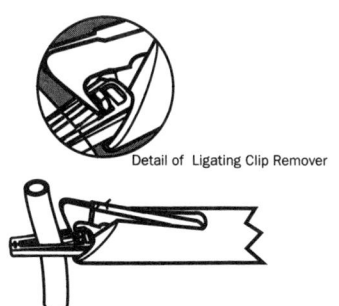

2. Close handle slightly to hold clip in position. As needed, rotate shaft for visual inspection to ensure tissue has not been captured between grasping hook and clip.
3. Firmly squeeze handle for complete actuation of grasping hook, this spreads the clip for removal.

STERILIZATION GUIDELINES: For specific instructions on cleaning and sterilization see Laparoscopic Clip Applier.

SPECIFICATIONS/HOW SUPPLIED: The Lapro-Clip Ligating Clip Remover is supplied non-sterile (order number 8487-99). Lapro-Clip Ligating Clips and Appliers are sold separately.

Consort Pvba
Parklaan 36
B-2300 Turnhout
Belgium
014/411279

Cory Brothers Co.
4 Dollis Pk.
London, N3 1HG
United Kingdom
081/349/1081

Electro Surgical Instrument Co.
37 Centennial St.
Rochester, NY 14611-1732
716-235-1430

Elpac Power Systems
1562 Reynolds Ave.
Irvine, CA 92714
714-476-6070

Hoekloos Medical Equipment
Kabelweg 44
P.O. Box 663
NL-1000 AR Amsterdam
Netherlands
020/5811470

Medicon Eg
15 Gansacker
Postfach 4455
D-78532 Tuttlingen
Germany
07462/20090

Medicon Instruments, Inc.
4405 International Blvd.
Norcross, GA 30093-3013
404-381-2858

Welch Allyn, Inc.
4341 State Street Rd.
P.O. Box 220
Skaneateles Falls, NY 13153-0220
315-685-4100

Abco Dealers, Inc.
6601 W. Mill Rd.
P.O. Box 23090
Milwaukee, WI 53218-0090
414-358-5420

Baxter Healthcare Corp.
Operating Room Div.
1500 Waukegan Rd.
McGaw Park, IL 60085-8210
708-473-1500

Davis & Geck Div.
American Cyanamid Company
One Cyanamid Plaza
Wayne, NJ 07470-2012
201-831-2000

Design Standards Corp.
643 North Ave.
Bridgeport, CT 06606-5745
203-366-7046

Design Standards Corp., Charlestown Div.
Ceda Industrial Park
P.O. Box 996
Charlestown, NH 03603-0996
603-826-7744

Dittmar, Inc.
101 E. Laurel Ave.
P.O. Box 66
Cheltenham, PA 19012-2125
215-379-5533

Ethicon, Inc.
U.S. Route 22
P.O. Box 151
Somerville, NJ 08876
908-218-0707

Medicon Eg
15 Gansacker
Postfach 4455
D-78532 Tuttlingen
Germany
07462/20090

Medicon Instruments, Inc.
4405 International Blvd.
Norcross, GA 30093-3013
404-381-2858

REMOVER, CLIP (cont'd)

Surgical Instrument Co. of America
1185 Edgewater Ave.
Ridgefield, NJ 07657-2102
201-941-6500

Weck & Co. Inc., Edward
1 Weck Dr.
P.O. Box 12600
Research Triangle Park, NC 27709
919-544-8000

REMOVER, STAPLE, SURGICAL

Ethicon Endo-Surgery
4545 Creek Rd.
Cincinnati, OH 45242
513-786-7000

PROXIMATE RHX

INSTRUCTIONS FOR USE:
Use of PROXIMATE* RHX extractor:

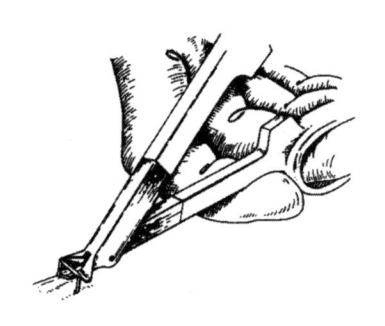

1. Position the lower jaw of the extractor beneath the staple crown.
PROXIMATE RH stapler contains coated staples, which facilitate extraction and minimize pain.

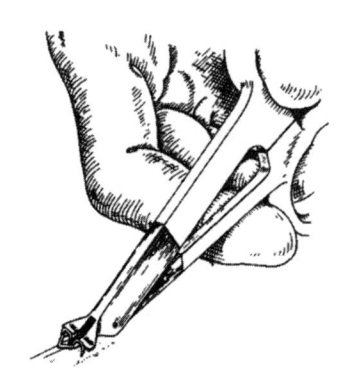

2. Squeeze down with the thumb until handles are firmly touching. The staple will reform.

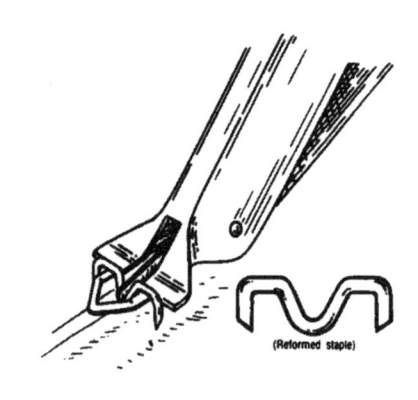

3. Ensure staple is completely reformed before lifting extractor from skin. Never pull up before extractor is fully closed. Turn extractor upside down and open handles. The staple will fall out.

Accurate Surgical & Scientific
Instrument Corp.
300 Shames Dr.
Westbury, NY 11590-1736
516-333-2570

Acme United Corporation, Medical Div.
75 Kings Highway Cutoff
Fairfield, CT 06430-5340
203-332-7330

Davis & Geck Div.
American Cyanamid Company
One Cyanamid Plaza
Wayne, NJ 07470-2012
201-831-2000

Design Standards Corp.
643 North Ave.
Bridgeport, CT 06606-5745
203-366-7046

Pollak Ltd.
6 Hasadna St., Industrial Zone
Kfar Sava 44100
Israel
972-9-9548

Retractor

RETRACTOR, FAN-TYPE, LAPAROSCOPY

Davis & Geck Endosurgery
1 Casper St.
Danbury, CT 06810
203-743-4451

LAPAROSCOPIC ASSIST DEVICES 8369 SERIES

INDICATIONS: The single-use **fan retractor** device is indicated wherever retraction is necessary to expose vital structures during endoscopic procedures.

CONTRAINDICATIONS: There are no contraindications except for the judgmental considerations of the endoscopist, just as these same considerations are necessary for retraction in open operative procedures.

PRECAUTIONS: This device should only be used by physicians trained in the performance of laparoscopic procedures.

INSTRUCTIONS FOR USE:
1. Based upon laparoscopic surgical trocar diameter, select either the 5mm or 10mm fan retractor. The 5mm fan retractor will fit a 5mm trocar and the 10mm fan retractor will fit a 10mm trocar. The actual shaft diameters on the retractors are 4.5mm and 9.5mm, respectively.
2. Prior to use, wet the shaft of the fan retractor with sterile saline or water.
3. Insert the fan retractor into and through the port while the fan retractor is in the collapsed state. Visualize the distal end of the fan retractor as it emerges from the port into the cavity.
4. Once inserted into the cavity, open the fan retractor to the desired span. All manipulation of the fan retractor should be under visualization.
5. Collapse the fan retractor prior to removing the retractor.

STERILIZATION GUIDELINES: For single-patient use only. Do not attempt to resterilize by any method.

SPECIFICATIONS/HOW SUPPLIED: Sterile if package is unopened and undamaged. Order number 8369-05 for 5mm fan retractor, and 8369-10 for 10mm fan retractor.
CAUTION: Federal (USA) law restricts this device to sale by or on the order of a physician.

Access Surgical International, Inc.
15 Caswell Ln.
Boat Yard Square
Plymouth, MA 02360
508-747-6006

Advanced Surgical, Inc.
305 College Rd. East
Princeton, NJ 08540
609-987-2340

Automated Medical Products Corp.
2315 Broadway, Ste. 410
New York, NY 10024-4332
212-874-0236

Birtcher Medical Systems, Inc.
50 Technology Dr.
Irvine, CA 92718-2301
714-753-9400

Boss Instruments, Ltd.
1310 Central Ct.
Hermitage, TN 37076
615-885-2231

Bryan Corp.
4 Plympton St.
Woburn, MA 01801-2908
617-935-0004

Cabot Medical Corp.
2021 Cabot Blvd. West
Langhorne, PA 19047-1875
215-752-8300

Coopersurgical, Inc.
15 Forest Pkwy.
Shelton, CT 06484-5458
203-929-6321

Davis & Geck Div.
American Cyanamid Company
One Cyanamid Plaza
Wayne, NJ 07470-2012
201-831-2000

Elekta Instruments, Inc.
8 Executive Park West, Ste. 809
Atlanta, GA 30329
404-315-1225

Elmed, Inc.
60 W. Fay Ave.
Addison, IL 60101-5198
708-543-2792

Leisegang Medical, Inc.
6401 Congress Ave.
Boca Raton, FL 33487-2883
407-994-0202

Medicon Instruments, Inc.
4405 International Blvd.
Norcross, GA 30093-3013
404-381-2858

Mist, Inc.
6307 E. Angus Dr.
Raleigh, NC 27613
919-787-8377

Origin Medsystems, Inc.
135 Constitution Dr.
Menlo Park, CA 94025
415-617-5000

United States Surgical Corp.
150 Glover Ave.
Norwalk, CT 06856-5080
203-845-1000

RETRACTOR, LAPAROSCOPY, OTHER

Access Surgical International, Inc.
15 Caswell Ln.
Boat Yard Square
Plymouth, MA 02360
508-747-6006

Advanced Surgical, Inc.
305 College Rd. East
Princeton, NJ 08540
609-987-2340

Automated Medical Products Corp.
2315 Broadway, Ste. 410
New York, NY 10024-4332
212-874-0236

Boss Instruments, Ltd.
1310 Central Ct.
Hermitage, TN 37076
615-885-2231

Cabot Medical Corp.
2021 Cabot Blvd. West
Langhorne, PA 19047-1875
215-752-8300

Electro Surgical Instrument Co.
37 Centennial St.
Rochester, NY 14611-1732
716-235-1430

Elekta Instruments, Inc.
8 Executive Park West, Ste. 809
Atlanta, GA 30329
404-315-1225

Ethicon Endo-Surgery
4545 Creek Road
Cincinnati, OH 45242
513-786-7000

Kensey Nash Corporation
55 E. Uwchlan Ave., Ste. 204
Exton, PA 19341-1247
215-524-0188

Laparomed Corp.
9272 Jeronimo Rd., Unit 109
Irvine, CA 92718-1914
714-768-1155

Leisegang Medical, Inc.
6401 Congress Ave.
Boca Raton, FL 33487-2883
407-994-0202

Origin Medsystems, Inc.
135 Constitution Dr.
Menlo Park, CA 94025
415-617-5000

Ranfac Corp.
Avon Indus. Pk./30 Doherty Ave., Box 635
Avon, MA 02322-1125
508-588-4400

United States Surgical Corp.
150 Glover Ave.
Norwalk, CT 06856-5080
203-845-1000

Scissors

During the early years of laparoscopic surgery, the use of scissors was limited to cutting an occasional adhesion or suture. However, with the advent of more advanced procedures, scissors have assumed an increasingly important role. Extensive adhesiolysis, the opening of ducts and organs, the cutting of sutures, and the dissection of tissue planes have all made the need for sharp scissors imperative. Unfortunately, the small blades required for laparoscopy frequently loose their edge or fail to reapproximate, making a very expensive pair of scissors into a useless artifact.

To keep their scissors sharp, manufacturers have tried tightening the blades, adding approximation washers between them, decreasing the opening of the blades, fitting them with disposable tips, and, finally, making completely disposable instruments.

Tightening the blades makes them approximate more closely and therefore cut better; but it also increases the force needed to open and close them. With greater force comes greater difficulty in holding the scissors still, so the tighter blades can reduce accuracy, as well as increasing the surgeon's fatigue.

The approximation washer overcomes these problems, but creates another one of its own. Placed in the joint of the scissors, this washer expands as the instrument wears, pushing the blades into constant approximation. However, the looseness of the blades in this arrangement makes it difficult to cut large pieces of tissue, so the design is best suited for small dissecting scissors.

Since most scissors are sharpest at the tip, reducing the opening of the blades forces the surgeon to use only the instrument's most effective portion. The narrower opening also improves approximation. Because scissors with wider openings encompass more tissue, their blades can be forced further apart, impairing the cut.

No matter which of these strategies a manufacturer employs, the blades are eventually bound to get dull and fail to approximate; and when this happens, the only remedy is to throw the scissors away and get a new pair. Hence the disposable scissor. Since the instrument is intended for one-time use, it will always be sharp. And even if it does lose its edge during a procedure, it can simply be tossed and replaced with a new one.

The cost of the disposables is of course a concern; but when faced with a choice between economy or effectiveness, most surgeons will opt for the most effective instrument available. To reduce cost, some manufacturers offer scissors with reusable handles and disposable tips; and these have met with moderate success. Nevertheless, the completely disposable scissor remains the workhorse of laparoscopy.

To increase their versatility, most scissors are now fitted with a cautery attachment that permits coagulation during cutting. The attachment can be used in two ways. The cut can be made and energy then applied as if using a cautery spatula, or the blades can be placed around the structure to be cut, current applied, and transection then performed on the desiccated tissue. The latter technique is sometimes employed as if the scissors were bipolar. However, each blade is in fact monopolar and can cause a burn. Bipolar scissors have been developed to overcome the disadvantages of monopolar current; but they are bulkier than standard scissors and have failed to gain popularity in the U.S.

The choice of blade configuration depends on the application. For fine dissection, Metzenbaum-type scissor blades are best. Heavier Mayo-type blades are needed for cutting fascia and heavy adhesions. Microscissors are the best choice for opening small ducts and performing extremely delicate dissection. A laparoscopic version of Potts scissors is available for angled cutting. And when precise cuts into ducts and tubes are needed, hook scissors permit the surgeon to fix mobile tissue with the hook tips prior to cutting, thus forcing the tissue into contact with the advancing blades and controlling the depth of the cut. Hook scissors or Mayo blades also should be used when cutting suture.

When selecting a scissor, it's important to consider application and price, as well as ease of cleaning and required source of energy. But above all, consider sharpness. Without it, the whole purpose of the scissor is lost.

SCISSORS/151

SCISSORS WITH REMOVABLE TIPS, LAPAROSCOPY

Access Surgical International, Inc.
15 Caswell Ln.
Boat Yard Square
Plymouth, MA 02360
508-747-6006

Davis & Geck Div.
American Cyanamid Company
One Cyanamid Plaza
Wayne, NJ 07470-2012
201-831-2000

Heraeus Surgical, Inc.
575 Cottonwood Dr.
Milpitas, CA 95035-7402
408-954-4000

Innovative Surgical, Inc.
3071 Continental Dr., Ste. 102
West Palm Beach, FL 33407
407-697-5051

Marlow Surgical Technologies, Inc.
1810 Joseph Lloyd Pkwy.
Willoughby, OH 44094-8030
216-946-2453

Microsurge, Inc.
150 A St.
Needham, MA 02194
617-444-2300

Mist, Inc.
6307 E. Angus Dr.
Raleigh, NC 27613
919-787-8377

Origin Medsystems, Inc.
135 Constitution Dr.
Menlo Park, CA 94025
415-617-5000

Smith & Nephew Dyonics, Inc.
160 Dascomb Rd.
Andover, MA 01810-5893
508-470-2800

Synectic Engineering, Inc.
4 Oxford Rd.
Milford, CT 06460-7007
203-877-8488

Ximed Medical Systems
2195 Trade Zone Blvd.
San Jose, CA 95131
408-945-4040

SCISSORS, LAPAROSCOPY

Davis & Geck Endosurgery
1 Casper St.
Danbury, CT 06810
203-743-4451

PROFESSIONAL LINE 8374 SERIES

DESCRIPTION:

Metzenbaum Scissors:
Tungsten carbide blade inserts, color coded orange. For tissue dissection with simultaneous control of bleeding:

METZENBAUM SCISSORS

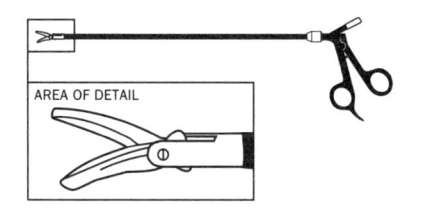

INSTRUMENT KNOB

Hook Scissors:
Blunt, color coded orange. For severing strand-like structures with simultaneous control of bleeding:

HOOK SCISSORS

360° ROTATION

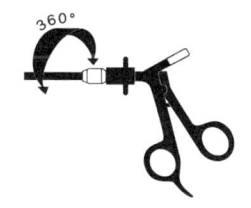

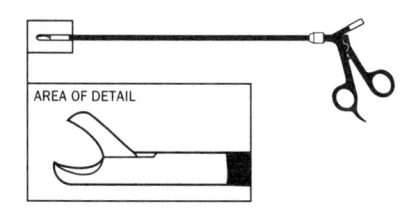

METZENBAUM SCISSORS

PRODUCT CODE	DIAMETER MM	SHAFT LENGTH CM	360° ROTATION	INSULATED MONOPOLAR	CURVED SHAFT	FLUSH PORT	D-TACH
8374-06	5	33	No	Yes	No	No	No
8374-07	10	33	Yes	Yes	No	No	No
8374-08	5	33	Yes	Yes	No	No	No
8390-04	5	35	Yes	Yes	No	No	Yes
8390-05	10	35	Yes	Yes	No	No	Yes
8390-07	5	26	Yes	Yes	No	No	Yes
8450-07	5	33	Yes	Yes	Yes	No	No
8450-08	5	26	Yes	Yes	No	No	No
8451-01	5	45	No	Yes	No	Yes	No

HOOK SCISSORS

PRODUCT CODE	DIAMETER MM	SHAFT LENGTH CM	360° ROTATION	INSULATED MONOPOLAR	FLUSH PORT	D-TACH
8374-01	5	33	No	No	No	No
8374-04	5	33	No	Yes	No	No
8374-10	10	33	No	Yes	No	No
8374-11	10	40	No	Yes	No	No
8390-02	5	35	Yes	Yes	No	Yes
8451-02	5	45	No	Yes	Yes	No

PRODUCT DIRECTORY

PERITONEAL SCISSORS

PRODUCT CODE	DIAMETER MM	SHAFT LENGTH CM	360° ROTATION	INSULATED MONOPOLAR	CURVED SHAFT	D-TACH
8374-02	5	33	No	No	No	No
8374-05	5	33	No	Yes	No	No
8374-12	10	33	No	Yes	No	No
8374-13	10	40	No	Yes	No	No
8390-03	5	35	Yes	Yes	No	Yes
8450-09	5	33	Yes	Yes	Yes	No

MICRO-DISSECTING SCISSORS

PRODUCT CODE	DIAMETER MM	SHAFT LENGTH CM	360° ROTATION	INSULATED MONOPOLAR	D-TACH
8374-03	5	33	No	No	No
8374-19	10	33	No	No	No
8374-20	10	40	No	Yes	No
8390-01	5	35	Yes	Yes	Yes
8390-06	5	26	Yes	Yes	Yes
8450-10	5	26	Yes	Yes	No

Peritoneal Scissors:
Serrated jaws, color coded orange. For severing and cutting tissue and organs with simultaneous control of bleeding:

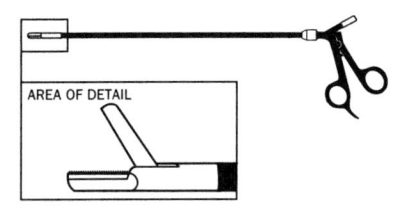

Micro-Dissecting Scissors:
Curved left, color coded orange. For dissecting small structures such as the bile duct:

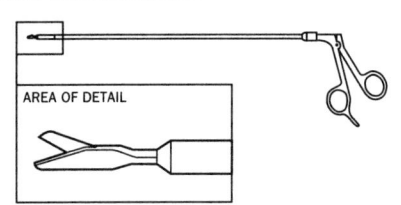

Macro-Dissecting Scissors:
10mm diameter, non-insulated, working length 33cm (order number 8374-09). 40cm length, insulated (order number 8374-21). For severing coarse structures: straps, cyst sacs, and myoma enucleations:

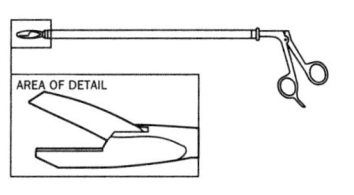

Bard Gynecology
25 Computer Dr.
Haverhill, MA 01832
508-373-1000

Baxter Healthcare Corp., V. Mueller Div.
6600 W. Touhy
Niles, IL 60714
708-647-9383

Chirurgische Instrumente
Hauptstrasse 18
D-78582 Balgheim
Germany
7424/501319

Circon Acmi
300 Stillwater Ave.
Stamford, CT 06902-3640
203-328-8689

Davis & Geck Div.
American Cyanamid Company
One Cyanamid Plaza
Wayne, NJ 07470-2012
201-831-2000

Ethicon Endo-Surgery
4545 Creek Road
Cincinnati, OH 45242
513-786-7000

Innovative Surgical, Inc.
3071 Continental Dr., Ste. 102
West Palm Beach, FL 33407
407-697-5051

Koros Surgical Instruments
610 Flinn Ave.
Moorpark, CA 93021-2008
818-889-5077

Leisegang Medical, Inc.
6401 Congress Ave.
Boca Raton, FL 33487-2883
407-994-0202

Origin Medsystems, Inc.
135 Constitution Dr.
Menlo Park, CA 94025
415-617-5000

Performance Surgical Instruments
40 Norfolk Ave.
Easton, MA 023334
508-230-0010

Schwarz Medical
Kirchstrasse 24
D-86935 Rott
Germany
8869/1881

T.A.G. Medical Products
Kibbutz Gaaton 25130
Israel
4-859810

Unisurge, Inc.
10231 Bubb Rd.
Cupertino, CA 95014
408-996-4700

SCISSORS, LAPAROSCOPY, ELECTROSURGICAL

Davis & Geck Div.
American Cyanamid Company
One Cyanamid Plaza
Wayne, NJ 07470-2012
201-831-2000

Everest Medical Corp.
13755 First Avenue. N.
Minneapolis, MN 55441-5454
612-473-6262

Leisegang Medical, Inc.
6401 Congress Ave.
Boca Raton, FL 33487-2883
407-994-0202

Solution

Fogging of the laparoscope not only adds to the risk of surgery, it costs valuable operating time as well. It is a constant threat to visibility; and the need to continually clean the scope can prolong the operation. A few simple preventive measures are well worth the effort.

Scopes can fog at any glass surface. For instance, after soaking the scope, it is not unusual for fog to develop at the eyepiece interface with the camera. This can be eliminated simply through careful drying, plus application of an antifogging solution. Heat at the camera/scope connection can cause the camera interface to fog as well. This can be corrected by holding the scope at a different position.

Most fogging, however, occurs at the distal end of the scope. The abdominal cavity is warm, and the scope is generally cooler. Upon initial insertion, this temperature gradient can cause condensation on the lens. Prewarmers are available to bring the scope to body temperature prior to insertion. In the absence of one of these, placing the scope in a pan of warm water will get the job done. Once the scope's temperature is in equilibrium with the body, the fogging problem diminishes.

At the opposite end of the scale is the temperature gradient between a warm scope and the cool CO_2 used to maintain pneumoperitoneum. Fogging due to this can usually be prevented by insufflating through a separate trocar. Some scopes have washing ports that allow the surgeon to remove condensation with a spray of water. The fog can also be cleared by touching a warm organ with the scope or washing the lens with an irrigating cannula.

Blood and grease within the abdominal cavity are other potential fogging agents. Obviously, their impact can't be completely eliminated; but anti-fogging solutions can decrease the incidence and severity of the problem. These solutions coat the lens with a protective layer that reduces condensation and helps keep grease from sticking to the surface. Many of the solutions come packaged with an applicator sponge. Since the solutions are water-soluble, many applications are needed during the course of a procedure.

If a scope continues to fog despite every precaution, moisture may be accumulating within the scope through a hairline crack in the distal lens. If you suspect this problem, return the scope to the factory for examination.

SOLUTION, INSTRUMENT, LAPAROSCOPIC, ANTI-FOG

American Hydro-Surgical Instruments, Inc.
430 Commerce Dr., Ste. 50E
Delray Beach, FL 33445
407-278-5664

Baxter Healthcare Corp.
Operating Room Div.
1500 Waukegan Rd.
McGaw Park, IL 60085-8210
708-473-1500

Dexide, Inc.
7509 Flagstone Dr.
P.O. Box 185789
Fort Worth, TX 76118-6953
817-589-1454

Marlow Surgical Technologies, Inc.
1810 Joseph Lloyd Pkwy.
Willoughby, OH 44094-8030
216-946-2453

Merocel Corporation
950 Flanders Rd.
P.O. Box 334
Mystic, CT 06355-1300
203-572-9586

O.R. Concepts, Inc.
12250 Nicollet Ave. South
Burnsville, MN 55337
612-894-7523

Wolf Medical Instruments Corp., Richard
353 Corporate Woods Pkwy.
Vernon Hills, IL 60061-3110
708-913-1113

Suture

While most any suture can be employed laparoscopically, some are specifically designed for it. For instance, laparoscopic suture intended for extracorporeal tying is supplied in lengths of at least 30 inches, preferably 36. The extra length permits the surgeon to pass the strand down through a trocar sleeve and around or through a structure, then pull both ends back through the sleeve for tying outside the abdomen. Since most knots tied extra-abdominally are either slip knots or must be advanced with a push rod, it is imperative that the suture present minimal friction. Some manufacturers employ a special coating for this purpose.

Sutures with a pre-tied knot and attached push rod are an important element in laparoscopic surgery. The suture is tied into a loop and passed into the abdomen through an introducer supplied with the product. The target organ or tissue within the abdomen is pulled into the loop and the loop tightened with the push rod.

This is one of the commonest approaches to laparoscopic suturing; but there are alternatives. Among them are straight sutures with curved, straight, or ski-tipped needles attached, accompanied by a push rod. The needle and suture are passed into the abdomen, through the target tissue, and back out of the abdomen. The needle is removed from the suture and a slip knot tied. The push rod is then used to advance the knot and tighten the loop.

For intra-abdominal tying, suture should be no more than seven inches long. Greater lengths tend to become tangled and knotted during tying. Although longer strands can be cut to size, short lengths are currently being packaged and sold specifically for laparoscopy.

Needle size should be determined by the job. However, needles with a curve greater than 18mm diameter cannot be easily advanced through a 10mm trocar. If a larger needle is necessary, a larger trocar can be inserted, or the needle can be passed directly through the abdominal wall. All laparoscopic needles should be permanently affixed to the suture. 'Pop off' needles have no place in laparoscopic surgery. If lost, they are too difficult to find and retrieve.

For running sutures, some manufacturers now supply a pre-tied loop at the free end of the strand. The surgeon passes the needle through tissue and then through the loop, eliminating the need for an initial knot. A similar design does away with the initial knot by incorporating a small bead at the free end.

For all laparoscopic work, braided suture generally works better than monofilament. It is more pliable, has less memory, and doesn't require as many knots.

SUTURE, LAPAROSCOPY

Davis & Geck Endosurgery
1 Casper St.
Danbury, CT 06810
203-743-4451

DEXON II

DESCRIPTION: DEXON* II Polyglycolic Acid Synthetic Absorbable Suture; USP is a homopolymer of glycolic acid.

DEXON II suture, in addition, is coated with polycaprolate, which is inert, non-collagenous, non-antigenic and non-pyrogenic.

The suture is sterile, inert, non-collagenous, non-antigenic, non-pyrogenic and flexible. The braided suture is colored green to enhance visibility in tissue. DEXON II braided sutures are also available undyed, with a natural beige color. It is uniform in size and tensile strength, but is smaller in diameter than other absorbable surgical sutures of equivalent tensile strength.

ACTIONS: When DEXON II sutures are placed in tissues, a minimal tissue reaction occurs, which is followed by a microscopic layer of fibrous connective tissue which grows into the suture material.

Absorption studies in animals show DEXON II sutures to be equivalent to DEXON "S" sutures. Studies in rabbits revealed minimal absorption at 7 to 15 days, significant absorption at 30 days, and maximum resorption after 60 to 90 days. In an animal model (rat), 99% of the coating was excreted as metabolites within 22 days following implantation.

Tensile strength, not being a function of the absorption rate, may vary from tissue to tissue, depending in part on the rate of hydrolysis. In animal studies (subcutaneous tissue in rats), it has been shown that at two weeks post-implantation, approximately 65% of the original tensile strength of DEXON II suture remains, while at three weeks approximately 35% of its original tensile strength is retained.

INDICATIONS: DEXON II sutures are indicated for use in all types of soft tissue approximation, including ophthalmic surgery, but not in cardiovascular, microsurgery or in neural tissue. DEXON II suture may also be used as a ligature.

CONTRAINDICATIONS: DEXON II sutures are contraindicated where extended approximation of tissue under stress must be maintained.

WARNINGS: Under certain circumstances, notably orthopaedic procedures, immobilization by external support may be employed at the discretion of the surgeon. Do not resterilize. Discard opened, unused sutures.

PRECAUTIONS: Acceptable surgical practice should be followed with respect to drainage and closure of infected wounds.

DEXON II sutures require the standard surgical technique of flat and square ties, with additional throws if indicated by surgical circumstances and the experience of the surgeon.

Skin sutures which remain in place for periods of longer than seven days may cause localized topical irritation, and the extended portion of the suture may be snipped off after five to seven days, as indicated.

ADVERSE REACTIONS: Those reactions that have been reported include tissue reactions or inflammation, fibrous or granulation tissue, wound separation and bleeding, and accumulation of fluid around subcuticular stitches.

INSTRUCTIONS FOR USE: Use as required.

SPECIFICATIONS/HOW SUPPLIED: DEXON II sutures braided sizes 6-0 through 2 (metric size 0.7 through 5) dyed green and/or natural beige. Supplied in cut lengths or ligating reels, non-needled or affixed to various DAVIS & GECK ATRAUMATIC* needles or D-TACH* removable needles USP in one, two and three dozen boxes.

0 DEXON II Green, 1x18in. (45cm)/TT-20 Needle, 5/8 Circle 27mm (Order No. 9451-61):

TT-20 NEEDLE, 5/8 CIRCLE 27MM

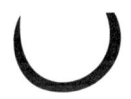

4-0 DEXON II Green, 1x12in. (30cm)/TH-2 Needle, Taper Ski (Order No. 9457-31),
3-0 DEXON II Green, 1x12in. (30cm)/TH-2 Needle, Taper Ski (Order No. 9457-41),
4-0 DEXON II Green, 1x48in. (1.2m)/TH-2 Needle, Taper Ski (Order No. 9459-31),
3-0 DEXON II Green, 1x48in. (1.2m)/TH-2 Needle, Taper Ski (Order No. 9459-41):

TH-2 NEEDLE, TAPER SKI

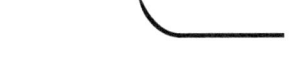

4-0 DEXON II Green, 1x12in. (30cm)/TE-7 Needle, 3/8 Circle 18mm (Order No. 9461-31),
3-0 DEXON II Green, 1x12in. (30cm)/TE-7 Needle, 3/8 Circle 18mm (Order No. 9461-41):

TE-7 NEEDLE, 3/8 CIRCLE 18MM

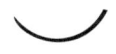

Davis & Geck Endosurgery
1 Casper St.
Danbury, CT 06810
203-743-4451

MAXON

DESCRIPTION: MAXON* Monofilament Polyglyconate Synthetic Absorbable Suture (clear or green) is prepared from a copolymer of glycolic acid and trimethylene carbonate. The dyed suture contains D&C Green No. 6, an inert green dye.

MAXON sutures are sterile, noncollagenous, nonantigenic, and nonpyrogenic and elicit only a slight tissue reaction during absorption.

MAXON suture exceeds USP maximum diameter limits (see table below).

MAXIMUM SUTURE OVERSIZING
IN DIAMETERS (MM) FROM USP

USP SUTURE SIZE	MAXIMUM (MM) OVERSIZE
2	0.070
1	0.070
0	0.070
2-0	0.055
3-0	0.055
4-0	0.040
5-0	0.035
6-0	0.025
7-0	0.015

ACTIONS: Three characteristics describe the in vivo performance of absorbable sutures: tensile strength retention, absorption of mass, and tissue reaction.

MAXON synthetic absorbable suture has been formulated to provide predictable wound support and absorption through the wound healing period, as shown by implantation studies in animals.

The table below represents the approximate percentage of the original suture strength remaining after implantation in animals.

TIME (IN DAYS)	% SUTURE STRENGTH
7	80
14	75
21	65
28	50
42	25

Animal data indicate that suture absorption is minimal until about the 60th day after implantation. Absorption is substantially complete within six months.

When implanted in animal tissue, MAXON suture elicits a minimal tissue reaction characteristic of foreign body response to a substance. The tissue reaction resolves as the suture is absorbed.

Experimental studies with MAXON suture produced no evidence of antigenicity, systemic toxicity, carcinogenicity, mutagenicity, teratogenicity, or adverse effects on reproductive performance.

INDICATIONS: MAXON is indicated for use in all types of soft tissue approximation, but not in cardiovascular, ophthalmic, or microsurgery, and not in neural tissue. MAXON suture may also be used as a ligature.

CONTRAINDICATIONS: Since MAXON suture is absorbable, it should not be used where prolonged approximation of tissues under stress is required.

WARNINGS: Under certain circumstances, notably orthopedic procedures, immobilization by external support may be employed at the discretion of the surgeon. Do not resterilize. Discard open, unused sutures.

PRECAUTIONS: Avoid damage when handling. Do not grip the strand with surgical instruments, such as needle holders or forceps, except when grasping the free end of the suture during an instrument tie.

Care should be exercised when knotting sutures used in continuous mass or layered closure of the abdomen, i.e., non-slip locking knots should be used at both ends of the continuous closure.

Vaginal mucosa sutures and skin sutures remaining in place for extended periods may be associated with localized irritation and should be removed as indicated.

Since any foreign material in the presence of bacterial contamination may enhance bacterial infectivity, standard surgical practice should be followed with respect to drainage and closure of infected wounds. MAXON did not enhance infection in animal and in vitro studies.

CAUTION: Federal (USA) law restricts this device to sale, distribution, and use by or on the order of a physician or veterinarian.

ADVERSE REACTIONS: Due to prolonged suture absorption, mild irritation could occur in the vaginal mucosa and skin.

INSTRUCTIONS FOR USE: The suture knots must be properly placed to be secure. As with other synthetic sutures, knot security requires the standard surgical technique of flat and square ties with additional throws as indicated by surgical circumstances and the experience of the surgeon.

Dosage and administration: Use as required per surgical procedure.

SPECIFICATIONS/HOW SUPPLIED: MAXON sutures are available as sterile, monofilament green (green with D&C Green No. 6 dye) and undyed (clear) sutures in sizes 7-0 through 2 (metric size 0.5-5) in a variety of lengths and with a variety of ATRAUMATIC* and D-TACH* needles (36 envelopes per box).

SUTURE, LAPAROSCOPY (cont'd)

4-0 MAXON Green, 1x12in. (30cm)/TS-20 Needle, Straight (Order No. 6451-31):

TS-20 NEEDLE, STRAIGHT

4-0 MAXON Green, 1x18in. (45cm)/TS-20 Needle, Double Armed (Order No. 6453-31):

TS-20 NEEDLE, DOUBLE ARMED

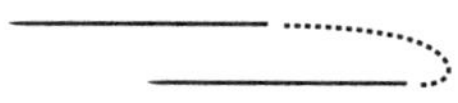

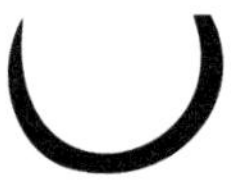

0 MAXON Green, 1x18in. (45cm)/TT-20 Needle, 5/8 Circle 27mm (Order No. 6455-61):

TT-20 NEEDLE, 5/8 CIRCLE 27 MM

4-0 MAXON Green, 1x12in. (30cm)/TH-2 Needle, Double Armed, Taper Ski (Order No. 6461-31),
3-0 MAXON Green, 1x12in. (30cm)/TH-2 Needle, Double Armed, Taper Ski (Order No. 6461-41):

TH-2 NEEDLE, DOUBLE ARMED, TAPER SKI

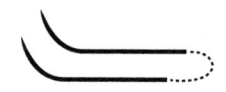

4-0 MAXON Green, 1x48in. (1.2m)/TH-2 Needle (Order No. 6463-31),
3-0 MAXON Green, 1x48in. (1.2m)/TH-2 Needle (Order No. 6463-41):

TH-2 NEEDLE

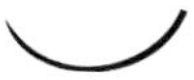

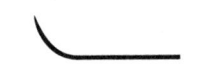

4-0 MAXON Green, 1x12in. (30cm)/TE-7 Needle, 3/8 Circle 18 mm (Order No. 6465-31),
3-0 MAXON Green, 1x12in. (30cm)/TE-7 Needle, 3/8 Circle 18 mm (Order No. 6465-41):

TE-7 NEEDLE, 3/8 CIRCLE 18 MM

Davis & Geck Endosurgery
1 Casper St.
Danbury, CT 06810
203-743-4451

SILK SUTURES

SPECIFICATIONS/HOW SUPPLIED: 3-0 Silk, Black Braided, 1x12in. (30cm)/TH-2 Needle, Taper Ski (Order No. 1404-41),
2-0 Silk, Black Braided, 1x12in. (30cm)/TH-2 Needle, Taper Ski (Order No. 1404-51),
3-0 Silk, Black Braided, 1x48in. (1.2m)/TH-2 Needle, Taper Ski (Order No. 1405-41),
2-0 Silk, Black Braided, 1x48in. (1.2m)/TH-2 Needle, Taper Ski (Order No. 1405-51):

TH-2 NEEDLE, TAPER SKI

3-0 Silk, Black Braided, 1x12in. (30cm)/TE-7 Needle, 3/8 Circle 18mm (Order No. 1406-41):

TE-7 NEEDLE, 3/8 CIRCLE 18 MM

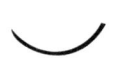

Sutures supplied in boxes containing 36 envelopes each.

Davis & Geck Div.
American Cyanamid Company
One Cyanamid Plaza
Wayne, NJ 07470-2012
201-831-2000

Deknatel Division
600 Airport Rd.
Fall River, MA 02720-4703
508-677-6600

Ethicon, Inc.
U.S. Route 22
P.O. Box 151
Somerville, NJ 08876
908-218-0707

Resorba Surgical Sutures
Schonerstr. 7
D-90443 Nuernburg
Germany
0911/442344

United States Surgical Corp.
150 Glover Ave.
Norwalk, CT 06856-5080
203-845-1000

Trainer

Surgeons preparing for laparoscopic work must learn to manipulate tissue with long instruments while watching the maneuvers on a video screen. While live animal procedures and supervised operations in humans remain an essential part of the learning process, less expensive training devices now permit would-be laparoscopists to practice their procedures without endangering lives or spending large amounts of time and money in the animal lab.

The first of these trainers was a sealed 'black box' with holes cut for trocar sleeves. The surgeon would insert a laparascope in the box, then practice various manipulations. However, this method tied up an entire expensive laparoscopic system; so later designs included a small video camera mounted inside the box. This eliminated the need not only for scarce laparascopic equipment, but also for a camera holder. Still later versions offered adjustable cameras and tops that could be replaced after repeated trocar punctures.

In early trainers, chicken breasts provided the practice. In a procedure called 'Chickensize,' the surgeon would cut and tie the skin and muscle of the raw chicken breast to sharpen his skills. With the advent of more difficult operations, plastic and rubber mockups *of human anatomy have been designed to give the surgeon a more realistic practice session.*

When selecting a trainer, keep these three requirements in mind: It should be workable by one person; it should have a built-in adjustable camera; and it should provide for easy access to the inside of the box.

TRAINER, LAPAROSCOPY

Advanced Surgical, Inc.
305 College Rd. East
Princeton, NJ 08540
609-987-2340

Cabot Medical Corp.
2021 Cabot Blvd. West
Langhorne, PA 19047-1875
215-752-8300

Davis & Geck Div.
American Cyanamid Company
One Cyanamid Plaza
Wayne, NJ 07470-2012
201-831-2000

Ethicon Endo-Surgery
4545 Creek Road
Cincinnati, OH 45242
513-786-7000

Leisegang Medical, Inc.
6401 Congress Ave.
Boca Raton, FL 33487-2883
407-994-0202

Marlow Surgical Technologies, Inc.
1810 Joseph Lloyd Pkwy.
Willoughby, OH 44094-8030
216-946-2453

United States Surgical Corp.
150 Glover Ave.
Norwalk, CT 06856-5080
203-845-1000

Wolf Medical Instruments Corp., Richard
353 Corporate Woods Pkwy.
Vernon Hills, IL 60061-3110
708-913-1113

Trocar

Trocars and trocar sleeves give access to the abdominal cavity while maintaining pneumoperitoneum. While the basic concept is simple, over the past five years the devices themselves have become increasingly complex and varied.

The trocar must be sharp to cut through and separate the muscle and fascia surrounding the abdominal cavity. A pyramidal cutting tip is preferred by most surgeons, but a conical tip is also available. The pyramidal tip tends to injure more muscle than the conical one, but it also requires considerably less pressure to insert, theoretically making it safer to use. The trocar may be hollow or solid. Hollow trocars may have a hole near the tip to allow peritoneal gases to escape, signaling entry of the device into the cavity.

Safety has become the major selling point for trocars in recent years. The original safety shield was developed by U.S. Surgical. It provided a spring-loaded plastic sheath that came forward over the penetrating tip immediately after it entered the peritoneal cavity. Many variations of this design appeared throughout the late 1980's. For greater safety, some trocars now employ a retracting tip that pulls back into the sheath as soon as the negative pressure of the intra-abdominal cavity is sensed. Irrespective of whether the shield advances or the tip retracts, these mechanisms not only isolate the tip from vulnerable organs, but also give audible and visible confirmation that the trocar has entered the abdominal cavity, alerting the surgeon to release pressure on the instrument.

Surgeons generally agree that safety-shield trocars are a safer choice for novice laparoscopists. It is less clear that this is the case for experienced laparoscopic surgeons. There is universal agreement, however, that a sharp trocar can be inserted with less pressure than a dull one. For this reason, the always-sharp, single-use, disposable trocars are generally preferred to reusable ones.

Since control over the trocar increases as the pressure required for insertion declines, electric trocars have recently been introduced. When energized by the surgeon, the tips of these trocars burn through the tissue of the abdominal wall, dramatically reducing the pressure needed to advance the instrument. To prevent intestinal injury from the hot tip, one design features a feedback mechanism that shuts off the electric current as soon as the instrument has penetrated the abdominal wall. Though electric trocars have seen far less clinical use than the nonburning variety, they have so far maintained a low injury rate.

Another approach is the dilation trocar. This device allows the surgeon to first place a small needle, then dilate the tract to accommodate a larger trocar. Because this procedure is time-consuming, dilation trocars are not used extensively.

Whatever the type of trocar in use, its sheath must seal the pneumoperitoneum while allowing entry and exit of instrumentation.

TROCAR (cont'd)

The first sheaths had no valve system, requiring a perfect fit for each instrument and forcing the surgeon to cover the hole with a finger each time an instrument was removed. Then small rubber tips were fashioned which, when placed over the mouth of the sheath, would seal around instruments of varying sizes. These tips, which tended to tear easily, often allowed gas to escape and had to be replaced frequently.

Later, the trumpet valve was introduced. This mechanism completely sealed the sheath when an instrument was removed, but required a free hand to work the valve. As advances in laparoscopic surgery began to demand use of both the surgeon's hands, the trumpet valve became a steadily less appealing solution. It also proved traumatic to electrical laparoscopic instrumentation, damaging the insulation and causing electrical injury at some distance from the instrument's tip. Nevertheless, this type of valve can still be found in many reusable trocars.

The most prevalent approach today is the automatic flapper valve, which appeared when disposable trocars were first introduced. This 'trap door' valve opens with the pressure of the laparoscopic instrument passing through it and closes with spring tension when the instrument is removed. A newer approach, just now available, is a membrane-type valve that closes around the instrument, providing a better seal than the flapper valve while causing less trauma to instruments.

The need to seal the sheath around a variety of instruments has led to the development of inserts that downsize a sheath to create a close fit with smaller devices. The inserts are built into some sheaths in a rotating or sliding fashion, while others snap on and off. Either approach requires some effort by the surgeon, so strategies for sealing the sheath with multiple diaphragms are currently under study.

To keep sleeves from slipping out of the abdomen during surgery, screw-in grips have now gained widespread acceptance. These hollow tubes fit around the sheath, while threads on the outer surface anchor them to the abdominal wall. Although some trocars have permanently attached anchors, many surgeons feel that detachable grips offer more versatility during trocar insertion. Two other methods of attachment have been devised: a trocar sheath with a mechanically expanding tip, and a sheath with a balloon attachment that, when inflated, blocks egress from the abdominal cavity.

Specialized trocars are also needed in modern laparoscopy, the most notable being the open trocar and the thoracic trocar. The open trocar was initially designed by Hasson to permit open entry into the abdomen in cases of inflammation or previous surgery, or as a desired method of initial entry. It included a trumpet-valved sheath modified with flanges to accommodate anchoring sutures and a sliding expansion sheath to seal the fascial defect. A blunt-tipped trocar replaced the sharp design. Although bulky, this arrangement proved excellent, and is still in use today. More recently, disposable open trocars have also been developed, and have met with some success. However, their design reduces the effective length of laparoscopic instruments, which can be detrimental at times.

Thoracoscopy does not require maintenance of pressure in the operative cavity, so a simpler, less expensive device can be used. These trocars are usually disposable, consisting of little more than a short plastic sheath with attached screw grips. With no valves or seals, they allow unobstructed access to the thoracic cavity.

Given the wide variety of options available today, choosing a trocar might seem like a major undertaking. In the end, though, the decision still hangs on three basic concerns: safety, ease of use, and ease of cleaning.

DILATOR, PORT, LAPAROSCOPIC

Davis & Geck Endosurgery
1 Casper St.
Danbury, CT 06810
203-743-4451

PROFESSIONAL LINE 8385 & 8388 SERIES

DESCRIPTION: Dilation set and replacement sealing caps to increase the size of a port from 5.5mm to 10mm (requires the use of a 10mm trocar):

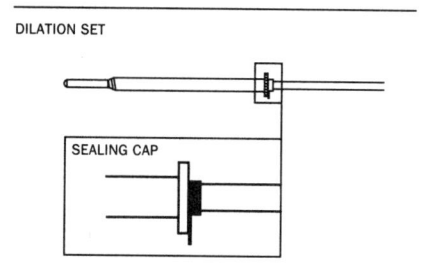

DILATION SET

SEALING CAP

SPECIFICATIONS/HOW SUPPLIED: Order number 8385-01 for dilation set (5.5mm to 10mm) and 8388-01 for sealing caps with center holes.

Davis & Geck Div.
American Cyanamid Company
One Cyanamid Plaza
Wayne, NJ 07470-2012
201-831-2000

Leisegang Medical, Inc.
6401 Congress Ave.
Boca Raton, FL 33487-2883
407-994-0202

OBTURATOR, ENDOSCOPIC

Aesculap
1000 Gateway Blvd.
South San Francisco, CA 94080-7030
415-876-7000

Bioteque America, Inc.
340 E. Maple Ave.
Langhorne, PA 19047
215-750-8071

Cabot Medical Corp.
2021 Cabot Blvd. West
Langhorne, PA 19047-1875
215-752-8300

Cal-Swiss Manufacturing Co., Inc.
390 S. Fair Oaks Ave.
P.O. Box 50430
Pasadena, CA 91105-0430
818-793-8661

Chirurgische Instrumente
Hauptstrasse 18
D-78582 Balgheim
Germany
7424/501319

Circon Acmi
300 Stillwater Ave.
Stamford, CT 06902-3640
203-328-8689

Coopersurgical, Inc.
15 Forest Pkwy.
Shelton, CT 06484-5458
203-929-6321

Ethicon Endo-Surgery
4545 Creek Road
Cincinnati, OH 45242
513-786-7000

Dexide, Inc.
7509 Flagstone Dr.
P.O. Box 185789
Fort Worth, TX 76118-6953
817-589-1454

Frantz Medical Development Ltd.
7740 Metric Drive
Mentor, OH 44060-4862
216-255-1155

Marlow Surgical Technologies, Inc.
1810 Joseph Lloyd Pkwy.
Willoughby, OH 44094-8030
216-946-2453

Martin, Gebr. GmbH & Co. KG
Ludwigstaler Str. 132
Postf. 60
D-78532 Tuttlingen
Germany
07461/7060

Schwarz Medical
Kirchstrasse 24
D-86935 Rott
Germany
8869/1881

Smith & Nephew Dyonics, Inc.
160 Dascomb Rd.
Andover, MA 01810-5893
508-470-2800

Storz Endoscopy-America Inc., Karl
10111 W. Jefferson Blvd.
Culver City, CA 90232-3509
310-558-1500

Storz GmbH & Co., Karl
Mittelstr. 8
Postfach 230
D-78532 Tuttlingen
Germany
07461/7080

UMC Incorporated
22510 Highway 55 West
Hamel, MN 55340
612-478-6609

United States Surgical Corp.
150 Glover Ave.
Norwalk, CT 06856-5080
203-845-1000

Wect Instrument Company, Inc.
5645 N. Ravenswood
Chicago, IL 60660-3922
312-769-1944

Wid-Med, Inc.
111 N. Wabash Ave.
Chicago, IL 60602-1903
312-236-8586

Wolf Medical Instruments Corp., Richard
353 Corporate Woods Pkwy.
Vernon Hills, IL 60061-3110
708-913-1113

SLEEVE, TROCAR

Davis & Geck Endosurgery
1 Casper St.
Danbury, CT 06810
203-743-4451

PROFESSIONAL LINE 8384 & 8386 SERIES

DESCRIPTION: Reducing sleeve and sealing cap to avoid loss of CO_2, when using a smaller diameter instrument with a larger diameter trocar:

REDUCING SLEEVE

SEALING CAP

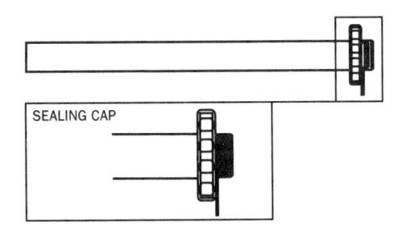

SPECIFICATIONS/HOW SUPPLIED: Order number 8384-01 for reducing sleeve (10mm to 5.5mm), 8386-01 for sealing caps with center holes. Disposable sealing caps supplied in boxes of 20 each.

Chirurgische Instrumente
Hauptstrasse 18
D-78582 Balgheim
Germany
7424/501319

Davis & Geck Div.
American Cyanamid Company
One Cyanamid Plaza
Wayne, NJ 07470-2012
201-831-2000

Ethicon Endo-Surgery
4545 Creek Road
Cincinnati, OH 45242
513-786-7000

Leisegang Medical, Inc.
6401 Congress Ave.
Boca Raton, FL 33487-2883
407-994-0202

TROCAR, ABDOMINAL

A&A Medical, Inc.
11485 Mountain Laurel Dr.
Roswell, GA 30075
800-424-1234

Access Surgical International, Inc.
15 Caswell Ln.
Boat Yard Square
Plymouth, MA 02360
508-747-6006

TROCAR, ABDOMINAL (cont'd)

Apple Medical Corp.
93 Nashaway Rd.
Bolton, MA 01740
508-779-2926

Austin Biomedical, Inc.
4211 Medical Pkwy
Austin, TX 78756-3309
512-459-6611

Bard Urological
8195 Industrial Blvd.
Covington, GA 30209-2656
404-784-6113

Baxter Healthcare Corp.
Operating Room Div.
1500 Waukegan Rd.
McGaw Park, IL 60085-8210
708-473-1500

Boss Instruments, Ltd.
1310 Central Ct.
Hermitage, TN 37076
615-885-2231

Bryan Corp.
4 Plympton St.
Woburn, MA 01801-2908
617-935-0004

Cabot Medical Corp.
2021 Cabot Blvd. West
Langhorne, PA 19047-1875
215-752-8300

Circon Acmi
300 Stillwater Ave.
Stamford, CT 06902-3640
203-328-8689

Conmed Corp.
310 Broad Street
Utica, NY 13501
315-797-8375

Coopersurgical, Inc.
15 Forest Pkwy.
Shelton, CT 06484-5458
203-929-6321

Cuda Products Corporation
6000 Powers Ave.
Jacksonville, FL 32217-2212
904-737-7611

Davis & Geck Div.
American Cyanamid Company
One Cyanamid Plaza
Wayne, NJ 07470-2012
201-831-2000

Dexide, Inc.
7509 Flagstone Dr.
P.O. Box 185789
Fort Worth, TX 76118-6953
817-589-1454

Disposable Instrument Co., Inc.
P.O. Box 14248
Shawnee Mission, KS 66285-4248
913-492-6492

Dittmar, Inc.
101 E. Laurel Ave.
P.O. Box 66
Cheltenham, PA 19012-2125
215-379-5533

Dynamic Industries (PVT) Ltd.
Wazirabad Rd. Ugoki
P.O. Box 1919
Sialkot
Pakistan
0432/62268

Elmed, Inc.
60 W. Fay Ave.
Addison, IL 60101-5198
708-543-2792

Ethicon Endo-Surgery
4545 Creek Road
Cincinnati, OH 45242
513-786-7000

Heraeus Surgical, Inc.
575 Cottonwood Dr.
Milpitas, CA 95035-7402
408-954-4000

Himalaya Trading Co., (PVT) Ltd.
Wazirabad Rd.
P.O. Box No. 59
Sialkot
Pakistan
(0432) 552249

Leisegang Medical, Inc.
6401 Congress Ave.
Boca Raton, FL 33487-2883
407-994-0202

Marlow Surgical Technologies, Inc.
1810 Joseph Lloyd Pkwy.
Willoughby, OH 44094-8030
216-946-2453

Medicon Eg
15 Gansacker
Postfach 4455
D-78532 Tuttlingen
Germany
07462/20090

Medicon Instruments, Inc.
4405 International Blvd.
Norcross, GA 30093-3013
404-381-2858

Mist, Inc.
6307 E. Angus Dr.
Raleigh, NC 27613
919-787-8377

Nopa Instruments Medizintechnik GmbH
Gansacker 9 - Postfach 4554
D-78532 Tuttlingen
Germany
07462/7801

Origin Medsystems, Inc.
135 Constitution Dr.
Menlo Park, CA 94025
415-617-5000

Pilling-Rusch
420 Delaware Dr.
Fort Washington, PA 19034-2711
215-643-2600

Pioneer Medical, Inc.
34 Laurelcrest Rd.
Madison, CT 06443
203-245-9337

Sherwood Medical Company
1915 Olive St.
St. Louis, MO 63103-1625
314-621-7788

Sklar Instrument Company
889 South Matlack St.
West Chester, PA 19380
215-430-3200

Smith & Nephew Dyonics, Inc.
160 Dascomb Rd.
Andover, MA 01810-5893
508-470-2800

Star Guide Corp.
6666 Stapleton Dr. S.
Denver, CO 80216
303-333-2100

Storz Endoscopy-America Inc., Karl
10111 W. Jefferson Blvd.
Culver City, CA 90232-3509
310-558-1500

Storz GmbH & Co., Karl
Mittelstr. 8
Postfach 230
D-78532 Tuttlingen
Germany
07461/7080

Surgical Instrument Co. of America
1185 Edgewater Ave.
Ridgefield, NJ 07657-2102
201-941-6500

Synectic Engineering, Inc.
4 Oxford Rd.
Milford, CT 06460-7007
203-877-8488

Technalytics, Inc.
210 Summit Ave.
Montvale, NJ 07645-1526
201-391-0494

Unisurge, Inc.
10231 Bubb Rd.
Cupertino, CA 95014
408-996-4700

United States Surgical Corp.
150 Glover Ave.
Norwalk, CT 06856-5080
203-845-1000

Weck & Co. Inc., Edward
1 Weck Dr.
P.O. Box 12600
Research Triangle Park, NC 27709
919-544-8000

Wect Instrument Company, Inc.
5645 N. Ravenswood
Chicago, IL 60660-3922
312-769-1944

Wolf Medical Instruments Corp., Richard
353 Corporate Woods Pkwy.
Vernon Hills, IL 60061-3110
708-913-1113

TROCAR, AMNIOTIC

Codman & Shurtleff, Inc.
41 Pacella Park Dr.
Randolph, MA 02368-1755
617-961-2300

Disposable Instrument Co., Inc.
P.O. Box 14248
Shawnee Mission, KS 66285-4248
913-492-6492

Dittmar, Inc.
101 E. Laurel Ave.
P.O. Box 66
Cheltenham, PA 19012-2125
215-379-5533

Pilling-Rusch
420 Delaware Dr.
Fort Washington, PA 19034-2711
215-643-2600

Scan-Med, Inc.
P.O. Box 128
Middle Grove, NY 12850-0128
518-893-2800

Star Guide Corp.
6666 Stapleton Dr. S.
Denver, CO 80216
303-333-2100

Storz Endoscopy-America Inc., Karl
10111 W. Jefferson Blvd.
Culver City, CA 90232-3509
310-558-1500

Storz GmbH & Co., Karl
Mittelstr. 8
Postfach 230
D-78532 Tuttlingen
Germany
07461/7080

Surgical Instrument Co. of America
1185 Edgewater Ave.
Ridgefield, NJ 07657-2102
201-941-6500

Swemed Lab International Ab
P. O. Box 4014
S-42104 V. Frolunda
Sweden

Wolf Medical Instruments Corp., Richard
353 Corporate Woods Pkwy.
Vernon Hills, IL 60061-3110
708-913-1113

TROCAR, CARDIOVASCULAR

Aesculap AG
Moehringerstr. 125
Postfach 40
D-78532 Tuttlingen
Germany
00149/0746951

Applied Medical Resources
26051 Merit Circle #104
Laguna Hills, CA 92653-7008
714-582-6120

Arbo Medizin Technologie GmbH
Wendenstr. 2-3 - Postfach 1204
D-38100 Braunschweig
Germany
0531/44516

Bashir, Jamil & Bros. (PVT). Ltd.
Khadim Ali Rd.
P.O. Box 7
Sialkot
Pakistan
0432-553862

Bauer & Haselbarth GmbH
Sauerbruchstr. 7 - Postfach
D-25479 Elleran bei Hamburg
Germany
04106/72091

Baxter Healthcare Corp.
Operating Room Div.
1500 Waukegan Rd.
McGaw Park, IL 60085-8210
708-473-1500

Deknatel Division
600 Airport Rd.
Fall River, MA 02720-4703
508-677-6600

Disposable Instrument Co., Inc.
P.O. Box 14248
Shawnee Mission, KS 66285-4248
913-492-6492

Dittmar, Inc.
101 E. Laurel Ave.
P.O. Box 66
Cheltenham, PA 19012-2125
215-379-5533

Hammacher GmbH, Karl
Steinendorferstr. 27
D-42699 Solingen
Germany
0212/66047

Kendall Co., The
15 Hampshire St.
Mansfield, MA 02048-1113
508-261-8000

Mader Instrument Corp.
25 Lamington Dr.
Succasunna, NJ 07876-2048
201-584-0816

Martin, Gebr. GmbH & Co. KG
Ludwigstaler Str. 132
Postf. 60
D-78532 Tuttlingen
Germany
07461/7060

Miltex Instrument Co., Inc.
6 Ohio Dr.
CB 5006
Lake Success, NY 11042-0006
516-775-7100

TROCAR, CARDIOVASCULAR (cont'd)

Nopa Instruments Medizintechnik GmbH
Gansacker 9 - Postfach 4554
D-78532 Tuttlingen
Germany
07462/7801

Pilling-Rusch
420 Delaware Dr.
Fort Washington, PA 19034-2711
215-643-2600

Sherwood Medical Company
1915 Olive St.
St. Louis, MO 63103-1625
314-621-7788

Sklar Instrument Company
889 South Matlack St.
West Chester, PA 19380
215-430-3200

Sklar-Witte GmbH
Mankhauser Str. 1
Solingen Nrw 5650,
Germany

Surgical Instrument Co. of America
1185 Edgewater Ave.
Ridgefield, NJ 07657-2102
201-941-6500

Ueth & Haug GmbH
Stockacher Str. 41/45
D-78532 Tuttlingen
Germany

TROCAR, GALLBLADDER

Aesculap
1000 Gateway Blvd.
South San Francisco, CA 94080-7030
415-876-7000

Apple Medical Corp.
93 Nashaway Rd.
Bolton, MA 01740
508-779-2926

Arrow International, Inc.
3000 Bernville Rd.
Reading, PA 19605
215-378-0131

Baxter Healthcare Corp.
Operating Room Div.
1500 Waukegan Rd.
McGaw Park, IL 60085-8210
708-473-1500

Boss Instruments, Ltd.
1310 Central Ct.
Hermitage, TN 37076
615-885-2231

Bryan Corp.
4 Plympton St.
Woburn, MA 01801-2908
617-935-0004

Codman & Shurtleff, Inc.
41 Pacella Park Dr.
Randolph, MA 02368-1755
617-961-2300

Conmed Corp.
310 Broad Street
Utica, NY 13501
315-797-8375

Core Dynamics, Inc.
11222-4 St. Johns Indust. Pkwy.
Jacksonville, FL 32216
904-641-6611

Davis & Geck Endosurgery
1 Casper Street
Danbury, CT 06810
203-743-4451

DCG Precision Manufacturing Corp.
9 Trowbridge Dr.
Bethel, CT 06801
203-743-5525

Disposable Instrument Co., Inc.
P.O. Box 14248
Shawnee Mission, KS 66285-4248
913-492-6492

Dittmar, Inc.
101 E. Laurel Ave.
P.O. Box 66
Cheltenham, PA 19012-2125
215-379-5533

Elmed, Inc.
60 W. Fay Ave.
Addison, IL 60101-5198
708-543-2792

Ethicon Endo-Surgery
4545 Creek Road
Cincinnati, OH 45242
513-786-7000

Herwig Surgical Instrument Co.
8741 Landmark Rd.
Richmond, VA 23228-2801
804-264-7585

Leisegang Medical, Inc.
6401 Congress Ave.
Boca Raton, FL 33487-2883
407-994-0202

Marlow Surgical Technologies, Inc.
1810 Joseph Lloyd Pkwy.
Willoughby, OH 44094-8030
216-946-2453

Medicon Instruments, Inc.
4405 International Blvd.
Norcross, GA 30093-3013
404-381-2858

Mist, Inc.
6307 E. Angus Dr.
Raleigh, NC 27613
919-787-8377

Nopa Instruments Medizintechnik GmbH
Gansacker 9 - Postfach 4554
D-78532 Tuttlingen
Germany
07462/7801

Phillips & Jones (U.S.A.), Inc.
P.O. Box 7246
Newark, DE 19714-7246
302-737-7987

Pilling-Rusch
420 Delaware Dr.
Fort Washington, PA 19034-2711
215-643-2600

Sklar Instrument Company
889 South Matlack St.
West Chester, PA 19380
215-430-3200

Smith & Nephew Dyonics, Inc.
160 Dascomb Rd.
Andover, MA 01810-5893
508-470-2800

Star Guide Corp.
6666 Stapleton Dr. S.
Denver, CO 80216
303-333-2100

Surgical Instrument Co. of America
1185 Edgewater Ave.
Ridgefield, NJ 07657-2102
201-941-6500

United States Surgical Corp.
150 Glover Ave.
Norwalk, CT 06856-5080
203-845-1000

Weck & Co. Inc., Edward
1 Weck Dr.
P.O. Box 12600
Research Triangle Park, NC 27709
919-544-8000

Wolf Medical Instruments Corp., Richard
353 Corporate Woods Pkwy.
Vernon Hills, IL 60061-3110
708-913-1113

TROCAR, GASTRO-UROLOGY

A&A Medical, Inc.
11485 Mountain Laurel Dr.
Roswell, GA 30075

Aesculap AG
Moehringerstr. 125
Postfach 40
D-78532 Tuttlingen
Germany
00149/0746951

Apple Medical Corp.
93 Nashaway Rd.
Bolton, MA 01740
508-779-2926

Baxter Healthcare Corp.
Operating Room Div.
1500 Waukegan Rd.
McGaw Park, IL 60085-8210
708-473-1500

Boss Instruments, Ltd.
1310 Central Ct.
Hermitage, TN 37076
615-885-2231

Bryan Corp.
4 Plympton St.
Woburn, MA 01801-2908
617-935-0004

Cabot Medical Corp.
2021 Cabot Blvd. West
Langhorne, PA 19047-1875
215-752-8300

DCG Precision Manufacturing Corp.
9 Trowbridge Dr.
Bethel, CT 06801
203-743-5525

Disposable Instrument Co., Inc.
P.O. Box 14248
Shawnee Mission, KS 66285-4248
913-492-6492

Lawton USA Surgical Instruments
6341 S. Troy Cir.
Englewood, CO 80111-6415
303-790-9416

Martin, Gebr. GmbH & Co. KG
Ludwigstaler Str. 132
Postf. 60
D-78532 Tuttlingen
Germany
07461/7060

Nopa Instruments Medizintechnik GmbH
Gansacker 9 - Postfach 4554
D-78532 Tuttlingen
Germany
07462/7801

Pioneer Medical, Inc.
34 Laurelcrest Rd.
Madison, CT 06443
203-245-9337

Smith & Nephew Dyonics, Inc.
160 Dascomb Rd.
Andover, MA 01810-5893
508-470-2800

Star Guide Corp.
6666 Stapleton Dr. S.
Denver, CO 80216
303-333-2100

Synectic Engineering, Inc.
4 Oxford Rd.
Milford, CT 06460-7007
203-877-8488

Ueth & Haug GmbH
Stockacher Str. 41/45
D-78532 Tuttlingen
Germany

Unisurge, Inc.
10231 Bubb Rd.
Cupertino, CA 95014
408-996-4700

Wolf Medical Instruments Corp., Richard
353 Corporate Woods Pkwy.
Vernon Hills, IL 60061-3110
708-913-1113

TROCAR, LAPAROSCOPIC

Conmed Corp.
310 Broad St.
Utica, NY 13501
315-797-8375

TROGARD ELECTRONIC TROCAR

DESCRIPTION: TroGARD™ is a single-patient use, electronically controlled trocar system that incorporates a blunt, conical electrosurgical trocar tip and an Electronic Trocar Monitor, for placement of cannula/sleeves into a body cavity. The TroGARD Electronic Trocar Monitor measures the impedance at the tip of the trocar and immediately deactivates the electrosurgical current when the trocar tip clears the tissue of the body wall.

The TroGARD trocar is a 5mm blunt, conical tip utilizing pure cut electrosurgical current for incising body wall tissue. The 5mm trocar fits into a 10/11 or 12mm obturator for use in a 10/11 or 10/12mm trocar sleeve. The obturator is removed for use in a 5mm sleeve. The 5mm puncture is automatically dilated by the obturator and cannula sleeve when inserted, to accommodate 10/11mm or 10/12mm cannulas. One trocar does *all* punctures for a procedure.

The body of the 10/11 and 10/12mm trocar sleeve has a built-in sliding gasket with 5mm "step-down" to seal around 5mm endoscopic instruments. The sleeve has an internal valve system to prevent gas leakage. Additionally, a conical tip (Hasson type) Trocar & 10/11 sleeve is available.

TroGARD must be used with the TroGARD Electronic Trocar Monitor, which will adapt to most isolated circuitry electrosurgical generators. All components are sterile, for single-patient use.

INDICATIONS: For use in establishing and maintaining surgical access to the body cavity in surgical endoscopy including laparoscopy, pelviscopy and thoracoscopy.

CONTRAINDICATIONS: TroGARD should only be used by surgeons trained in surgical endoscopy and the methods of safe trocar placement.

A "closed" method of trocar placement for the initial trocar is often contraindicated for patients with previous history of surgery, which may indicate a potential for abdominal adhesions.

See package insert for use directions, cautions, warnings, and detailed product descriptions.

TROCAR, LAPAROSCOPIC
(cont'd)

Davis & Geck Endosurgery
1 Casper St.
Danbury, CT 06810
203-743-4451

PROFESSIONAL LINE 8445 SERIES

DESCRIPTION: Trocar with non-locking trumpet valve:

NON-LOCKING TRUMPET VALVE TROCAR

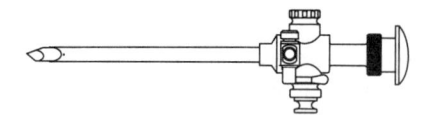

INSTRUCTIONS FOR USE: The DAVIS & GECK Reusable Endoscopic Trocar is supplied non-sterile. Sterilize the device in accordance with approved hospital sterilization methods, following the guidelines listed below under "Sterilization".

ASSEMBLY GUIDELINES:
1. Immediately after the completion of the surgical use of the endoscopic trocar, separate the trocar (obturator) from the trocar sleeve (cannula), and remove the trumpet valve sealing caps by unscrewing them from the valve assembly.
2. Remove the spring from the valve assembly and pull the piston sleeve from the housing in a straight line. Do not use force. Clean the entire piston and housing with a soft bristle brush and a mild soap.
3. To reassemble the trocar, replace the rear sealing cap on the valve assembly. Insert the spring into the piston and guide the entire piston assembly into its housing by aligning the slot on the piston with the screw guide on the trocar sleeve. Completely compress the plunger of the pistol, and hold it in place until the forward sealing cap is replaced. After complete assembly, activate the pistol plunger several times to ensure the movement of the piston.

CARE & MAINTENANCE: Do not use any solvent. Also, do not pile or store instruments on the top of the reusable trocar as inadvertent damage and dulling to the cutting edge may be caused.
Cleaning Guidelines:
1. Disassemble the trocar and clean all parts of the instrument thoroughly with a soft brush and a non-abrasive soap in warm water.
2. Flush the interior channels on the trocar, inclusive of the insufflation cocks, with a cleaning pistol or an appropriately sized brush.
3. Rinse the instrument and components thoroughly with warm water.
Lubrication:
After every use, the instrument should be dipped in an antimicrobial instrument lubricant. The lubricant forms a fine film over the instrument which prevents blood, debris and proteins from bonding to the instrument, as well as improving the action on moving parts.

STERILIZATION GUIDELINES:
1. The reusable endoscopic trocar should be placed in an approved sterilization container, such as the DAVIS & GECK instrument tray (product code number 8482-00).
2. If the instruments are placed in a perforated metal tray, gauze or approved instrument wraps should be folded about each instrument.
3. Contact of bare metal with plastic must be avoided at all times.
4. Sterilize product before use. Steam sterilize at a minimum temperature of 250°F (121°C). Use the steam sterilization guidelines as provided by the manufacturer.
  a. Do not disinfect or sterilize in EtO/Freon.
  b. Do not disinfect or sterilize in liquid solutions.
  c. Do not sterilize at temperatures greater than 275°F (135°C).
5. After removal of the instruments from the autoclave, they should be allowed to cool naturally to room temperature. Do not cold quench instruments in cold water or any other liquid following sterilization.

SPECIFICATIONS/HOW SUPPLIED: Order number 8445-01 for 5.5mm, 8445-02 for 10mm, and 8445-03 for 12mm diameter instrument (all with insufflation connection).

Davis & Geck Endosurgery
1 Casper St.
Danbury, CT 06810
203-743-4451

PROFESSIONAL LINE 8445 SERIES

DESCRIPTION: Trocars with locking trumpet valve:

LOCKING TRUMPET VALVE TROCAR
DETAIL OF LOCKING DEVICE
TOP VIEW

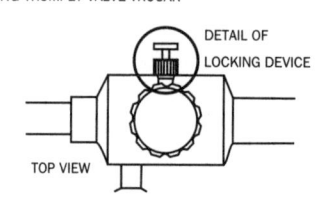

LOCKING TRUMPET VALVE TROCAR
SIDE VIEW

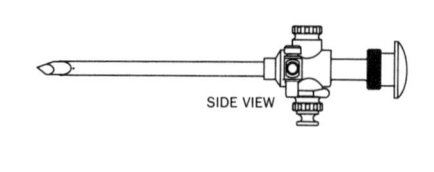

OBTURATOR (TAPER TIP)

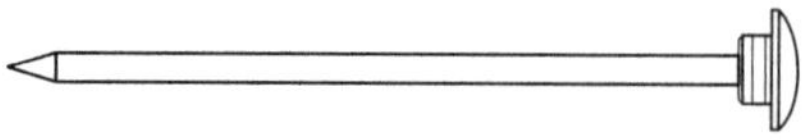

OBTURATOR (PYRAMID TIP)

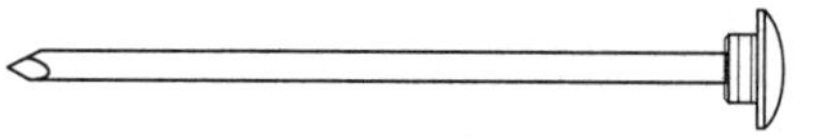

Trocars include a trocar sleeve and two obturators: One obturator has a pyramid ground tip, the other has a taper ground tip. Trocar sleeves have bevelled, elliptical ends, matte finish to reduce glare, and lockable trumpet valves to reduce instrument friction.

The trocars, 8445-09, 8445-10, 8445-11, and 8445-12, with a locking mechanism are designed for laparoscopic operations. Their purpose is to receive tubular shaft instruments or endoscopes and to introduce them through the abdominal wall into the abdomen.

INSTRUCTIONS FOR USE: On introducing the instrument into the trocar, the piston (2) should be fully depressed. The piston is automatically locked so that frictionless instrument introduction is guaranteed. To avoid a loss of CO_2 after removal of the instrument from the trocar, push-button (8) must be pressed. The lock is released and the piston (2) ensures a secure CO_2 seal.

LOCKING TRUMPET VALVE TROCAR

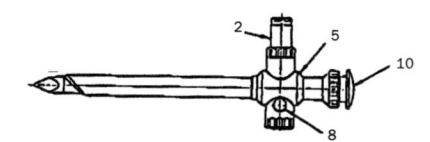

ASSEMBLY GUIDELINES: To dismantle the instrument, pull the obturator (10) out of the trocar body (5). Press push-button (8) to release the piston (2).
Then unscrew open valve cap (1) and pull piston (2) and spring (4) out of the trocar body (5). Unscrew closed valve cap (9) and sealing cap (7) and remove the seal (6). Unscrew push-button (8).

LOCKING TRUMPET VALVE TROCAR

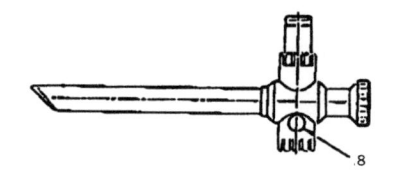

TROCAR/165

LOCKING TRUMPET VALVE TROCAR

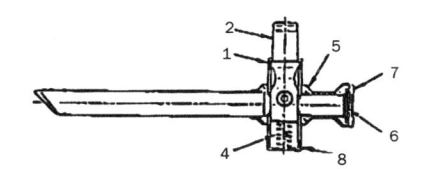

To assemble the instrument, insert seal (6) in the trocar body (5) and screw on sealing cap (7). Screw on push-button (8). Screw closed valve cap (9) onto trocar body. Then insert spring (4) into trocar body (5). Insert piston (2) into trocar body (5) so that marks on the piston (2) and trocar body (5) coincide [ensure that the retaining pin (3) is pushed in when inserting the piston (2)]. Push in piston (2) until it snaps in audibly. Screw on open valve cap (1) and insert required obturator (10) into the trocar.

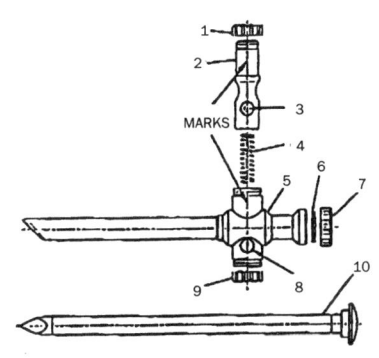

CARE & MAINTENANCE: The instrument should be cleaned immediately after use. For this purpose, the instrument must be dismantled and the individual parts cleaned with a soft sponge or cloth (outside) and brush (inside) under flowing water (in the case of extremely soiled instruments, manual cleaning or ultrasonic treatment is preferred). Dry thoroughly with a soft cloth or compressed air.

STERILIZATION GUIDELINES: Before sterilization, the instrument in the dry and dismantled state must be sprayed with oil spray. The instrument is preferably sterilized with steam at max. 275°F (135°C). The trocar is assembled at the operating table.

SPECIFICATIONS/HOW SUPPLIED:

LOCKING TRUMPET VALVE TROCAR PRODUCT CODE	DIAMETER	INSUFFLATOR CONNECTION
8445-09	5.5 mm	Yes
8445-10	10.0 mm	Yes
8445-11	12.5 mm	No
8445-12	7.0 mm	Yes

Davis & Geck Endosurgery
1 Casper St.
Danbury, CT 06810
203-743-4451

PROFESSIONAL LINE 8447 & 8448 SERIES

DESCRIPTION: Replacement parts for non-locking trumpet valve trocars.

Davis & Geck Endosurgery
1 Casper St.
Danbury, CT 06810
203-743-4451

PROFESSIONAL LINE 8449 SERIES

DESCRIPTION: Replacement parts for trocars with locking trumpet valve.

SPECIFICATIONS/HOW SUPPLIED:

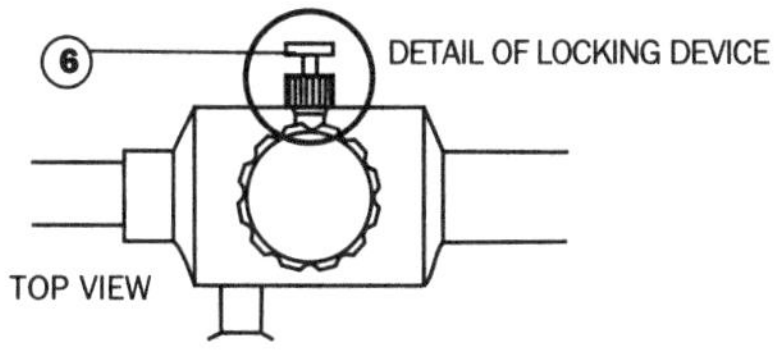

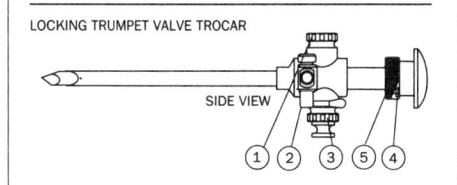

LOCKING TRUMPET VALVE TROCAR	5.5 mm	7 mm	10 mm	12.5 mm
1 - Valve Cap (closed end)	8449-21	8449-22	8449-23	8449-24
2 - Valve Spring	8449-25	8449-26	8449-27	8449-28
3 - Valve Cap (open end)	8449-29	8449-30	8449-31	8449-32
4 - Sealing Membrane	8449-33	8449-34	8449-35	8449-36
5 - Sealing Cap	8449-37	8449-38	8449-39	8449-40
6 - Locking Button and Spring	8449-42	8449-42	8449-44	8449-44

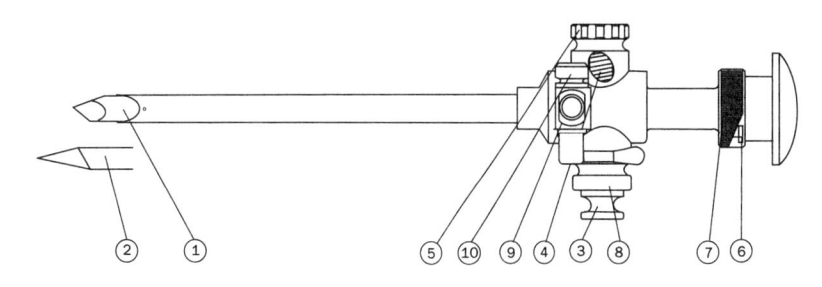

SPECIFICATIONS/HOW SUPPLIED:

NON-LOCKING TRUMPET VALVE TROCAR	5.5 mm	10 mm	12 mm
1 - Replacement Pyramidal Obturator	8447-03	8447-02	8447-01
2 - Replacement Conical Obturator	8447-06	8447-05	8447-04
3 - Trumpet Valve Piston	8448-03	8448-02	8448-01
4 - Trumpet Valve Spring	8448-06	8448-05	8448-04
5 - Trumpet Valve Retainer Button	8448-09	8448-08	8448-07
6 - Trocar Top Gasket	8448-12	8448-11	8448-10
7 - Top Gasket Retaining Ring	8448-20	8448-19	8448-18
8 - Valve Retaining Caps	8448-23	8448-22	8448-21
9 - Insufflation Valve	8448-24	8448-24	8448-24
10 - Insufflation Valve Retainer	8448-25	8448-25	8448-25

TROCAR, LAPAROSCOPIC
(cont'd)

Ethicon Endo-Surgery
4545 Creek Rd.
Cincinnati, OH 45242
513-786-7000

ENDOPATH BLUNT TIP TROCAR

DESCRIPTION: The ENDOPATH* Disposable Surgical Trocar with Blunt Tip Obturator is available with a radiolucent 10/11mm diameter sleeve. The sleeve is 100mm long and contains a stopcock. The trocar sleeve contains an external gasket and an internal flapper valve with a seal to prevent gas leakage when instruments are inserted or withdrawn. The obturator has a blunt plastic tip, which gently moves aside any internal viscera that may be adjacent to the abdominal wall. There is a stopcock valve for gas insufflation and a desufflation lever for gas evacuation.

INDICATIONS: The ENDOPATH Disposable Surgical Trocar with Blunt Tip Obturator has application in gynecologic and general surgery laparoscopy to establish a port of entry for endoscopic instruments.

CONTRAINDICATIONS: The device is not intended for use when endoscopic techniques are contraindicated.

WARNINGS:

1. Endoscopic procedures should be performed only by persons having adequate training and familiarity with endoscopic techniques. Consult medical literature relative to techniques, complications, and hazards prior to performance of any endoscopic procedure.

2. Use caution when introducing or removing instruments through the trocar sleeve in order to prevent inadvertent damage to the gasket, which could result in loss of pneumoperitoneum.

3. After removing the ENDOPATH Disposable Trocar Obturator from the abdominal cavity, always inspect the site for hemostasis. If hemostasis is not present, appropriate techniques should be utilized to achieve hemostasis.

4. Using endoscopic instruments with a smaller diameter than that found on the label of the ENDOPATH Trocar may result in desufflation of the abdominal cavity. For example, only 11mm down to 10mm endoscopic instruments can be used with the ENDOPATH Trocar with Blunt Tip.

5. Endoscopic instruments may vary in diameter from manufacturer to manufacturer. When endoscopic instruments and accessories from different manufacturers are employed together in a procedure, verify compatibility prior to initiation of procedure and ensure that electrical isolation or grounding is not compromised.

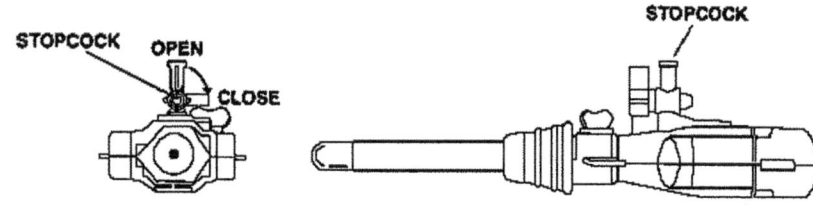

6. A thorough understanding of the principles and techniques involved in laparoscopic laser and electrosurgical procedures is essential to avoid shock and burn hazards to both patient and medical personnel and damage to the device or other medical instruments.

7. Dispose of all opened trocar products whether used or unused. DO NOT RESTERILIZE the trocar sleeve and/or obturator. Resterilization may compromise the integrity of the product, which may result in unintended injury.

Read all instructions carefully. Failure to properly follow the instructions may lead to serious surgical consequences.

INSTRUCTIONS FOR USE: Please read all information carefully. Failure to properly follow the instructions may lead to serious surgical consequences.

IMPORTANT: This package insert is designed to provide instructions for use of the ENDOPATH Disposable Surgical Trocar with Blunt Tip. It is not a reference to trocar insertion techniques.

Verify compatibility of all endoscopic instruments and accessories prior to using the ENDOPATH trocar with Blunt Tip (refer to paragraphs 4 and 5 under WARNINGS).

Prepare the abdominal cavity in accordance with proper surgical technique prior to insertion of the trocar.

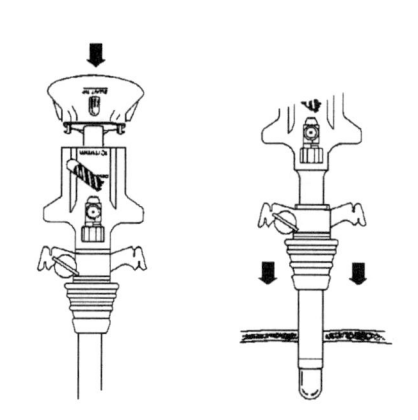

1. The trocar is packaged with the stopcock in the open position. Lock the blunt obturator handle assembly to the sleeve of the instrument. An audible "click" will be heard.

2. A finger is placed into the previously created umbilical incision to ensure that the free peritoneal cavity has been entered. Two size 0, Coated VICRYL* (polyglactin 910) sutures are passed, one through each fascial edge, and tagged. The sutures are then held upward and apart.

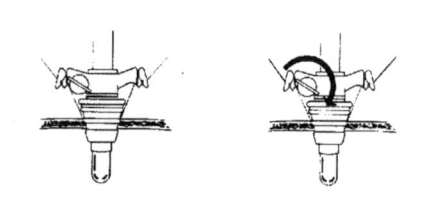

3. Insert the blunt tip trocar into the incision with the adjustable plug secured against the bottom of the trocar sleeve housing. Loosen and slide the adjustable plug down the trocar sleeve and into the incision. Pull and wrap the sutures snuggly around the tieposts on the adjustable plug. This forces the plug firmly into the incision to help seal it and prevent gas leakage later in the procedure. Position the desired amount of trocar sleeve in the abdomen by sliding it up or down accordingly. Once the desired sleeve position has been established, secure the plug to the sleeve by tightening the wingnut.

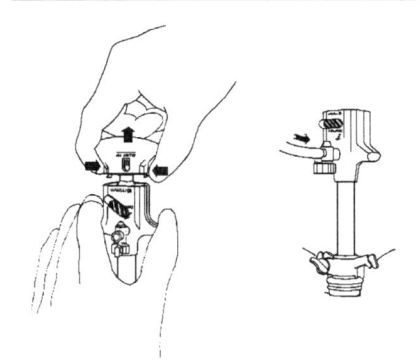

4. Remove the blunt tip obturator by squeezing the black locking handle buttons located on the sides of the obturator handle assembly.

5. Insufflation can be attained by attaching a gas line to the stopcock on the trocar sleeve. Instruments of appropriate size can be easily introduced and removed through the sleeve of the ENDOPATH Disposable Trocar with Blunt Tip. An internal flapper valve will open and close to maintain abdominal cavity insufflation. The flapper valve can be opened by rotating the desufflation lever clockwise.

6. Upon completion of the procedure, the abdominal cavity is rapidly deflated by using the desufflation lever. The ENDOPATH Trocar with Blunt Tip is removed and the abdominal wall is closed.

STERILIZATION GUIDELINES: Sterility is guaranteed unless the package is opened or damaged. DO NOT RESTERILIZE.

SPECIFICATIONS/HOW SUPPLIED: The ENDOPATH Disposable Surgical Trocar with Blunt Tip in the 10/11mm size with stopcock is for single use only. Discard after use.

CAUTION: Federal (USA) law restricts this device to sale by or on the order of a physician.

Ethicon Endo-Surgery
4545 Creek Rd.
Cincinnati, OH 45242
513-786-7000

ENDOPATH TRISTAR
DESCRIPTION:

1. Obturator Handle
2. Locking Buttons (housed in obturator handle)
3. Trcar Sleeve
4. Desufflation Lever
5. Stopcock
6. Safety Shield
7. Safety Shield Reset Button (Red) (housed in obturator handle)
8. Retracted Safety Shield

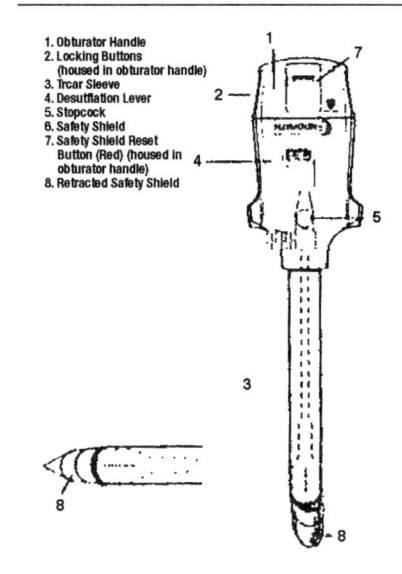

The ENDOPATH* TriStar Surgical Trocar in the 5mm, 11mm, and 12mm diameter sizes with stopcock, consists of a sharp pyramidal tip and spring-loaded safety shield. The safety shield is designed to cover the pyramidal tip to protect internal structures from puncture or laceration once the abdominal cavity has been entered. Due to reduced force to penetrate, excessive force to insert the trocar is not required.

The trocar sleeve contains an outer gasket and internal flapper valve with a seal to minimize gas leakage when instruments are inserted or withdrawn. The size of the trocar corresponds to the maximum size of the instrument that can be used in that trocar. There is a stopcock valve for gas insufflation and a desufflation lever for gas evacuation.

INDICATIONS: The ENDOPATH TriStar Surgical Trocar has application in thoracic, gynecologic laparoscopy, and other abdominal procedures to establish a path of entry for endoscopic instruments.

CONTRAINDICATIONS: The device is not intended for use when endoscopic techniques are contraindicated.

WARNINGS:

1. Endoscopic procedures should be performed only by persons having adequate training and familiarity with endoscopic techniques. Consult medical literature relative to techniques, complications, and hazards prior to performance of any endoscopic procedure.

2. Endoscopic instruments may vary in diameter from manufacturer to manufacturer. When endoscopic instruments and accessories from different manufacturers are employed together in a procedure, verify compatibility prior to initiation of the procedure, and ensure that electrical isolation or grounding is not compromised.

3. Using endoscopic instruments with a smaller diameter than that found on the label of the ENDOPATH TriStar Surgical Trocar may result in desufflation of the abdominal cavity. If smaller instruments are to be passed through the trocar sleeve, an ENDOPATH Multiseal Cap must be employed.

4. A thorough understanding of the principles and techniques involved in laparoscopic laser and electrosurgical procedures is essential to avoid shock and burn hazards to both patient and medical personnel and damage to the device or other medical instruments.

5. The incorporation of the safety shield feature in the trocar design is intended to minimize the likelihood of penetrating injury to intra-abdominal structures. However, because the trocar tip will be briefly unprotected prior to safety shield advancement, the standard precautionary measures employed in all trocar insertions must be observed.

6. Although the ENDOPATH TriStar Surgical Trocar is designed with a safety shield, care must still be taken, as with all trocars, to avoid damage to major vessels and other anatomic structures (such as bowel or mesentery). To minimize the risk of such injury, be sure to:
- Establish adequate pneumoperitoneum
- Properly position the patient to help displace organs out of the area of penetration
- Note important anatomical landmarks
- Direct the trocar tip away from major vessels and structures
- Avoid excessive force.

7. Do not attempt to insert the trocar if the red safety shield reset button does not stay in the activated position.

8. Once entry has been made into the abdominal cavity, the ENDOPATH TriStar Surgical Trocar should not be inadvertently reactivated for additional penetration. Continued entry of the exposed pyramidal tip at this point could cause injury to intra-abdominal structures.

9. Use caution when introducing or removing instruments through the trocar sleeve in order to prevent inadvertent damage to the gaskets, which could result in loss of pneumoperitoneum.

10. After removing the ENDOPATH TriStar Surgical Trocar Obturator from the abdominal cavity, always inspect the site for hemostasis. If hemostasis is not present, appropriate techniques should be used to achieve hemostasis.

11. During insertion of obturator into the sleeve housing, the obturator should not be in the activated position.

TROCAR, LAPAROSCOPIC
(cont'd)

12. Dispose of all opened trocar products, whether used or unused. DO NOT RESTERILIZE the trocar sleeve and/or obturator. Resterilization may compromise the integrity of this product, which may result in unintended injury.

INSTRUCTIONS FOR USE: Read all instructions carefully. Failure to properly follow the instructions may lead to serious surgical consequences.

IMPORTANT: This package insert is designed to provide instructions for the use of the ENDOPATH TriStar Surgical Trocar. It is not a reference to trocar insertion techniques.

Verify compatibility of all endoscopic instruments and accessories prior to using the ENDOPATH TriStar Surgical Trocar (Refer to paragraphs 2 and 3 under Warnings).

The ENDOPATH TriStar Surgical Trocar is packaged with the handle assemblies locked together and with the stopcock in the open position. Close the stopcock before use.

Prepare the abdominal cavity in accordance with proper laparoscopic technique prior to insertion of the trocar.

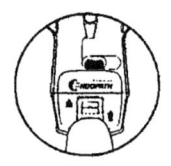

1. *Important: Push the reset button forward to the activated position to allow retraction of the safety shield. The trocar cannot be deactivated by forcing the reset button to the original position.*

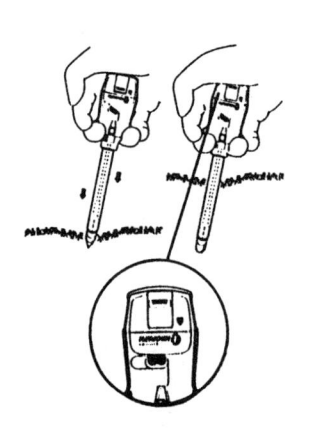

2. Incise the selected area adequately to accommodate the trocar sleeve. Introduce the trocar through the skin incision and apply continuous downward pressure on the trocar. When this pressure is applied, the safety shield will begin to retract. As the safety shield retracts, the sharp pyramidal tip is exposed to create the passage through the abdominal wall. Once the retracted safety shield has passed through the abdominal wall, it will advance forward and cover the exposed pyramidal tip. As the safety shield retracts, the red safety shield reset button returns to the original position.

NOTE: Trocar safety mechanisms are activated according to tissue resistance. Where there is insufficient tissue resistance to activate the safety mechanism, the red safety shield reset button will remain in the activated position.

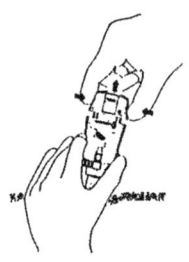

3. When the trocar is in the abdominal cavity, press the locking buttons to remove the obturator handle assembly, leaving the sleeve in place. Instruments of appropriate size can be easily introduced and removed through the sleeve of the trocar.

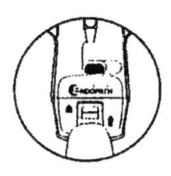

Important: If entry into the abdominal cavity is incomplete, the instrument must be reactivated. In order to reactivate the instrument, push the red safety shield reset button forward to the activated position. The safety shield will again be free to retract when pressure is applied.

4. To attain insufflation, attach a gas line to the stopcock on the handle, and open the stopcock. An internal flapper valve will open and close to maintain abdominal cavity insufflation. To open the flapper valve, rotate the desufflation lever clockwise. Upon completion of the procedure, use the desufflation lever to rapidly deflate the abdominal cavity.

If using an ENDOPATH Laparoscopic Kit which contains an additional sleeve, follow steps 1 through 4 under Instructions For Use for additional insertions.

STERILIZATION GUIDELINES: Sterility is guaranteed unless the package is opened or damaged. DO NOT RESTERILIZE.

SPECIFICATIONS/HOW SUPPLIED: The ENDOPATH TriStar Surgical Trocar in the 5mm, 11mm and 12mm diameter sizes with stopcock are for single-patient use only. Discard after use.

CAUTION: Federal (USA) law restricts this device to sale by or on the order of a physician.

Apple Medical Corp.
93 Nashaway Rd.
Bolton, MA 01740
508-779-2926

Cabot Medical Corp.
2021 Cabot Blvd. West
Langhorne, PA 19047-1875
215-752-8300

Chirurgische Instrumente
Hauptstrasse 18
D-78582 Balgheim
Germany
7424/501319

Chirurgisches Nahtmaterial
Franz Hiltner GmbH
Schonerstrabe 7
D-90443 Nurnberg
Germany
911/2068-850

Conmed Corp.
310 Broad Street
Utica, NY 13501
315-797-8375

Dexide, Inc.
7509 Flagstone Dr.
P.O. Box 185789
Fort Worth, TX 76118-6953
817-589-1454

Disposable Instrument Co., Inc.
P.O. Box 14248
Shawnee Mission, KS 66285-4248
913-492-6492

Leisegang Medical, Inc.
6401 Congress Ave.
Boca Raton, FL 33487-2883
407-994-0202

Minorax Corp.
7015 147th St. SW
Edmonds, WA 98026
206-743-0178

Nova Endoscopy Corp.
Route 29
P.O. Box 97
Palm, PA 18070
215-679-7404

United States Surgical Corp.
150 Glover Ave.
Norwalk, CT 06856-5080
203-845-1000

TROCAR, LARYNGEAL

Aesculap
1000 Gateway Blvd.
South San Francisco, CA 94080-7030
415-876-7000

Aesculap AG
Moehringerstr. 125
Postfach 40
D-78532 Tuttlingen
Germany
00149/0746951

Disposable Instrument Co., Inc.
P.O. Box 14248
Shawnee Mission, KS 66285-4248
913-492-6492

Elmed, Inc.
60 W. Fay Ave.
Addison, IL 60101-5198
708-543-2792

Lawton USA Surgical Instruments
6341 S. Troy Cir.
Englewood, CO 80111-6415
303-790-9416

Martin, Gebr. GmbH & Co. KG
Ludwigstaler Str. 132
Postf. 60
D-78532 Tuttlingen
Germany
07461/7060

Nopa Instruments Medizintechnik GmbH
Gansacker 9 - Postfach 4554
D-78532 Tuttlingen
Germany
07462/7801

Popper & Sons, Inc.
300 Denton Ave.
New Hyde Park, NY 11040-3437
516-248-0300

Star Guide Corp.
6666 Stapleton Dr. S.
Denver, CO 80216
303-333-2100

Storz Endoscopy-America Inc., Karl
10111 W. Jefferson Blvd.
Culver City, CA 90232-3509
310-558-1500

Storz GmbH & Co., Karl
Mittelstr. 8
Postfach 230
D-78532 Tuttlingen
Germany
07461/7080

Storz Instrument Company
3365 Tree Ct. Indust. Blvd.
St. Louis, MO 63122-6615
314-225-5051

Surgical Instrument Co. of America
1185 Edgewater Ave.
Ridgefield, NJ 07657-2102
201-941-6500

Wolf Medical Instruments Corp., Richard
353 Corporate Woods Pkwy.
Vernon Hills, IL 60061-3110
708-913-1113

TROCAR, OTHER

A&A Medical, Inc.
11485 Mountain Laurel Dr.
Roswell, GA 30075
800-424-1234

Aesculap
1000 Gateway Blvd.
South San Francisco, CA 94080-7030
415-876-7000

Apple Medical Corp.
93 Nashaway Rd.
Bolton, MA 01740
508-779-2926

Bryan Corp.
4 Plympton St.
Woburn, MA 01801-2908
617-935-0004

Cabot Medical Corp.
2021 Cabot Blvd. West
Langhorne, PA 19047-1875
215-752-8300

Conmed Corp.
310 Broad Street
Utica, NY 13501
315-797-8375

Core Dynamics, Inc.
11222-4 St. Johns Indust. Pkwy.
Jacksonville, FL 32216
904-641-6611

Disposable Instrument Co., Inc.
P.O. Box 14248
Shawnee Mission, KS 66285-4248
913-492-6492

Geister Medizintechnik GmbH
Foehrenstr. 2
Postfach 4228
D-78532 Tuttlingen
Germany
7461-8084

Instrument Makar, Inc.
2950 E. Mt. Hope
Okemos, MI 48864-1910
517-332-3593

Kensey Nash Corporation
55 E. Uwchlan Ave., Ste. 204
Exton, PA 19341-1247
215-524-0188

Leisegang Medical, Inc.
6401 Congress Ave.
Boca Raton, FL 33487-2883
407-994-0202

Lorenz Surgical, Walter
1520 Tradeport Dr.
Jacksonville, FL 32229-8009
904-741-4400

Marlow Surgical Technologies, Inc.
1810 Joseph Lloyd Pkwy.
Willoughby, OH 44094-8030
216-946-2453

Northgate Technologies, Inc.
3930 Ventura Dr., Ste. 150
Arlington Heights, IL 60004
708-506-9872

O.R. Concepts, Inc.
12250 Nicollet Ave. South
Burnsville, MN 55337
612-894-7523

Optical Micro Systems, Inc.
300 Willow St. S
North Andover, MA 01845-5920
508-681-0992

Pioneer Medical, Inc.
34 Laurelcrest Rd.
Madison, CT 06443
203-245-9337

Popper & Sons, Inc.
300 Denton Ave.
New Hyde Park, NY 11040-3437
516-248-0300

Precision Wire
Div. of New England Precision Grinding
459-B Fortune Blvd.
Milford, MA 01757
508-634-3050

TROCAR, OTHER (cont'd)

Premier Medical Manufacturing
10090 Sandmeyer Lane
Philadelphia, PA 19116-3502
215-676-9090

Sippex
Usine de la Giraudiere
F-69690 Courzieu
France
7470/9800

Smith & Nephew - Avon Medicals
Moons Moat Dr., Moons Moat N.
Redditch Worcester
United Kingdom
0527/64901

Technalytics, Inc.
210 Summit Ave.
Montvale, NJ 07645-1526
201-391-0494

United States Surgical Corp.
150 Glover Ave.
Norwalk, CT 06856-5080
203-845-1000

Wisap USA
P.O. Box 324
Tomball, TX 77377-0324
713-351-2629

Wolf Medical Instruments Corp., Richard
353 Corporate Woods Pkwy.
Vernon Hills, IL 60061-3110
708-913-1113

TROCAR, SHORT

Apple Medical Corp.
93 Nashaway Rd.
Bolton, MA 01740
508-779-2926

Bryan Corp.
4 Plympton St.
Woburn, MA 01801-2908
617-935-0004

Davis & Geck Div.
American Cyanamid Company
One Cyanamid Plaza
Wayne, NJ 07470-2012
201-831-2000

Ethicon Endo-Surgery
4545 Creek Road
Cincinnati, OH 45242
513-786-7000

Leisegang Medical, Inc.
6401 Congress Ave.
Boca Raton, FL 33487-2883
407-994-0202

Marlow Surgical Technologies, Inc.
1810 Joseph Lloyd Pkwy.
Willoughby, OH 44094-8030
216-946-2453

Origin Medsystems, Inc.
135 Constitution Dr.
Menlo Park, CA 94025
415-617-5000

Skye Precision Inc.
55 Florence Ave.
Plainesville, OH 44077
216-352-0020

United States Surgical Corp.
150 Glover Ave.
Norwalk, CT 06856-5080
203-845-1000

Wolf Medical Instruments Corp., Richard
353 Corporate Woods Pkwy.
Vernon Hills, IL 60061-3110
708-913-1113

TROCAR, SINUS

Aesculap
1000 Gateway Blvd.
South San Francisco, CA 94080-7030
415-876-7000

Aesculap AG
Moehringerstr. 125
Postfach 40
D-78532 Tuttlingen
Germany
00149/0746951

Baxter Healthcare Corp.
Operating Room Div.
1500 Waukegan Rd.
McGaw Park, IL 60085-8210
708-473-1500

Dieter Oertel Medizintechnik
Nendinger Str. 1
D-78532 Tuttlingen
Germany
07461/72426

Disposable Instrument Co., Inc.
P.O. Box 14248
Shawnee Mission, KS 66285-4248
913-492-6492

Leibinger GmbH
Botzinger Strasse 41
D-70437 Freiburg
Germany
0761/49058-0

Martin, Gebr. GmbH & Co. KG
Ludwigstaler Str. 132
Postf. 60
D-78532 Tuttlingen
Germany
07461/7060

Nopa Instruments Medizintechnik GmbH
Gansacker 9 - Postfach 4554
D-78532 Tuttlingen
Germany
07462/7801

Storz Endoscopy-America Inc., Karl
10111 W. Jefferson Blvd.
Culver City, CA 90232-3509
310-558-1500

Storz GmbH & Co., Karl
Mittelstr. 8
Postfach 230
D-78532 Tuttlingen
Germany
07461/7080

Ueth & Haug GmbH
Stockacher Str. 41/45
D-78532 Tuttlingen
Germany

TROCAR, SURGICAL

Ethicon, Inc.
U.S. Route 22
P.O. Box 151
Somerville, NJ 08876
908-218-0707

TROCAR, THORACIC

Apple Medical Corp.
93 Nashaway Rd.
Bolton, MA 01740
508-779-2926

Axiom Medical, Inc.
2377 Crenshaw Blvd., Ste. 330
Torrance, CA 90501
310-898-1779

Bashir, Jamil & Bros. PVT. Ltd.
Khadim Ali Rd.
P.O. Box 7
Sialkot
Pakistan
0432-553862

Baxter Healthcare Corp.
Operating Room Div.
1500 Waukegan Rd.
McGaw Park, IL 60085-8210
708-473-1500

Boss Instruments, Ltd.
1310 Central Ct.
Hermitage, TN 37076
615-885-2231

Bryan Corp.
4 Plympton St.
Woburn, MA 01801-2908
617-935-0004

Cabot Medical Corp.
2021 Cabot Blvd. West
Langhorne, PA 19047-1875
215-752-8300

Core Dynamics, Inc.
11222-4 St. Johns Indust. Pkwy.
Jacksonville, FL 32216
904-641-6611

Davis & Geck Div.
American Cyanamid Company
One Cyanamid Plaza
Wayne, NJ 07470-2012
201-831-2000

Disposable Instrument Co., Inc.
P.O. Box 14248
Shawnee Mission, KS 66285-4248
913-492-6492

Dittmar, Inc.
101 E. Laurel Ave.
P.O. Box 66
Cheltenham, PA 19012-2125
215-379-5533

Ethicon, Inc.
U.S. Route 22
P.O. Box 151
Somerville, NJ 08876
908-218-0707

Mader Instrument Corp.
25 Lamington Dr.
Succasunna, NJ 07876-2048
201-584-0816

Medicon Eg
15 Gansacker
Postfach 4455
D-78532 Tuttlingen
Germany
07462/20090

Medicon Instruments, Inc.
4405 International Blvd.
Norcross, GA 30093-3013
404-381-2858

Medovations, Inc.
102 East Keefe Ave.
Milwaukee, WI 53212-1535
414-265-7620

Miltex Instrument Co., Inc.
6 Ohio Dr.
CB 5006
Lake Success, NY 11042-0006
516-775-7100

Mist, Inc.
6307 E. Angus Dr.
Raleigh, NC 27613
919-787-8377

Nopa Instruments Medizintechnik GmbH
Gansacker 9 - Postfach 4554
D-78532 Tuttlingen
Germany
07462/7801

Origin Medsystems, Inc.
135 Constitution Dr.
Menlo Park, CA 94025
415-617-5000

Pilling-Rusch
420 Delaware Dr.
Fort Washington, PA 19034-2711
215-643-2600

Productes Clinics S.A.
C. Vic. 24
E-La Llagosta (Barcelona)
Spain
93/5603652

Sherwood Medical Company
1915 Olive St.
St. Louis, MO 63103-1625
314-621-7788

Sklar Instrument Company
889 South Matlack St.
West Chester, PA 19380
215-430-3200

Star Guide Corp.
6666 Stapleton Dr. S.
Denver, CO 80216
303-333-2100

Storz Endoscopy-America Inc., Karl
10111 W. Jefferson Blvd.
Culver City, CA 90232-3509
310-558-1500

Storz GmbH & Co., Karl
Mittelstr. 8
Postfach 230
D-78532 Tuttlingen
Germany
07461/7080

Surgical Instrument Co. of America
1185 Edgewater Ave.
Ridgefield, NJ 07657-2102
201-941-6500

Surgico Ltd., A.D.
P.O. Box 270
Sialkot 1
Pakistan
0432/88143

United States Surgical Corp.
150 Glover Ave.
Norwalk, CT 06856-5080
203-845-1000

Wolf Medical Instruments Corp., Richard
353 Corporate Woods Pkwy.
Vernon Hills, IL 60061-3110
708-913-1113

TROCAR, TRACHEAL

Aesculap
1000 Gateway Blvd.
South San Francisco, CA 94080-7030
415-876-7000

Aesculap AG
Moehringerstr. 125
Postfach 40
D-78532 Tuttlingen
Germany
00149/0746951

Bashir, Jamil & Bros. PVT. Ltd.
Khadim Ali Rd.
P.O. Box 7
Sialkot
Pakistan
0432-553862

TROCAR, TRACHEAL (cont'd)

Dieter Oertel Medizintechnik
Nendinger Str. 1
D-78532 Tuttlingen
Germany
07461/72426

Disposable Instrument Co., Inc.
P.O. Box 14248
Shawnee Mission, KS 66285-4248
913-492-6492

Graham-Field, Inc.
400 Rabro Dr. East
Hauppauge, NY 11788-4226
516-582-5900

Lawton USA Surgical Instruments
6341 S. Troy Cir.
Englewood, CO 80111-6415
303-790-9416

Medicon Eg
15 Gansacker
Postfach 4455
D-78532 Tuttlingen
Germany
07462/20090

Medicon Instruments, Inc.
4405 International Blvd.
Norcross, GA 30093-3013
404-381-2858

Mediplast Instruments, Inc.
P.O. Box 1126
New Castle, DE 19720
302-737-0237

Miltex Instrument Co., Inc.
6 Ohio Dr.
CB 5006
Lake Success, NY 11042-0006
516-775-7100

Nopa Instruments Medizintechnik GmbH
Gansacker 9 - Postfach 4554
D-78532 Tuttlingen
Germany
07462/7801

Pilling-Rusch
420 Delaware Dr.
Fort Washington, PA 19034-2711
215-643-2600

Sherwood Medical Company
1915 Olive St.
St. Louis, MO 63103-1625
314-621-7788

Star Guide Corp.
6666 Stapleton Dr. S.
Denver, CO 80216
303-333-2100

Surgical Instrument Co. of America
1185 Edgewater Ave.
Ridgefield, NJ 07657-2102
201-941-6500

Surgico Ltd., A.D.
P.O. Box 270
Sialkot 1
Pakistan
0432/88143

Ueth & Haug GmbH
Stockacher Str. 41/45
D-78532 Tuttlingen
Germany

Warmer

WARMER, ENDOSCOPE

Elmed, Inc.
60 W. Fay Ave.
Addison, IL 60101-5198
708-543-2792

Wolf Medical Instruments Corp., Richard
353 Corporate Woods Pkwy.
Vernon Hills, IL 60061-3110
708-913-1113

3
SUPPLIER PROFILES

In this section you'll find information on each of the suppliers—domestic and foreign alike—appearing in the Product Directory. Companies are listed alphabetically. Included in each entry are toll-free, Telex, TWX, and fax numbers and, when available, information on the company's sales volume, number of employees, and size of sales and marketing staff. For publicly owned companies, annual revenues and net income are also listed. Included in each entry is the company's primary method of distribution, its Federal Procurement Eligibility, and the names of several key executives, enabling you to more easily contact the appropriate individual or department for further information or quotations.

Listed in the profile are all minimally invasive surgery products supplied by the company. Products from the company that fall outside the scope of minimally invasive surgery can be found in *Medical Device Register*™.

A&A Medical, Inc. Tel: 800-424-1234
11485 Mountain Laurel Dr.
Roswell, GA 30075
CEO: Cedric Bernberg
Marketing: Keith Fuchs
Federal Procurement Eligibility: Small Business
Device Category:
Forceps, Endoscopic..GASTRO/UROLOGY
Trocar, Abdominal..GASTRO/UROLOGY
Trocar, Gastro-Urology...GASTRO/UROLOGY
Trocar, Other..GENERAL

Aaron Medical Industries, Inc. Tel: 813-384-2323
7100 30th Ave. North Tel: 800-537-2790
St. Petersburg, FL 33710-2902 Fax: 813-347-9144
CEO: J. Robert Saron, President
  Delton N. Cunningham, CFO
  Joseph Valenti, VP Int'l
Marketing: Dennis Daire, Natl. Sales Mgr.
Production: Richard Tilton, VP Oper.
Federal Procurement Eligibility: Small Business
Device Category:
Power Supply, Endoscopic, Battery Operated....................GENERAL

Abco Dealers, Inc. Tel: 414-358-5420
6601 W. Mill Rd. Tel: 800-327-1401
P.O. Box 23090 Fax: 414-358-5451
Milwaukee, WI 53218-0090
CEO: Joel W. Smith, Jr., President
  Michael Lemke, VP Fin. & Admin.
Marketing: Jim Ruderer, VP Mktg.
  Debby Klug, VP Sales
Production: Michael Spina, VP Oper.
Device Category:
Anoscope, Non-Powered.......................................GASTRO/UROLOGY
Holder, Leg, Arthroscopy...ORTHOPEDICS
Proctosigmoidoscope..GASTRO/UROLOGY
Remover, Clip..SURGERY
Sigmoidoscope, Rigid, Non-Electrical...................GASTRO/UROLOGY

Access Surgical International, Inc. Tel: 508-747-6006
15 Caswell Ln. Tel: 800-435-3126
Boat Yard Square Fax: 508-747-5118
Plymouth, MA 02360
CEO: Wayne Knupp, CEO
  Steve Stephens, President
  Pamela Myette, VP Personnel
Marketing: Mike Thorp, Dir. Mktg.
Federal Procurement Eligibility: Small Business
Device Category:
Blade, Knife, Laparoscopic..............................MIN. INV. SURGERY
Cannula, Extraction, Appendix........................MIN. INV. SURGERY
Clamp, Fixation, Cholangiography..................MIN. INV. SURGERY
Clamp, Laparoscopy..MIN. INV. SURGERY
Coagulator/Cutter, Endoscopic, Bipolar................OBSTETRICS/GYN
Coagulator/Cutter, Endoscopic, Unipolar..............OBSTETRICS/GYN
Electrode, Electrosurgery, Laparoscopic.............MIN. INV. SURGERY
Forceps, Endoscopic..GASTRO/UROLOGY
Forceps, Grasping, Atraumatic.........................MIN. INV. SURGERY
Forceps, Grasping, Traumatic..........................MIN. INV. SURGERY
Generator, Power, Electrosurgical.................................SURGERY
Holder, Instrument, Laparoscopic...................MIN. INV. SURGERY
Holder, Laparoscope..OBSTETRICS/GYN
Holder, Needle, Curved, Laparoscopic.............MIN. INV. SURGERY
Holder, Needle, Laparoscopic...........................MIN. INV. SURGERY
Holder/Scissors, Needle, Laparoscopic............MIN. INV. SURGERY
Instrument, Dissecting, Laparoscopic..............MIN. INV. SURGERY
Instrument, Knot Tying, Suture, Laparoscopic.....MIN. INV. SURGERY
Instrument, Needle Holder/Knot Tying.............MIN. INV. SURGERY
Instrument, Passing, Suture, Laparoscopic......MIN. INV. SURGERY
Introducer, T-Tube..MIN. INV. SURGERY
Kit, Cholecystectomy..MIN. INV. SURGERY
Kit, Laparoscopy..GASTRO/UROLOGY
Needle, Insufflation, Laparoscopic...................MIN. INV. SURGERY
Peritoneoscope..GASTRO/UROLOGY
Probe, Electrocauterization, Multi-Use.............MIN. INV. SURGERY
Probe, Suction, Irrigator/Aspirator, Laparoscopic....MIN. INV. SURGERY
Retractor, Fan-Type, Laparoscopy....................MIN. INV. SURGERY
Retractor, Laparoscopy, Other..........................MIN. INV. SURGERY
Scissors with Removable Tips, Laparoscopy.....MIN. INV. SURGERY
Tape, Television & Video, Endoscopic..................GASTRO/UROLOGY
Thoracoscope..CARDIOVASCULAR
Trocar, Abdominal..GASTRO/UROLOGY

Access/God Loves You Tel: 303-688-1808
651 Topeka Way Tel: 800-526-1020
P.O. Box 1630 Fax: 303-688-1453
Castle Rock, CO 80104-1630
CEO: Robert A. Hasse, President
  Ann Hasse, Corp. Administrator
Marketing: Michael Gauthier, Customer Assurance Mgr.
Production: Gwen Reed, Production Mgr.
Federal Procurement Eligibility: Small Business
Device Category:
Box, Battery, Rechargeable (Endoscopic)...............GASTRO/UROLOGY

Accurate Surgical & Tel: 516-333-2570
Scientific Instrument Corp. Tel: 800-645-3569
300 Shames Dr. Fax: 516-997-4948
Westbury, NY 11590-1736
Medical Products Sales Volume: $4,000,000
Total Employees: 20
Ownership: Private
Distribution: Exclusive Distributor
CEO: Marie T. Bonazinga, President
Marketing: Lorraine Gruenfelder, Sales Dir.
Federal Procurement Eligibility: Small Business, Woman Owned
Device Category:
Forceps, Electrosurgical..SURGERY
Kit, Laparoscopy..GASTRO/UROLOGY
Remover, Staple, Surgical...SURGERY

Acme United Corporation Tel: 203-332-7330
Medical Div. Tel: 800-243-9852
75 Kings Highway Cutoff Fax: 203-576-0007
Fairfield, CT 06430-5340
Medical Products Sales Volume: $20,000,000
Total Employees: 600
Ownership: Public
CEO: James F. Farrington, EVP
  Henry C. Wheeler, COB
  Dwight C. Wheeler II, President
  Andrew Harrison, Sr. VP
Marketing: William F. O'Dell, VP Mktg.
  Kenneth S. Green, VP Sales
  Mark B. Ryan, Mktg. Svcs. Mgr.
  Frank Abramo, Sales Admin. Mgr.
Federal Procurement Eligibility: VA Contract
Device Category:
Remover, Staple, Surgical...SURGERY

Acufex Microsurgical, Inc.
130 Forbes Blvd.
Mansfield, MA 02048
CEO: Edward L. Stephens, President
Device Category:
Accessories, Arthroscope .... ORTHOPEDICS
Arthroscope .... ORTHOPEDICS

Tel: 508-339-9700
Tel: 800-343-1343
Fax: 508-339-8916

Advanced Surgical, Inc.
305 College Rd. East
Princeton, NJ 08540
Marketing: Harriet Schwartzman, Mktg. Mgr.
Device Category:
Bag, Specimen, Laparoscopic .... MIN. INV. SURGERY
Catheter, Cholangiography .... SURGERY
Instrument, Knot Tying, Suture, Laparoscopic ..... MIN. INV. SURGERY
Kit, Cholecystectomy .... MIN. INV. SURGERY
Needle, Insufflation, Laparoscopic .... MIN. INV. SURGERY
Peritoneoscope .... GASTRO/UROLOGY
Retractor, Fan-Type, Laparoscopy .... MIN. INV. SURGERY
Retractor, Laparoscopy, Other .... MIN. INV. SURGERY
Thoracoscope .... CARDIOVASCULAR
Trainer, Laparoscopy .... MIN. INV. SURGERY

Tel: 609-987-2340
Fax: 609-987-2342

Aesculap
1000 Gateway Blvd.
South San Francisco, CA 94080-7030
CEO: T. Robert Perrett, President
  Robin Bush, Dir. Regulatory Affairs
  Mario Bertucci, HR Dir.
Marketing: William Shaw, III, Mktg. VP
  Val Hernandez, Sales Admin. Mgr.
  Marty Myers, Dir. Hosp. Sales
  Brian Martini, Mgr. Commercial Sales
  Bob Thompson, Sales VP
  Bob Frisz, Mktg. Comm. Mgr.
Production: Gary Orton, Mfg. Mgr.
Research: Wayne Kong, Mgr. Purchasing & Planning
  Tony Meser, Mgr. R & D
Federal Procurement Eligibility: GSA Contract, VA Contract
Device Category:
Accessories, Cleaning, Endoscopic .... GASTRO/UROLOGY
Applier, Clip, Laparoscopic .... MIN. INV. SURGERY
Cannula, Suprapubic, With Trocar .... GASTRO/UROLOGY
Carrier, Sponge, Endoscopic .... GASTRO/UROLOGY
Clamp, Laparoscopy .... MIN. INV. SURGERY
Coagulator, Laparoscopic, Unipolar .... OBSTETRICS/GYN
Coagulator/Cutter, Endoscopic, Bipolar .... OBSTETRICS/GYN
Coagulator/Cutter, Endoscopic, Unipolar .... OBSTETRICS/GYN
Endoscope, Direct Vision .... SURGERY
Forceps, Endoscopic .... GASTRO/UROLOGY
Forceps, Grasping, Atraumatic .... MIN. INV. SURGERY
Forceps, Grasping, Traumatic .... MIN. INV. SURGERY
Holder, Instrument, Laparoscopic .... MIN. INV. SURGERY
Instrument, Dissecting, Laparoscopic .... MIN. INV. SURGERY
Instrument, Knot Tying, Suture, Laparoscopic ..... MIN. INV. SURGERY
Kit, Cholecystectomy .... MIN. INV. SURGERY
Laparoscope, General & Plastic Surgery .... SURGERY
Mirror, Endoscopic .... SURGERY
Needle, Insufflation, Laparoscopic .... MIN. INV. SURGERY
Obturator, Endoscopic .... GASTRO/UROLOGY
Peritoneoscope .... GASTRO/UROLOGY
Probe, Electrocauterization, Multi-Use .... MIN. INV. SURGERY
Thoracoscope .... CARDIOVASCULAR
Trocar, Abdominal .... GASTRO/UROLOGY
Trocar, Gallbladder .... GASTRO/UROLOGY
Trocar, Laryngeal .... EAR/NOSE/THROAT
Trocar, Other .... GENERAL
Trocar, Sinus .... EAR/NOSE/THROAT
Trocar, Tracheal .... EAR/NOSE/THROAT

Tel: 415-876-7000
Tel: 800-258-1946
Fax: 415-876-7028

Aesculap AG
Moehringerstr. 125
Postfach 40
D-78532 Tuttlingen
Germany
CEO: Michael Ungethuem
Marketing: V. Paulus
Device Category:
Forceps, Endoscopic .... GASTRO/UROLOGY
Forceps, Grasping, Flexible Endoscopic .... GASTRO/UROLOGY
Trocar, Cardiovascular .... CARDIOVASCULAR
Trocar, Gastro-Urology .... GASTRO/UROLOGY
Trocar, Laryngeal .... EAR/NOSE/THROAT
Trocar, Sinus .... EAR/NOSE/THROAT
Trocar, Tracheal .... EAR/NOSE/THROAT

Tel: 01149/746951
Fax: 01149/746195600

Ak Tech Corp.
2FL, Kukdong Bldg., 945-2
Pangbae-2 Dong, Socho-Ku
Seoul
Korea
CEO: Haelyung Hwang
Marketing: Ei Sang Park
Device Category:
Computer, Image, Endoscopic .... GENERAL
Laparoscope, General & Plastic Surgery .... SURGERY

Tel: 02/525-2031
Fax: 02/525-2033

Albert-Wetzlar GmbH
Kreisstrasse 120
D-35583 Wetzlar
Germany
Marketing: Hannelore Hiepe
  Boris F. Albert, Mktg. Mgr.
Device Category:
Colposcope .... OBSTETRICS/GYN

Tel: 06441/45688
Fax: 06441/45688

Alexander Batteries
New Product/OEM Div.
P.O. Box 1508
Mason City, IA 50402
Total Employees: 300
Ownership: Private
Distribution: OEM, Manufacturer Through Distributors, Exporter
Advertising: Sandra Hayworth, PR Coord.
  Les Selton, Adv. Coord.
CEO: Steve Alexandres, EVP
  Richard Alexandres, President
Production: Jon Alexandres, VP Int'l. Oper.
  Bob Williams, VP Battery Production
Federal Procurement Eligibility: GSA Contract
Device Category:
Box, Battery, Pocket (Endoscopic) .... GASTRO/UROLOGY
Box, Battery, Rechargeable (Endoscopic) .... GASTRO/UROLOGY

Tel: 515-423-8955
Tel: 800-526-ALEX
Fax: 515-423-1644

All Orthopedic Appliances
9690 Deereco Road, Suite 600
Timonium, MD 21093
CEO: Warren M. Gitt, Division Mgr.
Marketing: Nancy C. Feder, Mktg. Svcs. Admin. & Contracts Coord.
  Lawrence F. Shaffer, Sales & Mktg. Dir.
Production: Kay Fowler
Federal Procurement Eligibility: GSA Contract, VA Contract
Device Category:
Holder, Shoulder, Arthroscopy .... SURGERY

Tel: 410-560-3333
Tel: 800-327-3288
Fax: 410-252-9067

Allen Medical Systems, Inc.   Tel: 216-765-0990
5198 Richmond Rd.   Tel: 800-433-5774
Bedford Heights, OH 44146-1331   Fax: 216-765-1304
Advertising: Ann Lordeman, Adv. Mgr.
CEO: Jim McCourt, Financial Officer
Marketing: R. Dan Allen, Int'l Sales & Mktg. Mgr.
    Gary Lacinski, Nat'l Sales Mgr.
    Ann Lordeman, Mkt. Research Mgr.
Production: Jim McCourt, VP Mfg.
    Dave McDiffit, Materials Mgr.
Research: R. Dan Allen, VP R&D
Federal Procurement Eligibility: Small Business
Device Category:
Holder, Leg, Arthroscopy .... ORTHOPEDICS
Holder, Shoulder, Arthroscopy .... SURGERY
System, Traction, Arthroscopy .... ORTHOPEDICS

Allgaier Instrumente GmbH   Tel: 07426/1056
Teuchelgrube 6-10   Fax: 07426/7665
D-78665 Frittlingen
Germany
CEO: Roland Allgaier, Owner / President
Device Category:
Bronchoscope, Rigid .... EAR/NOSE/THROAT

Aloka (U.S. Headquarters)   Tel: 203-269-5088
10 Fairfield Blvd.   Fax: 203-269-6075
P.O. Box 5002
Wallingford, CT 06492-7502
CEO: Shoichi Nakai, President
Marketing: William Jennings, Natl. Sales Mgr.
    James Pietropaolo, VP Sales & Mktg.
Production: Paul Smolenski, QA & Reg. Affairs Mgr.
Device Category:
Kit, Cholecystectomy .... MIN. INV. SURGERY
Probe, Detector, Flow, Blood,
    Laparoscopy, Ultrasonic .... MIN. INV. SURGERY

American Hydro-Surgical Instruments,   Tel: 407-278-5664
Inc.   Tel: 800-527-5294
430 Commerce Dr., Ste. 50E   Fax: 407-278-5358
Delray Beach, FL 33445
Medical Products Sales Volume: $5,000,000
Total Employees: 35
Distribution: Manufacturer Direct, Through Distributors & Reps.
Advertising: Bryan McGurn
CEO: James H. Dorsey, III
Marketing: Vincent S. Fall, Mktg. Dir.
    Patrick J. Moyna, Product Mgr.
Federal Procurement Eligibility: Small Business
Device Category:
Coagulator, Laparoscopic, Unipolar .... OBSTETRICS/GYN
Coagulator/Cutter, Endoscopic, Unipolar .... OBSTETRICS/GYN
Electrode, Electrosurgery, Laparoscopic .... MIN. INV. SURGERY
Equipment, Suction/Irrigation, Laparoscopic ..... SURGERY
Peritoneoscope .... GASTRO/UROLOGY
Solution, Instrument, Laparoscopic, Anti-Fog .... GENERAL

American International Medicine,   Tel: 310-470-4844
Inc.   Fax: 310-470-2487
1917 Glendon Ave., Ste. 201
Los Angeles, CA 90025
Ownership: Private
Distribution: Importer & Exporter
CEO: Said F. Hakim, M.D., President & CEO
Marketing: Karine Davoudy, Regional Dir.
Device Category:
Endoscope And Accessories, AC-Powered .... SURGERY
Endoscope, Rigid .... SURGERY

American Medical Devices, Inc.   Tel: 714-381-4364
287 S. Stoddard Ave.   Fax: 714-888-7190
San Bernardino, CA 92401-2021
CEO: Sam Nannetti, VP
    Johannes R. Wiesbauer, CEO & President
    Cory Baehr, VP
    Agnes LaYarda, Ass't VP Fin.
Production: Vickie M. Bullock, Production Mgr.
Federal Procurement Eligibility: Small Business
Device Category:
Kit, Laparoscopy .... GASTRO/UROLOGY

Amsco   Tel: 814-452-3100
2424 West 23rd Street   Tel: 800-333-8838
P.O. Box 620   Fax: 814-870-8475
Erie, PA 16506
Advertising: Lynda Veshecco, Mktg. Comm.
CEO: Steven F. Kreger, Corp. VP & Controller
    Keith Stoneback, Corp. VP
    John R. Hamilton, Corp. VP HR
    David Nelson, President, CEO, & COB
    David L. Bellitt, President AMSCO Eng. Svc.
    Daniel Barry, VP Corp. Finance & Admin./CFO
    Carl Gatewood, Corp. VP
Marketing: Mark Lane, VP Distribution Mktg.
    James R. Murray, VP Mktg. Dev.
    Eugene Jennings, VP Mktg./Bus. Dev.
Production: Thomas Van Dyke, VP Mfg.
    Eugene Jennings, VP Int'l Oper.
Research: John R. Anke, Sec. & Treasurer
    Gary L. Graham, M.D., Corp. VP R&D
Device Category:
Accessories, Cleaning, Endoscopic .... GASTRO/UROLOGY
Sterilizer/Washer, Endoscope .... GENERAL

Amtec Med. Prod., Inc.   Tel: 310-946-8505
13007 E. Park Ave.   Fax: 310-941-6328
Santa Fe Springs, CA 90670-4005
CEO: Wonni Salerno, VP
    Albert Salerno, President
Device Category:
Laryngoscope .... EAR/NOSE/THROAT

Anesthesia Associates, Inc.   Tel: 619-744-6561
460 Enterprise St.   Fax: 619-744-0054
San Marcos, CA 92069-4363
CEO: George Jackson, President
    Donald Rowean, VP
Production: Mary Klein, Office Mgr.
Federal Procurement Eligibility: VA Contract
Device Category:
Laryngoscope .... EAR/NOSE/THROAT

Anesthesia Medical Specialties, Inc.   Tel: 310-946-8303
13007 E. Park Ave.   Tel: 800-445-0597
Santa Fe Springs, CA 90670-4005   Fax: 310-941-6328
CEO: Al Salerno, President
Marketing: Wonni Salerno, VP Sales
Production: Robert Salerno
Device Category:
Laryngoscope .... EAR/NOSE/THROAT
Laryngoscope, Rigid .... ANESTH/PUL MED

178 / SUPPLIER PROFILES

Annex Medical, Inc.   Tel: 612-942-7576
7098 Shady Oak Rd.
Eden Prairie, MN 55344-3505
CEO: Stuart J. Lind, President
Device Category:
Accessories, Cleaning, Endoscopic .... GASTRO/UROLOGY
Brush, Cytology, Endoscopic .... GASTRO/UROLOGY

Anspach Effort, Inc.   Tel: 407-627-1080
4500 Riverside Dr.   Tel: 800-327-6887
Palm Beach Gardens, FL 33410   Fax: 800-327-6661
CEO: W. E. Anspach, Jr., MD
Marketing: Eileen M. WIlkins, Marketing
    Charles E. McGarrity, Nat'l Sales Mgr.
Production: C. Dale Sharrock
Federal Procurement Eligibility: Small Business, GSA Contract, VA
    Contract
Device Category:
Accessories, Arthroscope .... ORTHOPEDICS

Anthro Corporation   Tel: 503-241-7113
3221 N.W. Yeon St.   Tel: 800-325-3841
Portland, OR 97210   Fax: 503-241-1619
CEO: Shoaib Tareen, CEO
Marketing: Cathy Filgas, VP Sales & Mktg.
Federal Procurement Eligibility: Small Business, GSA Contract
Device Category:
Cart, Equipment, Video .... GENERAL

Apple Medical Corp.   Tel: 508-779-2926
93 Nashaway Rd.   Tel: 800-255-2926
Bolton, MA 01740   Fax: 508-779-6927
CEO: Robert W. Schaefer, President
Marketing: Scott E. Coleridge, VP Mktg.
    Ian Stevenson, Intl. Sales/Mktg. Mgr.
    E.J. Jones, VP Sales
Federal Procurement Eligibility: Small Business
Device Category:
Cord, Electric, Endoscope .... GASTRO/UROLOGY
Drain, Suction, Closed .... MIN. INV. SURGERY
Electrocautery Unit, Endoscopic .... OBSTETRICS/GYN
Equipment, Suction/Irrigation, Laparoscopic .... SURGERY
Extractor, Gall Bladder .... MIN. INV. SURGERY
Forceps, Laparoscopy, Electrosurgical .... SURGERY
Holder, Instrument, Laparoscopic .... MIN. INV. SURGERY
Illuminator, Fiberoptic (For Endoscope) .... GASTRO/UROLOGY
Instrument, Electrosurgery, Laparoscopic .... MIN. INV. SURGERY
Needle, Insufflation, Laparoscopic .... MIN. INV. SURGERY
Probe, Electrocauterization, Single-Use .... MIN. INV. SURGERY
Probe, Suction, Irrigator/Aspirator, Laparoscopic .... MIN. INV. SURGERY
Trocar, Abdominal .... GASTRO/UROLOGY
Trocar, Gallbladder .... GASTRO/UROLOGY
Trocar, Gastro-Urology .... GASTRO/UROLOGY
Trocar, Laparoscopic .... SURGERY
Trocar, Other .... GENERAL
Trocar, Short .... MIN. INV. SURGERY
Trocar, Thoracic .... CARDIOVASCULAR

Applied Fiberoptics, Inc.   Tel: 508-765-9121
E. Main St.   Tel: 800-225-7486
Southbridge, MA 01550   Fax: 508-764-3639
Advertising: Peter Kelleher, Adv. Mgr.
CEO: J. Will Hicks
Marketing: Charles Kiritsy, Mktg. Mgr.
Production: James Noonan
Federal Procurement Eligibility: Small Business
Device Category:
Colposcope .... OBSTETRICS/GYN
Lamp, Endoscopic, Incandescent .... SURGERY
Light, Surgical, Endoscopic .... SURGERY

Applied Medical Resources   Tel: 714-582-6120
26051 Merit Circle #104   Tel: 800-282-2212
Laguna Hills, CA 92653-7008   Fax: 714-582-6134
Advertising: Signe Dunn, Adv. Mgr.
CEO: Said S. Hilal, President & CEO
    Nabil Hilal, Gen. Mgr.
    George Wallace, Gen. Mgr.
Production: Vaughn Whalen, VP Oper.
Device Category:
Catheter, Cholangiography .... SURGERY
Trocar, Cardiovascular .... CARDIOVASCULAR

Aran Technology Inc.   Tel: 714-951-7750
23061 La Cadena Dr.   Fax: 714-951-9370
Laguna Hills, CA 92653
CEO: Homayoun Archang, President
Device Category:
Camera, Videotape, Surgical .... SURGERY

Arbor Technologies   Tel: 313-665-3300
3728 Plaza Dr.   Fax: 313-665-3516
Ann Arbor, MI 48108-7354
CEO: Monty E. Vincent, President
Marketing: Mary Boomus, SVP
Production: Leonard Knoedler, SVP
Research: Dawn I. Moore, Dir. QA
Federal Procurement Eligibility: Small Business
Device Category:
Insufflator, Other .... SURGERY

Armstrong Medical Industries Inc.   Tel: 708-913-0101
575 Knightsbridge Pkwy.   Tel: 800-323-4220
P.O. Box 700   Fax: 708-913-0138
Lincolnshire, IL 60069-3616
Advertising: Nan Hughes
CEO: Warren G. Armstrong, President
Marketing: George Mede, VP Sales & Mktg.
Federal Procurement Eligibility: Small Business, GSA Contract
Device Category:
Cart, Equipment, Video .... GENERAL

Arrow International, Inc.   Tel: 215-378-0131
3000 Bernville Rd.   Tel: 800-523-8446
Reading, PA 19605   Fax: 215-374-5360
Advertising: Rick Yanchuleff, Mgr. Corp. Comm.
    Lynne David, Adv. Spvr./Media
CEO: Tom Nickel, VP Reg. Affairs
    Ray Neag, SVP
    Marlin Miller, President
    John Broadbent, VP Fin. & Treasurer
Marketing: Peter McGregor, Mgr. Tech. Prod.
    Paul L. Frankhouser, VP Mktg.
    Patty Johnson, Mgr. Prod. Support
    Nancy Fidler, CS Mgr.
    Linda Wegman, Nat'l. Sales Mgr.
    David Stuckert, Dir. U.S. Sales
    Chris Mennone, Int'l Sales Mgr.
Production: Ron Torrence, VP Mfg.
Research: Phil Fleck, VP Res. & Eng.
Federal Procurement Eligibility: GSA Contract, VA Contract
Device Category:
Catheter, Cholangiography .... SURGERY
Trocar, Gallbladder .... GASTRO/UROLOGY

Arthrex Arthroscopy Instrument Tel: 813-643-5553
3050 North Horseshoe Dr., Ste. 168 Tel: 800-933-7001
Naples, FL 33942-7909 Fax: 813-643-6218
CEO: Reinhold Schmieding, President
Marketing: Kathy L'Esperance, Customer Svc. Mgr.
  Dennis Donnermeyer, Nat'l. Sales Mgr.
  Dennis D. Meyer, VP Sales
Production: Don Grafton, VP Eng.
Federal Procurement Eligibility: Small Business
Device Category:
Accessories, Arthroscope .... ORTHOPEDICS
Arthroscope .... ORTHOPEDICS
Cannula, Drainage, Arthroscopy .... ORTHOPEDICS
Holder, Leg, Arthroscopy .... ORTHOPEDICS
Holder, Shoulder, Arthroscopy .... SURGERY

Arthrex Medical Instrument GmbH Tel: 89/142257
Von Kahr Str. 2
D-80997 Muenchen 50
Germany
CEO: Reinhold Schmieding, President
Production: Dieter Rapp, Controller
Device Category:
Accessories, Arthroscope .... ORTHOPEDICS
Arthroscope .... ORTHOPEDICS
Cannula, Drainage, Arthroscopy .... ORTHOPEDICS
Holder, Leg, Arthroscopy .... ORTHOPEDICS

Arthro-Medic, Inc. Tel: 904-296-1188
4203 Belfort Rd., Ste. 150 Tel: 800-827-8476
Jacksonville, FL 32216-5896 Fax: 904-296-1122
Advertising: Gloria Williams, Adv. Mgr.
  Brenda Williams
CEO: Susan Williams, President
  John Webster Williams, Jr., CEO
Marketing: Teresa Williams, VP Sales & Mktg.
  Linda Williams
Federal Procurement Eligibility: Small Business
Device Category:
Accessories, Arthroscope .... ORTHOPEDICS
Holder, Leg, Arthroscopy .... ORTHOPEDICS

Arthrotek, Inc. Tel: 909-988-5595
4861 E. Airport Dr. Tel: 800-348-9500
Ontario, CA 91761
CEO: Tom Prichard, President
  Jeanette Kleist, Admin. Mgr.
Marketing: Stuart Kleopfer, Dir. Mktg.
Production: Susan Steen, R&D Mgr.
  DeeAnne Weber
Device Category:
Accessories, Photographic, Endoscopic .... GASTRO/UROLOGY

Asahi Optical Co., Ltd. Tel: 03/3960-5155
2-36-9, Maeno-Cho, Itabashi-Ku Fax: 03/3960-5226
Tokyo 174
Japan
CEO: Tohru Matsumoto, President
Marketing: Kinhei Yajima, Managing Dir.
Device Category:
Bronchoscope, Flexible .... EAR/NOSE/THROAT
Choledochoscope, Flexible Or Rigid .... GASTRO/UROLOGY
Colonoscope, General & Plastic Surgery .... SURGERY
Cystoscope .... GASTRO/UROLOGY
Duodenoscope, Esophago/Gastro .... GASTRO/UROLOGY
Endoscope, Electronic (Videoendoscope) .... SURGERY
Esophagoscope (Flexible Or Rigid) .... EAR/NOSE/THROAT
Gastroscope, Flexible .... GASTRO/UROLOGY
Nasopharyngoscope (Flexible Or Rigid) .... EAR/NOSE/THROAT
Sigmoidoscope, Flexible .... GASTRO/UROLOGY

Aspen Laboratories, Inc. Tel: 303-798-5800
P.O. Box 3936 Tel: 800-552-0138
Englewood, CO 80155-3936 Fax: 303-797-1491
CEO: Russ Gill, VP Finance
  Richard Drew, EVP & Gen. Mgr.
Marketing: Greg Loshak, Mktg. Dir.
Production: Ron Cosens, VP Oper.
Federal Procurement Eligibility: Small Business, VA Contract
Device Category:
Component, Electrical .... GENERAL
Forceps, Electrosurgical .... SURGERY
Forceps, Grasping, Flexible Endoscopic .... GASTRO/UROLOGY

ATD-American Co., Furniture Div. Tel: 215-576-1000
143 Greenwood Ave. Tel: 800-523-2300
Wyncote, PA 19095-1337 Fax: 215-576-1827
Advertising: Arnold Zaslow, VP
Marketing: Lida Goodhart, Mktg. Co-ord.
  Janet Wischnia, Prod. Mgr.
Federal Procurement Eligibility: Small Business, GSA Contract
Device Category:
Cart, Equipment, Video .... GENERAL

ATD-American Co., Hospital Tel: 215-576-1000
Supply Div. Tel: 800-523-2300
115-149 Greenwood Ave. Fax: 215-576-1827
Wyncote, PA 19095-1325
Medical Products Sales Volume: $50,000,000
Total Employees: 120
Distribution: Manufacturer and Distributor
CEO: Jerome M. Zaslow, President
Marketing: Lida Goodhart, Med. Surg. Prod. Mgr.
  Bruce Rappaport, Gen. Mgr.
  Arnold Zaslow, EVP Mktg.
Production: Spencer Zaslow, EVP Prod.
Federal Procurement Eligibility: Small Business, GSA Contract, VA Contract
Device Category:
Cart, Equipment, Video .... GENERAL

Austin Biomedical, Inc. Tel: 512-459-6611
4211 Medical Pkwy Tel: 800-257-2284
Austin, TX 78756-3309 Fax: 512-454-1197
CEO: Jack W. Moncrief
  Christina Jonk, Office Mgr.
Marketing: Lisa Moncrief
Federal Procurement Eligibility: Small Business
Device Category:
Trocar, Abdominal .... GASTRO/UROLOGY

Automated Medical Products Corp. Tel: 212-874-0236
2315 Broadway, Ste. 410 Tel: 800-832-4567
New York, NY 10024-4332 Fax: 212-787-0488
CEO: Gregory Diamant, CEO
  Emil Eisenberg, VP
Federal Procurement Eligibility: Small Business, GSA Contract, VA Contract
Device Category:
Holder, Laparoscope .... OBSTETRICS/GYN
Peritoneoscope .... GASTRO/UROLOGY
Retractor, Fan-Type, Laparoscopy .... MIN. INV. SURGERY
Retractor, Laparoscopy, Other .... MIN. INV. SURGERY

SUPPLIER PROFILES

Axiom Medical, Inc.   Tel: 310-898-1779
2377 Crenshaw Blvd., Ste. 330   Tel: 800-221-8569
Torrance, CA 90501   Fax: 310-632-1326
CEO: J. Rae Walker, M.D., President
Marketing: James Stewart
Production: Don May
Research: R. Hardy, R&D
Federal Procurement Eligibility: Small Business, Woman Owned
Device Category:
Trocar, Thoracic..CARDIOVASCULAR

B.E.C. Medical Products   Tel: 419-693-5307
615 Front St.   Tel: 800-331-6561
Toledo, OH 43605-2105   Fax: 419-691-1227
CEO: Norman J. Huff, VP
    James P. Kulla, President
Marketing: James A. Quick, Nat'l. Sales Dir.
Production: William Sevey, Mfg. Dir.
Federal Procurement Eligibility: Small Business
Device Category:
Kit, Laparoscopy...GASTRO/UROLOGY

Bag   Tel: 57/810464
B.P. 68   Fax: 56/391909
M. Rue de Fieuzal
F-33523 Bruges, Cedex
France
CEO: Antoine Baggio, General Dir.
Device Category:
Endoscope And Accessories, Battery-Powered................SURGERY
Endoscope, Direct Vision...SURGERY
Endoscope, Fetal Blood Sampling.......................OBSTETRICS/GYN

Bard Urological   Tel: 404-784-6113
8195 Industrial Blvd.
Covington, GA 30209-2656
CEO: Phil Ehert, President
    N. Mulkeen, VP Personnel
    D. Mullis, Regulatory Affairs Mgr.
Marketing: T. Lemberg, Contract Sales Mgr.
    R. Dunford, Mkt. Res. Mgr.
    M.A. Brady, Sales Training Mgr.
    James Stevens, Mktg. Comm. Mgr.
    David Christianson, VP Sales
    Dave McKinley, VP Mktg.
    A. Iadaresa, Intl. Sales & Mktg. Mgr.
Research: W. Norton, VP R&D
    Robert Dunford
Federal Procurement Eligibility: GSA Contract
Device Category:
Trocar, Abdominal...GASTRO/UROLOGY
Ureteroscope..GASTRO/UROLOGY

Bashir, Jamil & Bros. Pvt. Ltd.   Tel: 0432-553862
Khadim Ali Rd.   Fax: 0432-553455
P.O. Box 7
Sialkot
Pakistan
CEO: Sarfaraz Bashir
    M. B. Chaudhry
Production: M. E. Chaudhry
Device Category:
Clip, Suture..SURGERY
Proctoscope...SURGERY
Trocar, Cardiovascular...CARDIOVASCULAR
Trocar, Thoracic..CARDIOVASCULAR
Trocar, Tracheal...EAR/NOSE/THROAT

Bauer & Haselbarth GmbH   Tel: 04106/72091
Sauerbruchstr. 7 - Postfach   Fax: 04106/71047
D-25479 Ellerau bei Hamburg
Germany
Advertising: Ulrich Krings
CEO: Erhard Lenz, Mg. Dir. & President
Marketing: Helga Luebbe
Production: Manfred Salamon
Device Category:
Laryngoscope..EAR/NOSE/THROAT
Trocar, Cardiovascular...CARDIOVASCULAR
Urethroscope..GASTRO/UROLOGY

Bauerfeind USA, Inc.   Tel: 404-429-8330
Suite 114   Fax: 404-429-8477
1590 North Roberts Rd.
Kennesaw, GA 30144-3679
Marketing: Bernard F. Beaulieu
Federal Procurement Eligibility: Small Business
Device Category:
Holder, Shoulder, Arthroscopy..................................SURGERY

Baxter Healthcare Corp.   Tel: 708-473-0400
Hospital Supply Div.   Fax: 708-473-3165
1450 Waukegan Road
McGaw Park, IL 60085-8205
Medical Products Sales Volume: $1,486,900,000
Total Employees: 35,000
Distribution: Exclusive Distributor
CEO: Charles Jones
Device Category:
Anoscope, Non-Powered......................................GASTRO/UROLOGY

Baxter Healthcare Corp.   Tel: 708-647-9383
V. Mueller Div.
6600 W. Touhy
Niles, IL 60714
Distribution: Manufacturer Direct
Marketing: Diane Evans-Fitts, Product Mgr.
Device Category:
Forceps, Biopsy..MIN. INV. SURGERY
Scissors, Laparoscopy..MIN. INV. SURGERY

Becton Dickinson And Co.   Tel: 201-847-6800
Becton Dickinson Div.   Fax: 201-847-6475
One Becton Dr.
Franklin Lakes, NJ 07417-1815
Medical Products Sales Volume: $160,000,000 (E)
Total Employees: 3,000
Distribution: Manufacturer Through Distributors
Advertising: Daniel C. Grimm, Mktg. Comm. Mgr.
CEO: Robert S. Mink, Mktg. Dir.
    Robert E. Flaherty, President
Marketing: Robert L. Jones Jr., VP Sales
    Gary Cohen, Mktg. Dir.
Production: Frank B. Calabrese
Research: John Kao
Federal Procurement Eligibility: GSA Contract, VA Contract
Device Category:
Arthrogram Kit..ORTHOPEDICS

Berchtold Corp.
2050 Mabeline Rd., Ste. C
North Charlestown, SC 29418-4643
CEO: William R. Apperson, President
Marketing: Wylie M. Faw III, VP Mktg. & Sales
Federal Procurement Eligibility: GSA Contract, VA Contract
Device Category:
Cart, Equipment, Video..GENERAL
Electrode, Electrosurgery, Laparoscopic .... MIN. INV. SURGERY
Forceps, Laparoscopy, Electrosurgical .... SURGERY
Peritoneoscope .... GASTRO/UROLOGY

Tel: 803-569-6100
Tel: 800-243-5135
Fax: 803-569-6133

Berkeley Medevices, Inc.
907 Camelia St.
Berkeley, CA 94710-1419
CEO: Donna Kubny, Sec'y & Treas.
    Dieter Kubny, President
Federal Procurement Eligibility: Small Business
Device Category:
Hysteroscope .... OBSTETRICS/GYN

Tel: 510-526-4046
Tel: 800-227-2388
Fax: 510-526-0149

Bilmar Enterprises, Inc.
1211 W. La Palma Ave. #707
Anaheim, CA 92801-2855
CEO: William Cohen, President & CEO
    Marvin Udjoff, VP
    Elia Udhoff, Secretary
    Daril Cotler, Treasurer
Federal Procurement Eligibility: Small Business
Device Category:
Sterilizer/Washer, Endoscope .... GENERAL

Tel: 714-991-9170

Bio Quantum Technologies, Inc.
10270 S. Progress Way
P.O. Box 646
Parker, CO 80134
CEO: John F. Thomas, President
Device Category:
Colposcope .... OBSTETRICS/GYN

Tel: 303-840-9981
Fax: 303-841-3360

Biocare International, Inc.
3375 Park Ave., Suite 2000A
Wantagh, NY 11793-3712
CEO: Steven H. Reichman, President
Marketing: M. Seamans
Federal Procurement Eligibility: Small Business, Woman Owned
Device Category:
Laparoscope, General & Plastic Surgery .... SURGERY
Laparoscope, Gynecologic .... OBSTETRICS/GYN

Tel: 516-781-5800
Fax: 516-781-4934

Biodynamic Technologies, Inc.
1425 E. Newport Center Dr.
Deerfield Beach, FL 33442
CEO: Stephen Roy, President
Production: H.L. Rutkin, VP
Federal Procurement Eligibility: Small Business
Device Category:
Holder, Shoulder, Arthroscopy .... SURGERY

Tel: 305-421-3166
Fax: 305-570-6368

Bioenterics Corporation
1035A Cindy Lane
Carpinteria, CA 93013
CEO: Jim McGhan, President
    Ellen Duke, Gen. Mgr.
Marketing: Keith Lowrey, Reg. Affairs Mgr.
Production: Lola Zazueta, Production Spvr.
Research: Frederick Coe, Eng. Mgr.
Device Category:
Bougie, Esophageal, And Gastrointestinal,
    Gastro-Urology .... GASTRO/UROLOGY
Bougie, Esophageal, ENT .... EAR/NOSE/THROAT
Thoracoscope .... CARDIOVASCULAR

Tel: 805-684-3045
Tel: 800-435-4353
Fax: 805-684-0812

Biomedical Exports, Inc.
8002 California Ave.
P.O. Box 740
Fair Oaks, CA 95628-7506
CEO: Mike Mooney
Device Category:
Camera, Videotape, Surgical .... SURGERY

Tel: 916-967-4917
Fax: 916-863-1206

Biosearch Medical Products, Inc.
P.O. Box 1700
35 Industrial Pkwy.
Somerville, NJ 08876-1276
Advertising: John Kovar, Product Mgr.
CEO: Robert H. Bea, VP QA & Reg. Affairs
    Manfred F. Dyck, President & CEO
    Edward J. Milnarich, CFO
Marketing: Ursula M. Dyck, VP Sales Admin.
    Joan Newman, Int'l Sales & Mktg. Mgr.
Production: Robert Moravsik, VP Law
    Michael P. Eldredge, Contr.
    Martin C. Dyck, VP Operations
    Jim Sullivan, Materials Mgr.
    Algred Patrick, VP Eng. & R&D
Research: Robert Shull, Regional Mgr.
Federal Procurement Eligibility: Small Business, GSA Contract, VA
    Contract
Device Category:
Equipment, Suction/Irrigation, Laparoscopic .... SURGERY

Tel: 908-722-5000
Tel: 800-326-5976
Fax: 908-722-5024

Birtcher Medical Systems Inc.
Endoscopy Div.
41 Brooks Dr.
Braintree, MA 02184
CEO: Robert L. Kane, President
Federal Procurement Eligibility: Small Business
Device Category:
Light Source, Endoscope, Xenon Arc .... SURGERY

Tel: 617-356-4830
Fax: 617-356-4841

Birtcher Medical Systems, Inc.
Tel: 714-753-9400
Tel: 800-888-1771
Fax: 714-753-9171
50 Technology Dr.
Irvine, CA 92718-2301
Advertising: Jill Bye, Adv. Mgr.
CEO: William E. Maya, President & CEO
  Elizabeth Stevens, Dir. Personnel
Marketing: William Meyer, Intl. Sales/Mktg. Mgr.
  James Stevens, VP Sales
  Brian Kenney, Sales Training Mgr.
Production: Robert Berger, VP Mfg.
  Eric Galcher, Materials Mgr.
  Doug Bueschel, Reg. Affairs Mgr.
  Amy Lehmann Adkisson, Sr. Product Mgr. Endoscopy
Research: Harold J. Walbrink, VP R&D
Federal Procurement Eligibility: Small Business, GSA Contract, VA Contract
Device Category:
Camera, Video, Endoscopic...GENERAL
Camera, Video, Multi-Image............................MIN. INV. SURGERY
Clamp, Laparoscopy.......................................MIN. INV. SURGERY
Coagulator, Laparoscopic, Unipolar.....................OBSTETRICS/GYN
Coagulator/Cutter, Endoscopic, Bipolar................OBSTETRICS/GYN
Coagulator/Cutter, Endoscopic, Unipolar..............OBSTETRICS/GYN
Electrocautery Unit, Endoscopic..........................OBSTETRICS/GYN
Electrode, Electrosurgery, Laparoscopic...............MIN. INV. SURGERY
Endoscope And Accessories, AC-Powered.........................SURGERY
Endoscope, Rigid..SURGERY
Equipment, Suction/Irrigation, Laparoscopic....................SURGERY
Forceps, Electrosurgical..SURGERY
Forceps, Endoscopic..GASTRO/UROLOGY
Forceps, Grasping, Atraumatic..........................MIN. INV. SURGERY
Forceps, Grasping, Traumatic............................MIN. INV. SURGERY
Generator, Power, Electrosurgical....................................SURGERY
Holder, Needle, Curved, Laparoscopic................MIN. INV. SURGERY
Holder, Needle, Laparoscopic...........................MIN. INV. SURGERY
Instrument, Dissecting, Laparoscopic................MIN. INV. SURGERY
Insufflator, Laparoscopic.....................................OBSTETRICS/GYN
Laparoscope, Flexible..SURGERY
Light Source, Endoscope, Xenon Arc...............................SURGERY
Light, Surgical, Endoscopic..SURGERY
Probe, Electrocauterization, Multi-Use..............MIN. INV. SURGERY
Probe, Electrocauterization, Single-Use.............MIN. INV. SURGERY
Probe, Suction, Irrigator/Aspirator, Laparoscopic....MIN. INV. SURGERY
Retractor, Fan-Type, Laparoscopy......................MIN. INV. SURGERY
Telescope, Rigid, Endoscopic..............................GASTRO/UROLOGY
Thoracoscope..CARDIOVASCULAR

Bissinger Guenter Medizintechnik GmbH
Tel: 07641/8038
Fax: 07641/54984
Gottlieb-Daimler Str.5
D-79331 Teningen 1
Germany
Ownership: Private
Distribution: Excl. Distributor
CEO: Guenter Bissinger, President
Device Category:
Coagulator/Cutter, Endoscopic, Bipolar................OBSTETRICS/GYN

Blickman Health Industries
Tel: 201-909-0807
Tel: 800-247-5070
Fax: 201-909-0832
39 Robinson Rd. (at Rt. 17S)
Lodi, NJ 07644
CEO: Fred Heisman, President
  Ben Freedman, CEO
  Paul Freedman, VP Finance & Admin.
Marketing: Judy Siboni, VP Sales
  Carol Heisman, VP Mktg.
Production: Robert Freedman, VP Manufacturing
Federal Procurement Eligibility: Small Business, Woman Owned, GSA Contract
Device Category:
Cart, Equipment, Video...GENERAL

Blue Bell Bio-Medical
Tel: 215-699-2266
Fax: 215-699-8596
P.O. Box 455
Blue Bell, PA 19422
Advertising: Ronnie Sensinger, Adv. Adm.
CEO: Lei Barry, President
  Frank Mahan, VP
Production: Thomas Ford, VP Fin.
Research: Frank Mahan, VP
Federal Procurement Eligibility: Small Business, Woman Owned, VA Contract
Device Category:
Cart, Equipment, Video...GENERAL

Blue Ridge Anesthesia & Critical Care
Tel: 804-846-2637
Tel: 800-843-9075
Fax: 804-846-2676
1201-1207 Jefferson St.
Lynchburg, VA 24504-1813
Total Employees: 25
Distribution: Exclusive Distributor & Distributor
CEO: Willie H. Morris, President
  Steven Morris, CFO
Marketing: Brett R. Smith, VP
Federal Procurement Eligibility: Small Business
Device Category:
Laryngoscope...EAR/NOSE/THROAT

Boehm Surgical Instrument Corp.
Tel: 716-436-6584
Fax: 716-436-6428
966 Chili Avenue
Rochester, NY 14611-2831
CEO: Richard J. Boehm, President
Production: Paul R. Boehm, Gen. Mgr.
Federal Procurement Eligibility: Small Business
Device Category:
Bronchoscope, Rigid..EAR/NOSE/THROAT
Cystoscope...GASTRO/UROLOGY
Esophagoscope (Flexible Or Rigid)....................EAR/NOSE/THROAT
Laryngoscope, Rigid...ANESTH/PUL MED
Proctoscope..SURGERY
Proctosigmoidoscope..GASTRO/UROLOGY
Sigmoidoscope, Rigid, Non-Electrical................GASTRO/UROLOGY

Boss Instruments, Ltd.
Tel: 615-885-2231
Fax: 615-885-2992
1310 Central Ct.
Hermitage, TN 37076
CEO: Burns Phillips, President
Federal Procurement Eligibility: Small Business
Device Category:
Cannula, Extraction, Appendix..........................MIN. INV. SURGERY
Clamp, Fixation, Cholangiography....................MIN. INV. SURGERY
Coagulator, Laparoscopic, Unipolar....................OBSTETRICS/GYN
Dilator, Blunt..MIN. INV. SURGERY
Equipment, Suction/Irrigation, Laparoscopic....................SURGERY
Forceps, Grasping, Atraumatic..........................MIN. INV. SURGERY
Holder, Needle, Laparoscopic...........................MIN. INV. SURGERY
Instrument, Dissecting, Laparoscopic................MIN. INV. SURGERY
Instrument, Knot Tying, Suture, Laparoscopic....MIN. INV. SURGERY
Instrument, Needle Holder/Knot Tying..............MIN. INV. SURGERY
Instrument, Passing, Suture, Laparoscopic........MIN. INV. SURGERY
Laparoscope, General & Plastic Surgery.........................SURGERY
Needle, Insufflation, Laparoscopic....................MIN. INV. SURGERY
Probe, Suction, Irrigator/Aspirator, Laparoscopic....MIN. INV. SURGERY

Retractor, Fan-Type, Laparoscopy......................MIN. INV. SURGERY
Retractor, Laparoscopy, Other............................MIN. INV. SURGERY
Trocar, Abdominal..GASTRO/UROLOGY
Trocar, Gallbladder...GASTRO/UROLOGY
Trocar, Gastro-Urology..GASTRO/UROLOGY
Trocar, Thoracic...CARDIOVASCULAR

Bristol-Myers Squibb Company
Australia
556 Princes Highway
P.O. Box 39
Noble Park, VIC 3174
Australia
Tel: 03/7953722
Tel: 008/335384
Fax: 03/7950968
Medical Products Sales Volume: $3,000,000
Total Employees: 11
Distribution: Excl. Distributor
CEO: John Burton, General Mgr.
Production: Leon Hoare, Group Prod. Mgr.
Device Category:
Insufflator, Hysteroscopic......................................OBSTETRICS/GYN
Kit, Laparoscopy..GASTRO/UROLOGY

Bryan Corp.
4 Plympton St.
Woburn, MA 01801-2908
Tel: 617-935-0004
Tel: 800-343-7711
Fax: 617-935-7602
CEO: Frank Abrano, President
Marketing: Nancy Barbieri, Dir. Mktg.
  John L. Sullivan, VP Sales & Mktg.
Federal Procurement Eligibility: Small Business, Woman Owned, GSA Contract
Device Category:
Applier, Clip, Laparoscopic...................................MIN. INV. SURGERY
Bronchoscope, Rigid..EAR/NOSE/THROAT
Bronchoscope, Rigid, Non-Ventilating................ANESTH/PUL MED
Bronchoscope, Rigid, Ventilating.........................ANESTH/PUL MED
Camera, Video, Endoscopic..................................GENERAL
Coagulator, Laparoscopic, Unipolar....................OBSTETRICS/GYN
Cord, Electric, Endoscope.....................................GASTRO/UROLOGY
Endoscope...GASTRO/UROLOGY
Endoscope, Direct Vision.......................................SURGERY
Endoscope, Rigid...SURGERY
Endoscope, Transcervical (Amnioscope)...........OBSTETRICS/GYN
Equipment, Suction/Irrigation, Laparoscopic....SURGERY
Forceps, Endoscopic..GASTRO/UROLOGY
Forceps, Grasping, Atraumatic............................MIN. INV. SURGERY
Forceps, Grasping, Traumatic..............................MIN. INV. SURGERY
Holder, Needle, Laparoscopic..............................MIN. INV. SURGERY
Hysteroscope..OBSTETRICS/GYN
Illuminator, Fiberoptic (For Endoscope)............GASTRO/UROLOGY
Instrument, Dissecting, Laparoscopic.................MIN. INV. SURGERY
*Insufflator, Carbon-Dioxide, Automatic
  (For Endoscope)*..GASTRO/UROLOGY
Insufflator, Hysteroscopic......................................OBSTETRICS/GYN
Insufflator, Laparoscopic..OBSTETRICS/GYN
Insufflator, Other..SURGERY
Kit, Laparoscopy..GASTRO/UROLOGY
Light Source, Endoscope, Xenon Arc.................SURGERY
Monitor, Video, Endoscope...................................GENERAL
Needle, Endoscopic..GASTRO/UROLOGY
Needle, Insufflation, Laparoscopic......................MIN. INV. SURGERY
Probe, Suction, Irrigator/Aspirator, Laparoscopic....MIN. INV. SURGERY
Retractor, Fan-Type, Laparoscopy......................MIN. INV. SURGERY
Sheath, Endoscopic..GASTRO/UROLOGY
Tape, Television & Video, Endoscopic..............GASTRO/UROLOGY
Telescope, Rigid, Endoscopic...............................GASTRO/UROLOGY
Thoracoscope...CARDIOVASCULAR
Trocar, Abdominal..GASTRO/UROLOGY
Trocar, ENT...EAR/NOSE/THROAT
Trocar, Gallbladder...GASTRO/UROLOGY

Trocar, Gastro-Urology..GASTRO/UROLOGY
Trocar, Other..GENERAL
Trocar, Short...MIN. INV. SURGERY
Trocar, Thoracic...CARDIOVASCULAR

Buck GmbH, Rudolf
Obere Hauptstr. 40/1
D-78573 Wurmlingen-Tuttlingen
Germany
Tel: 07/461-3535
Fax: 07/461-14182
CEO: Herbert Schmid, Mgr.
Research: Michael Berger
Device Category:
Laryngoscope..EAR/NOSE/THROAT
Laryngoscope, Surgical..SURGERY
Transformer, Endoscope..SURGERY

Bulbtronics
45 Banfi Plaza
P.O. Box 306
Farmingdale, NY 11735-1539
Tel: 516-249-2272
Tel: 800-654-8542
Fax: 516-249-6066
Advertising: John V. Roberts
CEO: Mark Winter, CFO
  Frances Thaw
Marketing: Elayne Gray, VP Sales
Federal Procurement Eligibility: Small Business, Woman Owned, VA Contract
Device Category:
Lamp, Endoscopic, Incandescent.........................SURGERY
Light Source, Endoscope, Xenon Arc.................SURGERY

Burton Medical Products, Inc.
7922 Haskell Avenue
Van Nuys, CA 91406-1923
Tel: 818-989-4700
Fax: 818-989-3250
CEO: Robert D. Christianson, Gen. Mgr.
Marketing: Judy A. Thomas, Mktg. Mgr.
Production: Joe Engle, Operations Mgr.
Federal Procurement Eligibility: VA Contract
Device Category:
Laryngoscope..EAR/NOSE/THROAT

C.R. Bard Inc.
Interventional Products Div.
6091 Heisley Rd.
Mentor, OH 44060-1835
Tel: 216-352-2935
Fax: 216-352-0880
Ownership: Public
Distribution: Manufacturer Direct
CEO: John Delucia, Reg. Affairs Mgr.
  Brad Ciley, Bus. Dev. Mgr.
  Amy Paul, President
Marketing: Michael Barra, Dir. Mktg.
  Chuck Gerlowski, Natl. Sales Mgr.
Production: Paul Mucci, Oper. Mgr.
Device Category:
Endoscope...GASTRO/UROLOGY
Sterilizer/Washer, Endoscope...............................GENERAL

Cabot Medical Corp.
2021 Cabot Blvd. West
Langhorne, PA 19047-1875
Tel: 215-752-8300
Tel: 800-523-6078
Fax: 215-750-0161
CEO: Warren G. Wood, COB & CEO
  Noel Wray, VP & Finance Admin.
  John Mordock, President & COO
  Gary Pond, President, Surgitek, Inc.
Marketing: Jack Addicks, VP Sales
  Glenn Stahl, VP Mktg.
Production: Paul Helms, VP Oper.
  Adam Meyers, Mfg. Dir.
Federal Procurement Eligibility: Small Business
Device Category:

Accessories, Cleaning, Endoscopic	GASTRO/UROLOGY
Accessories, Photographic, Endoscopic	GASTRO/UROLOGY
Accessories, Surgical Camera	SURGERY
Adapter, Bulb, Endoscope, Miscellaneous	GASTRO/UROLOGY
Anoscope, Non-Powered	GASTRO/UROLOGY
Applier, Clip, Laparoscopic	MIN. INV. SURGERY
Bag, Specimen, Laparoscopic	MIN. INV. SURGERY
Balloon, Manipulation, Tissue	MIN. INV. SURGERY
Camera, Television, Endoscopic, Without Audio	SURGERY
Camera, Video, Endoscopic	GENERAL
Camera, Videotape, Surgical	SURGERY
Cannula, Suction/Irrigation, Laparoscopic	SURGERY
Cart, Equipment, Video	GENERAL
Coagulator, Hysteroscopic (With Accessories)	OBSTETRICS/GYN
Coagulator, Laparoscopic, Unipolar	OBSTETRICS/GYN
Coagulator/Cutter, Endoscopic, Bipolar	OBSTETRICS/GYN
Coagulator/Cutter, Endoscopic, Unipolar	OBSTETRICS/GYN
Colposcope	OBSTETRICS/GYN
Container, Specimen, Laparoscopic	SURGERY
Cystoscope	GASTRO/UROLOGY
Electrocautery Unit, Endoscopic	OBSTETRICS/GYN
Endoscope	GASTRO/UROLOGY
Equipment, Suction/Irrigation, Laparoscopic	SURGERY
Forceps, Electrosurgical	SURGERY
Forceps, Endoscopic	GASTRO/UROLOGY
Forceps, Grasping, Atraumatic	MIN. INV. SURGERY
Forceps, Grasping, Flexible Endoscopic	GASTRO/UROLOGY
Holder, Needle, Curved, Laparoscopic	MIN. INV. SURGERY
Hysteroscope	OBSTETRICS/GYN
Instrument, Dissecting, Laparoscopic	MIN. INV. SURGERY
Instrument, Knot Tying, Suture, Laparoscopic	MIN. INV. SURGERY
Instrument, Needle Holder/Knot Tying	MIN. INV. SURGERY
Instrument, Passing, Suture, Laparoscopic	MIN. INV. SURGERY
Insufflator, Carbon-Dioxide, Automatic (For Endoscope)	GASTRO/UROLOGY
Insufflator, Hysteroscopic	OBSTETRICS/GYN
Insufflator, Laparoscopic	OBSTETRICS/GYN
Lamp, Endoscopic, Incandescent	SURGERY
Laparoscope, General & Plastic Surgery	SURGERY
Laparoscope, Gynecologic	OBSTETRICS/GYN
Light Source, Endoscope, Xenon Arc	SURGERY
Monitor, Video, Endoscope	GENERAL
Needle, Aspiration, Cyst, Laparoscopic	MIN. INV. SURGERY
Needle, Insufflation, Laparoscopic	MIN. INV. SURGERY
Obturator, Endoscopic	GASTRO/UROLOGY
Peritoneoscope	GASTRO/UROLOGY
Probe, Suction, Irrigator/Aspirator, Laparoscopic	MIN. INV. SURGERY
Resectoscope	GASTRO/UROLOGY
Retractor, Fan-Type, Laparoscopy	MIN. INV. SURGERY
Retractor, Laparoscopy, Other	MIN. INV. SURGERY
Telescope, Rigid, Endoscopic	GASTRO/UROLOGY
Thoracoscope	CARDIOVASCULAR
Trainer, Laparoscopy	MIN. INV. SURGERY
Trocar, Abdominal	GASTRO/UROLOGY
Trocar, Gastro-Urology	GASTRO/UROLOGY
Trocar, Laparoscopic	SURGERY
Trocar, Other	GENERAL
Trocar, Thoracic	CARDIOVASCULAR

Cameron-Miller, Inc.
3949 S. Racine Ave.
Chicago, IL 60609-2523
Tel: 312-523-6360
Tel: 800-621-0142
Fax: 312-523-9495
CEO: John W. Martin, President
Marketing: Robert E. Peterson, Sales Mgr.
Federal Procurement Eligibility: Small Business
Device Category:

Anoscope, Non-Powered	GASTRO/UROLOGY
Coagulator/Cutter, Endoscopic, Bipolar	OBSTETRICS/GYN
Electrocautery Unit, Endoscopic	OBSTETRICS/GYN
Forceps, Electrosurgical	SURGERY
Forceps, Endoscopic	GASTRO/UROLOGY
Power Supply, Endoscopic, Line Operated	GENERAL
Proctoscope	SURGERY
Proctosigmoidoscope	GASTRO/UROLOGY
Sigmoidoscope, Rigid, Non-Electrical	GASTRO/UROLOGY
Snare, Endoscopic	SURGERY

Carley Lamps
1502 West 228th St.
Torrance, CA 90501-5105
Tel: 310-325-8474
Fax: 310-534-2912
Advertising: Sobedia De Lamoa, Adv. Mgr.
CEO: Margarette Tsang, V.P. Personnel
  James A. Carley, President
Marketing: Roberta R. Patton, Factory Sales & Service
  Legion Becket Carley, Bus. Dev. Mgr.
  Joe Sandoval, V.P. Sales & Mktg.
  Craig Carley, Natl. & Intl. Sales Mgr.
Research: Chuck Steinhoff, V.P. R & D
Federal Procurement Eligibility: Small Business, GSA Contract
Device Category:

Lamp, Endoscopic, Incandescent	SURGERY
Laryngoscope	EAR/NOSE/THROAT
Laryngoscope, Rigid	ANESTH/PUL MED
Laryngoscope, Surgical	SURGERY

Carsen Group Inc.
151 Telson Rd.
Markham, ONT L3R 1E7
Canada
Tel: 416-479-4100
Fax: 416-479-2595
Advertising: M. L. Little, Adv. Dir.
CEO: William J. Vella, VP & Gen. Mgr.
  Edward E. Meltz, President
Marketing: D. Rolfe, VP Sales & Mktg.
Device Category:

Arthroscope	ORTHOPEDICS
Bougie, Esophageal, ENT	EAR/NOSE/THROAT
Bronchoscope, Flexible	EAR/NOSE/THROAT
Brush, Cytology, Endoscopic	GASTRO/UROLOGY
Camera, Television, Surgical, With Audio	SURGERY
Choledochoscope, Flexible Or Rigid	GASTRO/UROLOGY
Colonoscope, General & Plastic Surgery	SURGERY
Colposcope	OBSTETRICS/GYN
Culdoscope	OBSTETRICS/GYN
Cystoscope	GASTRO/UROLOGY
Cystourethroscope	GASTRO/UROLOGY
Duodenoscope, Esophago/Gastro	GASTRO/UROLOGY
Esophagoscope (Flexible Or Rigid)	EAR/NOSE/THROAT
Gastroduodenoscope	GASTRO/UROLOGY
Gastroscope, Flexible	GASTRO/UROLOGY
Hysteroscope	OBSTETRICS/GYN
Laparoscope, General & Plastic Surgery	SURGERY

Laryngoscope .... EAR/NOSE/THROAT
Laryngoscope, Flexible .... ANESTH/PUL MED
Monitor, Video, Endoscope .... GENERAL
Nephroscope, Flexible .... GASTRO/UROLOGY
Nephroscope, Rigid .... GASTRO/UROLOGY
Pharyngoscope .... EAR/NOSE/THROAT
Power Supply, Endoscopic, Line Operated .... GENERAL
Proctosigmoidoscope .... GASTRO/UROLOGY
Prosthesis, Esophageal .... EAR/NOSE/THROAT
Resectoscope .... GASTRO/UROLOGY
Sigmoidoscope, Flexible .... GASTRO/UROLOGY
Snare, Endoscopic .... SURGERY
Trocar, Abdominal .... GASTRO/UROLOGY
Urethroscope .... GASTRO/UROLOGY

Chirurgische Instrumente   Tel: 7424/501319
Hauptstrasse 18   Fax: 7424/502303
D-78582 Balgheim
Germany
CEO: Hubert Wenzler
   Gebhard Wenzler
   Edwin Wenzler
Marketing: Edwin Wenzler
Device Category:
Arthroscope .... ORTHOPEDICS
Clamp, Fixation, Cholangiography .... MIN. INV. SURGERY
Equipment, Suction/Irrigation, Laparoscopic .... SURGERY
Forceps, Biopsy .... MIN. INV. SURGERY
Forceps, Grasping, Atraumatic .... MIN. INV. SURGERY
Forceps, Grasping, Traumatic .... MIN. INV. SURGERY
Holder, Needle, Laparoscopic .... MIN. INV. SURGERY
Hysteroscope .... OBSTETRICS/GYN
Laparoscope, General & Plastic Surgery .... SURGERY
Needle, Insufflation, Laparoscopic .... MIN. INV. SURGERY
Needle, Puncture .... MIN. INV. SURGERY
Obturator, Endoscopic .... GASTRO/UROLOGY
Scissors, Laparoscopy .... MIN. INV. SURGERY
Sleeve, Trocar .... MIN. INV. SURGERY
Trocar, Laparoscopic .... SURGERY

Chiu Technical Corp.   Tel: 516-544-0606
252 Indian Head Rd.   Fax: 516-544-0809
Kings Park, NY 11754-4814
CEO: David Chiu, President
Marketing: Frank A. Denny, VP Mktg.
Production: Bob Kirzl, Eng. Coord.
Federal Procurement Eligibility: Small Business, Minority Owned
Device Category:
Illuminator, Fiberoptic (For Endoscope) .... GASTRO/UROLOGY
Light Source, Endoscope, Xenon Arc .... SURGERY
Power Supply, Endoscopic, Battery Operated .... GENERAL

Chris Lutz Medical, Inc.   Tel: 714-830-2472
23011 Houlton Pkwy. B-3   Tel: 800-444-4729
Laguna Hills, CA 92653   Fax: 714-830-2316
Advertising: Bonnie Lutz
CEO: Chris Lutz
Research: Bonnie Lutz, Mkt. Res. Mgr.
Federal Procurement Eligibility: Small Business, Woman Owned
Device Category:
Cabinet, Storage, Endoscope .... GASTRO/UROLOGY

Circon Acmi   Tel: 203-328-8689
300 Stillwater Ave.   Tel: 800-325-7107
Stamford, CT 06902-3640   Fax: 203-328-8789
CEO: Michael Lorenz, President
Marketing: Nancy Caffiero
Production: David Zielinski
Device Category:
Bronchoscope, Flexible .... EAR/NOSE/THROAT
Brush, Cytology, Endoscopic .... GASTRO/UROLOGY
Choledochoscope, Flexible Or Rigid .... GASTRO/UROLOGY
Colonoscope, Gastro-Urology .... GASTRO/UROLOGY
Cord, Electric, Endoscope .... GASTRO/UROLOGY
Cystoscope .... GASTRO/UROLOGY
Cystourethroscope .... GASTRO/UROLOGY
Electrode, Electrosurgery, Laparoscopic .... MIN. INV. SURGERY
Endoscope .... GASTRO/UROLOGY
Forceps, Endoscopic .... GASTRO/UROLOGY
Forceps, Grasping, Flexible Endoscopic .... GASTRO/UROLOGY
Forceps, Grasping, Traumatic .... MIN. INV. SURGERY
Gastroscope, Gastro-Urology .... GASTRO/UROLOGY
Instrument, Dissecting, Laparoscopic .... MIN. INV. SURGERY
Kit, Laparoscopy .... GASTRO/UROLOGY
Laparoscope, Gynecologic .... OBSTETRICS/GYN
Nephroscope, Flexible .... GASTRO/UROLOGY
Nephroscope, Rigid .... GASTRO/UROLOGY
Obturator, Endoscopic .... GASTRO/UROLOGY
Peritoneoscope .... GASTRO/UROLOGY
Pump, Air, Non-Manual, Endoscopic .... GASTRO/UROLOGY
Resectoscope .... GASTRO/UROLOGY
Scissors, Laparoscopy .... MIN. INV. SURGERY
Sheath, Endoscopic .... GASTRO/UROLOGY
Sigmoidoscope, Flexible .... GASTRO/UROLOGY
Teaching Attachment, Endoscopic .... GASTRO/UROLOGY
Telescope, Rigid, Endoscopic .... GASTRO/UROLOGY
Thoracoscope .... CARDIOVASCULAR
Trocar, Abdominal .... GASTRO/UROLOGY
Ureteroscope .... GASTRO/UROLOGY

Circon Corporation   Tel: 805-967-0404
460 Ward Drive   Tel: 800-654-1263
Santa Barbara, CA 93111-2310   Fax: 805-683-2600
Advertising: Gloria Peyrat, Comm. Mgr.
CEO: Wayne Colahan, EVP & GM of Video Div.
   Richard Auhll, President
   Bruce Thompson, CFO
Marketing: Valerie Case, Mktg. Supv.
   Chris Pollock, Mktg. Mgr., Video Div.
Production: Eric Sluyter, VP Mfg.
Federal Procurement Eligibility: VA Contract
Device Category:
Camera, Video, Endoscopic .... GENERAL
Endoscope .... GASTRO/UROLOGY

Citation Medical Corp.
Tel: 702-324-1212
Tel: 800-343-4345
Fax: 702-856-0100
230 Edison Way
Reno, NV 89502
CEO: Douglas P. Rumberger, President
Device Category:
Accessories, Arthroscope .... ORTHOPEDICS
Arthroscope .... ORTHOPEDICS

Civco Medical Instruments Co., Inc.
Tel: 319-656-4447
Tel: 800-445-6741
Fax: 319-656-4451
Medical Pkwy.
102 Hwy. 1 South
Kalona, IA 52247
Advertising: Julie L. Meyer, Adv. Specialist
CEO: Victor J. Wedel, President & CEO
Marketing: Robin L. Therme, Mktg. Mgr.
Production: Rick Pruter, VP Eng.
Federal Procurement Eligibility: Small Business
Device Category:
Cover, Laparoscope .... MIN. INV. SURGERY

Clarus Medical Systems, Inc.
Tel: 612-559-8640
Fax: 612-559-5645
2605 Fernbrook Lane
Minneapolis, MN 55447-4736
CEO: Whitney A. McFarlin
   Monty K. Allen, VP & CFO
   Dave Meyer, Finance
Marketing: James Phillips
   Dave Van Hoof
   Brian McIntee, Mkt. Dev. Mgr.
Production: Thomas Barthel
Federal Procurement Eligibility: Small Business
Device Category:
Accessories, Arthroscope .... ORTHOPEDICS
Arthroscope .... ORTHOPEDICS
Cart, Equipment, Video .... GENERAL
Cart, Instrument/Equipment, Laparoscopy .... MIN. INV. SURGERY
Choledochoscope, Mini-Diameter (5mm or Less) ..... MIN. INV. SURGERY
Endoscope .... GASTRO/UROLOGY
Endoscope, Electronic (Videoendoscope) .... SURGERY
Endoscope, Flexible .... GASTRO/UROLOGY
Endoscope, Rigid .... SURGERY
Equipment, Suction/Irrigation, Laparoscopic .... SURGERY
Laparoscope, Flexible .... SURGERY
Laparoscope, Semi-Flexible .... MIN. INV. SURGERY
Sheath, Endoscopic .... GASTRO/UROLOGY

Clinipad Corp. (The)
Tel: 203-453-6543
Tel: 800-243-6548
Fax: 203-453-8347
66 High St.
P.O. Box 387
Guilford, CT 06437
Advertising: Melinda Winchell, Advertising Mgr.
CEO: Stephen N. Young, Sr. VP
   David A Greenberg, President
Marketing: David Salazar, National Sales Mgr.
Federal Procurement Eligibility: Small Business, GSA Contract
Device Category:
Kit, Laparoscopy .... GASTRO/UROLOGY

CMT, Inc.
Tel: 508-468-5640
Fax: 508-468-5640
648 Bay Road
P.O. Box 297
Hamilton, MA 01936
CEO: David C. de Sieyes, President
Federal Procurement Eligibility: Small Business
Device Category:
*Insufflator, Carbon-Dioxide, Automatic
   (For Endoscope)* .... GASTRO/UROLOGY
Insufflator, Hysteroscopic .... OBSTETRICS/GYN
Insufflator, Laparoscopic .... OBSTETRICS/GYN
Insufflator, Vaginal .... OBSTETRICS/GYN

Condor D.C. Power Supplies, Inc.
Tel: 805-486-4565
Tel: 800-235-5929
Fax: 805-487-8911
2311 Statham Pkwy.
Oxnard, CA 93033-3911
Advertising: Ken Eastman
CEO: Tom Ingman, President
Marketing: Michael F. Kirkowski, Exec. VP Sales & Mktg.
Production: Steve Miller, Eng. Mgr.
   Mark Goldberg, Materials Mgr.
   Geary Green
Research: Suzanne Roedl, VP Finance
Device Category:
Power Supply, Endoscopic, Line Operated .... GENERAL

Conmed Corp.
Tel: 315-797-8375
Tel: 800-448-6506
Fax: 315-797-0321
310 Broad St.
Utica, NY 13501
CEO: William W. Abraham, EVP
   Eugene R. Corasanti, President & Chairman
Marketing: William Andrus, Natl. Accts. Dir.
   Scott Dillenback, Mktg. Dir.
   Jeffrey H. Palmer, VP Sales
   Frank R. Williams, VP Business Dev.
   Alan Fink, VP Intl. Sales
Production: William W. Abraham, VP Mfg. & Eng.
   Martin Forte, Reg. Affairs Mgr.
   Joe Gross, V.P. of Operations
Research: John Gentilia, VP R&D
Federal Procurement Eligibility: Small Business, GSA Contract, VA
   Contract
Device Category:
Coagulator/Cutter, Endoscopic, Unipolar .... OBSTETRICS/GYN
Electrocautery Unit, Endoscopic .... OBSTETRICS/GYN
Electrode, Electrosurgery, Laparoscopic .... MIN. INV. SURGERY
Endoscope And Accessories, AC-Powered .... SURGERY
Equipment, Suction/Irrigation, Laparoscopic .... SURGERY
Module, Control, Electrosurgery .... MIN. INV. SURGERY
Needle, Insufflation, Laparoscopic .... MIN. INV. SURGERY
Probe, Electrocauterization, Single-Use .... MIN. INV. SURGERY
Probe, Suction, Irrigator/Aspirator, Laparoscopic .... MIN. INV. SURGERY
Trocar, Abdominal .... GASTRO/UROLOGY
Trocar, Gallbladder .... GASTRO/UROLOGY
Trocar, Laparoscopic .... SURGERY
Trocar, Other .... GENERAL
Tube, Smoke Removal, Endoscopic .... GASTRO/UROLOGY

Conrac Display Products, Inc.　　　Tel: 818-303-0095
1724 S. Mountain Ave.　　　　　　　　Fax: 818-303-5484
Duarte, CA 91010-2746
CEO: V. Hewitt, President
Marketing: G. Ives, Mktg. & Sales Dir.
Federal Procurement Eligibility: Small Business
Device Category:
Monitor, Video, Endoscope .... GENERAL

Contec Medical Ltd.　　　　　　　Tel: 03/5491153
11 Haroshet Street　　　　　　　　　Fax: 03/5491095
P.O. Box 1400
Ramat Hasharon, 47113
Israel
CEO: S. Rabiner, VP Personnel
　Nitzan Sneh
Marketing: Orly Sharon-Hass, VP Sales & Mktg.
　Ari Hoffman, Product Dir.
Production: David Cohen
Research: Ofer Dvir
Device Category:
Arthroscope .... ORTHOPEDICS
Aspirator, Arthroscopy .... ORTHOPEDICS
Camera, Still, Endoscopic ....SURGERY
Cannula, Drainage, Arthroscopy .... ORTHOPEDICS
Cart, Equipment, Video .... GENERAL
Electrocautery Unit, Endoscopic ....OBSTETRICS/GYN
Holder, Leg, Arthroscopy .... ORTHOPEDICS
Laparoscope, Flexible ....SURGERY
Laparoscope, General & Plastic Surgery ....SURGERY
Light, Surgical, Endoscopic ....SURGERY

Continuum Biomedical Inc.　　　Tel: 510-606-6118
547 Rhea Way　　　　　　　　　　Fax: 510-447-8378
Livermore, CA 94550
CEO: Robert S. Anderson, President
Marketing: Dianne Anderson, Mktg. Mgr.
Device Category:
Laser, Nd:YAG, Laparoscopy .... MIN. INV. SURGERY

Cook Urological, Inc.　　　　　　Tel: 812-829-4891
1100 West Morgan St.　　　　　　　Tel: 800-457-4448
P.O. Box 227　　　　　　　　　　　Fax: 812-829-1801
Spencer, IN 47460-9426
CEO: Jeffrey D. McGough, President
Marketing: Kelly Wikle, VP
　Jerry French, VP
　Fred Roemer, VP
Production: Carol Waldrip
Federal Procurement Eligibility: Small Business
Device Category:
Brush, Cytology, Endoscopic .... GASTRO/UROLOGY
Forceps, Grasping, Flexible Endoscopic .... GASTRO/UROLOGY
Needle, Endoscopic .... GASTRO/UROLOGY

Coopersurgical, Inc.　　　　　　　Tel: 203-929-6321
15 Forest Pkwy.　　　　　　　　　　Tel: 800-243-2974
Shelton, CT 06484-5458　　　　　　Fax: 203-926-9435
CEO: Nick Pichotta, CEO
Marketing: Stephen Albrecht, VP Mktg.
Federal Procurement Eligibility: VA Contract
Device Category:
Accessories, Cleaning, Endoscopic .... GASTRO/UROLOGY
Accessories, Photographic, Endoscopic .... GASTRO/UROLOGY
Adapter, Bulb, Endoscope, Miscellaneous .... GASTRO/UROLOGY
Brush, Cytology, Endoscopic .... GASTRO/UROLOGY
Camera, Cine, Endoscopic, Without Audio .... SURGERY
Camera, Still, Endoscopic .... SURGERY
Camera, Television, Endoscopic, Without Audio .... SURGERY
Camera, Television, Microsurgical, Without Audio .... SURGERY
Camera, Television, Surgical, Without Audio .... SURGERY
Camera, Video, Endoscopic .... GENERAL
Cart, Equipment, Video .... GENERAL
Colposcope .... OBSTETRICS/GYN
Cover, Laparoscope .... MIN. INV. SURGERY
Endoscope .... GASTRO/UROLOGY
Endoscope, Direct Vision .... SURGERY
Endoscope, Rigid .... SURGERY
Eyepiece, Lens, Non-Prescription, Endoscopic .... GASTRO/UROLOGY
Forceps, Endoscopic .... GASTRO/UROLOGY
Forceps, Grasping, Atraumatic .... MIN. INV. SURGERY
Forceps, Grasping, Flexible Endoscopic .... GASTRO/UROLOGY
Forceps, Grasping, Traumatic .... MIN. INV. SURGERY
Holder, Instrument, Laparoscopic .... MIN. INV. SURGERY
Holder, Needle, Curved, Laparoscopic .... MIN. INV. SURGERY
Holder, Needle, Laparoscopic .... MIN. INV. SURGERY
Hysteroscope .... OBSTETRICS/GYN
Insufflator, Carbon-Dioxide, Automatic
　(For Endoscope) .... GASTRO/UROLOGY
Insufflator, Hysteroscopic .... OBSTETRICS/GYN
Insufflator, Laparoscopic .... OBSTETRICS/GYN
Insufflator, Other .... SURGERY
Kit, Cholecystectomy .... MIN. INV. SURGERY
Kit, Laparoscopy .... GASTRO/UROLOGY
Laparoscope, General & Plastic Surgery .... SURGERY
Laparoscope, Gynecologic .... OBSTETRICS/GYN
Light Source, Endoscope, Xenon Arc .... SURGERY
Light, Surgical, Endoscopic .... SURGERY
Monitor, Video, Endoscope .... GENERAL
Needle, Insufflation, Laparoscopic .... MIN. INV. SURGERY
Obturator, Endoscopic .... GASTRO/UROLOGY
Peritoneoscope .... GASTRO/UROLOGY
Resectoscope .... GASTRO/UROLOGY
Retractor, Fan-Type, Laparoscopy .... MIN. INV. SURGERY
Sheath, Endoscopic .... GASTRO/UROLOGY
Telescope, Rigid, Endoscopic .... GASTRO/UROLOGY
Trocar, Abdominal .... GASTRO/UROLOGY
Videointerface, Laparoscopic, Non-Removable Rod . MIN. INV. SURGERY

Core Dynamics, Inc.
11222-4 St. Johns Indust. Pkwy.
Jacksonville, FL 32216
Tel: 904-641-6611
Fax: 904-641-6467
CEO: William G. Dennis, CEO
  Tim Reis, President
  George Dennis, VP
Federal Procurement Eligibility: Small Business
Device Category:
Cannula, Suprapubic, With Trocar .... GASTRO/UROLOGY
Coagulator, Laparoscopic, Unipolar .... OBSTETRICS/GYN
Endoscope And Accessories, AC-Powered .... SURGERY
Equipment, Suction/Irrigation, Laparoscopic................... SURGERY
Forceps, Endoscopic.. GASTRO/UROLOGY
Forceps, Grasping, Atraumatic .... MIN. INV. SURGERY
Forceps, Grasping, Traumatic .... MIN. INV. SURGERY
Instrument, Dissecting, Laparoscopic................. MIN. INV. SURGERY
Instrument, Knot Tying, Suture, Laparoscopic .... MIN. INV. SURGERY
Instrument, Needle Holder/Knot Tying................ MIN. INV. SURGERY
Kit, Cholecystectomy .... MIN. INV. SURGERY
Needle, Insufflation, Laparoscopic..................... MIN. INV. SURGERY
Probe, Electrocauterization, Multi-Use .... MIN. INV. SURGERY
Probe, Suction, Irrigator/Aspirator, Laparoscopic.... MIN. INV. SURGERY
Trocar, Abdominal .... GASTRO/UROLOGY
Trocar, Gallbladder .... GASTRO/UROLOGY
Trocar, Other .... GENERAL
Trocar, Thoracic .... CARDIOVASCULAR

Corpak, Inc.
100 Chaddick Dr.
Wheeling, IL 60090-6006
Tel: 708-537-4601
Tel: 800-323-6305
Fax: 708-541-9526
CEO: Thomas Kuhn, President
Marketing: Robert McVey, VP Mktg.
  Michael Shaughnessy, VP Sales
  Carole Schwager, Mktg. Mgr.
  Barbara Griggs, Market Dev. Mgr.
Research: Erik Anderson
Federal Procurement Eligibility: GSA Contract, VA Contract
Device Category:
Forceps, Grasping, Flexible Endoscopic................ GASTRO/UROLOGY

Cory Brothers Co.
4 Dollis Pk.
London, N3 1HG,
United Kingdom
Tel: 081/349/1081
Fax: 081/349/1962
CEO: D.N. Sharpe
Marketing: R. Sharpe, Sales & Mktg. Dir.
  J. Hawkins, Sales Training Mgr.
Production: L. Ridgewell, Operations Dir.
Research: P.E. Moignaro
Device Category:
Camera, Videotape, Surgical............................. SURGERY
Electrocautery Unit, Endoscopic..................... OBSTETRICS/GYN
Light, Surgical, Endoscopic................................. SURGERY
Power Supply, Endoscopic, Line Operated .... GENERAL
Teaching Attachment, Endoscopic..................... GASTRO/UROLOGY

Cuda Products Corporation
6000 Powers Ave.
Jacksonville, FL 32217-2212
Tel: 904-737-7611
Fax: 904-733-4832
CEO: Joseph Cuda, President
Marketing: Sherry Brooker
  Kim Reed, Mktg. Mgr.
  Kim Mixson
Production: Steve Long, Chief Eng.
  Mark Frederick, Application Eng.
  Antonio Galarza, Prod. Mgr.
Research: Cindy Arcusa
Federal Procurement Eligibility: Small Business
Device Category:
Accessories, Arthroscope .... ORTHOPEDICS
Endoscope.. GASTRO/UROLOGY
Endoscope, Direct Vision .... SURGERY
Endoscope, Rigid .... SURGERY
Illuminator, Fiberoptic (For Endoscope) .... GASTRO/UROLOGY
Kit, Laparoscopy .... GASTRO/UROLOGY
Lamp, Endoscopic, Incandescent......................... SURGERY
Laparoscope, General & Plastic Surgery .... SURGERY
Laparoscope, Gynecologic .... OBSTETRICS/GYN
Light Source, Endoscope, Xenon Arc .... SURGERY
Light, Surgical, Endoscopic................................. SURGERY
Telescope, Rigid, Endoscopic........................ GASTRO/UROLOGY
Trocar, Abdominal .... GASTRO/UROLOGY

Custom Ultrasonics, Inc.
P.O. Box 850
Buckingham, PA 18912-0850
Tel: 215-364-1477
Fax: 215-364-7674
CEO: Frank Weber, President
Marketing: George A. Innis, Mktg. Dir.
Federal Procurement Eligibility: Small Business, GSA Contract
Device Category:
Cabinet, Storage, Endoscope .... GASTRO/UROLOGY
Sterilizer/Washer, Endoscope............................. GENERAL

Dahlhausen & Co. Gmbh, P.J.
Oberbuschweg 76
Postfach 501269
D-5000 Koeln 50
Germany
Tel: 02236/39130
Fax: 02236/391349
Advertising: H. Schipper
CEO: P.J. Dalhausen
Marketing: J. Tueshaus
Device Category:
Laryngoscope... EAR/NOSE/THROAT

Daiichi Medical Co. Ltd.
2-27-16, Hongo, Bunkyo-Ku
Tokyo 113
Japan
Tel: 03/8140111
CEO: Shigeaki Hayashi, President
Device Category:
Bronchoscope, Flexible .... EAR/NOSE/THROAT
Laryngoscope, Surgical................................ SURGERY

Danek Medical, Inc.
3092 Directors Row
Memphis, TN 38131-0401
Tel: 901-396-3133
Tel: 800-876-3133
Fax: 901-332-3920
CEO: Jeff Horn, Group Dir.
  Alex Lukianov, President
Marketing: Lew Bennett, Sr. VP
  Bruce Chip Stevens, VP Sales
Production: Richard Treharne, Vp Regulatory/Clinical Affairs
  John Pafford, VP Product Dev.
Federal Procurement Eligibility: Small Business
Device Category:
Arthroscope.. ORTHOPEDICS

Datel Medical Storage Systems, Inc.   Tel: 616-791-7675
2748 Courier Ct. NW   Tel: 800-922-5966
P.O. Box 3740 ZIP 49501-3740   Fax: 616-791-7361
Grand Rapids, MI 49504
CEO: Dick Quartel, President
Federal Procurement Eligibility: Small Business, GSA Contract
Device Category:
Cart, Equipment, Video .... GENERAL

DaVinci Medical, Inc.   Tel: 612-473-4245
13700 First Ave. North   Fax: 612-473-3203
Minneapolis, MN 55441
CEO: Thom Murphy, VP Fin.
   Mark Dana, President
Production: Mike Pontius, VP Mfg.
Research: Arlen Johnson, VP R&D
Device Category:
Forceps, Grasping, Atraumatic .... MIN. INV. SURGERY
Forceps, Grasping, Traumatic .... MIN. INV. SURGERY
Instrument, Dissecting, Laparoscopic .... MIN. INV. SURGERY
Knife, Laparoscopic .... MIN. INV. SURGERY

Davis & Geck Div.   Tel: 201-831-2000
American Cyanamid Company   Tel: 800-225-5341
One Cyanamid Plaza   Fax: 201-831-3590
Wayne, NJ 07470-2012
Medical Products Sales Volume: $2,640,000,000
Total Employees: 32,000
Ownership: Public
Distribution: Manufacturer Through Distributor
Advertising: L. Cronin, Adv. Mgr. USA
CEO: W.S. Poole, President, D&G Div.
   S. Aichele, Dir. Natl. Accts.
   J. Schaefer, Reg. Affairs Mgr.
   J. Clifford, VP, D&G Div.
Marketing: T. Sanko, Mktg. Dir.
   M.G. Woosley, Mktg. Dir.
   J. D'Antonio, Sales Training Mgr.
   D. Jacobs, Natl. Sales Mgr.
Production: P. Southworth, VP Mfg.
Research: G.A. Dede, Group Mgr. Mkt. Res.
Federal Procurement Eligibility: VA Contract
Device Category:
Accessories, Cleaning, Endoscopic .... GASTRO/UROLOGY
Accessories, Electrical Power (Electrocautery) .... SURGERY
Applier, Clip, Laparoscopic .... MIN. INV. SURGERY
Applier, Ligature Clip .... SURGERY
Cannula, Suction/Irrigation, Laparoscopic .... SURGERY
Clamp, Fixation, Cholangiography .... MIN. INV. SURGERY
Clamp, Laparoscopy .... MIN. INV. SURGERY
Clip, Ligature .... SURGERY
Clip, Suture .... SURGERY
Coagulator, Laparoscopic, Unipolar .... OBSTETRICS/GYN
Coagulator/Cutter, Endoscopic, Bipolar .... OBSTETRICS/GYN
Coagulator/Cutter, Endoscopic, Unipolar .... OBSTETRICS/GYN
Component, Electrical .... GENERAL
Connector, Suction/Irrigation .... MIN. INV. SURGERY
Device, Anastomosis, Biofragmentable .... SURGERY
Dilator, Port, Laparoscopic .... MIN. INV. SURGERY
Endoscope, Direct Vision .... SURGERY
Endoscope, Rigid .... SURGERY
Equipment, Suction/Irrigation, Laparoscopic .... SURGERY
Equipment/Accessories, Laser, Laparoscopy .... MIN. INV. SURGERY
Extractor, Gall Bladder .... MIN. INV. SURGERY
Forceps, Biopsy .... MIN. INV. SURGERY
Forceps, Endoscopic .... GASTRO/UROLOGY
Forceps, Grasping, Atraumatic .... MIN. INV. SURGERY
Forceps, Grasping, Traumatic .... MIN. INV. SURGERY
Forceps, Laparoscopy, Electrosurgical .... SURGERY
Handle, Instrument, Laparoscopic (Electrocautery) .. MIN. INV. SURGERY
Handle, Instrument, Laparoscopic (Irrigation) .... MIN. INV. SURGERY
Holder, Needle, Laparoscopic .... MIN. INV. SURGERY
Forceps, Grasping, Flexible Endoscopic .... GASTRO/UROLOGY
Instrument, Dissecting, Laparoscopic .... MIN. INV. SURGERY
Instrument, Dissecting, Myoma, Laparoscopic .... MIN. INV. SURGERY
Instrument, Knot Tying, Suture, Laparoscopic ...... MIN. INV. SURGERY
Instrument, Passing, Suture, Laparoscopic .... MIN. INV. SURGERY
Knob, Instrument, Rotating .... MIN. INV. SURGERY
Laparoscope, General & Plastic Surgery .... SURGERY
Ligature, Laparoscopic .... MIN. INV. SURGERY
Needle, Insufflation, Laparoscopic .... MIN. INV. SURGERY
Needle, Puncture .... MIN. INV. SURGERY
Probe, Electrocauterization, Multi-Use .... MIN. INV. SURGERY
Probe, Electrocauterization, Single-Use .... MIN. INV. SURGERY
Probe, Suction, Irrigator/Aspirator, Laparoscopic .... MIN. INV. SURGERY
Rack, Instrument, Laparoscopy .... MIN. INV. SURGERY
Remover, Clip .... SURGERY
Remover, Staple, Surgical .... SURGERY
Retractor, Fan-Type, Laparoscopy .... MIN. INV. SURGERY
Scissors with Removable Tips, Laparoscopy .... MIN. INV. SURGERY
Scissors, Laparoscopy .... MIN. INV. SURGERY
Scissors, Laparoscopy, Electrosurgical .... SURGERY
Sizer, Device, Anastomosis .... SURGERY
Sleeve, Trocar .... MIN. INV. SURGERY
Stapler, Laparoscopic .... MIN. INV. SURGERY
Stapler, Surgical .... SURGERY
Suture, Laparoscopy .... MIN. INV. SURGERY
Telescope, Rigid, Endoscopic .... GASTRO/UROLOGY
Trainer, Laparoscopy .... MIN. INV. SURGERY
Tray, Sterilization, Instrument .... SURGERY
Trocar, Abdominal .... GASTRO/UROLOGY
Trocar, Gallbladder .... GASTRO/UROLOGY
Trocar, Laparoscopic .... SURGERY
Trocar, Short .... MIN. INV. SURGERY
Trocar, Thoracic .... CARDIOVASCULAR
Tubing, Irrigation .... MIN. INV. SURGERY

Davis & Geck Endosurgery
1 Casper St.
Danbury, CT 06810
Tel: 203-743-4451
Tel: 800-225-5341

Product	Category
Accessories, Electrical Power (Electrocautery)	SURGERY
Applier, Clip, Laparoscopic	MIN. INV. SURGERY
Applier, Ligature Clip	SURGERY
Cannula, Suction/Irrigation, Laparoscopic	SURGERY
Clamp, Fixation, Cholangiography	MIN. INV. SURGERY
Clamp, Laparoscopy	MIN. INV. SURGERY
Clip, Ligature	SURGERY
Clip, Suture	SURGERY
Coagulator, Laparoscopic, Unipolar	OBSTETRICS/GYN
Connector, Suction/Irrigation	MIN. INV. SURGERY
Dilator, Port, Laparoscopic	MIN. INV. SURGERY
Endoscope, Rigid	SURGERY
Equipment/Accessories, Laser, Laparoscopy	MIN. INV. SURGERY
Extractor, Gall Bladder	MIN. INV. SURGERY
Forceps, Biopsy	MIN. INV. SURGERY
Forceps, Grasping, Atraumatic	MIN. INV. SURGERY
Forceps, Grasping, Flexible Endoscopic	GASTRO/UROLOGY
Forceps, Grasping, Traumatic	MIN. INV. SURGERY
Forceps, Laparoscopy, Electrosurgical	SURGERY
Handle, Instrument, Laparoscopic (Electrocautery)	MIN. INV. SURGERY
Handle, Instrument, Laparoscopic (Irrigation)	MIN. INV. SURGERY
Holder, Needle, Laparoscopic	MIN. INV. SURGERY
Forceps, Grasping, Flexible Endoscopic	GASTRO/UROLOGY
Holder, Ring, Arthroscopic	MIN. INV. SURGERY
Instrument, Dissecting, Laparoscopic	MIN. INV. SURGERY
Instrument, Electrosurgery, Laparoscopic	MIN. INV. SURGERY
Instrument, Knot Tying, Suture, Laparoscopic	MIN. INV. SURGERY
Ligature, Laparoscopic	MIN. INV. SURGERY
Needle, Insufflation, Laparoscopic	MIN. INV. SURGERY
Needle, Puncture	MIN. INV. SURGERY
Probe, Electrocauterization, Multi-Use	MIN. INV. SURGERY
Probe, Electrocauterization, Single-Use	MIN. INV. SURGERY
Probe, Suction, Irrigator/Aspirator, Laparoscopic	MIN. INV. SURGERY
Rack, Instrument, Laparoscopy	MIN. INV. SURGERY
Remover, Clip	SURGERY
Retractor, Fan-Type, Laparoscopy	MIN. INV. SURGERY
Scissors, Laparoscopy	MIN. INV. SURGERY
Sizer, Device, Anastomosis	SURGERY
Sleeve, Trocar	MIN. INV. SURGERY
Stapler, Laparoscopic	MIN. INV. SURGERY
Stapler, Surgical	SURGERY
Suture, Laparoscopy	MIN. INV. SURGERY
Tray, Sterilization, Instrument	SURGERY
Trocar, Laparoscopic	SURGERY
Tubing, Irrigation	MIN. INV. SURGERY

Davol, Inc.
100 Sockanossett
P.O. Box 8500
Cranston, RI 02920-0500
Tel: 401-463-7000
Tel: 800-556-6756
Fax: 401-463-7224

CEO: William A. Lancellotta, VP Controller
  Ted Watson, Dir. Natl. Accts.
  Richard Daigle, VP Employee Relations
  Perry R. Clough, VP Davol Laparoscopic Prod.
  Edward W. Kelly, President
  Dale L. Richardson, VP Davol Blood Mgmt. Prod.
  Annette Fagnant, Mgr. Reg. Affairs
Marketing: Thomas W. Byrne, Dir. Mktg., Davol Laparoscopic
  Susan DiNapoli, Mgr. Sales Training
  Robin Ciardiello, Mktg. Mgr., Davol Laparoscopic
  Richard Longo, Mgr. Mktg. Res.
  Marshall K. Chalmers, Mgr. Intl. Mktg.
  Kim Netter, Mktg. Mgr.
  John Uhoch, Mktg. Mgr.
  Gary Halick, Mktg. Mgr.
  David Hahn, Mgr. Mktg. Comm.
  Cecil O. Sewell III, Natl. Sales Mgr.
  Annmarie Garceau, Mgr. Sales Admin.
Production: Leonard A. DiLorenzo, VP QA/Reg. Affairs
  Gregory Butterfield, Mgr. Matl. Ctrl.
  Edward T. Doorley, III, VP Mfg.
Research: Albert Solis, VP R&D
Federal Procurement Eligibility: GSA Contract
Device Category:

Product	Category
Aspirator, Arthroscopy	ORTHOPEDICS
Cannula, Drainage, Arthroscopy	ORTHOPEDICS
Catheter, Cholangiography	SURGERY
Clamp, Laparoscopy	MIN. INV. SURGERY
Coagulator, Laparoscopic, Unipolar	OBSTETRICS/GYN
Drain, Suction, Closed	MIN. INV. SURGERY
Equipment, Suction/Irrigation, Laparoscopic	SURGERY
Forceps, Endoscopic	GASTRO/UROLOGY
Forceps, Grasping, Atraumatic	MIN. INV. SURGERY
Forceps, Grasping, Traumatic	MIN. INV. SURGERY
Instrument, Dissecting, Laparoscopic	MIN. INV. SURGERY
Instrument, Dissecting, Myoma, Laparoscopic	MIN. INV. SURGERY
Instrument, Knot Tying, Suture, Laparoscopic	MIN. INV. SURGERY
Kit, Laparoscopy	GASTRO/UROLOGY
Probe, Electrocauterization, Multi-Use	MIN. INV. SURGERY
Probe, Suction, Irrigator/Aspirator, Laparoscopic	MIN. INV. SURGERY
Snare, Endoscopic	SURGERY

DCG Precision Manufacturing Corp.
9 Trowbridge Dr.
Bethel, CT 06801
Tel: 203-743-5525
Fax: 203-791-1737

CEO: John V. Valluzzo, President
Marketing: Dolores R. Levy, Mktg. Exec.
Production: Bernie R. Sherwill, Prod. Exec.
Federal Procurement Eligibility: Small Business
Device Category:

Product	Category
Cannula, Suprapubic, With Trocar	GASTRO/UROLOGY
Laparoscope, General & Plastic Surgery	SURGERY
Trocar, Gallbladder	GASTRO/UROLOGY
Trocar, Gastro-Urology	GASTRO/UROLOGY

Deknatel Division
600 Airport Rd.
Fall River, MA 02720-4703
Tel: 508-677-6600
Fax: 508-677-6666

Advertising: Carole Fiola
CEO: Robert Giggey, VP & Gen. Mgr.
Marketing: Steve Schiess
Federal Procurement Eligibility: GSA Contract
Device Category:

Product	Category
Suture, Laparoscopy	MIN. INV. SURGERY
Trocar, Cardiovascular	CARDIOVASCULAR

Depuy, Inc. Tel: 219-267-8143
700 Orthopaedic Dr. Tel: 800-366-8143
P.O. Box 988 Fax: 219-267-7640
Warsaw, IN 46581-0988
Advertising: Dawn Callahan
CEO: Michael McCaffrey, Financial Officer
   Jim Lent
Marketing: Roger Boggs
   Pete Wehrly, VP Mktg.
   Bob Purcell, VP Sales
Research: Dick Tarr, VP
Device Category:
Accessories, Arthroscope .... ORTHOPEDICS
Accessories, Cleaning, Endoscopic .... GASTRO/UROLOGY
Arthroscope .... ORTHOPEDICS
Cover, Laparoscope .... MIN. INV. SURGERY
Cystoscope .... GASTRO/UROLOGY
Endoscope, Direct Vision .... SURGERY
Endoscope, Rigid .... SURGERY
Forceps, Endoscopic .... GASTRO/UROLOGY
Laparoscope, General & Plastic Surgery .... SURGERY
Light Source, Endoscope, Xenon Arc .... SURGERY
Light, Surgical, Endoscopic .... SURGERY
System, Traction, Arthroscopy .... ORTHOPEDICS
Thoracoscope .... CARDIOVASCULAR

Dermalase Inc. Tel: 508-435-0277
3 Main St. Fax: 508-435-2663
Hopkinton, MA 01748
CEO: Michael L. Barretti, President
   Iain D. Miller, VP
Device Category:
Laser, Nd:YAG, Laparoscopy .... MIN. INV. SURGERY

DeRoyal Industries, Inc. Tel: 615-938-7828
200 DeBusk Lane Tel: 800-251-9864
Powell, TN 37849-4703 Fax: 615-938-6655
Advertising: Kathy Meyer, Adv. Mgr.
CEO: Pete DeBusk, President
   Jack Payne, DeRoyal Critical Care
Marketing: Wayne Walters, VP Mktg.
   Tracy Thompson, VP Sales
   Larry Jordan, Corp. Svcs.
   Dennis Crowley, VP Int'l Mktg.
   Charles Neal, VP Mktg. DeRoyal Orth. Group
   Angie Evans, Mktg. Coord.
Production: Susan Hevey, VP QC & RA
   Mike Mabry, VP Operations
   Mickey Wormsley, VP Mat'l. Mgmt.
   Gary Burchett, VP Mfg.
Federal Procurement Eligibility: GSA Contract, VA Contract
Device Category:
Kit, Laparoscopy .... GASTRO/UROLOGY

Design Standards Corp. Tel: 203-366-7046
643 North Ave. Fax: 203-335-0701
Bridgeport, CT 06606-5745
CEO: Lawrence Crainich, President
Marketing: Domenic Federici, Sales Mgr.
Production: Frank Lopez, Plant Mgr.
Federal Procurement Eligibility: Small Business
Device Category:
Coagulator, Laparoscopic, Unipolar .... OBSTETRICS/GYN
Coagulator/Cutter, Endoscopic, Bipolar .... OBSTETRICS/GYN
Coagulator/Cutter, Endoscopic, Unipolar .... OBSTETRICS/GYN
Forceps, Grasping, Flexible Endoscopic .... GASTRO/UROLOGY
Remover, Clip .... SURGERY
Remover, Staple, Surgical .... SURGERY
Stapler, Laparoscopic .... MIN. INV. SURGERY
Stapler, Surgical .... SURGERY

Design Standards Corp. Tel: 603-826-7744
Charlestown Div. Fax: 603-826-4406
Ceda Industrial Park
P.O. Box 996
Charlestown, NH 03603-0996
Medical Products Sales Volume: $2,000,000
Total Employees: 25
Distribution: OEM Manufacturer
CEO: Lawrence Crainich, President
Marketing: Irene Houle, Sales Mgr.
Production: Thomas Carignan, Plant Mgr.
Federal Procurement Eligibility: Small Business
Device Category:
Coagulator, Laparoscopic, Unipolar .... OBSTETRICS/GYN
Coagulator/Cutter, Endoscopic, Bipolar .... OBSTETRICS/GYN
Coagulator/Cutter, Endoscopic, Unipolar .... OBSTETRICS/GYN
Forceps, Grasping, Flexible Endoscopic .... GASTRO/UROLOGY
Remover, Clip .... SURGERY
Remover, Staple, Surgical .... SURGERY
Stapler, Surgical .... SURGERY

Designs For Vision, Inc. Tel: 516-585-3300
760 Koehler Ave. Tel: 800-345-4009
Ronkonkoma, NY 11779-7405 Fax: 516-585-3404
CEO: Richard E. Feinbloom, President
   Peter J. Murphy, EVP Sales & Mktg.
   Herb Schwartz, VP Finance
Marketing: Susan Dalton, Dir. Mktg.
Federal Procurement Eligibility: Small Business
Device Category:
Telescope, Rigid, Endoscopic .... GASTRO/UROLOGY

Dexide, Inc. Tel: 817-589-1454
7509 Flagstone Dr. Tel: 800-645-3378
P.O. Box 185789 Fax: 817-595-3300
Fort Worth, TX 76118-6953
CEO: William Hanson, President
   Jerry L. Tims
Marketing: Jay Tims, VP Mktg.
   Gene Burchfield, Exec. VP Sales
Federal Procurement Eligibility: Small Business
Device Category:
Bag, Specimen, Laparoscopic .... MIN. INV. SURGERY
Container, Specimen, Laparoscopic .... SURGERY
Equipment, Suction/Irrigation, Laparoscopic .... SURGERY
Needle, Insufflation, Laparoscopic .... MIN. INV. SURGERY
Obturator, Endoscopic .... GASTRO/UROLOGY
Solution, Instrument, Laparoscopic, Anti-Fog .... GENERAL
Trocar, Abdominal .... GASTRO/UROLOGY
Trocar, Laparoscopic .... SURGERY

Diefenbach Ing. Buero
Am Saaelnbusch 24-26
D-60386 Frankfurt 61
Germany
Tel: 069/412950
CEO: Helmut Heinemann
Research: Hans Sabo
Device Category:
Monitor, Video, Endoscope .... GENERAL

Diener, Christian
Rudolf Diesel Str. 18
D-78532 Tuttlingen
Germany
Tel: 7461/71067
Fax: 7461/78884
Marketing: Helmut Diener, Mktg. Mgr.
Device Category:
Endoscope, Rigid .... SURGERY
Forceps, Endoscopic .... GASTRO/UROLOGY
Forceps, Grasping, Flexible Endoscopic .... GASTRO/UROLOGY

Dieter Oertel Medizintechnik
Nendinger Str. 1
D-78532 Tuttlingen
Germany
Tel: 07461/72426
Fax: 07461/73320
CEO: Dieter Oertel
Device Category:
Trocar, Sinus .... EAR/NOSE/THROAT
Trocar, Tracheal .... EAR/NOSE/THROAT

Diez, Kurt
Mohringerstr. 65
D-78532 Tuttlingen
Germany
Tel: 07461-3318
CEO: Kurt Diez
Federal Procurement Eligibility: Small Business
Device Category:
Laryngoscope, Rigid .... ANESTH/PUL MED

Disposable Instrument Co., Inc.
P.O. Box 14248
Shawnee Mission, KS 66285-4248
Tel: 913-492-6492
Fax: 913-888-1762
CEO: Robert B. Clipsham, President
Marketing: Trisha Putthoff, Marketing
   Barb Aldrige
Production: Sandy A. Clipsham, VP
   Keith Holder, Mfg. Engr.
   D. Rose, QA Mgr.
   Connie Hawkins, Sales Training Mgr.
   Brad Bruss, Production Spv.
Federal Procurement Eligibility: Small Business
Device Category:
Trocar, Abdominal .... GASTRO/UROLOGY
Trocar, Amniotic .... OBSTETRICS/GYN
Trocar, Cardiovascular .... CARDIOVASCULAR
Trocar, Gallbladder .... GASTRO/UROLOGY
Trocar, Gastro-Urology .... GASTRO/UROLOGY
Trocar, Laparoscopic .... SURGERY
Trocar, Laryngeal .... EAR/NOSE/THROAT
Trocar, Other .... GENERAL
Trocar, Sinus .... EAR/NOSE/THROAT
Trocar, Thoracic .... CARDIOVASCULAR
Trocar, Tracheal .... EAR/NOSE/THROAT

Dittmar, Inc.
101 E. Laurel Ave.
P.O. Box 66
Cheltenham, PA 19012-2125
Tel: 215-379-5533
Tel: 800-523-0850
Fax: 215-663-0163
Advertising: David C. Santaspirt, Mktg. Dir.
CEO: Thomas W. Gross, Bus. Devel. Mgr.
   Joseph J. Nowak, President
Marketing: Dorothy Z. Grant, VP Sales
Production: RoseMary Heine, Materials Mgr.
   Frank Kowalski
Federal Procurement Eligibility: Small Business, VA Contract
Device Category:
Anoscope, Non-Powered .... GASTRO/UROLOGY
Proctoscope .... SURGERY
Remover, Clip .... SURGERY
Trocar, Abdominal .... GASTRO/UROLOGY
Trocar, Amniotic .... OBSTETRICS/GYN
Trocar, Cardiovascular .... CARDIOVASCULAR
Trocar, Gallbladder .... GASTRO/UROLOGY
Trocar, Thoracic .... CARDIOVASCULAR

Dixie USA, Inc.
7800 Amelia, P.O. Box 55549
Houston, TX 77255-5549
Tel: 713-688-4993
Tel: 800-347-3494
Fax: 713-688-5932
CEO: Robert A. Beeley, President
   Brenda K. Oswalt, EVP
Marketing: Brenda Oswalt, VP
Production: James A. Oswalt, VP
Federal Procurement Eligibility: Small Business, Woman Owned
Device Category:
Laryngoscope .... EAR/NOSE/THROAT

DMA Med-Chem Corporation
60 Cutter Mill Rd.
Great Neck, NY 11021-3104
Tel: 516-829-1200
Fax: 516-487-1239
CEO: Susan Mindick, Bus. Dev. Mgr.
   Leo R. Mindick, President
   Joelle D. Hochberg, VP Contract Adm.
Marketing: Sheryl Chow, Sales Training Mgr.
   Bart J. Tarulli, VP Sales & Mktg.
Production: Susan Mindick
Federal Procurement Eligibility: Small Business, VA Contract
Device Category:
Laryngoscope, Rigid .... ANESTH/PUL MED

Downs Surgical Ltd.
Parkway Industrial Estate
Parkway Close
Sheffield, S9 4WJ
United Kingdom
Tel: 0742/730346
Fax: 0742/701840
CEO: G. Watters
   C. Michelfelder, M.D.
Marketing: P.E. Gliddon
Production: A. Magree
Device Category:
Cystoscope .... GASTRO/UROLOGY

DRG Instruments GmbH
Postfach 644
D-35018 Marburg
Germany
CEO: W. Saenger, Gen. Mgr.
   Cyril E. Geacintov, CEO
Marketing: Dr. Bernd Roder, Sales & Mktg. Mgr.
   D. Lange, Mktg. Mgr.
Production: Dr. R. Fiedler, Prod. Mgr.
Research: J. Saenger, Mktg. Res. Mgr.
Tel: 06421/23005
Fax: 06421/24155
Device Category:
Laparoscope, Gynecologic .... OBSTETRICS/GYN

Dufner Instrumente
Foehrenstr. 9 - Postfach 4149
D-78532 Tuttlingen
Germany
CEO: Helmut Dufner
Tel: 07461/3697
Fax: 07461/79419
Device Category:
Accessories, Arthroscope .... ORTHOPEDICS

Dynamic Industries (PVT) Ltd.
Wazirabad Rd. Ugoki
P.O. Box 1919
Sialkot
Pakistan
Advertising: Khalida Zahid Khan
   Gulshan Zahid Khan
CEO: M. Zahid Khan, CEO
Marketing: Zafar Mahmood Bhatti
Production: M. Tahir Khan
Research: M. A. Toor
Tel: 0432/62268
Fax: 0432/558742
Device Category:
Trocar, Abdominal .... GASTRO/UROLOGY

Dyonics Video Division
4533 Enterprise Drive
Oklahoma City, OK 73128
CEO: Gary Henley, General Mgr.
Tel: 405-949-0171
Fax: 405-947-8029
Device Category:
Accessories, Arthroscope .... ORTHOPEDICS

Electro Fiberoptics Corporation
56 Hudson St.
Northborough, MA 01532-1922
Advertising: Elizabeth Cusanello
CEO: Konrad A. Lisi, President
   Bradley S. Goodrich, CFO
Marketing: Jean Chiniara, Intl. Sales & Mktg. Mgr.
Production: Tim Haley
   Kenneth Durbin, Reg. Affairs Mgr.
   Henry J. Kelly, Eng. Mgr.
Federal Procurement Eligibility: Small Business
Tel: 508-393-3753
Tel: 800-445-7016
Fax: 508-393-7360
Device Category:
Accessories, Photographic, Endoscopic .... GASTRO/UROLOGY
Arthroscope .... ORTHOPEDICS
Camera, Television, Endoscopic, Without Audio .... SURGERY
Camera, Video, Endoscopic .... GENERAL
Choledochoscope, Flexible Or Rigid .... GASTRO/UROLOGY
Cystoscope .... GASTRO/UROLOGY
Endoscope, Flexible .... GASTRO/UROLOGY
Endoscope, Neurological .... NEUROLOGY
Endoscope, Rigid .... SURGERY
Illuminator, Fiberoptic (For Endoscope) .... GASTRO/UROLOGY
Laparoscope, General & Plastic Surgery .... SURGERY
Ureteroscope .... GASTRO/UROLOGY

Electro Surgical Instrument Co.
37 Centennial St.
Rochester, NY 14611-1732
Advertising: Eleanor Phelps, VP
CEO: Anthony J. McAndrews, President
Federal Procurement Eligibility: Small Business
Tel: 716-235-1430
Device Category:
Cord, Electric, Endoscope .... GASTRO/UROLOGY
Endoscope, Direct Vision .... SURGERY
Endoscope, Rigid .... SURGERY
Lamp, Endoscopic, Incandescent .... SURGERY
Light, Surgical, Endoscopic .... SURGERY
Power Supply, Endoscopic, Line Operated .... GENERAL
Proctoscope .... SURGERY
Proctosigmoidoscope .... GASTRO/UROLOGY
Retractor, Laparoscopy, Other .... MIN. INV. SURGERY
Snare, Endoscopic .... SURGERY
Tube, Smoke Removal, Endoscopic .... GASTRO/UROLOGY

Electroscope, Inc.
4890 Sterling Dr.
Boulder, CO 80301
CEO: Roger C. Odell, President
Tel: 303-444-2600
Fax: 303-444-2693
Device Category:
Cover, Laparoscope .... MIN. INV. SURGERY
Electrode, Electrosurgery, Laparoscopic .... MIN. INV. SURGERY
Endoscope And Accessories, AC-Powered .... SURGERY
Kit, Laparoscopy .... GASTRO/UROLOGY
Peritoneoscope .... GASTRO/UROLOGY
Sheath, Endoscopic .... GASTRO/UROLOGY

Elekta Instruments, Inc.
8 Executive Park West, Ste. 809
Atlanta, GA 30329
CEO: Marc Buntaine, President
   Earl DeCarli, EVP
Federal Procurement Eligibility: Small Business
Tel: 404-315-1225
Tel: 800-535-7355
Fax: 404-315-7850
Device Category:
Forceps, Endoscopic .... GASTRO/UROLOGY
Forceps, Grasping, Atraumatic .... MIN. INV. SURGERY
Forceps, Grasping, Traumatic .... MIN. INV. SURGERY
Holder, Needle, Laparoscopic .... MIN. INV. SURGERY
Holder/Scissors, Needle, Laparoscopic .... MIN. INV. SURGERY
Instrument, Dissecting, Laparoscopic .... MIN. INV. SURGERY
Retractor, Fan-Type, Laparoscopy .... MIN. INV. SURGERY
Retractor, Laparoscopy, Other .... MIN. INV. SURGERY

Elmed, Inc.
60 W. Fay Ave.
Addison, IL 60101-5198
Tel: 708-543-2792
Fax: 708-543-2102
CEO: Karl Hausner, President
Production: Werner Hausner, Product Mgr.
Federal Procurement Eligibility: Small Business
Device Category:
Blade, Knife, Laparoscopic .... MIN. INV. SURGERY
Cabinet, Storage, Endoscope .... GASTRO/UROLOGY
Camera, Video, Endoscopic .... GENERAL
Cannula, Suction, Pool-Tip .... MIN. INV. SURGERY
Cart, Equipment, Video .... GENERAL
Cart, Instrument/Equipment, Laparoscopy .... MIN. INV. SURGERY
Clamp, Fixation, Cholangiography .... MIN. INV. SURGERY
Clamp, Laparoscopy .... MIN. INV. SURGERY
Coagulator, Hysteroscopic (With Accessories) .... OBSTETRICS/GYN
Coagulator, Laparoscopic, Unipolar .... OBSTETRICS/GYN
Coagulator/Cutter, Endoscopic, Bipolar .... OBSTETRICS/GYN
Coagulator/Cutter, Endoscopic, Unipolar .... OBSTETRICS/GYN
Colposcope .... OBSTETRICS/GYN
Cord, Electric, Endoscope .... GASTRO/UROLOGY
Cover, Laparoscope .... MIN. INV. SURGERY
Dilator, Blunt .... MIN. INV. SURGERY
Electrocautery Unit, Endoscopic .... OBSTETRICS/GYN
Endoscope, Rigid .... SURGERY
Equipment, Suction/Irrigation, Laparoscopic .... SURGERY
Forceps, Electrosurgical .... SURGERY
Forceps, Endoscopic .... GASTRO/UROLOGY
Forceps, Grasping, Atraumatic .... MIN. INV. SURGERY
Forceps, Grasping, Flexible Endoscopic .... GASTRO/UROLOGY
Forceps, Grasping, Traumatic .... MIN. INV. SURGERY
Holder, Laparoscope .... OBSTETRICS/GYN
Holder, Needle, Curved, Laparoscopic .... MIN. INV. SURGERY
Holder, Needle, Laparoscopic .... MIN. INV. SURGERY
Holder/Scissors, Needle, Laparoscopic .... MIN. INV. SURGERY
Illuminator, Fiberoptic (For Endoscope) .... GASTRO/UROLOGY
Instrument, Dissecting, Laparoscopic .... MIN. INV. SURGERY
Instrument, Dissecting, Myoma, Laparoscopic .... MIN. INV. SURGERY
Instrument, Knot Tying, Suture, Laparoscopic .... MIN. INV. SURGERY
Instrument, Needle Holder/Knot Tying .... MIN. INV. SURGERY
Instrument, Passing, Suture, Laparoscopic .... MIN. INV. SURGERY
*Insufflator, Carbon-Dioxide, Automatic
   (For Endoscope)* .... GASTRO/UROLOGY
Insufflator, Hysteroscopic .... OBSTETRICS/GYN
Insufflator, Laparoscopic .... OBSTETRICS/GYN
Kit, Cholecystectomy .... MIN. INV. SURGERY
Kit, Laparoscopy .... GASTRO/UROLOGY
Laparoscope, General & Plastic Surgery .... SURGERY
Laparoscope, Gynecologic .... OBSTETRICS/GYN
Light Source, Endoscope, Xenon Arc .... SURGERY
Monitor, Video, Endoscope .... GENERAL
Needle, Insufflation, Laparoscopic .... MIN. INV. SURGERY
Probe, Suction, Irrigator/Aspirator, Laparoscopic .... MIN. INV. SURGERY
Retractor, Fan-Type, Laparoscopy .... MIN. INV. SURGERY
Snare, Endoscopic .... SURGERY
Trocar, Abdominal .... GASTRO/UROLOGY
Trocar, Gallbladder .... GASTRO/UROLOGY
Trocar, Laryngeal .... EAR/NOSE/THROAT
Warmer, Endoscope .... MIN. INV. SURGERY

Encompas Unlimited, Inc.
1110 Pinellas Bayway, Ste. 104
Tierra Verde, FL 33715-8281
Tel: 813-867-7701
Tel: 800-825-7701
Fax: 813-866-6740
CEO: Neil Thomas Flynn, Finance
   Mary E. Flynn, President
Marketing: Michael B. Capelli, VP Sales & Mktg.
Federal Procurement Eligibility: Small Business, Woman Owned
Device Category:
Accessories, Cleaning, Endoscopic .... GASTRO/UROLOGY
Cabinet, Storage, Endoscope .... GASTRO/UROLOGY
Carrier, Sponge, Endoscopic .... GASTRO/UROLOGY
Cart, Equipment, Video .... GENERAL
Container, Specimen, Laparoscopic .... SURGERY
Cystoscope .... GASTRO/UROLOGY
Sterilizer/Washer, Endoscope .... GENERAL

Endo Image Corporation
1370 Blair Dr.
Odenton, MD 21113
Tel: 410-551-9700
Tel: 800-638-0440
Fax: 410-551-9702
CEO: John Ahern
   Eileen Ramage, VP Oper.
   Dick Wheeler, VP & Gen. Mgr.
Production: Peter Christiansen, Mfg. Dir.
Federal Procurement Eligibility: Small Business
Device Category:
Camera, Video, Endoscopic .... GENERAL
Endoscope .... GASTRO/UROLOGY
Endoscope And Accessories, AC-Powered .... SURGERY

Endoflush, Inc.
6420 Carter
Shawnee Mission, KS 66203
Tel: 913-432-7200
Tel: 800-945-4767
Fax: 913-432-7767
CEO: Mike Bowman, President & CEO
   Keith Odehnal, VP Personnel
Research: Mike Armentrout, VP R&D
Federal Procurement Eligibility: Small Business
Device Category:
Accessories, Cleaning, Endoscopic .... GASTRO/UROLOGY

Endomedix Corp.
2162 Michelson Dr.
Irvine, CA 92715
Tel: 714-253-1000
Tel: 800-553-6331
Bag, Specimen, Laparoscopic .... MIN. INV. SURGERY
Choledochoscope, Flexible Or Rigid .... GASTRO/UROLOGY
Endoscope .... GASTRO/UROLOGY
Laparoscope, General & Plastic Surgery .... SURGERY
Lithotriptor, Laparoscopic .... MIN. INV. SURGERY
Peritoneoscope .... GASTRO/UROLOGY
*Probe, Detector, Flow, Blood,
   Laparoscopy, Ultrasonic* .... MIN. INV. SURGERY
System, Imaging, Laparoscopy, Ultrasonic .... MIN. INV. SURGERY
Ureteroscope .... GASTRO/UROLOGY

Endovations, Inc.
Hill & George Avenues
Reading, PA 19610
Tel: 215-378-1606
Tel: 800-255-4848
Fax: 215-374-1160
CEO: T. Jerome Holleran, President
Marketing: Norman C. Mitchell
Production: Darnall Daley
Federal Procurement Eligibility: Small Business
Device Category:
Brush, Cytology, Endoscopic .... GASTRO/UROLOGY
Insufflator, Other .... SURGERY
Needle, Endoscopic .... GASTRO/UROLOGY
Sheath, Endoscopic .... GASTRO/UROLOGY

Engstrom Mie Ltd.
Sowton Industrial Estate
Falcon Rd.
Exeter, EX2 7NA
United Kingdom
Tel: 0392/431331
Fax: 0392/439927
CEO: R.G. Coates, Fin. Dir.
 I. Pursell, Managing Dir.
Marketing: J. Effer, Mktg. Mgr.
Production: T. Longman, Dir. Techn. Sales
 LE Bray, Prod. Dir.
Federal Procurement Eligibility: Small Business
Device Category:
Laryngoscope, Rigid .... ANESTH/PUL MED

Envirosurgical, Inc.
7195 E. Kemper Rd.
Cincinnati, OH 45249-1030
Tel: 513-489-6074
Tel: 800-879-5273
Fax: 513-489-8083
CEO: Robert Garner, General Manager
 Paul Rogers, CEO
Federal Procurement Eligibility: Small Business
Device Category:
Cart, Equipment, Video .... GENERAL

Erbe Elektromedizin GmbH
Waldhoernle Str. 17
D-72072 Tuebingen,
Germany
Tel: 07071/70010
Fax: 07071/700179
Advertising: Monika Koslowski
CEO: Helmut Erbe, Managing Dir.
Marketing: J. Klein, Mktg. Dir.
Production: D. Augustin
Research: T. Frauendiener
 G. Farin, R&D
Device Category:
Coagulator, Laparoscopic, Unipolar .... OBSTETRICS/GYN
Coagulator/Cutter, Endoscopic, Bipolar .... OBSTETRICS/GYN
Coagulator/Cutter, Endoscopic, Unipolar .... OBSTETRICS/GYN
Forceps, Electrosurgical .... SURGERY

Erbe USA, Inc.
2225 NW Parkway, Ste. 105
Marietta, GA 30067
Tel: 404-955-4400
Fax: 404-955-2577
CEO: Helmut Erbe, President
Marketing: David Blakey, VP Mktg.
Federal Procurement Eligibility: Small Business
Device Category:
Coagulator, Laparoscopic, Unipolar .... OBSTETRICS/GYN
Coagulator/Cutter, Endoscopic, Bipolar .... OBSTETRICS/GYN
Coagulator/Cutter, Endoscopic, Unipolar .... OBSTETRICS/GYN
Cord, Electric, Endoscope .... GASTRO/UROLOGY
Electrocautery Unit, Endoscopic .... OBSTETRICS/GYN
Needle, Endoscopic .... GASTRO/UROLOGY
Probe, Electrocauterization, Multi-Use .... MIN. INV. SURGERY
Probe, Electrocauterization, Single-Use .... MIN. INV. SURGERY

Escalon Ophthalmics
182 Tamarack Circle
Skillman, NJ 08558-9662
Tel: 609-497-9141
Fax: 609-497-0948
CEO: Sterling C. Johnson, President
 Ron Huneneke, VP Reg. Affairs
Marketing: David Belt, Mktg. Dir.
 Charles Mullen, VP Mktg.
Production: Kevin Sinnett, VP Prod.
Research: Alan Weiner, VP R&D
Federal Procurement Eligibility: Small Business
Device Category:
Insufflator, Other .... SURGERY

Ethicon Endo-Surgery
4545 Creek Rd.
Cincinnati, OH 45242
Tel: 513-786-7000
Fax: 513-786-7080
Marketing: Nicholas J. Valeriani, VP Mktg.
Research: Steve Napiecek, Market Res.Dir.
Device Category:
Applier, Clip, Laparoscopic .... MIN. INV. SURGERY
Applier, Clip, Repair, Hernia, Laparoscopic .... MIN. INV. SURGERY
Bag, Specimen, Laparoscopic .... MIN. INV. SURGERY
Camera, Video, Endoscopic .... GENERAL
Cannula, Extraction, Appendix .... MIN. INV. SURGERY
Cannula, Suction, Pool-Tip .... MIN. INV. SURGERY
Coagulator, Laparoscopic, Unipolar .... OBSTETRICS/GYN
Coagulator/Cutter, Endoscopic, Bipolar .... OBSTETRICS/GYN
Coagulator/Cutter, Endoscopic, Unipolar .... OBSTETRICS/GYN
Cutter, Linear, Laparoscopic .... MIN. INV. SURGERY
Dilator, Blunt .... MIN. INV. SURGERY
Electrode, Electrosurgery, Laparoscopic .... MIN. INV. SURGERY
Equipment, Suction/Irrigation, Laparoscopic .... SURGERY
Forceps, Endoscopic .... GASTRO/UROLOGY
Forceps, Grasping, Atraumatic .... MIN. INV. SURGERY
Forceps, Grasping, Flexible Endoscopic .... GASTRO/UROLOGY
Handle, Instrument, Laparoscopic (Electrocautery) .. MIN. INV. SURGERY
Handle, Instrument, Laparoscopic (Irrigation) .... MIN. INV. SURGERY
Holder, Needle, Laparoscopic .... MIN. INV. SURGERY
Instrument, Dissecting, Laparoscopic .... MIN. INV. SURGERY
Kit, Bowel .... MIN. INV. SURGERY
Kit, Laparoscopy .... GASTRO/UROLOGY
Kit, Pelviscopy .... MIN. INV. SURGERY
Kit, Trocar .... MIN. INV. SURGERY
Laparoscope, Gynecologic .... OBSTETRICS/GYN
Ligature, Laparoscopic .... MIN. INV. SURGERY
Needle, Insufflation, Laparoscopic .... MIN. INV. SURGERY
Obturator, Endoscopic .... GASTRO/UROLOGY
Peritoneoscope .... GASTRO/UROLOGY
Probe, Electrocauterization, Single-Use .... MIN. INV. SURGERY
Probe, Electrosurgery, Endoscopy .... MIN. INV. SURGERY
Probe, Suction, Irrigator/Aspirator, Laparoscopic .... MIN. INV. SURGERY
Remover, Staple, Surgical .... SURGERY
Retractor, Laparoscopic, Other .... MIN. INV. SURGERY
Scissors, Laparoscopy .... MIN. INV. SURGERY
Sleeve, Trocar .... MIN. INV. SURGERY
Stapler, Laparoscopic .... MIN. INV. SURGERY
Stapler, Surgical .... SURGERY
Teaching Attachment, Endoscopic .... GASTRO/UROLOGY
Trainer, Laparoscopy .... MIN. INV. SURGERY
Tray, Sterilization, Instrument .... SURGERY
Trocar, Abdominal .... GASTRO/UROLOGY
Trocar, Gallbladder .... GASTRO/UROLOGY
Trocar, Laparoscopic .... SURGERY
Trocar, Short .... MIN. INV. SURGERY

Ethnor
192 Ave. Charles De Gaulle
F-92523 Neuilly S/Seine Cedex
France
CEO: Jacques Dumont
Device Category:
Clip, Suture..SURGERY
Power Supply, Endoscopic, Battery Operated...............GENERAL
Stapler, Surgical..SURGERY

Tel: 1/47382233
Fax: 1/46241447

Everest Medical Corp.
13755 First Ave. N.
Minneapolis, MN 55441-5454
CEO: John L. Shannon, Jr., President & CEO
   David D. Koentopf, COB
   Brian J. Jackson, CFO
Marketing: R. Keith Poppe, VP Sales
   Keith Poppe, Nat. Sales Dir.
   Janet Shanedling, Mktg. Dir.
   David Parins, VP Bus. Dev.
Production: Steven M. Blakemore, VP Operations
Research: Brian Jackson, CFO
Federal Procurement Eligibility: Small Business
Device Category:
Coagulator/Cutter, Endoscopic, Bipolar.............OBSTETRICS/GYN
Coagulator/Cutter, Endoscopic, Unipolar............OBSTETRICS/GYN
Forceps, Electrosurgical...SURGERY
Forceps, Endoscopic..GASTRO/UROLOGY
Forceps, Laparoscopy, Electrosurgical......................SURGERY
Probe, Electrocauterization, Multi-Use...............MIN. INV. SURGERY
Scissors, Laparoscopy, Electrosurgical....................SURGERY

Tel: 612-473-6262
Tel: 800-852-9361
Fax: 612-473-6465

Eximed, Inc.
198-03 Hillside Ave.
Hollis, NY 11423-2128
CEO: Roseann Grogan, VP
Device Category:
Endoscope And Accessories, AC-Powered......................SURGERY

Tel: 718-479-0020
Fax: 718-479-1116

Expanded Optics, Inc.
7382 Bolsa Ave.
Westminster, CA 92683-5212
CEO: William Charneski, President & CEO
   Ralph Thorne, CFO
   Jerry McMahon, COB & COO
Marketing: John Dawoodjee, VP Mktg. & Sales
Federal Procurement Eligibility: Small Business, VA Contract
Device Category:
Arthroscope...ORTHOPEDICS
Camera, Video, Endoscopic...................................GENERAL
Cystoscope...GASTRO/UROLOGY
Endoscope..GASTRO/UROLOGY
Laparoscope, General & Plastic Surgery.....................SURGERY
Laparoscope, Gynecologic.............................OBSTETRICS/GYN
Light, Surgical, Endoscopic...................................SURGERY

Tel: 714-891-3996
Tel: 800-942-9144
Fax: 714-898-2228

Faro Technologies, Inc.
125 Technology Park
Lake Mary, FL 32746-6204
CEO: Gregory A. Fraser, CEO
Device Category:
Camera, Television, Surgical, Without Audio................SURGERY
Holder, Leg, Arthroscopy.................................ORTHOPEDICS

Tel: 407-333-9911
Tel: 800-736-6063
Fax: 407-333-4181

Fiber-Tech Medical, Inc.
5020 Campbell Blvd., Ste. K.
Baltimore, MD 21236
CEO: Lloyd Shue, VP
   Frank Majerowicz, President
Federal Procurement Eligibility: Small Business
Device Category:
Endoscope, Flexible...GASTRO/UROLOGY

Tel: 410-931-4411
Tel: 800-736-9876
Fax: 410-931-4414

Flexmedics Corp.
12400 Whitewater Dr. #2040
Minnetonka, MN 55343
CEO: James Stice, President
Marketing: Steve Nuss, Mktg. Mgr.
Production: Diana Vaman, Oper. Mgr.
   Chet Sievert, New Prod. Mgr.
Device Category:
Needle, Suture, Arthroscopy...............................ORTHOPEDICS

Tel: 612-939-0900
Tel: 800-338-0305
Fax: 612-939-0739

Frankignoul & Cie. S.A.
Zoning Industriel
B-4330 Grace-Hollogne
Belgium
CEO: L. Legros
Marketing: Marc Vujasin
Production: Pol Damanet
Device Category:
Power Supply, Endoscopic, Battery Operated...............GENERAL

Tel: 41/633920

Frantz Medical Development Ltd.
7740 Metric Drive
Mentor, OH 44060-4862
CEO: Mark G. Frantz, President
Production: Paul Hanson, Oper. VP
   Michael Litscher, V.P. Mauf. Oper.
Research: Mark R. Honard, Engineering Dir.
Device Category:
Forceps, Endoscopic..GASTRO/UROLOGY
Obturator, Endoscopic.....................................GASTRO/UROLOGY
Pump, Air, Non-Manual, Endoscopic....................GASTRO/UROLOGY

Tel: 216-255-1155
Tel: 800-522-6518
Fax: 216-255-6975

Frontline Medical Supplies
1601 S.W. 37th St.
Ocala, FL 34474
Advertising: Kevin P. Connell
CEO: C. P. Foster Jr., CEO
Marketing: C. J. Phillips II, VP Sales & Mktg.
Federal Procurement Eligibility: Small Business
Device Category:
Laryngoscope..EAR/NOSE/THROAT

Tel: 904-237-1122
Tel: 800-237-5131

Fuji Photo Optical Co. Ltd.
1-324, Uetake-Machi, Omiya
Saitama 330
Japan
CEO: Minoru Mori, President
   H. Kawamura, Gen. Mgr.
Device Category:
Bronchoscope, Flexible....................................EAR/NOSE/THROAT
Colonoscope, Gastro-Urology..............................GASTRO/UROLOGY

Tel: 048/668-2153
Fax: 048/651-8517

Esophagoscope (Flexible Or Rigid).....................EAR/NOSE/THROAT
Gastroscope, Flexible ....GASTRO/UROLOGY
Laparoscope, Flexible...SURGERY
Light Source, Endoscope, Xenon Arc ....SURGERY
Panendoscope ....GASTRO/UROLOGY
Pharyngoscope...................................EAR/NOSE/THROAT
Sigmoidoscope, Flexible ....GASTRO/UROLOGY

Fujinon, Inc.
10 High Point Dr.
Wayne, NJ 07470-7434
Tel: 201-633-5600
Tel: 800-872-0196
Fax: 201-633-8818
CEO: S. Takada, President
   Mark Lehmann, Bus. Dev. Mgr.
Marketing: Karl Weydig, Dir. Mktg. & New Products
Federal Procurement Eligibility: Small Business, GSA Contract
Device Category:
Basket, Biliary Stone Retrieval.........................GASTRO/UROLOGY
Bottle, Endoscopic Wash ....GASTRO/UROLOGY
Bronchoscope, Flexible ....EAR/NOSE/THROAT
Brush, Cytology, Endoscopic ....GASTRO/UROLOGY
Camera, Still, Endoscopic......................................SURGERY
Choledochoscope, Flexible Or Rigid ....GASTRO/UROLOGY
Colonoscope, Gastro-Urology........................GASTRO/UROLOGY
Duodenoscope, Esophago/Gastro....................GASTRO/UROLOGY
Endoscope ....GASTRO/UROLOGY
Endoscope, Electronic (Videoendoscope).......................SURGERY
Gastroduodenoscope.................................GASTRO/UROLOGY
Gastroscope, Flexible ....GASTRO/UROLOGY
Gastroscope, Gastro-Urology.........................GASTRO/UROLOGY
Kit, Laparoscopy ....GASTRO/UROLOGY
Laparoscope, Flexible...SURGERY
Laparoscope, General & Plastic Surgery ....SURGERY
Light Source, Endoscope, Xenon Arc ....SURGERY
Module, Control, Electrosurgery ....MIN. INV. SURGERY
Monitor, Video, Endoscope ....GENERAL
Panendoscope ....GASTRO/UROLOGY
Sigmoidoscope, Flexible ....GASTRO/UROLOGY
Thoracoscope..CARDIOVASCULAR

Galileo Electro-Optics Corp.
Galileo Park, Rte. 20
P.O. Box 550
Sturbridge, MA 01566
Tel: 508-347-9191
Tel: 800-648-1800
Fax: 508-347-3849
CEO: William T. Hanley, President & CEO
Marketing: Laurie Placella, Mktg. Comm. Specialist
   David Skiles, VP Sales & Mktg.
Production: David Byrne, VP Mfg.
Federal Procurement Eligibility: Small Business
Device Category:
Illuminator, Fiberoptic (For Endoscope) ....GASTRO/UROLOGY

Geister Medizintechnik GmbH
Foehrenstr. 2
Postfach 4228
D-78532 Tuttlingen
Germany
Tel: 7461-8084
Fax: 7461-77587
CEO: Guenter Geister
Marketing: Carsten Geister
Device Category:
Camera, Video, Endoscopic ....GENERAL
Forceps, Electrosurgical ....SURGERY
Forceps, Endoscopic.................................GASTRO/UROLOGY
Forceps, Grasping, Flexible Endoscopic................GASTRO/UROLOGY
Insufflator, Laparoscopic................................OBSTETRICS/GYN
Laparoscope, General & Plastic Surgery ....SURGERY
Laparoscope, Gynecologic ....OBSTETRICS/GYN
Laryngoscope, Surgical..SURGERY
Trocar, Other..GENERAL

Glaser & Co. GmbH Medizintechnik
Eisenbahnstrasse 61
D-82110 Germering
Germany
Tel: 089/847125
Fax: 089/840-2274
Advertising: Verena Glaser
CEO: Paul Glaser
Federal Procurement Eligibility: GSA Contract
Device Category:
Tape, Television & Video, Endoscopic.................GASTRO/UROLOGY

Globe Medical, Inc. (Endo Scientific)
9291 130th Ave. N., Ste. 410
Largo, FL 34643
Tel: 813-585-9700
Tel: 800-237-4456
Fax: 813-585-4930
Ownership: Private
Distribution: Manufacturer Through Distributors & Reps., Importer
CEO: H.P. Zinnecker, President
Marketing: R.O. Zinnecker, Dir. Mktg.
   D.L. Zinnecker, VP Sales
Federal Procurement Eligibility: Small Business
Device Category:
Forceps, Endoscopic.................................GASTRO/UROLOGY

GM Engineering, Inc.
2549 Sierra Way #B
La Verna, CA 91750-5800
Tel: 909-596-5065
Fax: 909-596-4267
CEO: Gregory M. Miles, President
Federal Procurement Eligibility: Small Business
Device Category:
Kit, Laparoscopy ....GASTRO/UROLOGY

Gowllands Limited
176 Morland Rd.
Croydon,
United Kingdom
Tel: 081/654-3011
Fax: 081/655-1839
CEO: John Gowlland
Device Category:
Laryngoscope, Rigid......................................ANESTH/PUL MED

Graham-Field, Inc.
400 Rabro Dr. East
Hauppauge, NY 11788-4226
Tel: 516-582-5900
Tel: 800-645-8176
Fax: 516-234-7584
Advertising: Stan Fox, VP Sales
   Kerrin Ernst, Dir. Cust. Relations
CEO: Wayne Merdinger, Exec. VP
   Irwin Selinger, President
Marketing: Ed Link, Mktg. Dir.
Federal Procurement Eligibility: Small Business, GSA Contract
Device Category:
Bulb, Inflation (Endoscope)............................GASTRO/UROLOGY
Trocar, Tracheal....................................EAR/NOSE/THROAT

Greenwald Surgical Co., Inc.
Tel: 219-962-1604
Fax: 219-962-4009
2688 Dekalb Street
Lake Station, IN 46405-1519
CEO: Christopher Reynolds, General Manager
Federal Procurement Eligibility: Small Business
Device Category:
Cannula, Suprapubic, With Trocar .... GASTRO/UROLOGY
Coagulator/Cutter, Endoscopic, Bipolar .... OBSTETRICS/GYN
Needle, Endoscopic .... GASTRO/UROLOGY
Sheath, Endoscopic .... GASTRO/UROLOGY

Grieshaber & Co. AG
Tel: 053/248121
Fax: 053/245608
Winkelriedstr. 52
CH-8203 Schaffhausen
Switzerland
Advertising: J. van Loon, VP Customer Svc.
CEO: Hans R. Grieshaber, President
Marketing: B. Wicki, VP Mktg. & Sales
Production: W. Steinmann, VP & Prod. Mgr.
Research: R. Demmerle, R&D Head
Device Category:
Cannula, Suprapubic, With Trocar .... GASTRO/UROLOGY

Gyne-Tech Instrument Corp.
Tel: 213-849-1512
Tel: 818-842-2199
Fax: 818-848-8067
1111 Chestnut Street
Burbank, CA 91506-1624
CEO: J. Kermit Floyd, President
Federal Procurement Eligibility: Small Business
Device Category:
Colposcope .... OBSTETRICS/GYN

Hall Surgical
Tel: 805-684-0456
Fax: 805-684-3185
1170 Mark Ave.
Carpinteria, CA 93013-2918
Advertising: Brooke Rye, Advertising Mgr.
CEO: George Kempsell, Pres.
Marketing: Jim Robson, Mktg. VP
  Brenda Acosta, Mktg. Analyst
Device Category:
Accessories, Arthroscope .... ORTHOPEDICS

Hammacher GmbH, Karl
Tel: 0212/66047
Fax: 0212/67135
Steinendorferstr. 27
D-42699 Solingen
Germany
CEO: Rolf Hammacher
Production: Karl-Willi Hammacher
Device Category:
Trocar, Cardiovascular .... CARDIOVASCULAR

Harloff Company
Tel: 719-637-0300
Tel: 800-433-4064
Fax: 719-597-8273
650 Ford St.
Colorado Springs, CO 80915-3712
CEO: Tom Mosteller, CEO
Marketing: Nancy Quinata, Telemktg. Mgr.
  James Dausch, VP Mktg.
Federal Procurement Eligibility: Small Business, GSA Contract, VA Contract
Device Category:
Cabinet, Storage, Endoscope .... GASTRO/UROLOGY
Cart, Equipment, Video .... GENERAL

Hemox, Inc.
Tel: 407-777-4772
Tel: 800-323-4393
P.O. Box 362115
Melbourne, FL 32902-0115
CEO: Judith V. Simpson, President
  James L. Simpson, CEO
Federal Procurement Eligibility: Small Business
Device Category:
Insufflator, Other .... SURGERY

Henke-Sass GmbH, Wolf
Tel: 07461/189-0
Fax: 07461/189-181
Kronenstrasse 16
D-78532 Tuttlingen
Germany
CEO: Werner Sartorius
Marketing: Roland Keuffel, Sales Mgr.
  Gunther Schnell, Sales Mgr.
  Gerhard Gabel, Sales Mgr. Disp.
  Armin Scham, Prod. Mgr.
  Armin Lekitsch, VP Sales & Mktg.
Production: Peter Decker
Device Category:
Endoscope .... GASTRO/UROLOGY

Heraeus Surgical, Inc.
Tel: 408-954-4000
Tel: 800-227-8372
Fax: 408-954-4040
575 Cottonwood Dr.
Milpitas, CA 95035-7402
Advertising: Travis Lee, Adv. Mgr.
CEO: Tony Pollace, Controller
  Tom Ihlenfeldt, President
Marketing: John Morley, VP Mktg.
  Alan Polish, Mktg. Mgr.
Device Category:
Accessories, Photographic, Endoscopic .... GASTRO/UROLOGY
Camera, Video, Endoscopic .... GENERAL
Camera, Video, Multi-Image .... MIN. INV. SURGERY
Camera, Videotape, Surgical .... SURGERY
Cart, Equipment, Video .... GENERAL
Endoscope And Accessories, AC-Powered .... SURGERY
Endoscope, Rigid .... SURGERY
Equipment/Accessories, Laser, Laparoscopy .... MIN. INV. SURGERY
Forceps, Endoscopic .... GASTRO/UROLOGY
Forceps, Grasping, Atraumatic .... MIN. INV. SURGERY
Forceps, Grasping, Traumatic .... MIN. INV. SURGERY
Illuminator, Fiberoptic (For Endoscope) .... GASTRO/UROLOGY
Instrument, Dissecting, Laparoscopic .... MIN. INV. SURGERY
Laparoscope, Gynecologic .... OBSTETRICS/GYN
Laser, Nd:YAG, Laparoscopy .... MIN. INV. SURGERY
Monitor, Video, Endoscope .... GENERAL
Needle, Insufflation, Laparoscopic .... MIN. INV. SURGERY
Scissors with Removable Tips, Laparoscopy .... MIN. INV. SURGERY
Trocar, Abdominal .... GASTRO/UROLOGY

Herger AG Tel: 61/354060
Dornacherstr. 89, Postfach 80
CH-4008 Basel,
Switzerland
CEO: M. Herger
Device Category:
Cannula, Drainage, Arthroscopy...................ORTHOPEDICS
Cannula, Suprapubic, With Trocar ....GASTRO/UROLOGY

Herwig Surgical Instrument Co. Tel: 804-264-7585
8741 Landmark Rd. Tel: 800-876-9898
Richmond, VA 23228-2801 Fax: 804-264-7631
CEO: Jerry Scheib, Gen. Mgr.
Marketing: Susan Worley, Cust. Svc. Supv.
Production: Buster Pugh, VP Mfg.
Device Category:
Trocar, Gallbladder......................................GASTRO/UROLOGY

Himalaya Trading Co., (PVT) Ltd. Tel: (0432) 552249
Wazirabad Rd. Fax: 432-552250
P.O. Box No. 59
Sialkot
Pakistan
Advertising: M. Ashraf Mirza, Adv. Mgr.
CEO: Manzoor Hussain, Accountant
    M. Farooq Qureshi
Marketing: Zubair Qureshi, Mktg/Accounts Dir.
    M. Farooq Qureshi, CEO
    Istiaq Ahmed Qadri, Local Purchase Mgr.
Production: Khalid Javed Qureshi, Production Dir.
    Ejaz Ahmed Qureshi, QC Dir.
Device Category:
Anoscope, Non-Powered ....GASTRO/UROLOGY
Laryngoscope, Surgical ....SURGERY
Proctoscope ....SURGERY
Sigmoidoscope, Rigid, Electrical ....GASTRO/UROLOGY
Sigmoidoscope, Rigid, Non-Electrical ....GASTRO/UROLOGY
Sphincteroscope...GASTRO/UROLOGY
Trocar, Abdominal ....GASTRO/UROLOGY

Hipp GmbH, Anton Tel: 07463/7776-5088
Annastr. 25/1 Fax: 07463/1708
Postfach 80
D-78567 Fridingen
Germany
CEO: Anton Hipp
Marketing: Gerhard Hipp
Production: Dieter Hipp
Device Category:
Arthroscope ....ORTHOPEDICS
Coagulator, Laparoscopic, Unipolar ....OBSTETRICS/GYN
Coagulator/Cutter, Endoscopic, Bipolar ....OBSTETRICS/GYN
Kit, Laparoscopy ....GASTRO/UROLOGY
Laparoscope, General & Plastic Surgery ....SURGERY
Laparoscope, Gynecologic ....OBSTETRICS/GYN

Hitachi Denshi America, Ltd. Tel: 516-921-7200
150 Crossways Park Drive Fax: 516-496-3718
Woodbury, NY 11797-2028
Advertising: Karen Sawyer
CEO: M. Matsuhashi, Gen. Mgr.
    A. Kobayashi, President
Marketing: Todd Yokomichi, Regional Sales Mgr.
    Nick Stamas, Regional Sales Mgr.
    Fred Posner, Nat'l Sales Mgr.
    Bernard V. Munzelle, VP Sales & Mktg.
Production: Fred Scott, Dir. Eng.
Device Category:
Camera, Television, Surgical, With Audio........SURGERY
Camera, Videotape, Surgical..........................SURGERY
Monitor, Video, Endoscope ....GENERAL

Hitachi Denshi Ltd. Tel: 03/2558411
1-23-2, Kanda Suda-Cho
Chiyoda-Ku
Tokyo 101
Japan
CEO: S. Ozawa, President
Marketing: Keiji Hara, Overseas Oper.
Device Category:
Camera, Television, Endoscopic, With Audio .....SURGERY
Camera, Television, Endoscopic, Without Audio ...SURGERY
Camera, Television, Microsurgical, With Audio ....SURGERY
Camera, Television, Microsurgical, Without Audio ..SURGERY
Camera, Television, Surgical, With Audio ....SURGERY
Camera, Television, Surgical, Without Audio ...SURGERY
Monitor, Video, Endoscope ....GENERAL

Hobbs Medical, Inc. Tel: 203-684-5875
P.O. Box 46 Tel: 800-344-6227
Stafford Springs, CT 06076-0046 Fax: 203-684-7574
CEO: George Pompeo, President
Marketing: John McGrath
Federal Procurement Eligibility: Small Business, Minority Owned
Device Category:
Basket, Biliary Stone Retrieval.......................GASTRO/UROLOGY
Brush, Cytology, Endoscopic ....GASTRO/UROLOGY
Forceps, Grasping, Flexible Endoscopic.........GASTRO/UROLOGY
Needle, Endoscopic ....GASTRO/UROLOGY

Hoekloos Medical Equipment Tel: 020/5811470
Kabelweg 44 Fax: 020/810016
P.O. Box 663
NL-1000 AR Amsterdam
Netherlands
CEO: J. Bakker, Gen. Mgr. Med. Equipment
Marketing: J. Ooykaas
Research: E. Palmboom
Device Category:
Power Supply, Endoscopic, Line Operated ....GENERAL

Horizon Medical Tel: 612-298-0843
324 State St. Tel: 800-367-6435
St. Paul, MN 55107-1608 Fax: 612-298-0018
CEO: Timothy M. Scanlan, President
Marketing: Walter J. Olson, VP Sales & Mktg.
    Mark Anderson, Mktg. Mgr.
    Frank Coolong, Nat'l. Sales Mgr.
Production: Sarah Burgwald, Asst. Operations Mgr.
    Julie Rielly, VP Oper.
Federal Procurement Eligibility: Small Business
Device Category:
Arthroscope ....ORTHOPEDICS

I.C. Medical, Inc.
Tel: 602-943-6162
Fax: 602-870-3755
2340 W. Shangri-La, Ste. 202
Phoenix, AZ 85029-4746
CEO: Ioan Cosmescu
Marketing: Elena Cosmescu, Mktg. Mgr.
Federal Procurement Eligibility: Small Business
Device Category:
Tube, Smoke Removal, Endoscopic......................GASTRO/UROLOGY

I.S.I. Manufacturing, Inc.
Tel: 412-863-4911
Tel: 800-827-4911
Fax: 412-863-9629
1947 Ivanhoe Dr.
Irwin, PA 15642-4454
Advertising: Sue Smith
CEO: Samuel Johnson, CEO
  Michael Shedlock, Controller
  Frances Johnson, Treasurer
Marketing: Sean C. Johnson
Production: A. Scott Johnson
Federal Procurement Eligibility: Small Business, Woman Owned, GSA Contract, VA Contract
Device Category:
Endoscope..GASTRO/UROLOGY
Endoscope, Rigid..SURGERY
Stapler, Surgical...SURGERY

Ibiom Instruments Ltd.
Tel: 514-678-5468
Fax: 514-445-9837
6640 Rue Barry
Brossard, QUE J4Z 1T8
Canada
CEO: Andre Choquette
Federal Procurement Eligibility: Small Business
Device Category:
Camera, Videotape, Surgical..SURGERY

Ideas For Medicine, Inc.
Tel: 813-576-2747
Tel: 800-768-4332
Fax: 813-573-7907
12167 49th St. N
Clearwater, FL 34622-4304
CEO: Bill McPherson, President
Marketing: Toshio Ihahara, VP
Federal Procurement Eligibility: Small Business
Device Category:
Catheter, Cholangiography..SURGERY
Holder, Instrument, Laparoscopic......................MIN. INV. SURGERY

Imagyn Medical, Inc.
Tel: 714-362-2500
Fax: 714-362-2520
27651 La Paz Rd.
Laguna Beach, CA 92656
CEO: Thomas Hazen, VP Personnel
  J. C. MacRae, VP & CFO
  Guy R. Lowery, President
  Glendon French, CEO
Marketing: Keith Tholin, VP, Mktg.
Research: Gary M. Woker, VP R & D
Device Category:
Camera, Video, Endoscopic..GENERAL

Inben Brothers Company
Tel: 312-286-7241
Fax: 312-286-5424
5250 N. Leamington Ave.
Chicago, IL 60630-1622
CEO: Duck S. Yim, President
Federal Procurement Eligibility: Small Business, Minority Owned
Device Category:
Brush, Cytology, Endoscopic...............................GASTRO/UROLOGY

Inlet Medical, Inc.
Tel: 612-942-5034
Fax: 612-942-5036
9951 Valley View Rd.
Eden Prairie, MN 55344
CEO: Thomas Parafinik, President
Marketing: John Cook, VP Mktg.
Federal Procurement Eligibility: Small Business
Device Category:
Equipment, Suction/Irrigation, Laparoscopic.....................SURGERY
Probe, Suction, Irrigator/Aspirator, Laparoscopic....MIN. INV. SURGERY
Tubing, Irrigation...MIN. INV. SURGERY

Innovative Surgical, Inc.
Tel: 407-697-5051
Tel: 800-940-2680
Fax: 407-697-4558
3071 Continental Dr., Ste. 102
West Palm Beach, FL 33407
Marketing: Warren Kirschbaum, Dir. Mktg.
  Chip Jones, Product Mgr.
Federal Procurement Eligibility: Small Business
Device Category:
Forceps, Endoscopic...GASTRO/UROLOGY
Forceps, Grasping, Atraumatic..........................MIN. INV. SURGERY
Instrument, Dissecting, Laparoscopic..................MIN. INV. SURGERY
Scissors with Removable Tips, Laparoscopy..........MIN. INV. SURGERY
Scissors, Laparoscopy......................................MIN. INV. SURGERY

Instrument Makar, Inc.
Tel: 517-332-3593
Tel: 800-248-4668
Fax: 517-332-2043
2950 E. Mt. Hope
Okemos, MI 48864-1910
CEO: Dean Z. Look, Director
Marketing: Rick Carrow, Sales
  Keith M. McGrath, Mktg. Dir.
Federal Procurement Eligibility: Small Business
Device Category:
Accessories, Arthroscope....................................... ORTHOPEDICS
Arthroscope... ORTHOPEDICS
Cannula, Drainage, Arthroscopy............................... ORTHOPEDICS
Coagulator/Cutter, Endoscopic, Bipolar.................OBSTETRICS/GYN
Forceps, Endoscopic...GASTRO/UROLOGY
Forceps, Grasping, Atraumatic..........................MIN. INV. SURGERY
Forceps, Grasping, Flexible Endoscopic................GASTRO/UROLOGY
Holder, Leg, Arthroscopy... ORTHOPEDICS
Holder, Shoulder, Arthroscopy...SURGERY
Instrument, Knot Tying, Suture, Laparoscopic........MIN. INV. SURGERY
Instrument, Needle Holder/Knot Tying..................MIN. INV. SURGERY
Needle, Suture, Arthroscopy.................................... ORTHOPEDICS
Probe, Electrocauterization, Single-Use................MIN. INV. SURGERY
Sheath, Endoscopic..GASTRO/UROLOGY
Trocar, Other... GENERAL

Instrument Technology, Inc.
33 Airport Rd.
P.O. Box 381
Westfield, MA 01086-1357
Tel: 413-562-3606
Fax: 413-568-9809
Advertising: Tracy Donovan, Adv. Mgr.
CEO: Jeffrey K. Carignan, President
Marketing: Denise Brethen
Production: Gregory Carignan, VP Mfg.
Research: Joseph Rose Warne, VP R&D
Federal Procurement Eligibility: Small Business, GSA Contract
Device Category:
Endoscope .... GASTRO/UROLOGY
Endoscope, Direct Vision .... SURGERY
Endoscope, Electronic (Videoendoscope) .... SURGERY
Endoscope, Flexible .... GASTRO/UROLOGY
Endoscope, Rigid .... SURGERY

International General Med. Sys. Ltd. Picker Div.
P.O. Box 2, East Lane
GB-Wembley, Middlesex HA9 7PR
United Kingdom
Tel: 01/904-1288
Fax: 01/908-4908
Total Employees: 600
Distribution: Manufacturer Direct
Advertising: J. Mitchell
CEO: G. Mandy, Managing Dir.
Marketing: J.K. Alderson
Device Category:
Arthrogram Kit .... ORTHOPEDICS

Intertech Resources, Inc.
300 Tri-State Int'l, Ste. 150
Lincolnshire, IL 60069-4446
Tel: 708-940-7789
Tel: 800-258-5361
Fax: 708-940-8119
CEO: Vito Manone, President & CEO
  Ed Murphy, CFO
Marketing: Chuck McGee
  Bill Odell
Federal Procurement Eligibility: GSA Contract, VA Contract
Device Category:
Laryngoscope .... EAR/NOSE/THROAT

Intramed Labs
11100 Roselle Street
San Diego, CA 92121-1210
Tel: 619-455-5000
Fax: 619-455-5033
CEO: Stuart Foster, President & CEO
  Steven McGowan, VP Finance
Marketing: Alan Schempp, VP Mktg. & Sales
Production: Stephen Sosnowski, VP Oper.
Device Category:
Choledochoscope, Flexible Or Rigid .... GASTRO/UROLOGY
Pump, Air, Non-Manual, Endoscopic .... GASTRO/UROLOGY
Ureteroscope .... GASTRO/UROLOGY

Izumo Rubber Manufacturing Co. Ltd.
7-13, Kitashinagawa 5 Chome
Shinagawa-ku
Tokyo 141
Japan
Tel: 03/3441-3105
Fax: 03/3445-5705
CEO: Atsuo Tazuke, Chairman
  Atsuhiko Unno
Marketing: H. Yokoi, Export Mgr.
Device Category:
Laryngoscope .... EAR/NOSE/THROAT

Jarit Instruments
9 Skyline Dr.
Hawthorne, NY 10532-2119
Tel: 914-592-9050
Tel: 800-431-1123
Fax: 914-592-8056
CEO: Jay Jamner
Marketing: Richard Kolar, Sales Mgr.
  Howard Jamner
Production: Mike Rubin
Federal Procurement Eligibility: Small Business
Device Category:
Forceps, Endoscopic .... GASTRO/UROLOGY
Kit, Cholecystectomy .... MIN. INV. SURGERY
Laparoscope, General & Plastic Surgery .... SURGERY

Jason Marketing Co.
P.O. Box 2608
Seal Beach, CA 90740
Tel: 714-891-5544
Fax: 714-891-5875
CEO: Hank Mancini, General Mgr.
Marketing: Michael Yale, Mktg. Mgr.
Federal Procurement Eligibility: Small Business, GSA Contract, VA Contract
Device Category:
Tape, Television & Video, Endoscopic .... GASTRO/UROLOGY

Javelin Electronics
19831 Magellan Dr.
Torrance, CA 90502
Tel: 310-327-7440
Tel: 800-421-2716
Fax: 310-327-5405
Advertising: Mary Perry, Adv. Mgr.
CEO: Ray Payne, EVP
  Patricia Smith, Human Res. Mgr.
  Graham Wallis, President
Marketing: Mike Wolpert, VP Sales
  Doug Gray, Intl. Sales/Mktg. Mgr.
  Arnie Newman, Natl. Sales Mgr.
Production: Mike Burton, Oper. Mgr.
Federal Procurement Eligibility: GSA Contract
Device Category:
Camera, Video, Endoscopic .... GENERAL

Jedmed Instruments Co.
6096 Lemay Ferry Rd.
St. Louis, MO 63129-2217
Tel: 314-845-3770
Fax: 314-845-3771
CEO: John E. Dull, President
Marketing: Thomas Schreiber, Customer Rel. Mgr.
  James Lankford, VP
Federal Procurement Eligibility: Small Business
Device Category:
Forceps, Electrosurgical .... SURGERY
Laryngostroboscope (Endoscope) .... EAR/NOSE/THROAT

Johnson Controls Inc. Tel: 414-961-6500
Specialty Battery Div. Fax: 414-961-6506
900 E. Keefe Ave.
Milwaukee, WI 53212-1709
Medical Products Sales Volume: $4,000,000
Total Employees: 250
Distribution: Manufacturer Direct, Through Distributors
CEO: Ray Kubis, VP & Gen. Mgr.
Marketing: Jim L. Winistorfer, Mktg. Dir.
Production: Tammy Kwiecinski, Dist. Mgr.
 T.E. Ruhlmann, Tech. Field Svc. Mgr.
Device Category:
Box, Battery, Rechargeable (Endoscopic)..............GASTRO/UROLOGY

JSB-Medizintechnik Tel: 07424/4303
Hauptstr. 24 Fax: 07424/4301
D-78549 Spaichingen
Germany
CEO: Joachim S. Braun
Device Category:
Needle, Suture, Arthroscopy........................ORTHOPEDICS

Justman Brush Co. Tel: 402-451-4420
P.O. Box 12364 Fax: 402-451-1473
Omaha, NE 68112-2216
CEO: John S. Matthews, President
Production: Robert E. Miller, Mgr.
Federal Procurement Eligibility: Small Business
Device Category:
Accessories, Cleaning, Endoscopic.................GASTRO/UROLOGY

JVC Professional Products Co. Tel: 201-794-3900
41 Slater Dr. Tel: 800-526-5308
Elmwood Park, NJ 07407-1348 Fax: 201-523-2077
CEO: Tom McCarthy, Gen. Mgr.
 Mike Yoshida
Marketing: David Walton
Federal Procurement Eligibility: GSA Contract
Device Category:
Camera, Cine, Endoscopic, Without Audio..............SURGERY
Camera, Videotape, Surgical..........................SURGERY

K+A Medical Tel: 904-767-0229
413 Oak Pl., Bldg. 6J Tel: 800-545-2633
Port Orange, FL 32127-4352 Fax: 904-767-0559
CEO: Louis L. Rudt, President
Marketing: Marilyn Willhoit, VP Mktg. & Sales
 Debbie Brown, Contract Sales Mgr.
Production: Meir Kozbusky, VP Operations
Federal Procurement Eligibility: Small Business, VA Contract
Device Category:
Kit, Cholecystectomy.........................MIN. INV. SURGERY
Thoracoscope..................................CARDIOVASCULAR

K-medic, Inc. Tel: 201-944-8731
117 Fort Lee Rd. Tel: 800-955-0559
Leonia, NJ 07605-2216 Fax: 201-944-9014
CEO: Helmut Kapczynski, President
Marketing: Colleen Neff
 Blair Engelken, VP Sales & Mktg.
Production: Patrice Schmitz, Purchasing Mgr.
 Holger Greunart, QA Mgr.
Federal Procurement Eligibility: Small Business
Device Category:
Laparoscope, General & Plastic Surgery..........................SURGERY

Karindo Alkestron P.T. Tel: 021/5600896
17 Tomang Raya Tel: 021/5600898
Jakarta 11440 Fax: 021/5600906
Indonesia
CEO: Tony Sirad
 I.R. Tugiman
Marketing: Kristanto Sidjono
 Joseph O. Mulia
Device Category:
Camera, Video, Endoscopic...............................GENERAL
Endoscope, Electronic (Videoendoscope)..................SURGERY

Kelleher Medical, Inc. Tel: 804-323-4040
9710 Farrar Court, Suite N Tel: 800-222-7577
Richmond, VA 23236 Fax: 804-323-4073
CEO: Nicole M. Kelleher
 Johana L. Kelleher
 Francis J. Kelleher, President
Marketing: Ana S. Kelleher
Federal Procurement Eligibility: Small Business, VA Contract
Device Category:
Accessories, Surgical Camera............................SURGERY
Bronchoscope, Rigid............................EAR/NOSE/THROAT
Camera, Still, Endoscopic...............................SURGERY
Esophagoscope, Rigid, Gastro-Urology..............GASTRO/UROLOGY
Laryngoscope...................................EAR/NOSE/THROAT
Laryngoscope, Rigid............................ANESTH/PUL MED
Laryngostroboscope (Endoscope)...................EAR/NOSE/THROAT
Nasopharyngoscope (Flexible Or Rigid)............EAR/NOSE/THROAT

Kendall Co., The Tel: 508-261-8000
15 Hampshire St. Tel: 800-346-7197
Mansfield, MA 02048-1113 Fax: 508-261-8145
CEO: Richard J. Meelia, President
 R.A. Gilleland, President & CEO
 K.H. Titlebaum, Controller
 A.R. Castaldi, Sr. VP & CFO
Marketing: John H. Hammergren, VP & Gen. Mgr. Med/Surg Div.
Production: K.J. Gould, VP & Gen. Mgr. Crit. Care Div.
Federal Procurement Eligibility: GSA Contract, VA Contract
Device Category:
Trocar, Cardiovascular..........................CARDIOVASCULAR

Kensey Nash Corporation Tel: 215-524-0188
55 E. Uwchlan Ave., Ste. 204 Fax: 215-524-0265
Exton, PA 19341-1247
CEO: K. Kensey, COB
  Joseph Kaufmann, CFO
  John Nash, EVP
  David W. Anderson, President & CEO
Federal Procurement Eligibility: Small Business
Device Category:
Cannula, Suprapubic, With Trocar .... GASTRO/UROLOGY
Drain, Suction, Closed .... MIN. INV. SURGERY
Forceps, Endoscopic .... GASTRO/UROLOGY
Forceps, Grasping, Atraumatic .... MIN. INV. SURGERY
Forceps, Grasping, Traumatic .... MIN. INV. SURGERY
Instrument, Dissecting, Laparoscopic .... MIN. INV. SURGERY
Probe, Electrocauterization, Multi-Use .... MIN. INV. SURGERY
Retractor, Laparoscopy, Other .... MIN. INV. SURGERY
Snare, Endoscopic .... SURGERY
Trocar, Other .... GENERAL

Kentek Corp., The Tel: 603-225-1117
4 Depot St. Fax: 603-225-6368
Pittsfield, NH 03263-1108
CEO: Mike Toepel, President
  Joe Jeng
Marketing: Laura Williams, Dir. Mktg.
Federal Procurement Eligibility: Small Business, Minority Owned, GSA Contract
Device Category:
Laser, Nd:YAG, Laparoscopy .... MIN. INV. SURGERY

Key Surgical, Inc. Tel: 612-831-7331
7101 York Ave. S. Tel: 800-541-7995
Edina, MN 55435-4450 Fax: 612-921-3298
Marketing: Gerry Barlage Lattimore
Federal Procurement Eligibility: Small Business, Woman Owned
Device Category:
Endoscope, Rigid .... SURGERY

Keymed Medical & Tel: 0702/616333
Industrial Equipment Ltd. Fax: 0702/465677
Keymed House, Stock Rd.
Southend-on-Sea, Essex SS2 5QH
United Kingdom
Medical Products Sales Volume: $60,000,000
Total Employees: 550
Distribution: Manufacturer & Exclusive Distributor
CEO: S.M. Greengrass, Products Dir.
  M.C. Woodford, Managing Dir.
  M. Kishimoto
  I. Kawahara
  B. Knight, Finance Dir.
Marketing: P.A. Hillman, Sales & Mktg. Dir.
Production: P. Virgo, Production Dir.
  G.C. Parker, Tech. Dir.

Device Category:
Accessories, Cleaning, Endoscopic .... GASTRO/UROLOGY
Arthroscope .... ORTHOPEDICS
Camera, Television, Endoscopic, With Audio .... SURGERY
Cystoscope .... GASTRO/UROLOGY
Cystourethroscope .... GASTRO/UROLOGY
Endoscope, Flexible .... GASTRO/UROLOGY
Laparoscope, Gynecologic .... OBSTETRICS/GYN
Prosthesis, Esophageal .... EAR/NOSE/THROAT
Resectoscope .... GASTRO/UROLOGY
Sheath, Endoscopic .... GASTRO/UROLOGY
Tape, Television & Video, Endoscopic .... GASTRO/UROLOGY
Urethroscope .... GASTRO/UROLOGY

Keymed, Inc. Tel: 914-425-3100
400 Airport Executive Park Fax: 914-425-2192
Spring Valley, NY 10977-7404
CEO: Peter Virgo, President
Marketing: James Trochanowski, VP
Production: Christine Noselli, Prod. Mgr.
Federal Procurement Eligibility: Small Business
Device Category:
Accessories, Cleaning, Endoscopic .... GASTRO/UROLOGY
Cabinet, Storage, Endoscope .... GASTRO/UROLOGY
Endoscope And Accessories, AC-Powered .... SURGERY
Prosthesis, Esophageal .... EAR/NOSE/THROAT
Sheath, Endoscopic .... GASTRO/UROLOGY
Sterilizer/Washer, Endoscope .... GENERAL
Tape, Television & Video, Endoscopic .... GASTRO/UROLOGY

Kimura Medical Instrument Co. Ltd. Tel: 03/3814-4481
17-5, 2-Chome, Yushima Fax: 03/3814-5304
Bunkyo-Ku
Tokyo 113
Japan
CEO: S. Kimura, President
Marketing: M. Tsushima, Director/Gen. Mgr., Int'l. Div.
Device Category:
Laryngoscope, Rigid .... ANESTH/PUL MED

Kirwan Surgical Products, Inc. Tel: 617-878-2706
83 East Water St. Tel: 800-752-8086
P.O. Box 545 Fax: 617-871-2816
Rockland, MA 02370-1837
Advertising: Ann Bailey
CEO: Lawrence T. Kirwan, Sr., President
  Lawrence T. Kirwan, Jr., Gen. Mgr.
Research: Christine Kirwan McGrath
Federal Procurement Eligibility: Small Business
Device Category:
Coagulator/Cutter, Endoscopic, Bipolar .... OBSTETRICS/GYN
Cord, Electric, Endoscope .... GASTRO/UROLOGY
Forceps, Electrosurgical .... SURGERY
Forceps, Endoscopic .... GASTRO/UROLOGY

Knight Instrument Co., J. Hugh Tel: 504-524-2797
226 S. Villere St. Tel: 800-535-5645
New Orleans, LA 70112-2816 Fax: 504-524-2798
CEO: Craig Simpson, Gen. Mgr.
Federal Procurement Eligibility: Small Business
Device Category:
Colonoscope, General & Plastic Surgery .... SURGERY

Komamura Photographic Co. Ltd.
Tel: 03/5618591
2-12-11, Kyobashi, Chuo-Ku
Tokyo 104
Japan
Advertising: Y. Kido
CEO: Tosh Komamura
Production: Jin Yamaguchi
Device Category:
Camera, Television, Surgical, Without Audio .... SURGERY

L&M Instruments, Inc.
Tel: 408-733-5858
Fax: 408-733-6251
P.O. Box 2070
Sunnyvale, CA 94087-0070
CEO: Gene Ritchey, General Mgr.
Federal Procurement Eligibility: Small Business
Device Category:
Forceps, Electrosurgical .... SURGERY
Forceps, Endoscopic .... GASTRO/UROLOGY

Lamp Technology, Inc.
Tel: 516-567-1800
Tel: 800-533-7548
Fax: 516-567-1806
1645 Sycamore Ave.
Bohemia, NY 11716-1729
CEO: Edith Reuter, President
Marketing: Janet Lang, Mktg. Res. Mgr.
Production: Neal Shupak, Prod. Mgr.
Federal Procurement Eligibility: Small Business, Woman Owned
Device Category:
Lamp, Endoscopic, Incandescent .... SURGERY

Lapac, Inc.
Tel: 201-646-0101
Fax: 201-646-1110
130 Overlook Ave.
Hackensack, NJ 07601-2225
CEO: Peter Fan
Federal Procurement Eligibility: Small Business
Device Category:
Kit, Laparoscopy .... GASTRO/UROLOGY

Laparomed Corp.
Tel: 714-768-1155
Tel: 800-336-1155
Fax: 714-768-0464
9272 Jeronimo Rd., Unit 109
Irvine, CA 92718-1914
CEO: Ed McDonald, President & CEO
Marketing: Stephen Bumb, Mktg. Dir.
Production: Paul Lubock
Device Category:
Catheter, Cholangiography .... SURGERY
Coagulator, Laparoscopic, Unipolar .... OBSTETRICS/GYN
Coagulator/Cutter, Endoscopic, Unipolar .... OBSTETRICS/GYN
Kit, Pelviscopy .... MIN. INV. SURGERY
Ligature, Laparoscopic .... MIN. INV. SURGERY
Peritoneoscope .... GASTRO/UROLOGY
Retractor, Laparoscopy, Other .... MIN. INV. SURGERY
Snare, Endoscopic .... SURGERY

Laser Technologies Group
Tel: 612-560-0433
Fax: 612-566-9303
6606 Bryant Ave. N.
Minneapolis, MN 55430-1805
CEO: L. Schultz
Marketing: D. Hewitt
Device Category:
Tube, Smoke Removal, Endoscopic .... GASTRO/UROLOGY

Laserscope
Tel: 408-943-0636
Tel: 800-356-7600
Fax: 408-428-0512
3052 Orchard Dr.
San Jose, CA 95134-2011
Advertising: Richard Wood, Adv. Mgr.
CEO: Robert V. McCormick, President & CEO
  Bonnie Jones, VP Personnel
  Alfred G. Merriweather, Fin. Dir.
Marketing: Susan Smith, Intl. Sales & Mktg. Mgr.
  Richard Wood, Dir. Corp. Comm.
  Michael Starmer, Dir. Natl. Accts.
  Michael Gioffredi, VP Mktg.
  Kevin Candio, Natl. Sales Mgr.
  Joseph Remy, Sales Training Mgr.
  Gary Melanson, Cust. Serv. Dir.
  Eli Wismer, VP Sales
Production: Robert Bogart, Eng. Dir.
  Mas Tsurada, VP Mfg.
  Donna Page, Reg. Affairs Mgr.
Research: Jeff Rondinone, VP R&D
Federal Procurement Eligibility: GSA Contract, VA Contract
Device Category:
Electrocautery Unit, Endoscopic .... OBSTETRICS/GYN
Equipment/Accessories, Laser, Laparoscopy .... MIN. INV. SURGERY
Laser, Nd:YAG, Laparoscopy .... MIN. INV. SURGERY
Probe, Electrocauterization, Multi-Use .... MIN. INV. SURGERY
Probe, Electrocauterization, Single-Use .... MIN. INV. SURGERY

Leibinger GmbH
Tel: 0761/49058-0
Fax: 0761/4905820
Botzinger Strasse 41
D-70437 Freiburg
Germany
CEO: Karl A. Leibinger
Marketing: Edgar Schule
Device Category:
Accessories, Arthroscope .... ORTHOPEDICS
Laryngoscope, Surgical .... SURGERY
Sigmoidoscope, Rigid, Non-Electrical .... GASTRO/UROLOGY
Trocar, Sinus .... EAR/NOSE/THROAT

Leibinger L.P.
Tel: 214-392-3636
Tel: 800-962-6558
Fax: 214-392-7258
14540 Beltwood Pkwy. E., Ste. 1
Dallas, TX 75244
CEO: Paul Stewart, President
  Karla Jorgensen, Controller
  Karl Leibinger, Chairman
Marketing: Ron Oberleitner, VP Prod. Dev.
  Rick Hawk, Reg. Sales Mgr.
  Jeff Simmons, Reg. Sales Mgr.
  Chris Pontikes, Reg Sales Mgr.
  Bob C. Young, VP Sales
Federal Procurement Eligibility: Small Business
Device Category:
Accessories, Arthroscope .... ORTHOPEDICS

Leisegang Medical, Inc.   Tel: 407-994-0202
6401 Congress Ave.   Tel: 800-448-4450
Boca Raton, FL 33487-2883   Fax: 407-998-0846
Advertising: Claudia Lozano, Advertising Mgr.
CEO: W. Kip Speyer, President
   Joseph DaSacco, Controller
Marketing: Jane Klaffer, Sales Mgr./Surgical Products
Production: Jonathan Thielmann, Service Mgr.
   Jeff Shelton, Prod. Mgr.
   Douglas Kwart, QA Mgr.
   B. Jay Epps, Eng. Mgr.
Federal Procurement Eligibility: Small Business, GSA Contract
Device Category:
Accessories, Cleaning, Endoscopic .... GASTRO/UROLOGY
Accessories, Photographic, Endoscopic .... GASTRO/UROLOGY
Applier, Clip, Laparoscopic .... MIN. INV. SURGERY
Applier, Clip, Repair, Hernia, Laparoscopic .... MIN. INV. SURGERY
Camera, Still, Endoscopic .... SURGERY
Camera, Television, Microsurgical, Without Audio .... SURGERY
Camera, Television, Surgical, Without Audio .... SURGERY
Camera, Video, Endoscopic .... GENERAL
Cart, Equipment, Video .... GENERAL
Cart, Instrument/Equipment, Laparoscopy .... MIN. INV. SURGERY
Clamp, Fixation, Cholangiography .... MIN. INV. SURGERY
Clamp, Laparoscopy .... MIN. INV. SURGERY
Coagulator, Hysteroscopic (With Accessories) .... OBSTETRICS/GYN
Coagulator, Laparoscopic, Unipolar .... OBSTETRICS/GYN
Coagulator/Cutter, Endoscopic, Bipolar .... OBSTETRICS/GYN
Coagulator/Cutter, Endoscopic, Unipolar .... OBSTETRICS/GYN
Colposcope .... OBSTETRICS/GYN
Cord, Electric, Endoscopic .... GASTRO/UROLOGY
Cover, Laparoscope .... MIN. INV. SURGERY
Dilator, Blunt .... MIN. INV. SURGERY
Dilator, Port, Laparoscopic .... MIN. INV. SURGERY
Electrocautery Unit, Endoscopic .... OBSTETRICS/GYN
Endoscope And Accessories, AC-Powered .... SURGERY
Endoscope, Flexible .... GASTRO/UROLOGY
Endoscope, Rigid .... SURGERY
Equipment, Suction/Irrigation, Laparoscopic .... SURGERY
Equipment/Accessories, Laser, Laparoscopy .... MIN. INV. SURGERY
Eyepiece, Lens, Non-Prescription, Endoscopic .... GASTRO/UROLOGY
Forceps, Biopsy .... MIN. INV. SURGERY
Forceps, Endoscopic .... GASTRO/UROLOGY
Forceps, Grasping, Atraumatic .... MIN. INV. SURGERY
Forceps, Grasping, Flexible Endoscopic .... GASTRO/UROLOGY
Forceps, Grasping, Traumatic .... MIN. INV. SURGERY
Generator, Power, Electrosurgical .... SURGERY
Holder, Instrument, Laparoscopic .... MIN. INV. SURGERY
Holder, Laparoscope .... OBSTETRICS/GYN
Holder, Needle, Curved, Laparoscopic .... MIN. INV. SURGERY
Holder, Needle, Laparoscopic .... MIN. INV. SURGERY
Holder/Scissors, Needle, Laparoscopic .... MIN. INV. SURGERY
Hysteroscope .... OBSTETRICS/GYN
Illuminator, Fiberoptic (For Endoscope) .... GASTRO/UROLOGY
Instrument, Dissecting, Laparoscopic .... MIN. INV. SURGERY
Instrument, Dissecting, Myoma, Laparoscopic .... MIN. INV. SURGERY
Instrument, Knot Tying, Suture, Laparoscopic .... MIN. INV. SURGERY
Instrument, Needle Holder/Knot Tying .... MIN. INV. SURGERY
*Insufflator, Carbon-Dioxide, Automatic
  (For Endoscope)* .... GASTRO/UROLOGY
Insufflator, Hysteroscopic .... OBSTETRICS/GYN
Insufflator, Laparoscopic .... OBSTETRICS/GYN
Insufflator, Vaginal .... OBSTETRICS/GYN
Kit, Laparoscopy .... GASTRO/UROLOGY
Lamp, Endoscopic, Incandescent .... SURGERY
Laparoscope, General & Plastic Surgery .... SURGERY

Laparoscope, Gynecologic .... OBSTETRICS/GYN
Light Source, Endoscope, Xenon Arc .... SURGERY
Light, Surgical, Endoscopic .... SURGERY
Monitor, Video, Endoscope .... GENERAL
Needle, Insufflation, Laparoscopic .... MIN. INV. SURGERY
Probe, Electrocauterization, Multi-Use .... MIN. INV. SURGERY
Probe, Electrocauterization, Single-Use .... MIN. INV. SURGERY
Probe, Suction, Irrigator/Aspirator, Laparoscopic .. MIN. INV. SURGERY
Resectoscope .... GASTRO/UROLOGY
Retractor, Fan-Type, Laparoscopy .... MIN. INV. SURGERY
Retractor, Laparoscopy, Other .... MIN. INV. SURGERY
Scissors, Laparoscopy .... MIN. INV. SURGERY
Scissors, Laparoscopy, Electrosurgical .... SURGERY
Sheath, Endoscopic .... GASTRO/UROLOGY
Sleeve, Trocar .... MIN. INV. SURGERY
Tape, Television & Video, Endoscopic .... GASTRO/UROLOGY
Telescope, Rigid, Endoscopic .... GASTRO/UROLOGY
Trainer, Laparoscopy .... MIN. INV. SURGERY
Trocar, Abdominal .... GASTRO/UROLOGY
Trocar, Gallbladder .... GASTRO/UROLOGY
Trocar, Laparoscopic .... SURGERY
Trocar, Other .... GENERAL
Trocar, Short .... MIN. INV. SURGERY
Tube, Smoke Removal, Endoscopic .... GASTRO/UROLOGY

Leonard Medical Inc.   Tel: 215-938-1499
1464 Holcomb Rd.   Tel: 800-227-0014
Huntingdon Valley, PA 19006   Fax: 215-938-1096
CEO: Leonard Bonnell, President
Marketing: Andrea Bergeron, Natl. Sales Mgr.
Federal Procurement Eligibility: Small Business
Device Category:
Holder, Laparoscope .... OBSTETRICS/GYN
Kit, Cholecystectomy .... MIN. INV. SURGERY
Peritoneoscope .... GASTRO/UROLOGY
Thoracoscope .... CARDIOVASCULAR

Li Medical Technologies, Inc.   Tel: 203-371-2227
7 Cambridge Dr.   Fax: 203-371-2241
Trumbull, CT 06611
CEO: Lehmann K. Li, President
Marketing: Rhodemann Li, Bus. Dev. Mgr.
Federal Procurement Eligibility: Small Business, GSA Contract
Device Category:
Laparoscope, General & Plastic Surgery .... SURGERY
Peritoneoscope .... GASTRO/UROLOGY

Lican Medical Products Ltd.   Tel: 519-737-1142
5120 Halford Dr., R.R. 1   Fax: 519-737-1528
Windsor, ONT N9A 6J3
Canada
CEO: Steve Livneh, President
   Deborah Livneh, VP Admin. & Finance
Federal Procurement Eligibility: Small Business
Device Category:
Coagulator, Laparoscopic, Unipolar .... OBSTETRICS/GYN
Laparoscope, Flexible .... SURGERY
Laparoscope, General & Plastic Surgery .... SURGERY
Laparoscope, Gynecologic .... OBSTETRICS/GYN

Life Medical Technologies, Inc.
3649 W. 1987 S.
Salt Lake City, UT 84104
Tel: 801-972-1900
Tel: 800-743-6153
Fax: 801-972-0123
CEO: David Vangeison, President & CEO
Marketing: R. Scott Bader, Natl. Sales Mgr.
Production: Mark Nelson, VP Mfg.
Research: Costas Diamantopoulos, VP R&D
Federal Procurement Eligibility: Small Business
Device Category:
Bronchoscope, Flexible .... EAR/NOSE/THROAT
Choledochoscope, Flexible Or Rigid .... GASTRO/UROLOGY
Choledochoscope, Mini-Diameter (5mm or Less) ..... MIN. INV. SURGERY
Endoscope, Flexible .... GASTRO/UROLOGY
Esophagoscope (Flexible Or Rigid) .... EAR/NOSE/THROAT
Eyepiece, Lens, Prescription, Endoscopic .... GASTRO/UROLOGY
Forceps, Endoscopic .... GASTRO/UROLOGY
Forceps, Grasping, Flexible Endoscopic .... GASTRO/UROLOGY
Gastroscope, Flexible .... GASTRO/UROLOGY
Kit, Laparoscopy .... GASTRO/UROLOGY
Nephroscope, Flexible .... GASTRO/UROLOGY
Snare, Endoscopic .... SURGERY
Ureteroscope .... GASTRO/UROLOGY

Linvatec Corporation
11311 Concept Blvd.
Largo, FL 34643-4908
Tel: 813-399-5344
Tel: 800-237-0169
Fax: 813-399-2603
Advertising: Eric Williams, Mktg. Svcs. Mgr.
CEO: Lawrence Hamilton, VP Personnel
    James Treace, President
    Cindy Swope, Dir. Sales Admin.
Marketing: Guy Williams, VP Mktg. & Int'l Opers.
Production: Mark Snyder, VP Mfg.
    Dick Naylor, VP Mfg. Oper.
Research: Jeff Roberts, VP R&D
Device Category:
Accessories, Arthroscope .... ORTHOPEDICS
Accessories, Photographic, Endoscopic .... GASTRO/UROLOGY
Accessories, Surgical Camera .... SURGERY
Arthroscope .... ORTHOPEDICS
Camera, Video, Endoscopic .... GENERAL
Cannula, Drainage, Arthroscopy .... ORTHOPEDICS
Choledochoscope, Flexible Or Rigid .... GASTRO/UROLOGY
Endoscope .... GASTRO/UROLOGY
Instrument, Knot Tying, Suture, Laparoscopic .... MIN. INV. SURGERY
Instrument, Passing, Suture, Laparoscopic .... MIN. INV. SURGERY
Insufflator, Other .... SURGERY
Peritoneoscope .... GASTRO/UROLOGY
Thoracoscope .... CARDIOVASCULAR

Linvatec
Div. of Zimmer of Canada Ltd.
2323 Argentia Rd.
Mississauga, ONT L5N 5N3
Canada
Tel: 905-858-8588
Tel: 800-387-9632
Fax: 905-858-0324
Distribution: Exclusive Distributor
Advertising: Gerry Pilon, Adv. Mgr.
CEO: Doug Thomson, President
Marketing: Michael Furgal, Dir. Sales, Western Canada
    Johanne Touchette, Mgr. Professional Dev.
    Gerry Pilon, VP Sales & Mktg.
    Denis Boutet, Dir. Sales, Eastern Canada
Production: Noel Baxter, Materials Mgr.
    Jim McDowell, Reg. Affairs Mgr.
Device Category:
Accessories, Arthroscope .... ORTHOPEDICS
Arthroscope .... ORTHOPEDICS
Cart, Equipment, Video .... GENERAL
Hysteroscope .... OBSTETRICS/GYN
Laparoscope, General & Plastic Surgery .... SURGERY
Laparoscope, Gynecologic .... OBSTETRICS/GYN
Needle, Insufflation, Laparoscopic .... MIN. INV. SURGERY

Lorenz Surgical, Walter
1520 Tradeport Dr.
Jacksonville, FL 32229-8009
Tel: 904-741-4400
Tel: 800-874-7711
Fax: 904-741-4500
CEO: Walter Lorenz, President
Marketing: Michael Teague, Sr. VP Sales & Mktg.
Production: Kurt Bucher, Production Mgr.
    Debra Powers, EVP
Federal Procurement Eligibility: Small Business
Device Category:
Accessories, Arthroscope .... ORTHOPEDICS
Trocar, Other .... GENERAL

Luxtec Corp.
326 Clark St.
Worcester, MA 01606
Tel: 508-856-9454
Tel: 800-325-8966
Fax: 508-856-9462
CEO: Sam Stein, CFO
    James Hobbs, President
Marketing: David Mutch, Dir. Sales & Mktg.
Production: Joseph Campbell, VP Operations
Federal Procurement Eligibility: Small Business
Device Category:
Endoscope And Accessories, AC-Powered .... SURGERY
Light Source, Endoscope, Xenon Arc .... SURGERY

M.D. Engineering
3464 Depot Rd.
Hayward, CA 94545-2714
Tel: 510-732-9950
Tel: 800-633-8423
Fax: 510-785-8182
Advertising: Tim Galen
CEO: Lawrence Ngm, CFO
    Andrew Halsey, President & CEO
Marketing: Ron Cerina, Sales Dir.
Production: Lynn Holloway, Oper. Dir.
    Donald A. Parker, Mfg. Dir.
Research: Robert Lash, R&D Dir.
Federal Procurement Eligibility: Small Business
Device Category:
Camera, Video, Endoscopic .... GENERAL
Insufflator, Other .... SURGERY
Tube, Smoke Removal, Endoscopic .... GASTRO/UROLOGY

Mabis Healthcare
28401 N. Ballard Dr., Unit H
Lake Forest, IL 60045
Tel: 708-680-6811
Tel: 800-728-6811
Fax: 708-680-9646
CEO: Steven M. Bisucla, VP
  Michael A. Mazza, President
Marketing: Jerry Lisman, VP Sales & Mktg.
Device Category:
Laryngoscope .... EAR/NOSE/THROAT

Machida Endoscope Co. Ltd.
6-13-8, Honkomagome, Bunkyo-Ku
Tokyo 113
Japan
Tel: 03/946-2151
Fax: 03/946-2620
CEO: Masashi Machida, President
Marketing: Takashi Kawasaki, Med. Sales Div. Mgr. Intl. Dept.
Device Category:
Arthroscope .... ORTHOPEDICS
Endoscope .... GASTRO/UROLOGY
Endoscope, Flexible .... GASTRO/UROLOGY
Endoscope, Rigid .... SURGERY

Machida, Inc.
40 Ramland Rd. South
Orangeburg, NY 10962-2617
Tel: 914-365-0600
Tel: 800-431-5420
Fax: 914-365-0620
CEO: Mik Okamoto, Gen. Mgr.
  Jim Bradley, Reg. Affairs Mgr.
  David Prigmore, President
Marketing: Ginger Ratsep, Adm. Sales Mgr.
  Bill Checkley, VP Sales & Mktg.
Production: Lsao Fujimoto, VP Mfg.
Federal Procurement Eligibility: Small Business
Device Category:
Accessories, Cleaning, Endoscopic .... GASTRO/UROLOGY
Camera, Still, Endoscopic .... SURGERY
Computer, Image, Endoscopic .... GENERAL
Laryngoscope, Flexible .... ANESTH/PUL MED
Nasopharyngoscope (Flexible Or Rigid) .... EAR/NOSE/THROAT

Mader Instrument Corp.
25 Lamington Dr.
Succasunna, NJ 07876-2048
Tel: 201-584-0816
Tel: 800-526-0872
Fax: 201-584-3318
CEO: Wolf Mader, President
Production: Hannelore Mader, VP
Federal Procurement Eligibility: Small Business, Woman Owned
Device Category:
Anoscope, Non-Powered .... GASTRO/UROLOGY
Clip, Suture .... SURGERY
Kit, Laparoscopy .... GASTRO/UROLOGY
Proctoscope .... SURGERY
Trocar, Cardiovascular .... CARDIOVASCULAR
Trocar, Thoracic .... CARDIOVASCULAR

Maramed Orthopedic Systems
2480 W. 82nd St.
Hialeah, FL 33016-2753
Tel: 305-823-8300
Tel: 800-327-5830
Fax: 305-823-8304
Advertising: Rand Johns, Adv. Mgr.
CEO: Alan R. Finnieston
Marketing: Russ Lafave, Natl. Sales Mgr.
  Arnold Bockar, Sales Mgr.
Production: Todd Tyrrell
  Chris Chase, Reg. Affairs Mgr.
Federal Procurement Eligibility: Small Business
Device Category:
Holder, Leg, Arthroscopy .... ORTHOPEDICS

Mark Medical Manufacturing, Inc.
484 Douglas Drive
West Chester, PA 19380-1120
Tel: 215-296-3020
Fax: 215-296-3020
CEO: Diana L. McBrinn
Marketing: Mark T. McBrinne
Federal Procurement Eligibility: Small Business, Woman Owned
Device Category:
Laparoscope, General & Plastic Surgery .... SURGERY

Marlow Surgical Technologies, Inc.
1810 Joseph Lloyd Pkwy.
Willoughby, OH 44094-8030
Tel: 216-946-2453
Tel: 800-992-5581
Fax: 216-946-1997
CEO: Rick Hart, CFO
  Kip Marlow, President
Marketing: D. Fred Herdman, VP Mktg. & Sales
  Craig Lanese, Sales Dir.
Research: Scott Marlow, VP R&D
Federal Procurement Eligibility: Small Business
Device Category:
Accessories, Cleaning, Endoscopic .... GASTRO/UROLOGY
Bag, Specimen, Laparoscopic .... MIN. INV. SURGERY
Cannula with Inflatable Balloon (Distal Tip) .... MIN. INV. SURGERY
Cannula, Suprapubic, With Trocar .... GASTRO/UROLOGY
Carrier, Sponge, Endoscopic .... GASTRO/UROLOGY
Endoscope, Rigid .... SURGERY
Equipment, Suction/Irrigation, Laparoscopic .... SURGERY
Forceps, Endoscopic .... GASTRO/UROLOGY
Forceps, Grasping, Atraumatic .... MIN. INV. SURGERY
Forceps, Grasping, Traumatic .... MIN. INV. SURGERY
Forceps, Laparoscopy, Electrosurgical .... SURGERY
Holder, Needle, Curved, Laparoscopic .... MIN. INV. SURGERY
Instrument, Dissecting, Laparoscopic .... MIN. INV. SURGERY
Instrument, Dissecting, Myoma, Laparoscopic .... MIN. INV. SURGERY
Instrument, Knot Tying, Suture, Laparoscopic .... MIN. INV. SURGERY
Instrument, Needle Holder/Knot Tying .... MIN. INV. SURGERY
Instrument, Passing, Suture, Laparoscopic .... MIN. INV. SURGERY
Insufflator, Carbon-Dioxide, Automatic
  (For Endoscope) .... GASTRO/UROLOGY
Insufflator, Laparoscopic .... OBSTETRICS/GYN
Insufflator, Other .... SURGERY
Kit, Cholecystectomy .... MIN. INV. SURGERY
Kit, Laparoscopy .... GASTRO/UROLOGY
Laparoscope, Gynecologic .... OBSTETRICS/GYN
Needle, Insufflation, Laparoscopic .... MIN. INV. SURGERY
Obturator, Endoscopic .... GASTRO/UROLOGY
Peritoneoscope .... GASTRO/UROLOGY
Probe, Electrocauterization, Multi-Use .... MIN. INV. SURGERY
Probe, Electrocauterization, Single-Use .... MIN. INV. SURGERY
Probe, Suction, Irrigator/Aspirator, Laparoscopic .... MIN. INV. SURGERY
Scissors with Removable Tips, Laparoscopy .... MIN. INV. SURGERY
Snare, Endoscopic .... SURGERY
Solution, Instrument, Laparoscopic, Anti-Fog .... GENERAL
Trainer, Laparoscopy .... MIN. INV. SURGERY
Trocar, Abdominal .... GASTRO/UROLOGY
Trocar, Gallbladder .... GASTRO/UROLOGY
Trocar, Other .... GENERAL
Trocar, Short .... MIN. INV. SURGERY

Martin, Gebr. GmbH & Co. KG

Tel: 07461/7060
Fax: 07461/706193

Ludwigstaler Str. 132
Postf. 60
D-78532 Tuttlingen
Germany
Advertising: Heinrich Herrmann
CEO: Friedhelm Schlotter
Marketing: Heiner Schroeder, Senior Sales Mgr.
Device Category:
Anoscope, Non-Powered .... GASTRO/UROLOGY
*Bougie, Esophageal, And
Gastrointestinal, Gastro-Urology* .... GASTRO/UROLOGY
Box, Battery, Pocket (Endoscopic) .... GASTRO/UROLOGY
Cannula, Suprapubic, With Trocar .... GASTRO/UROLOGY
Cord, Electric, Endoscope .... GASTRO/UROLOGY
Lamp, Endoscopic, Incandescent .... SURGERY
Laryngoscope .... EAR/NOSE/THROAT
Laryngoscope, Surgical .... SURGERY
Obturator, Endoscopic .... GASTRO/UROLOGY
Proctoscope .... SURGERY
Sheath, Endoscopic .... GASTRO/UROLOGY
Sigmoidoscope, Rigid, Electrical .... GASTRO/UROLOGY
Sigmoidoscope, Rigid, Non-Electrical .... GASTRO/UROLOGY
Stapler, Surgical .... SURGERY
Transformer, Endoscope .... SURGERY
Trocar, Cardiovascular .... CARDIOVASCULAR
Trocar, Gastro-Urology .... GASTRO/UROLOGY
Trocar, Laryngeal .... EAR/NOSE/THROAT
Trocar, Sinus .... EAR/NOSE/THROAT

Matrx Medical, Inc.

Tel: 716-662-6650
Tel: 800-847-1000
Fax: 716-662-7130

145 Mid County Dr.
Orchard Park, NY 14127-1726
CEO: William Burns, President & CEO
   Daniel Horrigan, Exec. VP
Marketing: Gary Kaczor, VP Mktg.
   Daniel Thomas, VP Sales
Production: Jesse Garringer, VP Operations
Federal Procurement Eligibility: Small Business
Device Category:
Laryngoscope, Rigid .... ANESTH/PUL MED

Mclean Medical Scientific, Inc.

Tel: 612-225-9295
Tel: 800-248-9295
Fax: 612-298-0018

328 State St.
St. Paul, MN 55107
Advertising: Mark Anderson, Advertising Mgr.
CEO: Timothy M. Scanlan, President & CEO
Marketing: Walter J. Olson, Sales & Mktg. VP
   Julie Brennan, National Sales Mgr.
Research: Kenneth R. Blake, R&D VP
Federal Procurement Eligibility: Small Business
Device Category:
Endoscope .... GASTRO/UROLOGY
Laparoscope, General & Plastic Surgery .... SURGERY

Med-Co Hospital Supplies Ltd.

Tel: 096/273-4629
Fax: 096/273-4577

7, Shelf House Ind. Est
New Farm Rd.
Alresford, Hampshire SO24 9QE
United Kingdom
Advertising: H.S. Thomson
CEO: C.D. Galpin
Device Category:
Insufflator, Other .... SURGERY

Med-Surg Industries, Inc.

Tel: 703-742-9700
Tel: 800-223-8481
Fax: 703-437-8469

251 Exchange Place
Herndon, VA 22070-4822
CEO: Micheal Sahady
Marketing: Tom Rody, VP Sales
   Mike Marano, Mktg. Dir.
   Kevin McMillen, Dir. Natl. Accts.
Production: Steven Plante, VP Mfg.
Federal Procurement Eligibility: Small Business
Device Category:
Arthrogram Kit .... ORTHOPEDICS
Kit, Laparoscopy .... GASTRO/UROLOGY

Medchem Products, Inc.

Tel: 617-938-9328
Tel: 800-451-4716
Fax: 617-938-0657

232 W. Cummings Pk.
Woburn, MA 01801-6333
CEO: P. O'Brien, Regulatory Affairs Mgr.
   J. Marten, Chairman
   J. Donaldson, Vice Chairman & CEO
Marketing: J. McConnell, VP Domestic Sales
   F. Brophy, VP Intl.
   Bradford R. Gay, Sr. VP Mktg. & Sales
Production: S. Severance, VP Mfg.
   M. McCartin, Product Mgr.
Research: A. Ferdman, Dir. Product Dev.
Federal Procurement Eligibility: GSA Contract, VA Contract
Device Category:
Endoscope And Accessories, AC-Powered .... SURGERY
Kit, Cholecystectomy .... MIN. INV. SURGERY
Peritoneoscope .... GASTRO/UROLOGY

Medesign GmbH

Tel: 089/769-5217
Fax: 089/769-8424

Partnachplatz 7-9
D-81373 Muenchen
Germany
CEO: Lothar Engel
Marketing: Monika Engel
Federal Procurement Eligibility: Small Business, Woman Owned
Device Category:
Coagulator/Cutter, Endoscopic, Bipolar .... OBSTETRICS/GYN

Medgyn Products, Inc.

Tel: 708-627-4105
Tel: 800-451-9667
Fax: 708-627-0127

328 Eisenhower Ln. #B
Lombard, IL 60148-5405
Advertising: Maria Wojciechowski, Adv. Mgr.
CEO: Lakshman M. Agadi, President
Marketing: Brian Milano, VP Sales & Mktg.
Production: Y.S. Knag, Prod. Mgr.
Federal Procurement Eligibility: Small Business, Minority Owned
Device Category:
Colposcope .... OBSTETRICS/GYN

Medi-Globe Corp.
6202 South Maple Ave. #131
Tempe, AZ 85283
Tel: 602-897-2772
Fax: 602-897-2878
CEO: Stefan Wohnhas, President & CEO
   Dr. Andreas Lindner, Vice Chairman
Production: Brian Karler, VP Oper.
Device Category:
Basket, Biliary Stone Retrieval .... GASTRO/UROLOGY
Endoscope, Flexible .... GASTRO/UROLOGY

Medi-Tech/Boston Scientific Corp.
480 Pleasant St.
Watertown, MA 02172-2414
Tel: 617-923-1720
Tel: 800-225-3238
Fax: 617-972-4540
CEO: Joseph Ciffolillo, COO
Marketing: Donald Woods, VP Mktg.
Device Category:
Forceps, Grasping, Flexible Endoscopic .... GASTRO/UROLOGY

Medical Concepts, Inc.
175 B Cremona Dr.
Goleta, CA 93117-5502
Tel: 805-968-5563
Fax: 805-968-2046
CEO: Stephen Kurtzer, President
   Kathy J. O'Dell, COO
Marketing: Mary Morton, Product Mgr.
   Jeffrey Kvrtzer, Mktg Svs. Coord.
   Angeli Mancuso, Product Mgr.
Production: David Chatenever, VP Eng.
   Daniel P. McGuire, VP Mfg.
Federal Procurement Eligibility: Small Business
Device Category:
Camera, Video, Endoscopic .... GENERAL

Medical Dynamics, Inc.
99 Inverness Dr. E.
Englewood, CO 80112-5115
Tel: 303-790-2990
Tel: 800-525-1294
Fax: 303-799-1378
CEO: Van A. Horsley, President
   John Adair, Controller
   Jo Brehm, VP
Federal Procurement Eligibility: Small Business
Device Category:
Accessories, Surgical Camera .... SURGERY
Camera, Still, Endoscopic .... SURGERY
Camera, Video, Endoscopic .... GENERAL
Camera, Videotape, Surgical .... SURGERY
Endoscope .... GASTRO/UROLOGY
Monitor, Video, Endoscope .... GENERAL

Medical Surgical Specialties Ltd.
5148 Lovers Lane
Kalamazoo, MI 49002
Tel: 616-385-5000
Tel: 800-527-5672
Fax: 616-385-3333
Advertising: Bill Kelley
CEO: Jim McCabe
Marketing: Richard Leder
Production: Dan Gagne
Federal Procurement Eligibility: Small Business, GSA Contract, VA Contract
Device Category:
Endoscope, Flexible .... GASTRO/UROLOGY
Endoscope, Rigid .... SURGERY

Medicon Eg
15 Gansacker
Postfach 4455
D-78532 Tuttlingen
Germany
Tel: 07462/20090
Fax: 07461/200950
Advertising: W. Enslin
CEO: Hubertus Scholz, Mg. Director
Marketing: K.L. Liebermann
   D. Raabe, Sales Dir.
Device Category:
Anoscope, Non-Powered .... GASTRO/UROLOGY
Bronchoscope, Rigid .... EAR/NOSE/THROAT
Esophagoscope (Flexible Or Rigid) .... EAR/NOSE/THROAT
Forceps, Endoscopic .... GASTRO/UROLOGY
Forceps, Grasping, Flexible Endoscopic .... GASTRO/UROLOGY
Laryngoscope .... EAR/NOSE/THROAT
Laryngoscope, Rigid .... ANESTH/PUL MED
Power Supply, Endoscopic, Line Operated .... GENERAL
Proctoscope .... SURGERY
Proctosigmoidoscope .... GASTRO/UROLOGY
Remover, Clip .... SURGERY
Trocar, Abdominal .... GASTRO/UROLOGY
Trocar, Gallbladder .... GASTRO/UROLOGY
Trocar, Thoracic .... CARDIOVASCULAR
Trocar, Tracheal .... EAR/NOSE/THROAT

Medicon Instruments, Inc.
4405 International Blvd.
Norcross, GA 30093-3013
Tel: 404-381-2858
Tel: 800-633-4266
Fax: 404-381-2861
CEO: Richard M. Harris, EVP & Gen. Mgr.
   Hubertus Scholz, President
Federal Procurement Eligibility: Small Business
Device Category:
Anoscope, Non-Powered .... GASTRO/UROLOGY
Bronchoscope, Rigid .... EAR/NOSE/THROAT
Esophagoscope, Rigid, Gastro-Urology .... GASTRO/UROLOGY
Forceps, Endoscopic .... GASTRO/UROLOGY
Forceps, Grasping, Atraumatic .... MIN. INV. SURGERY
Forceps, Grasping, Flexible Endoscopic .... GASTRO/UROLOGY
Forceps, Laparoscopy, Electrosurgical .... SURGERY
Holder, Needle, Curved, Laparoscopic .... MIN. INV. SURGERY
Holder, Needle, Laparoscopic .... MIN. INV. SURGERY
Instrument, Knot Tying, Suture, Laparoscopic .... MIN. INV. SURGERY
Kit, Cholecystectomy .... MIN. INV. SURGERY
Laryngoscope .... EAR/NOSE/THROAT
Laryngoscope, Rigid .... ANESTH/PUL MED
Needle, Insufflation, Laparoscopic .... MIN. INV. SURGERY
Power Supply, Endoscopic, Line Operated .... GENERAL
Proctoscope .... SURGERY
Proctosigmoidoscope .... GASTRO/UROLOGY
Remover, Clip .... SURGERY
Retractor, Fan-Type, Laparoscopy .... MIN. INV. SURGERY
Sigmoidoscope, Rigid, Non-Electrical .... GASTRO/UROLOGY
Trocar, Abdominal .... GASTRO/UROLOGY
Trocar, Gallbladder .... GASTRO/UROLOGY
Trocar, Thoracic .... CARDIOVASCULAR
Trocar, Tracheal .... EAR/NOSE/THROAT

Mediflex Surgical Products
250 Gibbs Rd.
Islandia, NY 11722-2697
Tel: 516-582-8440
Tel: 800-879-7575
Fax: 516-582-8487
Advertising: Wes Michele, Adv. Mgr.
CEO: John S. Adler, VP
   David T. Adler, President
Marketing: Wayne Bellen, Mktg. Mgr.
   Lawrence W. Murphy, Natl. Sales Dir.
Production: Terry Di Paulo, New Product Mgr.
   Bernd Ascher, QA Mgr.
Research: Greg Sonnen
Federal Procurement Eligibility: Small Business
Device Category:
Camera, Television, Endoscopic, Without Audio ....SURGERY
Forceps, Laparoscopy, Electrosurgical ....SURGERY
Holder, Laparoscope ....OBSTETRICS/GYN
Laparoscope, General & Plastic Surgery ....SURGERY
Light Source, Endoscope, Xenon Arc ....SURGERY
Peritoneoscope ....GASTRO/UROLOGY

Medin Corporation
111 Lester St.
Wallington, NJ 07057-1012
Tel: 201-779-2400
Tel: 800-925-0476
Fax: 201-779-2463
CEO: Jay Schainholz, VP
   Herbert Schainholz, Pres.
Production: N. Ramakrishinan, VP Mfg.
Federal Procurement Eligibility: Small Business
Device Category:
Holder, Leg, Arthroscopy ....ORTHOPEDICS
Holder, Shoulder, Arthroscopy ....SURGERY

Mediplast Instruments, Inc.
P.O. Box 1126
New Castle, DE 19720
Tel: 302-737-0237
Fax: 302-368-7104
Advertising: S. E. Billey
CEO: Taskeen Ellahi
Federal Procurement Eligibility: Small Business
Device Category:
Trocar, Tracheal..EAR/NOSE/THROAT

Meditron Devices, Inc.
83 Hobart St.
Hackensack, NJ 07601-3912
Tel: 201-489-4222
Tel: 800-527-3530
Fax: 201-489-6745
CEO: Milton Frank, President
Marketing: Larry Doll, VP Mktg. & Sales
Production: Samuel Dickstein, VP
Federal Procurement Eligibility: Small Business
Device Category:
Insufflator, Laparoscopic......................................OBSTETRICS/GYN
Insufflator, Other ....SURGERY
Snare, Endoscopic..SURGERY

Medizintechnik
Wurttemberger Str. 26
D-78567 Fridingen
Germany
Tel: 07/463-8076
Fax: 07/463-492
CEO: Hans Hermann
Marketing: Daniela Geiger, Mktg. Dir.
Production: Hans-Josef Hermann, Production Mgr.
Device Category:
Arthroscope ....ORTHOPEDICS
Endoscope ....GASTRO/UROLOGY
Kit, Laparoscopy ....GASTRO/UROLOGY

Medmetric Corp.
7542 Trade St.
San Diego, CA 92121-2412
Tel: 619-536-9122
Fax: 619-536-9303
CEO: Dick Watkins, President
Marketing: Tracy Van Every, Sales & Mktg. Dir.
Device Category:
Arthroscope ....ORTHOPEDICS

Medovations, Inc.
102 East Keefe Ave.
Milwaukee, WI 53212-1535
Tel: 414-265-7620
Tel: 800-558-6408
Fax: 414-265-7628
Advertising: Mark Stecker, Mktg. Manager
Marketing: Barbara Stanford, VP Sales
Federal Procurement Eligibility: Small Business
Device Category:
Bougie, Esophageal, ENT..............................EAR/NOSE/THROAT
Laryngoscope, Rigid..ANESTH/PUL MED
Trocar, Thoracic ....CARDIOVASCULAR

Medrecon, Inc.
257 South Ave.
Garwood, NJ 07027-1341
Tel: 908-789-2050
Tel: 800-526-4323
Fax: 908-789-3275
CEO: Gary P. Sitcer, President
Marketing: Victor Neumark, Mktg. Dir.
   Jim Druckenmiller, Sales & Service Mgr.
Production: Andy Kroszczynski, Plant Mgr.
Federal Procurement Eligibility: Small Business
Device Category:
Holder, Leg, Arthroscopy ....ORTHOPEDICS

Megadyne Medical Products, Inc.
11506 S. State St.
Draper, UT 84020
Tel: 801-576-9669
Tel: 800-747-6110
Fax: 801-576-9698
CEO: Matt Sansom, EVP
   Mardsen Blanch, M.D.
   Gary R. Kehl, President
Marketing: Theresa Vonk, Dir. PR
   H.J. Nicolas, Natl. Sales Mgr.
   H.J. Nicholas, Sales & Mktg.
Production: Nedra Etton
   Drew Weaver, Regulatory Affairs Mgr.
Research: Bill Nette-Koven, R&D Mgr.
Federal Procurement Eligibility: Small Business
Device Category:
Equipment, Suction/Irrigation, Laparoscopic.....................SURGERY
Probe, Suction, Irrigator/Aspirator, Laparoscopic....MIN. INV. SURGERY

Mercury Medical
11300 49th St. N #A
Clearwater, FL 34622-4800
Tel: 813-573-0088
Tel: 800-237-6418
Fax: 813-573-6040
Advertising: Garry Blount, Adv. Mgr.
CEO: Stanley G. Tangalakis, President & CEO
　Arthur Ward, COO
Marketing: Phillip D. Millman, VP Sales & Mktg.
　Joe Glymph, New Bus. Dev. Dir.
　Gary French, Natl. Sales Mgr.
　Garry P. Blount, Mercury Products
　Becky Hamm, Prod. Mgr.
Production: George E. Howe, Jr., VP Oper.
　Gary Schmoeger, Matls. Mgr.
Federal Procurement Eligibility: Small Business, GSA Contract
Device Category:
Laryngoscope .... EAR/NOSE/THROAT
Laryngoscope, Rigid .... ANESTH/PUL MED
Laryngoscope, Surgical .... SURGERY

Merocel Corporation
950 Flanders Rd.
P.O. Box 334
Mystic, CT 06355-1300
Tel: 203-572-9586
Tel: 800-637-6235
Fax: 203-572-7485
CEO: Mark Adams, CEO
Marketing: Scott Black, Natl. Sales Mgr.
　Joe Gassman, Intl. Sales & Mktg. Mgr.
　Dom L. Gatto, VP Mktg.
Production: Tom Drury, Bus. Dev. Mgr.
　Ron Cercone, VP Mfg.
Federal Procurement Eligibility: Small Business
Device Category:
Solution, Instrument, Laparoscopic, Anti-Fog .... GENERAL

Microlux, Inc.
6000-1 Powers Ave., Medical Bldg.
Jacksonville, FL 32217
Tel: 904-737-9660
Fax: 904-733-4832
Marketing: Cynthia Arcusa, Sales & Mktg. Mgr.
Federal Procurement Eligibility: Small Business, GSA Contract, VA Contract
Device Category:
Accessories, Arthroscope .... ORTHOPEDICS
Illuminator, Fiberoptic (For Endoscope) .... GASTRO/UROLOGY
Lamp, Endoscopic, Incandescent .... SURGERY
Light, Surgical, Endoscopic .... SURGERY

Micromedics, Inc.
1285 Corporate Center Dr., Ste. #150
Eagan, MN 55121-1236
Tel: 612-452-1977
Tel: 800-624-5662
Fax: 612-452-1787
CEO: Lorraine Ouchene, Finance
　Curtis H. Miller, President
Marketing: Stephen Hannes, Mktg. & Sales VP
　Jeff Johnson, Int'l Sales & Mktg. Mgr.
　David Hull
Production: Carrie Foley
Federal Procurement Eligibility: Small Business, GSA Contract, VA Contract
Device Category:
Endoscope And Accessories, AC-Powered .... SURGERY
Tray, Sterilization, Instrument .... SURGERY

Microsurge, Inc.
150 A St.
Needham, MA 02194
Tel: 617-444-2300
Tel: 800-229-5555
Fax: 617-444-2389
CEO: Jim Hutchens, President
Marketing: John T. Kilcoyne, Mktg. Dir.
　Bill Barrett, Intl. Sales & Mktg. Mgr.
Production: Rick Lariviere, Reg. Affairs Mgr.
　Carmine Sammarco, VP Mfg.
Research: Andy Levine, VP R&D
Device Category:
Endoscope And Accessories, AC-Powered .... SURGERY
Equipment, Suction/Irrigation, Laparoscopic .... SURGERY
Forceps, Laparoscopy, Electrosurgical .... SURGERY
Handle, Instrument, Laparoscopic (Electrocautery) .. MIN. INV. SURGERY
Instrument, Dissecting, Laparoscopic .... MIN. INV. SURGERY
Kit, Cholecystectomy .... MIN. INV. SURGERY
Kit, Pelviscopy .... MIN. INV. SURGERY
Peritoneoscope .... GASTRO/UROLOGY
Scissors with Removable Tips, Laparoscopy .... MIN. INV. SURGERY
Thoracoscope .... CARDIOVASCULAR

Microtek Medical, Inc.
602 Lehmberg Rd.
P.O. Box 2487
Columbus, MS 39702-2487
Tel: 601-327-1863
Tel: 800-274-1863
Fax: 800-642-0255
Advertising: Wesley Harmon
CEO: Tico Capote, VP Int'l
　Kim Vought, President
　Dan Lee, VP & COO
Marketing: Kathy W. Zachry, Mktg. Mgr.
Production: William D. Darnell, VP Mfg.
Device Category:
Accessories, Surgical Camera .... SURGERY

Microvasive/Boston Scientific Corp. Urology Div.
Tel: 617-923-1720
Tel: 800-225-3226
Fax: 617-972-4540
480 Pleasant St.
Watertown, MA 02172
Distribution: OEM, Manufacturer Direct
Advertising: Rob Levenson, Mktg. Comm. Dir.
CEO: Joseph Ciffolillo, CEO
   John Carnuccio, VP & Gen. Mgr.
Marketing: David Budreau, Nat'l Sales Mgr.
Federal Procurement Eligibility: Small Business
Device Category:
Basket, Biliary Stone Retrieval............................GASTRO/UROLOGY
Endoscope And Accessories, AC-Powered........................SURGERY
Kit, Cholecystectomy..MIN. INV. SURGERY
Peritoneoscope..GASTRO/UROLOGY

Midas Rex Institute
Tel: 817-831-2604
Tel: 800-433-7639
Fax: 817-834-4835
3000 Race Street
Fort Worth, TX 76111
CEO: Forest C. Barber, M.D., President
Federal Procurement Eligibility: Small Business
Device Category:
Arthroscope..ORTHOPEDICS

Midwest Dental Products Corp.
Tel: 708-640-4800
Tel: 800-800-2888
Fax: 708-640-6165
901 W. Oakton St.
Des Plaines, IL 60018-1884
CEO: John McDonough, CEO
   Gloria McFadden, VP Personnel
   Gary Neilsson, Bus. Dev. Mgr.
   Dawn Johnson, Dir. Mktg.
   Ann O'Connor, Dir. Natl. Accts.
   Al Brennan, President
Marketing: Gary Neilsson, Contract Sales Mgr.
Production: Mark Greenwood, VP Mfg.
Research: Gary Schneck, VP R&D
Federal Procurement Eligibility: GSA Contract
Device Category:
Illuminator, Fiberoptic (For Endoscope)................GASTRO/UROLOGY

Mill-Rose Laboratories
Tel: 216-255-7995
Tel: 800-321-1380
Fax: 216-255-5061
7310 Corporate Blvd.
Mentor, OH 44060-4856
Advertising: Nina Alban
CEO: Victor Miller, President
Marketing: Tom Lowrey, Sales Mgr.
Production: John Dombrosky, Production Mgr.
Research: Alan Poje, Dir. Regulatory Affairs
Federal Procurement Eligibility: Small Business
Device Category:
Accessories, Cleaning, Endoscopic........................GASTRO/UROLOGY
Basket, Biliary Stone Retrieval............................GASTRO/UROLOGY
Brush, Cytology, Endoscopic...............................GASTRO/UROLOGY
Forceps, Endoscopic..GASTRO/UROLOGY
Forceps, Grasping, Flexible Endoscopic.................GASTRO/UROLOGY
Needle, Endoscopic...GASTRO/UROLOGY
Snare, Endoscopic..SURGERY

Miltex Instrument Co., Inc.
Tel: 516-775-7100
Tel: 800-645-8000
Fax: 516-775-7185
6 Ohio Dr.
CB 5006
Lake Success, NY 11042-0006
Advertising: Linda Pujia, Promotional Mgr.
CEO: Saul Kleinkramer, President
   Irwin Goldman, EVP
Marketing: Sandra L. Bruschi, Customer Service
   Robert B. Pugliesi, Mktg. Dir.
   Orestes Fundora, Int'l Sales Dir.
   Marie Amato, Nat'l Sales Coord.
   Andrew L. Anmuth, Sales Dir.
Production: Karl Leber, Oper. Dir.
Federal Procurement Eligibility: Small Business
Device Category:
Anoscope, Non-Powered....................................GASTRO/UROLOGY
Clip, Suture...SURGERY
Proctoscope..SURGERY
Trocar, Cardiovascular.....................................CARDIOVASCULAR
Trocar, Thoracic..CARDIOVASCULAR
Trocar, Tracheal..EAR/NOSE/THROAT

Mitsubishi Cable America, Inc.
Tel: 212-888-2270
Fax: 212-888-2276
520 Madison Ave., 17th Fl.
New York, NY 10022
CEO: Yoshie Fukya, President
Device Category:
Endoscope, Flexible..GASTRO/UROLOGY

Mitsubishi Electronics Of America
Tel: 908-563-9889
Tel: 800-733-8439
Fax: 908-563-0713
800 Cottontail Lane
Somerset, NJ 08873-6759
Advertising: Russell Novy, Adv. Mgr.
CEO: David Bright, VP
Marketing: Frank Benna, Mktg. & Sales Mgr.
Device Category:
Monitor, Video, Endoscope..GENERAL

Mizuno Ika Kikai K.K.
Tel: 06/768-1454
7-18 Ajihara-cho, Tennoji-ku
Osaka 543
Japan
CEO: Shigeru Mizuno, President
Device Category:
Endoscope..GASTRO/UROLOGY

MP Video, Inc.
Tel: 508-435-2131
Tel: 800-624-6274
Fax: 508-435-2227
63 South St.
Hopkinton, MA 01748-2212
CEO: John Halt, CEO
   Fred Capallo, Finance
Marketing: Winnie Shannon, Sr. Product Mgr.
   Jim Torraco, Natl. Sales Mgr.
Production: Allan Dennison
Federal Procurement Eligibility: Small Business
Device Category:
Accessories, Photographic, Endoscopic................GASTRO/UROLOGY
Camera, Video, Endoscopic...GENERAL
Insufflator, Other...SURGERY
Monitor, Video, Endoscope..GENERAL

Multigon Industries, Inc.
Tel: 914-664-7300
Fax: 914-664-9502
559 Gramatan Ave.
Mt. Vernon, NY 10552-2155
CEO: Ruth Samuels
Device Category:
Kit, Laparoscopy...GASTRO/UROLOGY
Peritoneoscope..GASTRO/UROLOGY

Myriadlase, Inc.
Tel: 817-483-9237
Fax: 817-478-7016
4800 S.E. Loop 820
Forest Hill, TX 76140
CEO: H.A. Lawhon, President & CEO
Marketing: Robert Kripaitis, VP Mktg.
  Mike Geraghty, Natl. Sales Mgr.
Federal Procurement Eligibility: Small Business, GSA Contract
Device Category:
Cystoscope..GASTRO/UROLOGY
Endoscope, Rigid...SURGERY
Laser, Nd:YAG, Laparoscopy.............................MIN. INV. SURGERY
Sheath, Endoscopic.....................................GASTRO/UROLOGY

N.A.D., Inc.
Tel: 215-721-5400
Fax: 215-723-5935
1488 Quarry Rd.
Telford, PA 18969-1099
CEO: Peter Schreiber, President
Marketing: Thomas Caltabiano, Nat'l. Sales Mgr.
  Thomas Barford, VP Sales & Mktg.
  Joseph A. Condurso, Mktg. Mgr.
  J. Horvath, Int'l Sales Mgr.
Production: Joachim Schreiber, VP Eng.
  Charles Chew, VP Mfg. & Oper.
Federal Procurement Eligibility: Small Business, GSA Contract, VA Contract
Device Category:
Laryngoscope, Rigid............................ANESTH/PUL MED

Nagashima Medical Instrument Co. Ltd.
Tel: 03/3812-1271
Fax: 03/3816-2824
24-1 Hongo 5-Chome, Bunkyo-Ku
Tokyo 113
Japan
Medical Products Sales Volume: $20,000,000
Total Employees: 80
Distribution: Manufacturer Direct
CEO: Jiro Nagashima, President
Marketing: Chushichiro Nagashima
Production: Shinrokuro Nagashima
Device Category:
Laryngoscope...EAR/NOSE/THROAT

National Wire & Stamping, Inc.
Tel: 303-777-9441
Fax: 303-762-8213
2801 South Vallejo Street
Englewood, CO 80110
CEO: Peter J. Neidecker
Marketing: Thomas K. Richey
Production: Robert L. Brown
Research: James R. Chambers
Federal Procurement Eligibility: Small Business
Device Category:
Coagulator, Laparoscopic, Unipolar........................OBSTETRICS/GYN
Coagulator/Cutter, Endoscopic, Unipolar................OBSTETRICS/GYN

NDM Corporation
Tel: 513-294-1767
Fax: 513-294-8363
3040 E. River Rd.
Dayton, OH 45439-1436
CEO: William Shea, President
Marketing: Thomas Cycyota, Mktg. Dir.
  David Snider, Mktg. Dir.
  Austin Short, Mktg. Dir.
Production: Larry Pattee, Manufacturing VP
Research: James Cartmell, R & D VP
Federal Procurement Eligibility: GSA Contract, VA Contract
Device Category:
Endoscope And Accessories, AC-Powered........................SURGERY

Needletech Products, Inc.
Tel: 508-699-4148
Fax: 508-699-4187
428 Towne St.
North Attleborough, MA 02760-3407
CEO: Ronald G. Routhier, General Mgr.
Marketing: C. Russell Small, Sales & Mktg.
Federal Procurement Eligibility: Small Business
Device Category:
Kit, Laparoscopy..GASTRO/UROLOGY

Nesa Corp.
Tel: 203-775-0578
Fax: 203-775-0522
12 Silvermine Road
Brookfield Center, CT 06804-3316
Marketing: Harold R. Burke, Marketing Mgr.
Device Category:
Box, Battery, Rechargeable (Endoscopic)...............GASTRO/UROLOGY

Neutech Corporation
Tel: 201-731-2707
79 Fitzrandolph Road
West Orange, NJ 07052-3527
CEO: Barry P. Neustein
Device Category:
Laryngoscope...EAR/NOSE/THROAT

New Life Systems, Inc.
Tel: 305-972-4600
Fax: 305-968-1990
1870 N. State Road 7
Margate, FL 33063-5708
Advertising: Maxine Fineman
CEO: Edgar Bentolila, President
Device Category:
Endoscope...GASTRO/UROLOGY

Nextec Surgical Corp.
Tel: 813-643-2553
Fax: 813-643-1619
2629 South Horseshoe Dr.
Naples, FL 33942-6122
CEO: Jack Kloots
Production: Don Grafton
Federal Procurement Eligibility: Small Business, Woman Owned, GSA Contract, VA Contract
Device Category:
Accessories, Arthroscope..ORTHOPEDICS
Arthroscope...ORTHOPEDICS
Illuminator, Fiberoptic (For Endoscope)................GASTRO/UROLOGY
Laparoscope, General & Plastic Surgery..........................SURGERY

Nikon Inc., Instrument Group
Tel: 516-547-8500
Fax: 516-547-0306
1300 Walt Whitman Rd.
P.O. Box 9050
Melville, NY 11747-3012
Advertising: Barbara Loechner, Adv. Mgr.
CEO: Y. Imagawa, President
Marketing: Walter L. Buhrmann, EVP
  Stephen Stoll, Ophth. Insr. Sales Mgr.
  Lee Shuett, Scien. Insr. Sales Mgr.
Federal Procurement Eligibility: GSA Contract
Device Category:
Camera, Still, Endoscopic..SURGERY

Nopa Instruments Medizintechnik GmbH
Tel: 07462/7801
Fax: 07462/7822

Gansacker 9 - Postfach 4554
D-78532 Tuttlingen
Germany
CEO: Norbert Pauli
Marketing: Joe Schmid
Device Category:
Forceps, Electrosurgical .... SURGERY
Forceps, Endoscopic .... GASTRO/UROLOGY
Forceps, Grasping, Flexible Endoscopic .... GASTRO/UROLOGY
Laryngoscope .... EAR/NOSE/THROAT
Laryngoscope, Rigid .... ANESTH/PUL MED
Laryngoscope, Surgical .... SURGERY
Needle, Endoscopic .... GASTRO/UROLOGY
Trocar, Abdominal .... GASTRO/UROLOGY
Trocar, Cardiovascular .... CARDIOVASCULAR
Trocar, Gallbladder .... GASTRO/UROLOGY
Trocar, Gastro-Urology .... GASTRO/UROLOGY
Trocar, Laryngeal .... EAR/NOSE/THROAT
Trocar, Sinus .... EAR/NOSE/THROAT
Trocar, Thoracic .... CARDIOVASCULAR
Trocar, Tracheal .... EAR/NOSE/THROAT

North American Medical Products, Inc.
Tel: 518-347-1646
Tel: 800-488-6267
Fax: 518-347-1648

Rotterdam Ind. Pk. Bldg.
901 Vischer Ave.
Schenectady, NY 12306
Distribution: OEM Manufacturer Direct, Through Distributors & Reps., Exporter
CEO: Arthur Gianakos, President
Federal Procurement Eligibility: Small Business, GSA Contract, VA Contract
Device Category:
Laryngoscope .... EAR/NOSE/THROAT

North American Sterilization & Packaging
Tel: 201-579-1397
Fax: 201-579-1377

15 White Lake Rd.
P.O. Box 923
Sparta, NJ 07871-3206
Total Employees: 100
Distribution: Service Direct
CEO: Norman T. Reudt, President
   Charles E. Meisch, Corporate VP
Marketing: Kim Decker, Project Coord.
Production: William Giliam, Mktg. Dir.
Federal Procurement Eligibility: Small Business
Device Category:
Endoscope And Accessories, AC-Powered .... SURGERY

Northgate Technologies, Inc.
Tel: 708-506-9872
Tel: 800-348-0424
Fax: 708-506-9891

3930 Ventura Dr., Ste. 150
Arlington Heights, IL 60004
Advertising: Peter Manzie, Adv. Mgr.
CEO: Robert Baker, President
   Dan Washburn, VP Personnel
Marketing: Robert Sexauer, Mktg. Mgr.
   Robert Baker, VP Mktg.
   Peter Manzie, Mktg. Dir.
   Chris Lawson, Natl. Sales Mgr.
Production: Victor Schur, Reg. Affairs Mgr.
   Robert Mantell, VP Mfg.
Research: Scott Gilchrist, Research Mgr.
   Chuck Zander, VP R&D
Device Category:
Cart, Equipment, Video .... GENERAL
Coagulator, Laparoscopic, Unipolar .... OBSTETRICS/GYN
Equipment, Suction/Irrigation, Laparoscopic .... SURGERY
Insufflator, Laparoscopic .... OBSTETRICS/GYN
Laparoscope, Gynecologic .... OBSTETRICS/GYN
Trocar, Other .... GENERAL
Tube, Smoke Removal, Endoscopic .... GASTRO/UROLOGY

Nu Surg Medical, Inc.
Tel: 513-753-3633
Fax: 513-753-1075

4440 Glen Este-Withamsville Rd., Ste.780
Cincinnati, OH 45245
CEO: Dennis Knoepfler, M.D., CEO
Device Category:
Catheter, Cholangiography .... SURGERY
Dispenser, Laparoscopic .... MIN. INV. SURGERY
Dispenser, Thorascopic .... CARDIOVASCULAR
Electrode, Electrosurgery, Laparoscopic .... MIN. INV. SURGERY
Holder, Needle, Laparoscopic .... MIN. INV. SURGERY
Instrument, Separating, Nerve .... MIN. INV. SURGERY
Knife, Laparoscopic .... MIN. INV. SURGERY

O.R. Concepts, Inc.
Tel: 612-894-7523
Tel: 800-826-3723
Fax: 612-894-0546

12250 Nicollet Ave. South
Burnsville, MN 55337
CEO: Ron Williams, President
   Joe A. Staley, VP
Marketing: James Elder, VP Mktg.
Device Category:
Electrode, Electrosurgery, Laparoscopic .... MIN. INV. SURGERY
Kit, Laparoscopy .... GASTRO/UROLOGY
Peritoneoscope .... GASTRO/UROLOGY
Solution, Instrument, Laparoscopic, Anti-Fog .... GENERAL
Trocar, Other .... GENERAL

O.R. Surgical Co., Inc.
Tel: 919-855-6714
Fax: 919-855-9851

120 Montlieu Ave.
Greensboro, NC 27409-2620
CEO: W.J. Schwabenton, President
Device Category:
Accessories, Arthroscope .... ORTHOPEDICS
Arthroscope .... ORTHOPEDICS
Aspirator, Arthroscopy .... ORTHOPEDICS

Olsen Electrosurgical, Inc. Tel: 510-825-8151
2100 Meridian Park Blvd. Tel: 800-227-2814
Concord, CA 94520-5709 Fax: 510-685-6177
CEO: Shirley Shier, VP
　Maria Mursell, President
　Eugene Olsen, Chief Exec.
Production: Jack Stroski, Prod. Mgr.
Federal Procurement Eligibility: Small Business, Woman Owned, GSA Contract
Device Category:
Accessories, Arthroscope .... ORTHOPEDICS
Coagulator/Cutter, Endoscopic, Bipolar .... OBSTETRICS/GYN
Forceps, Electrosurgical .... SURGERY

Olympus America, Inc. Tel: 516-488-3880
4 Nevada Dr. Tel: 800-223-0130
Lake Success, NY 11042-1179 Fax: 516-222-0878
Advertising: Bob Gillis, Adv. Mgr.
CEO: Yasutoshi Watanabe, President
Marketing: Michael Oberstfeld, VP Med. Instr. Div.
Device Category:
Accessories, Surgical Camera .... SURGERY
Arthroscope .... ORTHOPEDICS
Bronchoscope, Flexible .... EAR/NOSE/THROAT
Brush, Cytology, Endoscopic .... GASTRO/UROLOGY
Camera, Video, Endoscopic .... GENERAL
Choledochoscope, Flexible Or Rigid .... GASTRO/UROLOGY
Choledochoscope, Mini-Diameter (5mm or Less) ..... MIN. INV. SURGERY
Colonoscope, Gastro-Urology .... GASTRO/UROLOGY
Colposcope .... OBSTETRICS/GYN
Cystoscope .... GASTRO/UROLOGY
Cystourethroscope .... GASTRO/UROLOGY
Duodenoscope, Esophago/Gastro .... GASTRO/UROLOGY
Endoscope .... GASTRO/UROLOGY
Esophagoscope (Flexible Or Rigid) .... EAR/NOSE/THROAT
Forceps, Endoscopic .... GASTRO/UROLOGY
Gastroduodenoscope .... GASTRO/UROLOGY
Gastroscope, Flexible .... GASTRO/UROLOGY
Hysteroscope .... OBSTETRICS/GYN
Laparoscope, General & Plastic Surgery .... SURGERY
Laparoscope, Gynecologic .... OBSTETRICS/GYN
Laryngoscope .... EAR/NOSE/THROAT
Monitor, Video, Endoscope .... GENERAL
Nasopharyngoscope (Flexible Or Rigid) .... EAR/NOSE/THROAT
Nephroscope, Flexible .... GASTRO/UROLOGY
Resectoscope .... GASTRO/UROLOGY
Sigmoidoscope, Flexible .... GASTRO/UROLOGY
System, Camera, 3-Dimensional .... MIN. INV. SURGERY
Telescope, Rigid, Endoscopic .... GASTRO/UROLOGY
Thoracoscope .... CARDIOVASCULAR
Ureteroscope .... GASTRO/UROLOGY

Olympus Optical Co. Ltd. Tel: 03/3402111
San-Ei Bldg.
1-22-2, Nishi-Shinjuku
Shinjuku-Ku, Tokyo 163-91
Japan
CEO: Toshiro Shimoyama, President
Device Category:
Arthroscope .... ORTHOPEDICS
Bronchoscope, Flexible .... EAR/NOSE/THROAT
Bronchoscope, Rigid .... EAR/NOSE/THROAT
Brush, Cytology, Endoscopic .... GASTRO/UROLOGY
Choledochoscope, Flexible Or Rigid .... GASTRO/UROLOGY
Colonoscope, Gastro-Urology .... GASTRO/UROLOGY
Colposcope .... OBSTETRICS/GYN
Cystoscope .... GASTRO/UROLOGY
Cystourethroscope .... GASTRO/UROLOGY
Duodenoscope, Esophago/Gastro .... GASTRO/UROLOGY
Esophagoscope (Flexible Or Rigid) .... EAR/NOSE/THROAT
Forceps, Endoscopic .... GASTRO/UROLOGY
Gastroduodenoscope .... GASTRO/UROLOGY
Gastroscope, Flexible .... GASTRO/UROLOGY
Gastroscope, Gastro-Urology .... GASTRO/UROLOGY
Hysteroscope .... OBSTETRICS/GYN
Laparoscope, General & Plastic Surgery .... SURGERY
Laparoscope, Gynecologic .... OBSTETRICS/GYN
Laryngoscope .... EAR/NOSE/THROAT
Laryngoscope, Flexible .... ANESTH/PUL MED
Laryngoscope, Rigid .... ANESTH/PUL MED
Nasopharyngoscope (Flexible Or Rigid) .... EAR/NOSE/THROAT
Nephroscope, Flexible .... GASTRO/UROLOGY
Resectoscope .... GASTRO/UROLOGY
Sigmoidoscope, Flexible .... GASTRO/UROLOGY
Ureteroscope .... GASTRO/UROLOGY

Olympus Winter & Ibe GmbH Tel: 040/66966-0
Kuehnstrasse 61, Postf. 701709 Fax: 040/6681591
D-22045 Hamburg 70
Germany
CEO: Heide Krohn, OWI Hamburg
Device Category:
Arthroscope .... ORTHOPEDICS
Bronchoscope, Rigid .... EAR/NOSE/THROAT
Choledochoscope, Flexible Or Rigid .... GASTRO/UROLOGY
Cystoscope .... GASTRO/UROLOGY
Cystourethroscope .... GASTRO/UROLOGY
Forceps, Endoscopic .... GASTRO/UROLOGY
Laparoscope, Flexible .... SURGERY
Laparoscope, General & Plastic Surgery .... SURGERY

Omega Universal Technologies Ltd. Tel: 71/490-1318
Omega House, 211 New North Rd. Fax: 71/490-1468
London, N1 6UT
United Kingdom
CEO: Costas Diamantopoulos, Director
Device Category:
Ureteroscope .... GASTRO/UROLOGY

Omni-Tract Surgical Div.
Minnesota Scientific Co.
Tel: 612-633-8448
Tel: 800-367-8657
Fax: 612-633-5133

403 County Rd. E2 West
St. Paul, MN 55112-6858
Total Employees: 26
Ownership: Private
Distribution: Manufacturer Direct, Exporter
CEO: Joan Anderson, Contr.
    Dale Stull, President
    Bruce LeVahn, CEO
Marketing: Larry Griffith, Sales & Mktg. Dir.
Production: Del Gorham, Mfg. Dir.
Federal Procurement Eligibility: Small Business
Device Category:
Holder, Laparoscope .... OBSTETRICS/GYN
Kit, Laparoscopy .... GASTRO/UROLOGY

Optical Micro Systems, Inc.
Tel: 508-681-0992
Tel: 800-777-6280
Fax: 508-686-2677

300 Willow St. S
North Andover, MA 01845-5920
CEO: B. J. Barwick, Jr., President
Marketing: Richard B. Packard, Natl. Sales Mgr.
    Michael J. Crocetta, Dir. of Mktg.
Production: John Gately, VP Operations
    Jerry Clay, Regulatory Affairs Mgr.
    Bob Houlden, Materials Mgr.
Federal Procurement Eligibility: Small Business
Device Category:
Trocar, Other .... GENERAL

Optical Radiation Corp.
Tel: 818-969-3344
Tel: 800-423-1887
Fax: 818-334-4168

1300 Optical Drive
Azusa, CA 91702-3251
Advertising: Robert Fleming, Comm. Dir.
CEO: Richard Wood, President
    Gary Patten, VP Finance
Marketing: Ginger Silva, VP Sales & Mktg. Opthalmic Surg. Prod. Div.
    Dan Meek, Group Prod. Mkt. Mgr.
    Bill Hanley, Mktg. Dir.
Production: Susan McSweeney, Prod. Mgr.
    Gregg Whitaker, VP & Div. Mgr. Opthalmic Surg. Prod. Div.
    David Zeffren, Prod. Mgr.
    Barry Ford, VP Oper.
Research: Patricia Krapf, Sr. Product Mgr.
Device Category:
Illuminator, Fiberoptic (For Endoscope) .... GASTRO/UROLOGY

Optical Resources, Inc.
Tel: 914-753-5309

15 Harriman Ave.
Sloatsburg, NY 10974-2628
CEO: Arnold Reif, President
Device Category:
Accessories, Arthroscope .... ORTHOPEDICS
Arthroscope .... ORTHOPEDICS

Optik, Inc.
Tel: 410-551-9700
Tel: 800-638-0440
Fax: 410-551-9702

1370 Blair Dr.
Odenton, MD 21113
CEO: John Ahern
    Gail Showalter
    Eileen Ramage, VP Oper.
Federal Procurement Eligibility: Small Business, GSA Contract, VA Contract
Device Category:
Accessories, Arthroscope .... ORTHOPEDICS
Insufflator, Laparoscopic .... OBSTETRICS/GYN
Insufflator, Other .... SURGERY

Origin Medsystems, Inc.
Tel: 415-617-5000
Tel: 800-457-8145
Fax: 415-617-5100

135 Constitution Dr.
Menlo Park, CA 94025
Advertising: Beth Ladd, Adv. Mgr.
CEO: Robert Klee, Personnel Dir.
    Joseph Mandato, President & CEO
Marketing: Thierry Thaure, Intl. Sales & Mktg. Mgr.
    Phil Hopper, VP Sales & Mktg.
    Joe Lima, Dir. Mfg.
    Jill Scheweiger, Reg. Affairs Dir.
    Dana Mead, Natl. Sales Mgr.
Production: Paul Penny, VP Mfg.
    James E. Reilly, Jr., Dir. Mfg.
Research: Al Chin, VP R&D
Device Category:
Amnioscope, Transabdominal (Fetoscope) .... OBSTETRICS/GYN
Applier, Clip, Laparoscopic .... MIN. INV. SURGERY
Camera, Cine, Endoscopic, Without Audio .... SURGERY
Camera, Television, Endoscopic, Without Audio .... SURGERY
Camera, Video, Endoscopic .... GENERAL
Cannula with Inflatable Balloon (Distal Tip) .... MIN. INV. SURGERY
Catheter, Cholangiography .... SURGERY
Coagulator/Cutter, Endoscopic, Bipolar .... OBSTETRICS/GYN
Endoscope, Rigid .... SURGERY
Equipment, Suction/Irrigation, Laparoscopic .... SURGERY
Forceps, Endoscopic .... GASTRO/UROLOGY
Forceps, Grasping, Atraumatic .... MIN. INV. SURGERY
Forceps, Grasping, Traumatic .... MIN. INV. SURGERY
Holder, Instrument, Laparoscopic .... MIN. INV. SURGERY
Holder, Needle, Laparoscopic .... MIN. INV. SURGERY
Holder/Scissors, Needle, Laparoscopic .... MIN. INV. SURGERY
Instrument, Dissecting, Laparoscopic .... MIN. INV. SURGERY
Instrument, Needle Holder/Knot Tying .... MIN. INV. SURGERY
Kit, Laparoscopy .... GASTRO/UROLOGY
Light Source, Endoscope, Xenon Arc .... SURGERY
Needle, Endoscopic .... GASTRO/UROLOGY
Needle, Insufflation, Laparoscopic .... MIN. INV. SURGERY
Probe, Suction, Irrigator/Aspirator, Laparoscopic .... MIN. INV. SURGERY
Retractor, Fan-Type, Laparoscopy .... MIN. INV. SURGERY
Retractor, Laparoscopy, Other .... MIN. INV. SURGERY
Scissors with Removable Tips, Laparoscopy .... MIN. INV. SURGERY
Scissors, Laparoscopy .... MIN. INV. SURGERY
Trocar, Abdominal .... GASTRO/UROLOGY
Trocar, Short .... MIN. INV. SURGERY
Trocar, Thoracic .... CARDIOVASCULAR

Orthopedic Systems, Inc.　　　　　　　　Tel: 510-785-1020
1897 National Ave.　　　　　　　　　　　　Tel: 800-777-4674
Hayward, CA 94545-1794　　　　　　　　　Fax: 510-785-9621
CEO: Robert R. Moore, Gen. Mgr.
　　Lois L. Moore, President
　　Jana B. Orear, VP
Federal Procurement Eligibility: Small Business, Woman Owned, GSA
　　Contract, VA Contract
Device Category:
Accessories, Arthroscope .... ORTHOPEDICS
Holder, Leg, Arthroscopy .... ORTHOPEDICS

Osram Corp.　　　　　　　　　　　　　　Tel: 914-457-4040
110 Bracken Road　　　　　　　　　　　　　Tel: 800-431-9980
Montgomery, NY 12549-2600　　　　　　　Fax: 914-457-4142
Advertising: R.D. Sipe
CEO: Paul Caramagna, VP
　　H. Peters, President
Marketing: David Olsen, Mkt. Mgr.
Device Category:
Lamp, Endoscopic, Incandescent .... SURGERY

Osram GmbH　　　　　　　　　　　　　　Tel: 089/62131
Hellabrunner Str. 1　　　　　　　　　　　　Fax: 089/6232018
Postfach 900 620
D-81543 Muenchen
Germany
Advertising: Hans Joern Schenkat
CEO: Wolf-Dieter Bopst
Marketing: Dr. Lepp
Production: D. Joerg Schafer
Device Category:
Lamp, Endoscopic, Incandescent .... SURGERY

Ovamed Corporation　　　　　　　　　Tel: 408-720-9876
111 W. Evelyn Ave. Ste. #214　　　　　　Tel: 800-526-4397
Sunnyvale, CA 94086-6129　　　　　　　Fax: 408-720-9875
CEO: Laurie Ayres, VP Regulatory Affairs
　　John Zink, President
Marketing: David Pruitt, Dir. Mktg.
　　Barbara Mark, VP Sales & Mktg.
Federal Procurement Eligibility: Small Business
Device Category:
Bronchoscope, Flexible .... EAR/NOSE/THROAT
Choledochoscope, Flexible Or Rigid .... GASTRO/UROLOGY
Ureteroscope .... GASTRO/UROLOGY

P.A.K. Orthopaedics, Inc.　　　　　　Tel: 201-939-6906
3 De Camp Ct.　　　　　　　　　　　　　　Fax: 201-939-0977
West Long Branch, NJ 07764-1165
CEO: Peter J. Scranton
Device Category:
Instrument, Dissecting, Laparoscopic .... MIN. INV. SURGERY

Pan Servico Surgical Ltd.　　　　　　Tel: 081-764-1806
436 Streatham High Rd.　　　　　　　　　Fax: 081-679-2489
London, SW16 1DA
United Kingdom
CEO: J. Thomas
Marketing: M. S. Khan
Production: P. Jewell
Research: M. M. Quinn
Device Category:
Endoscope .... GASTRO/UROLOGY
Needle, Biopsy, Mammary .... OBSTETRICS/GYN

Pentax Precision Instrument Corp.　　Tel: 914-365-0700
30 Ramland Rd.　　　　　　　　　　　　　　Tel: 800-431-5880
Orangeburg, NY 10962-2699　　　　　　　Fax: 914-365-0822
CEO: Paul Magrath, VP Controller
　　Ken Shirahata, President
Marketing: Paul Silva, Dir. Product Management
　　Mark Pierce, VP Mktg. & Sales
　　Laura Gartner, Comm. Coord.
Production: Keith Nelson, Dir. Tech. Svcs.
Federal Procurement Eligibility: GSA Contract, VA Contract
Device Category:
Accessories, Cleaning, Endoscopic .... GASTRO/UROLOGY
Adapter, Bulb, Endoscope, Miscellaneous .... GASTRO/UROLOGY
Bronchoscope, Flexible .... EAR/NOSE/THROAT
Brush, Cytology, Endoscopic .... GASTRO/UROLOGY
Camera, Still, Endoscopic .... SURGERY
Camera, Television, Endoscopic, Without Audio .... SURGERY
Camera, Videotape, Surgical .... SURGERY
Cart, Equipment, Video .... GENERAL
Choledochoscope, Flexible Or Rigid .... GASTRO/UROLOGY
Colonoscope, Gastro-Urology .... GASTRO/UROLOGY
Computer, Image, Endoscopic .... GENERAL
Cystoscope .... GASTRO/UROLOGY
Duodenoscope, Esophago/Gastro .... GASTRO/UROLOGY
Enteroscope .... GASTRO/UROLOGY
Gastroscope, Flexible .... GASTRO/UROLOGY
Laryngoscope, Flexible .... ANESTH/PUL MED
Light Source, Endoscope, Xenon Arc .... SURGERY
Nasopharyngoscope (Flexible Or Rigid) .... EAR/NOSE/THROAT
Needle, Endoscopic .... GASTRO/UROLOGY
Nephroscope, Flexible .... GASTRO/UROLOGY
Observerscope .... GENERAL
Sigmoidoscope, Flexible .... GASTRO/UROLOGY
Snare, Endoscopic .... SURGERY
Tape, Television & Video, Endoscopic .... GASTRO/UROLOGY
Teaching Attachment, Endoscopic .... GASTRO/UROLOGY
Ureteroscope .... GASTRO/UROLOGY

Performance Orthopedics　　　　　　　Tel: 804-270-0140
3971 Deep Rock Rd.　　　　　　　　　　　Fax: 804-270-0169
Richmond, VA 23233-1433
CEO: Broaddus, VP Chief Admin.
Federal Procurement Eligibility: Small Business
Device Category:
Holder, Leg, Arthroscopy .... ORTHOPEDICS

Performance Surgical Instruments   Tel: 508-230-0010
40 Norfolk Ave.   Tel: 800-622-1223
Easton, MA 023334   Fax: 508-238-3807
CEO: Russel P. Holmes
Marketing: Terry Rouvalis, Mktg. Dir.
Federal Procurement Eligibility: Small Business
Device Category:
Clamp, Laparoscopy .... MIN. INV. SURGERY
Forceps, Endoscopic .... GASTRO/UROLOGY
Forceps, Grasping, Atraumatic .... MIN. INV. SURGERY
Forceps, Grasping, Traumatic .... MIN. INV. SURGERY
Forceps, Laparoscopy, Electrosurgical .... SURGERY
Holder, Needle, Curved, Laparoscopic .... MIN. INV. SURGERY
Holder, Needle, Laparoscopic .... MIN. INV. SURGERY
Instrument, Dissecting, Laparoscopic .... MIN. INV. SURGERY
Instrument, Knot Tying, Suture, Laparoscopic .... MIN. INV. SURGERY
Instrument, Needle Holder/Knot Tying .... MIN. INV. SURGERY
Instrument, Passing, Suture, Laparoscopic .... MIN. INV. SURGERY
Introducer, T-Tube .... MIN. INV. SURGERY
Kit, Cholecystectomy .... MIN. INV. SURGERY
Kit, Laparoscopy .... GASTRO/UROLOGY
Peritoneoscope .... GASTRO/UROLOGY
Probe, Electrocauterization, Multi-Use .... MIN. INV. SURGERY
Scissors, Laparoscopy .... MIN. INV. SURGERY
Snare, Endoscopic .... SURGERY

Phillips & Jones (U.S.A.), Inc.   Tel: 302-737-7987
P.O. Box 7246   Fax: 302-737-9440
Newark, DE 19714-7246
CEO: Raina A. Ehsan, VP
    Abid Ehsan, President
Marketing: Jeff Samlock
Production: R.I. Mirza
Federal Procurement Eligibility: Small Business
Device Category:
Trocar, Gallbladder .... GASTRO/UROLOGY

Phillips Medical Group   Tel: 919-469-4641
562 East Chatham St.   Tel: 800-779-0370
Cary, NC 27511   Fax: 919-319-1200
CEO: John Duncan, President
    James Phillips, COO
    Fred Billetter, Administrator
Production: K. Smith
    John Duncan
    D. Duncan
Research: James Phillips
Federal Procurement Eligibility: Small Business, GSA Contract
Device Category:
Endoscope, Flexible .... GASTRO/UROLOGY
Endoscope, Rigid .... SURGERY
Forceps, Endoscopic .... GASTRO/UROLOGY

Picker International Inc.   Tel: 216-473-6787
Health Care Products Div.   Tel: 800-635-XRAY
6700 Beta Dr.   Fax: 216-473-7046
Mayfield Village, OH 44143-2321
Medical Products Sales Volume: $200,000,000
Total Employees: 500
Ownership: Private
Distribution: Manufacturer Through Distributor, OEM, Exclusive
    Distributor
Advertising: Judy Abelman
CEO: Joseph Largey, President
    J. W. Hiles, VP Nat'l & Fed. Accts.
    Carl Schwartzenberg, VP Human Resources & Quality
Marketing: Mike Carson, West Zone Sales Mgr.
    Michael Burke, VP Sales & Distr.
    Karl Wolcott, East Zone Sales Mgr.
    Jerry Cirino, VP Mktg.
    Dave Breen, Nat'l Training Mgr.
Production: Herb Myers, VP Manufacturing
Federal Procurement Eligibility: GSA Contract, VA Contract
Device Category:
Arthrogram Kit .... ORTHOPEDICS
Insufflator, Other .... SURGERY

Picker International, Inc.   Tel: 216-473-3000
595 Miner Rd.
Cleveland, OH 44143-2131
Advertising: Robert A. Spademan, Corp. Comm. Dir.
    Peterson, P.R. Mgr.
    Don Pavlov, Comm. Mgr.
CEO: Cary J. Nolan, CEO & President
Marketing: William Webb, President Sales & Service
    Joe Largey, President, Healthcare Products Div.
Production: Joe Cavaliere, Dir. Oper.
Federal Procurement Eligibility: GSA Contract, VA Contract
Device Category:
Arthrogram Kit .... ORTHOPEDICS

Pilling-Rusch   Tel: 215-643-2600
420 Delaware Dr.   Tel: 800-523-6507
Fort Washington, PA 19034-2711   Fax: 215-641-0971
CEO: John Chester, President
Marketing: Jim Davis, SVP Sales & Mktg.
Production: Lee Wimer, VP Oper.
    Diane Clemson, Dir. Purchasing
Research: William Pilling, VP Product Dev.
Federal Procurement Eligibility: Small Business, GSA Contract
Device Category:
Accessories, Cleaning, Endoscopic .... GASTRO/UROLOGY
Anoscope, Non-Powered .... GASTRO/UROLOGY
Bougie, Esophageal And Gastrointestinal .... GASTRO/UROLOGY
Bougie, Esophageal, ENT .... EAR/NOSE/THROAT
Bronchoscope, Rigid .... EAR/NOSE/THROAT
Bronchoscope, Rigid, Ventilating .... ANESTH/PUL MED
Carrier, Sponge, Endoscopic .... GASTRO/UROLOGY
Esophagoscope (Flexible Or Rigid) .... EAR/NOSE/THROAT
Eyepiece, Lens, Non-Prescription, Endoscopic ...... GASTRO/UROLOGY
Forceps, Electrosurgical .... SURGERY
Forceps, Endoscopic .... GASTRO/UROLOGY
Lamp, Endoscopic, Incandescent .... SURGERY
Laryngoscope .... EAR/NOSE/THROAT
Laryngoscope, Rigid .... ANESTH/PUL MED
Mediastinoscope .... SURGERY
Needle, Endoscopic .... GASTRO/UROLOGY
Telescope, Rigid, Endoscopic .... GASTRO/UROLOGY
Thoracoscope .... CARDIOVASCULAR
Trocar, Abdominal .... GASTRO/UROLOGY
Trocar, Amniotic .... OBSTETRICS/GYN
Trocar, Cardiovascular .... CARDIOVASCULAR
Trocar, Gallbladder .... GASTRO/UROLOGY
Trocar, Thoracic .... CARDIOVASCULAR
Trocar, Tracheal .... EAR/NOSE/THROAT

Pioneer Medical, Inc.
34 Laurelcrest Rd.
Madison, CT 06443
Tel: 203-245-9337
Tel: 800-966-6453
Fax: 203-245-5718
CEO: Michael D. Cecchi, President
Production: William Nye
Federal Procurement Eligibility: Small Business
Device Category:
Camera, Cine, Endoscopic, With Audio .... SURGERY
Endoscope, Rigid .... SURGERY
Laparoscope, Gynecologic .... OBSTETRICS/GYN
Light Source, Endoscope, Xenon Arc .... SURGERY
Telescope, Rigid, Endoscopic .... GASTRO/UROLOGY
Trocar, Abdominal .... GASTRO/UROLOGY
Trocar, Gastro-Urology .... GASTRO/UROLOGY
Trocar, Other .... GENERAL

Plastofilm Industries, Inc.
P.O. Box 531
Wheaton, IL 60189-0531
Tel: 708-668-2838
Tel: 800-937-4744
Fax: 708-668-5431
CEO: Stuart Benton, President
Marketing: Robert A. Moren, VP Nat'l Sales
  Rich Partlow, VP Sales & Mktg.
  Douglas B. Slomski, Dir. Mktg.
Production: Jon Beard, VP Mfg.
Federal Procurement Eligibility: GSA Contract
Device Category:
Carrier, Sponge, Endoscopic .... GASTRO/UROLOGY

PLC Systems Div.
Laser Engineering, Inc.
113 Cedar St.
Milford, MA 01757-1154
Tel: 508-478-5991
Tel: 800-232-8422
Fax: 508-478-6737
Medical Products Sales Volume: $6,000,000
Total Employees: 41
Ownership: Public
Distribution: Exclusive Distributor
CEO: Robert Rudko, President
  Pat Murphy, Controller
Marketing: Francis Martin, VP Mktg. & Sales
  Don Lankford, Product Mgr.
Production: Steve Linhares, Dir. Eng.
Federal Procurement Eligibility: Small Business, GSA Contract, VA Contract
Device Category:
Laparoscope, Flexible .... SURGERY

Popper & Sons, Inc.
300 Denton Ave.
New Hyde Park, NY 11040-3437
Tel: 516-248-0300
Fax: 516-747-1188
CEO: Zev Asch, Natl. Sales Mgr.
  Walter L. Popper, President
  Hilda Hoffman, VP Comptroller
  Burt W. Sheier, Admin. Dir.
Marketing: Stuart Carter, Mktg. Mgr.
  Joseph A. Popper, Exec. VP Mktg.
Production: Ira L. Zuckerman, Oper. Dir.
Federal Procurement Eligibility: Small Business
Device Category:
Trocar, Laryngeal .... EAR/NOSE/THROAT
Trocar, Other .... GENERAL

Portlyn Medical Products
Route 25
Moultonboro, NH 03254
Tel: 603-476-5538
Tel: 800-237-8248
Fax: 603-476-5019
CEO: Ronald V. Porter, CEO
  David E. Porter, President
Marketing: Kenneth V. Freeman, VP Sales & Mktg.
Federal Procurement Eligibility: Small Business
Device Category:
Accessories, Arthroscope .... ORTHOPEDICS
Forceps, Endoscopic .... GASTRO/UROLOGY
Forceps, Grasping, Flexible Endoscopic .... GASTRO/UROLOGY
Forceps, Grasping, Traumatic .... MIN. INV. SURGERY

Practical Design, Inc.
4711 126th Ave. North, Ste. J
Clearwater, FL 34622
Tel: 813-572-4820
Tel: 800-768-9447
Fax: 813-573-2218
CEO: Robert C. Gray, President
Marketing: Mary Holley, Mktg. Mgr.
Federal Procurement Eligibility: Small Business
Device Category:
Cart, Equipment, Video .... GENERAL

Precision Optics Corp.
22 E. Broadway
Gardner, MA 01440-3338
Tel: 508-630-1800
Fax: 508-630-1487
CEO: Richard E. Forkey, President
Marketing: Robert C. Meinhold, VP Sales & Mktg.
Federal Procurement Eligibility: Small Business
Device Category:
Endoscope .... GASTRO/UROLOGY
Laparoscope, General & Plastic Surgery .... SURGERY
Thoracoscope .... CARDIOVASCULAR

Premier Medical Manufacturing
10090 Sandmeyer Lane
Philadelphia, PA 19116-3502
Tel: 215-676-9090
Fax: 215-464-0917
CEO: William Frezel, General Mgr.
Production: Mark Fishman, Oper. Mgr.
Federal Procurement Eligibility: Small Business
Device Category:
Trocar, Other .... GENERAL

Proclinics
C/Vic. 24
E-La Llagosta (Barcelona)
Spain
Tel: 3/560-3652
Fax: 560-5771
CEO: Candido Gasco Seguir
Marketing: Joaquin Cabrero Roura
  Francere Cuxart Vaques
Production: Antonio Godes Adell
Device Category:
Trocar, Thoracic .... CARDIOVASCULAR

Professional Surgical Instrument Co.
Tel: 908-390-1133
Fax: 908-390-1112
102 Old Stage Rd.
East Brunswick, NJ 08816
CEO: Ragzi Mohammed Ellahi, Operations
Research: Zahur Mughal
Device Category:
Laryngoscope .... EAR/NOSE/THROAT

Progressive Dynamics, Inc.
Tel: 616-781-4241
Fax: 616-781-7802
507 Industrial Rd.
Marshall, MI 49068-1758
CEO: Eugene Kilbourn, President
Marketing: Joseph A. Namenye
Federal Procurement Eligibility: Small Business
Device Category:
Illuminator, Fiberoptic (For Endoscope) .... GASTRO/UROLOGY
Insufflator, Laparoscopic .... OBSTETRICS/GYN
Insufflator, Other .... SURGERY

Promedica, Inc.
Tel: 813-889-9250
Tel: 800-899-5278
Fax: 813-886-9342
5501 D Airport Blvd.
Tampa, FL 33634-5171
CEO: Michael K. Trout, President
John F. Spangler, COB
Marketing: Ann Doucette, Mktg. & Sales Dir.
Production: Barrie Carson, Plant Mgr.
Federal Procurement Eligibility: Small Business
Device Category:
Cart, Equipment, Video .... GENERAL
System, Traction, Arthroscopy .... ORTHOPEDICS

Propper Manufacturing Co., Inc.
Tel: 718-392-6650
Fax: 718-482-8909
36-04 Skillman Avenue
Long Isl. City, NY 11101-1730
CEO: Seymor Schuman, COB
Maxine Kaplan, Personnel
Ken Summer, President
Jane Schuman, VCOB
Marketing: Tom Lane, Nat'l Sales Mgr.
Mary DiSilvestri, Contract Sales Mgr.
Leon Yahes, Int'l Sales & Mktg. Mgr.
John E. McGinley, VP Mktg. & Sales
Bill Fitzgerald, Asst. to President
Production: Thomas Augurt, VP R&D
John Charles Toussaint, Dir. of Operations
Dr. Thomas Augert, Regulatory Affairs Mgr.
Federal Procurement Eligibility: Small Business, GSA Contract, VA Contract
Device Category:
Laryngoscope, Surgical .... SURGERY

Puritan-Bennett Corp.
Tel: 913-661-0444
Tel: 800-255-6773
Fax: 913-661-0234
9401 Indian Creek Pkwy.
P.O. Box 25905
Overland Park, KS 66210-2005
CEO: Tom Jones, SVP
John Morrow, COO & Exec. VP
Jim Reller, VP Human Relations
Burton A. Dole, President & Chairman
Marketing: Ron Richard, Prod. Mgr.
Nate Hope, VP Sales
Kumar Shahani, Sr. Prod. Mgr.
George Fagg, Prod. Mgr.
Caye Cross White, Corp. Comm. Mgr.
Bob Doyle, SVP Mktg.
Device Category:
Laryngoscope, Rigid .... ANESTH/PUL MED

Quantum Instruments Corp.
Tel: 214-733-6566
Fax: 214-733-6809
17304 Preston Rd., Ste. 800
Dallas, TX 75252
Advertising: Tom Bunce, Adv. Mgr.
CEO: Robert Frischer, M.D., Bus. Dev. Mgr.
Chris Crowe, CEO & COB
Carroll Shmidt, VP Personnel
Marketing: Robert Frischer, M.D., Mkt. Res. Mgr.
Mick Ward, VP Sales & Mktg.
Production: Jim Monti, VP Mfg.
Federal Procurement Eligibility: Small Business
Device Category:
Generator, Power, Electrosurgical .... SURGERY
Peritoneoscope .... GASTRO/UROLOGY

Questus Corp.
Tel: 617-639-1900
Fax: 617-639-1905
Lime St.
P.O. Box 9
Marblehead, MA 01945-0009
CEO: Allen H. DeSatnick, President
Marketing: Robert E. Brissette, VP
Federal Procurement Eligibility: Small Business
Device Category:
Accessories, Arthroscope .... ORTHOPEDICS
Arthroscope .... ORTHOPEDICS
Forceps, Grasping, Flexible Endoscopic .... GASTRO/UROLOGY

R-Group International
Tel: 904-378-3633
Fax: 904-378-3661
2321 N.W. 66th Court, Ste. W4
Gainesville, FL 32606
CEO: Henry J. Kahn
Marketing: Darren F. Kahn
Production: Mark J. Kahn
Federal Procurement Eligibility: Small Business
Device Category:
Accessories, Cleaning, Endoscopic .... GASTRO/UROLOGY
Brush, Cytology, Endoscopic .... GASTRO/UROLOGY

Radiographics
Tel: 301-460-1736
Fax: 301-460-2777
3013 Regina Dr. Ste. B
Silver Spring, MD 20906-5364
CEO: John Rauscher, Asst. Office Mgr.
James F. Rauch, President
Federal Procurement Eligibility: Small Business
Device Category:
Arthrogram Kit .... ORTHOPEDICS

Ranfac Corp.
Avon Indus. Pk./30 Doherty Ave., Box 635
Avon, MA 02322-1125
Advertising: Barry H. Zinble
CEO: Robert M. Adler, President
    John H. Hackett, Controller
    Barry H. Zimble, Dir. Bus. Dev.
Production: Christopher P. Whelan, Mfg. Dir.
Research: Marilyn Adler
Federal Procurement Eligibility: Small Business
Device Category:
Catheter, Cholangiography .... SURGERY
Instrument, Knot Tying, Suture, Laparoscopic .... MIN. INV. SURGERY
Instrument, Passing, Suture, Laparoscopic .... MIN. INV. SURGERY
Needle, Aspiration, Cyst, Laparoscopic .... MIN. INV. SURGERY
Needle, Biopsy, Mammary .... OBSTETRICS/GYN
Needle, Endoscopic .... GASTRO/UROLOGY
Needle, Insufflation, Laparoscopic .... MIN. INV. SURGERY
Retractor, Laparoscopy, Other .... MIN. INV. SURGERY

Tel: 508-588-4400
Tel: 800-2RANFAC
Fax: 508-584-8588

Redfield Corporation
210 Summit Ave.
Montvale, NJ 07645-1526
CEO: Ingram S. Chodorow, CEO
    Don Osur, President
Federal Procurement Eligibility: Small Business
Device Category:
Coagulator, Laparoscopic, Unipolar .... OBSTETRICS/GYN
Endoscope And Accessories, AC-Powered .... SURGERY
Light, Surgical, Endoscopic .... SURGERY
Peritoneoscope .... GASTRO/UROLOGY

Tel: 201-391-0494
Tel: 800-678-4472
Fax: 201-930-1495

Rema Medizintechnik GmbH
In Breiten 10
D-78589 Duerbheim-Tuttlingen
Germany
CEO: Reinhold Mattes, President
Device Category:
Arthroscope .... ORTHOPEDICS
Culdoscope .... OBSTETRICS/GYN
Endoscope, Fetal Blood Sampling .... OBSTETRICS/GYN
Endoscope, Rigid .... SURGERY
Endoscope, Transcervical (Amnioscope) .... OBSTETRICS/GYN
Hysteroscope .... OBSTETRICS/GYN
Laparoscope, General & Plastic Surgery .... SURGERY
Laparoscope, Gynecologic .... OBSTETRICS/GYN
Proctoscope .... SURGERY
Vaginoscope .... OBSTETRICS/GYN

Tel: 07424-4064
Fax: 07424-501590

Resorba Surgical Sutures
F. Hiltner Ltd. & Co.
Schonerstr. 7
D-90443 Nurnberg
Germany
Medical Products Sales Volume: $18,288,400
Total Employees: 100
Distribution: Manufacturer Direct
CEO: C. M. Hiltner
Marketing: Werner Hohlein
Production: Manfred Kruger
Device Category:
Holder, Instrument, Laparoscopic .... MIN. INV. SURGERY

Tel: 0911/442344
Fax: 0911/4467242

Richard-Allan Medical Industries, Inc.
8850 M-89
P.O. Box 351
Richland, MI 49083-0351
Medical Products Sales Volume: $15,000,000
Total Employees: 150
Distribution: Manufacturer Direct, Exporter
CEO: Susan Newhauser, VP Personnel
    Richard R. Newhauser, President
    Julie Powell, Reg. Affairs Mgr.
    Gary Thoma, Dir. Finance
Marketing: Tom Roberts, Mktg. Mgr.
    Rick Holmes, Contract Sales Mgr.
    Dana Williams, Mktg. Mgr.
    Chris Woods, Contract Sales Mgr.
Production: Kathy Gietzen, Product Team Dir.
    Hugh Melling, Co-Dir. Design & Eng.
    Denise Simon, Co-Dir. Design & Eng.
    Debbie Myers, Product Team Dir.
    Dan Richardson
    Andy Lenzeyski, Product Team Dir.
Research: Jerry Fredenburgh
Device Category:
Kit, Cholecystectomy .... MIN. INV. SURGERY
Peritoneoscope .... GASTRO/UROLOGY
Stapler, Surgical .... SURGERY

Tel: 616-629-5811
Tel: 800-253-7900
Fax: 616-629-9654

Richmond Products, Inc.
1021 S. Rogers Circle, Ste. 6
Boca Raton, FL 33487-2894
CEO: P. L. Powell
Federal Procurement Eligibility: Small Business
Device Category:
Accessories, Cleaning, Endoscopic .... GASTRO/UROLOGY

Tel: 407-994-2112
Tel: 800-448-4538
Fax: 407-994-2235

Riko Trading Co. Ltd.
34-6 Nishigoken-cho
Shinjuku-ku
Tokyo 162
Japan
CEO: Yoichi Yamamoto, President
Device Category:
Endoscope .... GASTRO/UROLOGY

Tel: 03/267-1211

Rose GmbH
Gottbillstr. 27-30
D-54294 Trier
Germany
CEO: Ewald Rose
Marketing: Wolfgang Kromus
Device Category:
Amniscope, Transabdominal (Fetoscope) .... OBSTETRICS/GYN
Proctoscope .... SURGERY

Tel: 0651/89051
Fax: 0651/800440

Rovers B.V.
Lekstraat 10
NL-5347 KV - Oss
Netherlands
CEO: Willem P.G. Rovers, President
Device Category:
Cannula, Drainage, Arthroscopy .... ORTHOPEDICS

Tel: 04120 - 48870
Fax: 04120 - 23835

Rudolf GmbH
Tuttlinger Str. 4
Postfach 28
D-78567 Fridingen
Germany
Marketing: Mr. Renner, Mktg. Mgr.
Device Category:
Choledochoscope, Flexible Or Rigid .... GASTRO/UROLOGY
Endoscope .... GASTRO/UROLOGY
Endoscope, Rigid .... SURGERY

Tel: 07463/1094
Fax: 07463/8864

Rusch Of Canada Ltd.
2000 Ellesmere Road Unit 12
Scarborough, ONT M1H 2W4
Canada
CEO: H. Greenberg
Device Category:
Basket, Biliary Stone Retrieval .... GASTRO/UROLOGY
Laryngoscope, Rigid .... ANESTH/PUL MED

Tel: 416-438-6317
Fax: 416-438-7542

Rusch, Inc.
2450 Meadowbrook Pkwy.
Duluth, GA 30136-4635
Advertising: Samantha Burns, Product Mgr.
CEO: David Emm, General Mgr.
Marketing: Charles Higgins, National Accts. Dir.
Production: Kathleen A. Lumberg, Regulatory Affairs Mgr.
Federal Procurement Eligibility: GSA Contract
Device Category:
Bougie, Esophageal And Gastrointestinal .... GASTRO/UROLOGY
Bougie, Esophageal, ENT .... EAR/NOSE/THROAT
Laryngoscope, Rigid .... ANESTH/PUL MED
Prosthesis, Esophageal .... EAR/NOSE/THROAT

Tel: 404-623-0816
Tel: 800-553-5214
Fax: 404-623-1829

Rx Honing Machine Corporation
1301 East Fifth St.
Mishawaka, IN 46544-2827
CEO: Robert E. Magnuson, President
Marketing: R. J. Watson, Sales Mgr.
Production: Marvin Yocum
Federal Procurement Eligibility: Small Business, Woman Owned
Device Category:
Arthroscope .... ORTHOPEDICS
Peritoneoscope .... GASTRO/UROLOGY

Tel: 219-259-1606
Tel: 800-346-6464
Fax: 219-259-9163

Sanderson-Macleod, Inc.
199 S. Main St.
P.O. Box 50
Palmer, MA 01069-1899
CEO: Eric Sanderson, EVP
Marketing: Ron Sohlgren, Sales Mgr.
Production: Jim Pascale, Mfg. Dir.
Federal Procurement Eligibility: Small Business
Device Category:
Brush, Cytology, Endoscopic .... GASTRO/UROLOGY

Tel: 413-283-3481
Fax: 413-289-1919

Scan-Med, Inc.
P.O. Box 128
Middle Grove, NY 12850-0128
CEO: Marianne I. Gage, President
Federal Procurement Eligibility: Small Business, Woman Owned
Device Category:
Trocar, Amniotic .... OBSTETRICS/GYN

Tel: 518-893-2800
Tel: 800-722-6016
Fax: 518-893-2878

Scanlan International, Inc.
One Scanlan Plaza
St. Paul, MN 55107-1629
Advertising: Elizabeth Bossart
CEO: Timothy M. Scanlan, President & CEO
Marketing: Walter Olson, SVP Mktg. & Sales
    Mark Anderson, Mktg. Mgr.
Production: Julie Reilly, VP Oper.
Federal Procurement Eligibility: Small Business, GSA Contract
Device Category:
Coagulator/Cutter, Endoscopic, Bipolar .... OBSTETRICS/GYN

Tel: 612-298-0997
Tel: 800-328-9458
Fax: 612-298-0018

Scherzer Medical Program
Franz Petterstr. 18
A-2560 Berndorf
Austria
Marketing: Wilhelm Scherzer, Exp. Dir.
Device Category:
Cannula, Drainage, Arthroscopy .... ORTHOPEDICS

Tel: 2672/7953-13
Fax: 2672/7983-14

Schoelly Fiberoptic GmbH
Robert Bosch Str. 1-3
Postfach 1280
D-79211 Denzlingen
Germany
Advertising: Daniel Lacher, Intl. Sales & Mktg. Mgr.
CEO: Werner Scholly, President
Production: Seigfried Schindler, VP Mfg.
    Berthold Reich, Materials Mgr.
Research: Edgar Shub, VP R&D
Device Category:
Arthroscope .... ORTHOPEDICS
Hysteroscope .... OBSTETRICS/GYN
Nasopharyngoscope (Flexible Or Rigid) .... EAR/NOSE/THROAT

Tel: 07666/1018/1019
Fax: 07666/7725

Schott Fiber Optics, Inc.
122 Charlton St.
Southbridge, MA 01550-1960
Advertising: Dee Mitchell
CEO: Richard Taylor, Regulatory Affairs Mgr.
    Donald Miller, VP Finance
    Brian A. Edney, President
Marketing: William Hill, Dir. Mktg/Sales Instruments
    Norm Allard, Dir. Mktg/Sales Fused Components
    John M. Smith, Dir. New Product Dev.
Production: David Gibson, VP Operations
Research: Paul W. Remijan, Ph.D.

Tel: 508-765-9744
Tel: 800-343-6120
Fax: 508-765-1680

Device Category:
Cystoscope .... GASTRO/UROLOGY
Endoscope .... GASTRO/UROLOGY
Hysteroscope .... OBSTETRICS/GYN
Illuminator, Fiberoptic (For Endoscope) .... GASTRO/UROLOGY
Lamp, Endoscopic, Incandescent .... SURGERY
Laparoscope, General & Plastic Surgery .... SURGERY
Laryngoscope .... EAR/NOSE/THROAT
Laryngoscope, Flexible .... ANESTH/PUL MED
Nasopharyngoscope (Flexible Or Rigid) .... EAR/NOSE/THROAT
Sigmoidoscope, Flexible .... GASTRO/UROLOGY
Ureteroscope .... GASTRO/UROLOGY

Schwarz Medical
Tel: 8869/1881
Kirchstrasse 24
Fax: 8869/765
D-86935 Rott
Germany
CEO: Berthold A. Schwarz, President
Device Category:
Accessories, Surgical Camera .... SURGERY
Applier, Clip, Repair, Hernia, Laparoscopic .... MIN. INV. SURGERY
Clamp, Fixation, Cholangiography .... MIN. INV. SURGERY
Connector, Suction/Irrigation .... MIN. INV. SURGERY
Extractor, Gall Bladder .... MIN. INV. SURGERY
Forceps, Grasping, Atraumatic .... MIN. INV. SURGERY
Forceps, Grasping, Traumatic .... MIN. INV. SURGERY
Holder, Needle, Laparoscopic .... MIN. INV. SURGERY
Needle, Puncture .... MIN. INV. SURGERY
Obturator, Endoscopic .... GASTRO/UROLOGY
Scissors, Laparoscopy .... MIN. INV. SURGERY

Seitz Technical Products, Inc.
Tel: 215-268-2228
111-C Newark Rd.
Fax: 215-268-2229
P.O. Box 338
Avondale, PA 19311-0338
CEO: John R. Seitz
Marketing: W. Patrick McVay
Federal Procurement Eligibility: Small Business
Device Category:
Camera, Television, Endoscopic, Without Audio .... SURGERY
Camera, Television, Microsurgical, Without Audio .... SURGERY

Select-Sutter GmbH
Tel: 0761/515510
Tullastr. 87
Fax: 0761/5155130
D-79108 Freiburg/Breisgau
Germany
CEO: Hermann Sutter
Marketing: Birgit Sutter
Device Category:
Coagulator/Cutter, Endoscopic, Bipolar .... OBSTETRICS/GYN
Laryngoscope .... EAR/NOSE/THROAT

Sharn, Inc.
Tel: 813-889-9614
4801 George Rd., Ste. 180
Tel: 800-325-3671
Tampa, FL 33634-6236
Fax: 813-886-2701
CEO: Bruce A. Tomlinson, President
Federal Procurement Eligibility: Small Business, GSA Contract, VA Contract
Device Category:
Cart, Equipment, Video .... GENERAL

Sharplan Lasers (Europe) Ltd.
Tel: 081/203-0006
141-155 Brent St.
Fax: 081/203-7159
London NW4 4DJ
United Kingdom
CEO: David Meridor
Marketing: D. Winterstein
Device Category:
Anoscope, Non-Powered .... GASTRO/UROLOGY
Bronchoscope, Rigid .... EAR/NOSE/THROAT
Laparoscope, Gynecologic .... OBSTETRICS/GYN
Proctoscope .... SURGERY
Proctosigmoidoscope .... GASTRO/UROLOGY
Sigmoidoscope, Rigid, Non-Electrical .... GASTRO/UROLOGY

Sharplan Lasers, Inc.
Tel: 201-327-1666
1 Pearl Ct.
Tel: 800-394-2000
Allendale, NJ 07401-1675
Fax: 201-445-4048
CEO: Yigal Baruch, Finance Dir.
     Eitan Nahum, President
Marketing: Michael Slatkine, Mktg. Development Dir.
     Karen Amburgey, Mktg. Mgr.
Production: Douglass Mead, Reg. Affairs Dir.
     Avi Farbstein, Oper. Dir.
Federal Procurement Eligibility: VA Contract
Device Category:
Colposcope .... OBSTETRICS/GYN
Equipment/Accessories, Laser, Laparoscopy .... MIN. INV. SURGERY
Laparoscope, General & Plastic Surgery .... SURGERY
Laser, Nd:YAG, Laparoscopy .... MIN. INV. SURGERY
Probe, Suction, Irrigator/Aspirator, Laparoscopic .... MIN. INV. SURGERY

Sherwood Medical Company
Tel: 314-621-7788
1915 Olive St.
Tel: 800-325-7472
St. Louis, MO 63103-1625
Fax: 314-241-1673
Advertising: Martin N. Farb, EVP Industry Svcs.
CEO: David A. Low, President
Marketing: R. C. Egan, EVP Mktg.
     J. Terry Broers, EVP Mktg.
Device Category:
Equipment, Suction/Irrigation, Laparoscopic .... SURGERY
Trocar, Abdominal .... GASTRO/UROLOGY
Trocar, Cardiovascular .... CARDIOVASCULAR
Trocar, Thoracic .... CARDIOVASCULAR
Trocar, Tracheal .... EAR/NOSE/THROAT

Siemens Medical Corp.
Tel: 908-321-4500
186 Wood Ave. South
Fax: 908-494-2250
Iselin, NJ 08830-2704
Advertising: Bruce Ellis, Adv. Mgr.
CEO: Robert V. Dumke, President & CEO
     H. Hirschmann, EVP Admin. & Fin.
     G. Westermann, SVP Tech. Div.
     F. Stuvek, VP Gov't & Nat'l Accts.
Marketing: I. Johansen, Jr., VP Mktg. Svcs.
Federal Procurement Eligibility: GSA Contract, VA Contract
Device Category:
Camera, Television, Microsurgical, With Audio .... SURGERY
Camera, Television, Microsurgical, Without Audio .... SURGERY
Camera, Videotape, Surgical .... SURGERY

Simal Belgium Instrument Co.
Tel: 800-638-0440
Fax: 301-261-0941
2131 Espey Court, Suite 7
Crofton, MD 21114-2424
CEO: Mary Margaret Ahern, CEO
  Elieen Ramage, VP Fin.
Marketing: Rob Stolar, Sales Mgr.
  E. J. Smith, Mktg.
  Bill Macfie
Production: John Augustine
Federal Procurement Eligibility: Small Business, Minority Owned, Woman Owned
Device Category:
Arthroscope .... ORTHOPEDICS
Aspirator, Arthroscopy .... ORTHOPEDICS
Cannula, Drainage, Arthroscopy .... ORTHOPEDICS
Choledochoscope, Flexible Or Rigid .... GASTRO/UROLOGY
Laparoscope, General & Plastic Surgery .... SURGERY
System, Traction, Arthroscopy .... ORTHOPEDICS

Sippex
Tel: 7470/9800
Fax: 7470/9793
Usine de la Giraudiere
F-69690 Courzieu
France
CEO: Yves Rabut, Manager
Device Category:
Trocar, Other .... GENERAL

Site Microsurgical Systems, Inc.
Tel: 215-674-5800
Tel: 800-445-SITE
Fax: 215-675-2461
135 Gibraltar Rd.
Horsham, PA 19044-0936
CEO: Richard Bechtold, CFO
  Marvin L. Woodall, President
Marketing: Don Todd, Mktg. Dir.
Research: Raymond Krauss, R&D Dir.
Device Category:
Coagulator/Cutter, Endoscopic, Bipolar .... OBSTETRICS/GYN

Sklar Instrument Company
Tel: 215-430-3200
Tel: 800-221-2166
Fax: 215-429-0500
889 South Matlack St.
West Chester, PA 19380
CEO: Don Taylor, President
Marketing: John W. Kane, VP Mktg.
Production: Mike Malinowski, EVP
Federal Procurement Eligibility: Small Business, GSA Contract, VA Contract
Device Category:
Anoscope, Non-Powered .... GASTRO/UROLOGY
Bougie, Esophageal, ENT .... EAR/NOSE/THROAT
Laparoscope, Flexible .... SURGERY
Laparoscope, General & Plastic Surgery .... SURGERY
Laparoscope, Gynecologic .... OBSTETRICS/GYN
Proctoscope .... SURGERY
Sphincteroscope .... GASTRO/UROLOGY
Trocar, Abdominal .... GASTRO/UROLOGY
Trocar, Cardiovascular .... CARDIOVASCULAR
Trocar, Gallbladder .... GASTRO/UROLOGY
Trocar, Thoracic .... CARDIOVASCULAR

Skye Precision Inc.
Tel: 216-352-0020
Fax: 216-352-0050
55 Florence Ave.
Plainesville, OH 44077
CEO: Robert Anthony, Reg. Affairs Mgr.
  John T. Nelson, President
Marketing: Bradley Hall
Production: Jack Hostutler
Federal Procurement Eligibility: Small Business
Device Category:
Trocar, Short .... MIN. INV. SURGERY

Smith & Nephew - Avon Medicals
Tel: 0527/64901
Moons Moat Dr., Moons Moat N.
Redditch Worcester
United Kingdom
Advertising: I.J. Crowe
CEO: P.A. Watson
  J.A. Foster, Fin.
Marketing: J.R. Howard, Export Mgr.
  J.A. Woolston
Production: H.K. Nasta
  D. Kay
Device Category:
Trocar, Other .... GENERAL

Smith & Nephew Donjoy, Inc.
Tel: 619-438-9091
Tel: 800-336-6569
Fax: 619-438-3210
2777 Loker West
Carlsbad, CA 92008-6601
CEO: Greg Nelson, President
Device Category:
Holder, Shoulder, Arthroscopy .... SURGERY

Smith & Nephew Dyonics, Inc.
Tel: 508-470-2800
Tel: 800-343-8386
Fax: 508-470-2227
160 Dascomb Rd.
Andover, MA 01810-5893
Advertising: Kathleen Higgins
CEO: Robert Parlady, VP Finance
  Charles W. Federico, President
Marketing: Lisa Curtis, Mktg. Dir.
Production: Hooks Johnston, VP Mfg.
Research: Glen Jorgensen, R&D Dir.
Device Category:
Accessories, Arthroscope .... ORTHOPEDICS
Arthroscope .... ORTHOPEDICS
Aspirator, Arthroscopy .... ORTHOPEDICS
Camera, Cine, Endoscopic, With Audio .... SURGERY
Camera, Cine, Endoscopic, Without Audio .... SURGERY
Camera, Still, Endoscopic .... SURGERY
Camera, Television, Endoscopic, With Audio .... SURGERY
Camera, Television, Endoscopic, Without Audio .... SURGERY
Camera, Television, Microsurgical, With Audio .... SURGERY
Camera, Television, Microsurgical, Without Audio ...... SURGERY
Camera, Television, Surgical, With Audio .... SURGERY
Camera, Television, Surgical, Without Audio .... SURGERY
Camera, Video, Endoscopic .... GENERAL
Camera, Video, Multi-Image .... MIN. INV. SURGERY
Cannula, Drainage, Arthroscopy .... ORTHOPEDICS
Cannula, Suprapubic, With Trocar .... GASTRO/UROLOGY
Cart, Equipment, Video .... GENERAL
Coagulator, Laparoscopic, Unipolar .... OBSTETRICS/GYN
Coagulator/Cutter, Endoscopic, Unipolar .... OBSTETRICS/GYN

Endoscope, Direct Vision . . . . SURGERY
Endoscope, Rigid . . . . SURGERY
Forceps, Endoscopic . . . . GASTRO/UROLOGY
Forceps, Grasping, Atraumatic . . . . MIN. INV. SURGERY
Forceps, Grasping, Traumatic . . . . MIN. INV. SURGERY
Holder, Leg, Arthroscopy . . . . ORTHOPEDICS
Holder, Needle, Curved, Laparoscopic . . . . MIN. INV. SURGERY
Holder, Needle, Laparoscopic . . . . MIN. INV. SURGERY
Holder, Shoulder, Arthroscopy . . . . SURGERY
Holder/Scissors, Needle, Laparoscopic . . . . MIN. INV. SURGERY
Hysteroscope . . . . OBSTETRICS/GYN
Illuminator, Fiberoptic (For Endoscope) . . . . GASTRO/UROLOGY
Instrument, Dissecting, Laparoscopic . . . . MIN. INV. SURGERY
Instrument, Needle Holder/Knot Tying . . . . MIN. INV. SURGERY
Insufflator, Carbon-Dioxide, Automatic
   (For Endoscope) . . . . GASTRO/UROLOGY
Insufflator, Laparoscopic . . . . OBSTETRICS/GYN
Insufflator, Other . . . . SURGERY
Laparoscope, General & Plastic Surgery . . . . SURGERY
Laparoscope, Gynecologic . . . . OBSTETRICS/GYN
Light Source, Endoscope, Xenon Arc . . . . SURGERY
Monitor, Video, Endoscope . . . . GENERAL
Needle, Insufflation, Laparoscopic . . . . MIN. INV. SURGERY
Obturator, Endoscopic . . . . GASTRO/UROLOGY
Probe, Electrocauterization, Single-Use . . . . MIN. INV. SURGERY
Scissors with Removable Tips, Laparoscopy . . . . MIN. INV. SURGERY
Thoracoscope . . . . CARDIOVASCULAR
Trocar, Abdominal . . . . GASTRO/UROLOGY
Trocar, Gallbladder . . . . GASTRO/UROLOGY
Trocar, Gastro-Urology . . . . GASTRO/UROLOGY

Smith & Nephew Richards Inc. Tel: 901-396-2121
1450 Brooks Road Tel: 800-821-5700
Memphis, TN 38116 Fax: 901-396-9929
Advertising: Lorraine Potocki, Adv. Dir.
CEO: Walter Grant, SVP & Gen. Counsel
   Tom Martin, VP Adm.
   Ruben Rosales, VP International
   Ron W. Sparks, VP Finance
   Larry Papasan, President, S & N Richards
   Joe Bagwell, SVP Reg. Affairs
   Jim Duncan, Pres. Med. Specialties Div.
   Jack R. Blair, President, Surgical Prod. Grp.
Marketing: William Scott, VP Sales & Mktg. Medical Specialties Div.
   George Howard, SVP Sales & Mktg. Orthopedics Div.
Device Category:
Camera, Television, Microsurgical, Without Audio . . . . SURGERY
Camera, Video, Endoscopic . . . . GENERAL
Cart, Equipment, Video . . . . GENERAL
Colposcope . . . . OBSTETRICS/GYN
Endoscope And Accessories, AC-Powered . . . . SURGERY
Endoscope, Rigid . . . . SURGERY
Forceps, Endoscopic . . . . GASTRO/UROLOGY
Holder, Needle, Laparoscopic . . . . MIN. INV. SURGERY
Holder/Scissors, Needle, Laparoscopic . . . . MIN. INV. SURGERY
Introducer, T-Tube . . . . MIN. INV. SURGERY

Snowden-Pencer Tel: 404-496-0952
5175 S. Royal Atlanta Dr. Tel: 800-367-7874
Tucker, GA 30084-3053 Fax: 404-934-4922
CEO: Norman Black III, CEO
   Jack Gilsdorf, President
Marketing: W. Alan Mock, VP Sales & Mktg.
Federal Procurement Eligibility: Small Business
Device Category:
Cart, Equipment, Video . . . . GENERAL
Endoscope And Accessories, AC-Powered . . . . SURGERY
Forceps, Endoscopic . . . . GASTRO/UROLOGY
Forceps, Grasping, Flexible Endoscopic . . . . GASTRO/UROLOGY
Insufflator, Other . . . . SURGERY
Kit, Laparoscopy . . . . GASTRO/UROLOGY
Thoracoscope . . . . CARDIOVASCULAR

Sodem Systems Tel: 22/794-9696
110, Chemin du Pont du Centenaire Fax: 22/794-4546
Pont-du-Centenaire
CH-1228 Plan-les-Quates/Geneva
Switzerland
CEO: G. Oltramare
   B.P. Legrand, President
Marketing: Eric Bouvier, Mktg. & Sales VP
Production: Bernard Pittet
Device Category:
Accessories, Arthroscope . . . . ORTHOPEDICS
Holder, Leg, Arthroscopy . . . . ORTHOPEDICS
Holder, Shoulder, Arthroscopy . . . . SURGERY

Sony Corporation Of America Tel: 201-930-7098
Medical Systems Div. Tel: 800-535-7669
3 Paragon Drive (S-200) Fax: 201-358-4977
Montvale, NJ 07645
Total Employees: 50
Distribution: OEM, Manufacturer Direct, Through Distr. & Reps,
   Exclusive Distr.
Advertising: Ron Grade, Sales Dir.
   Rick Kantor, Sales Dir.
   Louise Nardone, Adv. Mgr.
CEO: Tom Huban, Human Res. Mgr.
   Patrick Carpentieri, Controller
   Anthony A. Lombardo, Gen. Mgr.
Marketing: Thomas Danisiewicz, Mktg. Mgr.
   Terry Hartl, Mktg. Mgr. Pathology Systems
   Steve Schnitter, Sales Analyst, Intl. Sales
   Mitchell Goldburgh, Tech. Mktg. Mgr.
   Loralee Morales, Mktg. Adm.
   John Kefalos, Tech. Mktg. Specialist
   Jerry Mack, Mktg. Mgr. Medical Media
   Denis O'Connor, Sales & Mktg. Dir.
Production: Erwin Ishmael, VP Engineering
Device Category:
Endoscope And Accessories, AC-Powered . . . . SURGERY

Sparco, Inc. Tel: 619-727-8309
2141-A Industrial Court Tel: 415-785-2755
Vista, CA 92083-7960 Fax: 800-783-8309
CEO: Monica Sinler, Office Mgr.
   Diane Kuhnly, VP
   Beverly Sparks, President
Production: Kelly James Griffin
Federal Procurement Eligibility: Small Business, Minority Owned,
   Woman Owned
Device Category:
Sterilizer/Washer, Endoscope . . . . GENERAL

Spiess Design, Inc.
495 Lindberg Lane
Northbrook, IL 60062-2412
Tel: 708-564-1098
Fax: 708-564-0169
CEO: Joachim Spiess
Federal Procurement Eligibility: Small Business
Device Category:
*Insufflator, Carbon-Dioxide, Automatic
    (For Endoscope)* ....GASTRO/UROLOGY
Light Source, Endoscope, Xenon Arc ....SURGERY

Stackhouse, Inc.
2059 Atlanta Ave.
Riverside, CA 92507-2439
Tel: 909-276-4600
Tel: 800-325-0082
Fax: 909-275-9518
CEO: William Arsenault, Controller
    Martin Green, President
Marketing: Linda Ciccone, Mktg. Comm. Mgr.
    David Correale, Mktg. Mgr.
Production: Roger Ignon, VP Eng.
Federal Procurement Eligibility: Small Business
Device Category:
Endoscope And Accessories, AC-Powered ....SURGERY
Tube, Smoke Removal, Endoscopic ....GASTRO/UROLOGY

Sterling Stainless Tube
1400 W. Dartmouth Ave.
Englewood, CO 80110-1385
Tel: 303-789-0528
Fax: 303-781-5901
CEO: Robert J. Fulton, Gen. Mgr.
Marketing: Danielle Percival, Sales Rep.
    Bruce Meyer, Mktg. Mgr.
Device Category:
Cannula, Suction/Irrigation, Laparoscopic ....SURGERY

Storz Endoscopy-America Inc., Karl
10111 W. Jefferson Blvd.
Culver City, CA 90232-3509
Tel: 310-558-1500
Tel: 800-421-0837
Fax: 310-280-2504
Advertising: Marcie Geco
CEO: Karl Storz, President
    Norman Silbertrust, EVP
Marketing: Don Fraley, Exec. Dir. Mktg.
    Charlie Wilhelm, Exec. Dir. Sales
Production: Marshall Pearlman, Mfg. Mgr.
Federal Procurement Eligibility: Small Business, GSA Contract, VA Contract
Device Category:
Accessories, Cleaning, Endoscopic ....GASTRO/UROLOGY
Accessories, Photographic, Endoscopic ....GASTRO/UROLOGY
Anoscope, Non-Powered ....GASTRO/UROLOGY
Arthroscope ....ORTHOPEDICS
Bronchoscope, Rigid ....EAR/NOSE/THROAT
Bronchoscope, Rigid, Ventilating ....ANESTH/PUL MED
Camera, Still, Endoscopic ....SURGERY
Camera, Television, Surgical, With Audio ....SURGERY
Camera, Video, Endoscopic ....GENERAL
Cannula, Drainage, Arthroscopy ....ORTHOPEDICS
Cannula, Suprapubic, With Trocar ....GASTRO/UROLOGY
Cart, Equipment, Video ....GENERAL
Choledochoscope, Flexible Or Rigid ....GASTRO/UROLOGY
Coagulator/Cutter, Endoscopic, Bipolar ....OBSTETRICS/GYN
Colposcope ....OBSTETRICS/GYN
Culdoscope ....OBSTETRICS/GYN
Cystoscope ....GASTRO/UROLOGY
Cystourethroscope ....GASTRO/UROLOGY
Endoscope ....GASTRO/UROLOGY
Endoscope And Accessories, Battery-Powered ....SURGERY
Endoscope, Direct Vision ....SURGERY
Endoscope, Rigid ....SURGERY
Esophagoscope (Flexible Or Rigid) ....EAR/NOSE/THROAT
Eyepiece, Lens, Non-Prescription, Endoscopic ....GASTRO/UROLOGY
Eyepiece, Lens, Prescription, Endoscopic ....GASTRO/UROLOGY
Forceps, Electrosurgical ....SURGERY
Forceps, Endoscopic ....GASTRO/UROLOGY
Forceps, Grasping, Flexible Endoscopic ....GASTRO/UROLOGY
Hysteroscope ....OBSTETRICS/GYN
Illuminator, Fiberoptic (For Endoscope) ....GASTRO/UROLOGY
*Insufflator, Carbon-Dioxide, Automatic
    (For Endoscope)* ....GASTRO/UROLOGY
Insufflator, Carbon-Dioxide, Uterotubal ....OBSTETRICS/GYN
Insufflator, Laparoscopic ....OBSTETRICS/GYN
Insufflator, Other ....SURGERY
Kit, Cholecystectomy ....MIN. INV. SURGERY
Kit, Laparoscopy ....GASTRO/UROLOGY
Lamp, Endoscopic, Incandescent ....SURGERY
Laparoscope, General & Plastic Surgery ....SURGERY
Laparoscope, Gynecologic ....OBSTETRICS/GYN
Laryngoscope ....EAR/NOSE/THROAT
Laryngoscope, Rigid ....ANESTH/PUL MED
Laryngoscope, Surgical ....SURGERY
Light Source, Endoscope, Xenon Arc ....SURGERY
Monitor, Video, Endoscope ....GENERAL
Nasopharyngoscope (Flexible Or Rigid) ....EAR/NOSE/THROAT
Needle, Endoscopic ....GASTRO/UROLOGY
Nephroscope, Rigid ....GASTRO/UROLOGY
Observerscope ....GENERAL
Obturator, Endoscopic ....GASTRO/UROLOGY
Peritoneoscope ....GASTRO/UROLOGY
Pharyngoscope ....EAR/NOSE/THROAT
Power Supply, Endoscopic, Battery Operated ....GENERAL
Proctoscope ....SURGERY
Resectoscope ....GASTRO/UROLOGY
Sheath, Endoscopic ....GASTRO/UROLOGY
Sigmoidoscope, Rigid, Non-Electrical ....GASTRO/UROLOGY
Snare, Endoscopic ....SURGERY
Teaching Attachment, Endoscopic ....GASTRO/UROLOGY
Telescope, Rigid, Endoscopic ....GASTRO/UROLOGY
Thoracoscope ....CARDIOVASCULAR
Trocar, Abdominal ....GASTRO/UROLOGY
Trocar, Amniotic ....OBSTETRICS/GYN
Trocar, Laryngeal ....EAR/NOSE/THROAT
Trocar, Sinus ....EAR/NOSE/THROAT
Trocar, Thoracic ....CARDIOVASCULAR
Ureteroscope ....GASTRO/UROLOGY
Urethroscope ....GASTRO/UROLOGY
Vaginoscope ....OBSTETRICS/GYN

Storz GmbH & Co., Karl Tel: 07461/7080
Mittelstr. 8 Fax: 07461/708105
Postfach 230
D-78532 Tuttlingen
Germany
CEO: O. Schreiber
Device Category:
Accessories, Cleaning, Endoscopic .... GASTRO/UROLOGY
Accessories, Photographic, Endoscopic .... GASTRO/UROLOGY
Amnioscope, Transabdominal (Fetoscope) .... OBSTETRICS/GYN
Anoscope, Non-Powered .... GASTRO/UROLOGY
Arthroscope .... ORTHOPEDICS
Bronchoscope, Rigid .... EAR/NOSE/THROAT
Bronchoscope, Rigid, Ventilating .... ANESTH/PUL MED
Camera, Still, Endoscopic .... SURGERY
Camera, Television, Surgical, With Audio .... SURGERY
Cannula, Drainage, Arthroscopy .... ORTHOPEDICS
Cannula, Suprapubic, With Trocar .... GASTRO/UROLOGY
Choledochoscope, Flexible Or Rigid .... GASTRO/UROLOGY
Coagulator/Cutter, Endoscopic, Bipolar .... OBSTETRICS/GYN
Colposcope .... OBSTETRICS/GYN
Culdoscope .... OBSTETRICS/GYN
Cystoscope .... GASTRO/UROLOGY
Cystourethroscope .... GASTRO/UROLOGY
Endoscope And Accessories, Battery-Powered .... SURGERY
Endoscope, Direct Vision .... SURGERY
Endoscope, Rigid .... SURGERY
Endoscope, Transcervical (Amnioscope) .... OBSTETRICS/GYN
Esophagoscope (Flexible Or Rigid) .... EAR/NOSE/THROAT
Eyepiece, Lens, Non-Prescription, Endoscopic .... GASTRO/UROLOGY
Eyepiece, Lens, Prescription, Endoscopic .... GASTRO/UROLOGY
Forceps, Electrosurgical .... SURGERY
Forceps, Endoscopic .... GASTRO/UROLOGY
Forceps, Grasping, Flexible Endoscopic .... GASTRO/UROLOGY
Hysteroscope .... OBSTETRICS/GYN
Illuminator, Fiberoptic (For Endoscope) .... GASTRO/UROLOGY
Insufflator, Carbon-Dioxide, Automatic
  (For Endoscope) .... GASTRO/UROLOGY
Insufflator, Carbon-Dioxide, Uterotubal .... OBSTETRICS/GYN
Insufflator, Laparoscopic .... OBSTETRICS/GYN
Insufflator, Other .... SURGERY
Lamp, Endoscopic, Incandescent .... SURGERY
Laparoscope, General & Plastic Surgery .... SURGERY
Laparoscope, Gynecologic .... OBSTETRICS/GYN
Laryngoscope .... EAR/NOSE/THROAT
Laryngoscope, Rigid .... ANESTH/PUL MED
Laryngoscope, Surgical .... SURGERY
Light Source, Endoscope, Xenon Arc .... SURGERY
Monitor, Video, Endoscope .... GENERAL
Nasopharyngoscope (Flexible Or Rigid) .... EAR/NOSE/THROAT
Needle, Endoscopic .... GASTRO/UROLOGY
Nephroscope, Rigid .... GASTRO/UROLOGY
Observerscope .... GENERAL
Obturator, Endoscopic .... GASTRO/UROLOGY
Peritoneoscope .... GASTRO/UROLOGY
Pharyngoscope .... EAR/NOSE/THROAT
Power Supply, Endoscopic, Battery Operated .... GENERAL
Proctoscope .... SURGERY
Resectoscope .... GASTRO/UROLOGY
Sheath, Endoscopic .... GASTRO/UROLOGY
Sigmoidoscope, Rigid, Non-Electrical .... GASTRO/UROLOGY
Snare, Endoscopic .... SURGERY
Teaching Attachment, Endoscopic .... GASTRO/UROLOGY

Telescope, Rigid, Endoscopic .... GASTRO/UROLOGY
Thoracoscope .... CARDIOVASCULAR
Trocar, Abdominal .... GASTRO/UROLOGY
Trocar, Amniotic .... OBSTETRICS/GYN
Trocar, Laryngeal .... EAR/NOSE/THROAT
Trocar, Sinus .... EAR/NOSE/THROAT
Trocar, Thoracic .... CARDIOVASCULAR
Ureteroscope .... GASTRO/UROLOGY
Urethroscope .... GASTRO/UROLOGY
Vaginoscope .... OBSTETRICS/GYN

Storz Instrument Company Tel: 314-225-5051
3365 Tree Ct. Indust. Blvd. Tel: 800-325-9500
St. Louis, MO 63122-6615 Fax: 314-225-7365
CEO: Robert Blankemeyer, COO
  J. Donald Gaines, President
Marketing: Sam Alioto, VP Ophthalmics
  Dave Dallam, Mktg. Dir.
  Bill DeGrooat, VP Intl.
Production: Mike Nicoletta, VP Mfg.
Federal Procurement Eligibility: Small Business, GSA Contract
Device Category:
Trocar, Laryngeal .... EAR/NOSE/THROAT

Stryker B.V. Tel: 4132-61555
Industrielaan 1 - Postbox 118 Fax: 4132-61285
NL-5400 AC Uden
Netherlands
CEO: Hans Verleun
Marketing: Frank Wydeveld
Production: Frank Koopmans, Reg. Affairs Mgr.
Device Category:
Arthroscope .... ORTHOPEDICS

Stryker Corp., Surgical Div. Tel: 616-323-7700
4100 E. Milham Ave. Tel: 800-253-3210
Kalamazoo, MI 49003-6197 Fax: 616-323-2402
CEO: Si Johnson, VP & General Mgr.
  Ron Elenbaas, Group President
  John Brown, COB & President
Production: Pedro Martinez, Operations Dir.
Device Category:
Arthroscope .... ORTHOPEDICS
Monitor, Video, Endoscope .... GENERAL

Stryker Endoscopy Tel: 408-435-0220
210 Baypointe Pkwy. Tel: 800-624-4422
San Jose, CA 95134 Fax: 800-729-2917
Marketing: Paul Patriarco, Mktg. Mgr.
Device Category:
Camera, Television, Surgical, With Audio .... SURGERY
Camera, Videotape, Surgical .... SURGERY
Monitor, Video, Endoscope .... GENERAL
Tape, Television & Video, Endoscopic .... GASTRO/UROLOGY

Stryker Pacific
Tel: 852/5/538165

53 Wong Chuk Hang Rd
Sungib Ind Ctr. 7th
Aberdeen
Hong Kong
CEO: William Laube, President
Marketing: Edward Lee, Mktg. Dir.
Device Category:
Arthroscope .... ORTHOPEDICS

Stuemer GmbH & Co.
Tel: 0931/885350

Sieboldstrasse 2
D-97072 Wuerzburg 1
Germany
CEO: Herbert Bomba
    Charles Schraut
Device Category:
Laryngoscope .... EAR/NOSE/THROAT

Sun-Med, Inc.
Tel: 813-530-7099
Tel: 800-433-2797
Fax: 813-531-3991

5401 Tech Data Dr.
Clearwater, FL 34620-3106
Advertising: Ruth Alves, Adv. Dir.
CEO: John King, Gen. Mgr.
    George Cranton, President
Marketing: Gwen Matlock
    Barry L. Wall, Sales Mgr.
Production: Chuck Harstad, Purch.
Federal Procurement Eligibility: Small Business
Device Category:
Laryngoscope .... EAR/NOSE/THROAT
Laryngoscope, Rigid .... ANESTH/PUL MED

Surgical Instrument Co. Of America
Tel: 201-941-6500
Fax: 201-941-6656

1185 Edgewater Ave.
Ridgefield, NJ 07657-2102
CEO: Alfred G. Biberfeld, President
Marketing: Debra Dilkes, Contract Sales Mgr.
Production: Michael Rehak, Gen. Mgr.
Federal Procurement Eligibility: Small Business, GSA Contract
Device Category:
Anoscope, Non-Powered .... GASTRO/UROLOGY
Arthroscope .... ORTHOPEDICS
Bronchoscope, Rigid .... EAR/NOSE/THROAT
Clip, Suture .... SURGERY
Culdoscope .... OBSTETRICS/GYN
Forceps, Electrosurgical .... SURGERY
Forceps, Endoscopic .... GASTRO/UROLOGY
Laryngoscope, Flexible .... ANESTH/PUL MED
Laryngoscope, Rigid .... ANESTH/PUL MED
Proctoscope .... SURGERY
Proctosigmoidoscope .... GASTRO/UROLOGY
Remover, Clip .... SURGERY
Sigmoidoscope, Rigid, Non-Electrical .... GASTRO/UROLOGY
Trocar, Abdominal .... GASTRO/UROLOGY
Trocar, Amniotic .... OBSTETRICS/GYN
Trocar, Cardiovascular .... CARDIOVASCULAR
Trocar, Gallbladder .... GASTRO/UROLOGY
Trocar, Laryngeal .... EAR/NOSE/THROAT
Trocar, Thoracic .... CARDIOVASCULAR
Trocar, Tracheal .... EAR/NOSE/THROAT

Surgical Instrument Manufacturers, Inc.
Tel: 314-349-4960
Fax: 314-326-2417

1549 Fenpark Dr.
Fenton, MO 63026-2915
Total Employees: 18
Distribution: Manufacturer Through Distributors
CEO: Kurt Hensler, President
Device Category:
Coagulator/Cutter, Endoscopic, Bipolar .... OBSTETRICS/GYN

Surgical Service Of London, The
Tel: 0322/79772
Fax: 0322/91831

Darenth Mill, Darenth Road
Dartford, Kent
United Kingdom
CEO: Brian W. Mitchinson, Managing Dir.
Marketing: Michael White
Federal Procurement Eligibility: Small Business
Device Category:
Laryngoscope .... EAR/NOSE/THROAT

Surgico Ltd., A.D.
Tel: 0432/88143

P.O. Box 270
Sialkot 1
Pakistan
CEO: Rashid Ahmed Malik
Marketing: Ehsan Malik
Production: Inam Elahi Malik
Device Category:
Trocar, Thoracic .... CARDIOVASCULAR
Trocar, Tracheal .... EAR/NOSE/THROAT

Surgilase, Inc.
Tel: 401-732-6440
Tel: 800-537-5273
Fax: 401-732-6445

33 Plan Way
Warwick, RI 02886
CEO: Larry Levy, President
Marketing: Joseph Jay Houser, Mktg. & Sales Dir.
    John Ziegler, Mktg. & Sales VP
Production: Phil Prive, Production Mgr.
    Cliff Morrow, VP Technology
Research: Clifford Morrow, Technology VP
Federal Procurement Eligibility: Small Business
Device Category:
Equipment/Accessories, Laser, Laparoscopy .... MIN. INV. SURGERY
Laser, Nd:YAG, Laparoscopy .... MIN. INV. SURGERY

Surgimedics/SLP
Tel: 713-363-4949
Tel: 800-669-9001
Fax: 713-292-1269

2828 N. Crescent Ridge Dr.
The Woodlands, TX 77381
CEO: Thomas Early
Marketing: Donald F. Hijlts, VP Sales & Mktg.
Production: David Huff
Research: John Bruce, VP R&D
    Bryan Lynch, VP R&D
Device Category:
Catheter, Cholangiography .... SURGERY
Mirror, Endoscopic .... SURGERY

Surgin, Inc. Tel: 714-832-6300
14762 Bentley Circle Fax: 714-993-2372
Tustin, CA 92680
CEO: Ted Wortrich, VP
 Armand Maaskamp, President
Production: Sonia Gaeta
Federal Procurement Eligibility: GSA Contract
Device Category:
Cannula, Suction, Pool-Tip .... MIN. INV. SURGERY
Equipment, Suction/Irrigation, Laparoscopic .... SURGERY
Needle, Aspiration, Cyst, Laparoscopic .... MIN. INV. SURGERY
Probe, Suction, Irrigator/Aspirator, Laparoscopic .... MIN. INV. SURGERY

Surgitek Tel: 414-639-7205
3037 Mt. Pleasant St. Tel: 800-558-9494
Racine, WI 53404-1509 Fax: 414-681-4044
Advertising: Marilyn Lemsky, Mktg. Comm. Mgr.
Marketing: Nancy Caffiero, VP Sales & Mktg.
 Dick Zimmerman, VP Sales & Mktg., Plastic Surgery Div.
Production: Steve Aperavich, VP Mfg.
 Garry Carter, Gen. Mgr.
Research: Keith Hofmann, VP Human Resources
Federal Procurement Eligibility: GSA Contract
Device Category:
Cystoscope .... GASTRO/UROLOGY
Endoscope, Flexible .... GASTRO/UROLOGY
Forceps, Grasping, Flexible Endoscopic .... GASTRO/UROLOGY
Nephroscope, Flexible .... GASTRO/UROLOGY
Ureteroscope .... GASTRO/UROLOGY

Swemed Lab International AB
P.O. Box 4014
S-421 04 V. Frolunda
Sweden
CEO: Lars-Goran Itskowitz
Device Category:
Trocar, Amniotic .... OBSTETRICS/GYN

Synectic Engineering, Inc. Tel: 203-877-8488
4 Oxford Rd. Fax: 203-874-4290
Milford, CT 06460-7007
CEO: Jeffrey Slein, President
Marketing: Betsy Zeller, Mktg. Mgr.
Federal Procurement Eligibility: Small Business
Device Category:
Applier, Clip, Laparoscopic .... MIN. INV. SURGERY
Applier, Clip, Repair, Hernia, Laparoscopic .... MIN. INV. SURGERY
Bag, Specimen, Laparoscopic .... MIN. INV. SURGERY
Cannula, Suprapubic, With Trocar .... GASTRO/UROLOGY
Coagulator, Hysteroscopic (With Accessories) .... OBSTETRICS/GYN
Coagulator, Laparoscopic, Unipolar .... OBSTETRICS/GYN
Coagulator/Cutter, Endoscopic, Bipolar .... OBSTETRICS/GYN
Coagulator/Cutter, Endoscopic, Unipolar .... OBSTETRICS/GYN
Endoscope .... GASTRO/UROLOGY
Equipment, Suction/Irrigation, Laparoscopic .... SURGERY
Forceps, Endoscopic .... GASTRO/UROLOGY
Forceps, Grasping, Atraumatic .... MIN. INV. SURGERY
Forceps, Grasping, Flexible Endoscopic .... GASTRO/UROLOGY
Forceps, Grasping, Traumatic .... MIN. INV. SURGERY
Holder, Needle, Laparoscopic .... MIN. INV. SURGERY
Holder/Scissors, Needle, Laparoscopic .... MIN. INV. SURGERY
Instrument, Dissecting, Laparoscopic .... MIN. INV. SURGERY
Instrument, Needle Holder/Knot Tying .... MIN. INV. SURGERY
Insufflator, Laparoscopic .... OBSTETRICS/GYN
Needle, Insufflation, Laparoscopic .... MIN. INV. SURGERY
Probe, Electrocauterization, Multi-Use .... MIN. INV. SURGERY
Probe, Electrocauterization, Single-Use .... MIN. INV. SURGERY
Probe, Suction, Irrigator/Aspirator, Laparoscopic .... MIN. INV. SURGERY
Scissors with Removable Tips, Laparoscopy .... MIN. INV. SURGERY
Stapler, Surgical .... SURGERY
Trocar, Abdominal .... GASTRO/UROLOGY
Trocar, Gastro-Urology .... GASTRO/UROLOGY

Taut, Inc. Tel: 708-232-2507
2571 Kaneville Ct. Tel: 800-231-8288
Geneva, IL 60134-2505 Fax: 708-232-8005
CEO: R. H. McFarlane, President
 G. G. McFarlane, EVP
Marketing: R.N. Brizuela, Int'l Sales and Mktg. Mgr.
 M.S. Mc Farlane, Mktg. Mgr.
 G. G. McFarlane, EVP
Production: R. D. Kenseth, VP Oper.
Federal Procurement Eligibility: Small Business
Device Category:
Catheter, Cholangiography .... SURGERY

Technalytics, Inc. Tel: 201-391-0494
210 Summit Ave. Fax: 201-930-1495
Montvale, NJ 07645-1526
CEO: Myron Blatt, CFO
 Ingram Chodorow, President
Federal Procurement Eligibility: Small Business
Device Category:
Stapler, Surgical .... SURGERY
Trocar, Abdominal .... GASTRO/UROLOGY
Trocar, Other .... GENERAL

Technical Enterprises Tel: 904-495-9961
10023 S.W. 77th Court
Gainesville, FL 32608
CEO: Andris Taube
Federal Procurement Eligibility: Small Business
Device Category:
Colposcope .... OBSTETRICS/GYN

Tecnol, Inc. Tel: 817-581-6424
7201 Industrial Park Blvd. Tel: 800-832-6651
Fort Worth, TX 76180-6153 Fax: 817-284-0731
Advertising: Delania Truly, VP Corp. Comms.
CEO: Van Hubbard, President & CEO
 Valerie Hubbard, President Hosp. Prod. Div.
 Tom Sweatt, Dir. Natl. Accts.
 Leona Hammel, VP RA/QA
 David Radunsky, COO
Marketing: Tom Sweatt, Sales Training Mgr.
 Steve Langrein, Natl Sales Mgr.
 James Weaver, VP Business Dev.
 Craig D. Giovanni, Intl. Sales & Mktg. Mgr.
 Adrienne Stokes, Mktg. Dir.
Production: Paul Brost, President, Orthopedic Div.
 Kirk Brunson, EVP Eng.
 Jim Petty, VP Mfg.
 Derek Baird, Plant Mgr.
 Dan Reese, VP Engineering
 Bruce Korr, Materials Mgr.
Research: Kevin Brunson, VP Prod. Dev.
Federal Procurement Eligibility: Small Business, GSA Contract
Device Category:
Holder, Leg, Arthroscopy .... ORTHOPEDICS

Tekno-Medical Optik Chirur. GmbH & Co. KG
Tel: 07461/6067
Fax: 07461/78838

Sattlerstr. 11
D-78532 Tuttlingen 16
Germany
Medical Products Sales Volume: $5,000,000
Total Employees: 54 (E)
Distribution: OEM
CEO: Bruno Mattes, President
Marketing: Rainer Zubrod
Device Category:
Laryngoscope .... EAR/NOSE/THROAT
Laryngoscope, Rigid .... ANESTH/PUL MED
Laryngoscope, Surgical .... SURGERY

Thermotec, Inc.
Tel: 203-579-4300
Fax: 203-576-0409

575 Broad St.
Bridgeport, CT 06604-5122
CEO: Enzo Del Brocco, President
Device Category:
Colonoscope, Gastro-Urology .... GASTRO/UROLOGY
Colonoscope, General & Plastic Surgery .... SURGERY

Thompson Surgical Instruments, Inc.
Tel: 616-922-0177
Tel: 800-227-7543
Fax: 616-922-0174

10170 E. Cherry Bend Rd.
P.O. Box 1051
Traverse City, MI 49685
CEO: Daniel K. Farley, President
Federal Procurement Eligibility: Small Business
Device Category:
Camera, Video, Endoscopic .... GENERAL
Holder, Instrument, Laparoscopic .... MIN. INV. SURGERY
Holder, Laparoscope .... OBSTETRICS/GYN

Tiemann & Co., George
Tel: 516-273-0005
Tel: 800-843-6266
Fax: 516-273-6199

25 Plant Ave.
Hauppauge, NY 11788-3804
CEO: Richard Moriarty, President
Marketing: Kenneth Moriarty, VP
Federal Procurement Eligibility: Small Business
Device Category:
Electrocautery Unit, Endoscopic .... OBSTETRICS/GYN

Timesco of London
Tel: 071/278-0712-3
Fax: 071/278-0707

176 Pentonville Rd.
London N1 9JP
United Kingdom
CEO: S. Bhatti
  M. F. Bhatti
Marketing: S. J. Fayyaz
Federal Procurement Eligibility: Small Business
Device Category:
Laryngoscope .... EAR/NOSE/THROAT
Sigmoidoscope, Flexible .... GASTRO/UROLOGY

Tnco, Inc.
Tel: 617-447-6661
Fax: 617-447-2132

P.O. Box 231
Whitman, MA 02382-0231
CEO: Roger M. Burke, President
Production: G. P. Honkanen, R&D
  F. M. Reilly, Mfg. Mgr.
Federal Procurement Eligibility: Small Business
Device Category:
Accessories, Arthroscope .... ORTHOPEDICS

Toolmex Corporation
Tel: 508-653-8897
Tel: 800-992-4766
Fax: 508-653-5110

1075 Worchester Rd.
Natick, MA 01760-1510
CEO: Jan Dul, President
Marketing: Voytek Kucharski, VP Mktg.
  Andy Fijalkowski, Sales Mgr.
Device Category:
Kit, Laparoscopy .... GASTRO/UROLOGY

Toshiba Medical Systems Europe B.V.
Tel: 015/610121
Fax: 015/621338

Schieweg 1
NL-2627 An Delft, AN
Netherlands
Marketing: A.M. Ruis, Sr. Mktg. Mgr.
Device Category:
Tape, Television & Video, Endoscopic .... GASTRO/UROLOGY

Transamerican Technologies International
Tel: 510-484-0700
Tel: 800-322-7373 CA
Fax: 510-484-0826

7026 Koll Center Pkwy., Ste. 207
Pleasanton, CA 94566-3108
Medical Products Sales Volume: $4,000,000
Total Employees: 10
Distribution: OEM, Manufacturer through Distributor & Reps
CEO: Gregory Sutyak, Financial Officer
  Donna Hill Howes, VP
  Allen R. Howes, President
Marketing: Lowell Crow, VP Mktg. & Sales
Production: John E. Patton, Eng.
Federal Procurement Eligibility: Small Business
Device Category:
Accessories, Photographic, Endoscopic .... GASTRO/UROLOGY
Camera, Television, Microsurgical, Without Audio .... SURGERY
Camera, Video, Endoscopic .... GENERAL
Cannula, Suction, Pool-Tip .... MIN. INV. SURGERY
Coagulator, Laparoscopic, Unipolar .... OBSTETRICS/GYN
Coagulator/Cutter, Endoscopic, Unipolar .... OBSTETRICS/GYN
Electrode, Electrosurgery, Laparoscopic .... MIN. INV. SURGERY
Kit, Cholecystectomy .... MIN. INV. SURGERY
Light Source, Endoscope, Xenon Arc .... SURGERY
Probe, Electrocauterization, Multi-Use .... MIN. INV. SURGERY

Tri-Med Specialties, Inc.
Tel: 913-888-4440
Tel: 800-874-6331
Fax: 913-642-7418

P.O. Box 23306
Overland Park, KS 66223
CEO: Bill Fry
Marketing: Larry Scott, Mktg. Dir.
Federal Procurement Eligibility: Small Business
Device Category:
Endoscope .... GASTRO/UROLOGY

Truphatek International Ltd.
Tel: 09-851155
Fax: 09-851212

Park Poleg, Industrial Area
P.O. Box 8051
Netanya
Israel
CEO: David Grey
Marketing: Melissa Marks
Production: Avi Bhonkar
Research: Aaron Schulman, R&D VP
Device Category:
Laryngoscope .... EAR/NOSE/THROAT
Laryngoscope, Rigid .... ANESTH/PUL MED

U.S. Endoscopy Group
Tel: 216-269-8226
Tel: 800-269-8226
Fax: 216-269-8626

7123 Industrial Park Blvd.
Mentor, OH 44060
CEO: Rhonda Mansal, Personnel Dir.
    Marlin Younkers, President
Marketing: Mark Kozak, Sales Dir.
    Lynn Roman, VP Sales & Mktg.
    Cynthia Kraft, Nat'l. Sales Mgr.
Production: Jon Younker, Materials Mgr.
    Gretchen Younkers, Reg. Affairs Mgr.
Research: Dean Secrest, VP R&D
Federal Procurement Eligibility: Small Business, Woman Owned
Device Category:
Bag, Specimen, Laparoscopic .... MIN. INV. SURGERY
Brush, Cytology, Endoscopic .... GASTRO/UROLOGY
Catheter, Cholangiography .... SURGERY
Electrode, Electrosurgery, Laparoscopic .... MIN. INV. SURGERY
Forceps, Biopsy .... MIN. INV. SURGERY
Kit, Cholecystectomy .... MIN. INV. SURGERY
Needle, Endoscopic .... GASTRO/UROLOGY
Peritoneoscope .... GASTRO/UROLOGY
Snare, Endoscopic .... SURGERY

Ultracision Inc.
Tel: 401-232-7660
Tel: 800-333-9181
Fax: 401-232-7664

25 Thurber Blvd., Unit 3
Smithfield, RI 02917
Advertising: John Reid, VP Sales
CEO: Thomas W. Davison, President
    Catherine L. Conaty, Controller
Marketing: Bernard F. Galat, VP Mktg.
Production: Steve Galiker, VP & CFO
Device Category:
Scalpel, Ultrasonic .... SURGERY

UMC Incorporated
Tel: 612-478-6609
Fax: 612-478-6483

22510 Highway 55 West
Hamel, MN 55340
CEO: Terry Tomann
Federal Procurement Eligibility: Small Business
Device Category:
Endoscope .... GASTRO/UROLOGY
Obturator, Endoscopic .... GASTRO/UROLOGY

Uniflex Inc.
Medical Packaging Div.
Tel: 516-932-2000
Tel: 800-223-0564
Fax: 516-932-3129

383 W. John St.
P.O. Box 96
Hicksville, NY 11802
Ownership: Public
Distribution: Manufacturer Through Distributor
CEO: B. H. Barry, President
Marketing: J. Brink, Product Mgr.
    H. Brownstein, Mktg. Dir.
Production: H. Samuels, VP Mfg.
Federal Procurement Eligibility: GSA Contract, VA Contract
Device Category:
Bag, Specimen, Laparoscopic .... MIN. INV. SURGERY

Unimar, Inc.
Tel: 203-762-9550
Tel: 800-243-6608
Fax: 203-834-1123

475 Danbury Rd.
Wilton, CT 06897-2126
Advertising: Clarice DeRubeis, Nat'l. Sales Mgr.
CEO: James Boylan, Controller
    Anthony W. Hemming, President & CEO
Production: Phillip G. Moore, Oper. Mgr.
    Edward C. Vollmer, VP
Federal Procurement Eligibility: Small Business
Device Category:
Insufflator, Carbon-Dioxide, Uterotubal .... OBSTETRICS/GYN
Insufflator, Hysteroscopic .... OBSTETRICS/GYN

Unisurge, Inc.
Tel: 408-996-4700
Tel: 800-327-9555
Fax: 408-996-4774

10231 Bubb Rd.
Cupertino, CA 95014
CEO: Robert Berkowitz, President
    Linda O'Keefe, CFO
Marketing: Kent Richards, VP Mktg.
Device Category:
Equipment, Suction/Irrigation, Laparoscopic .... SURGERY
Forceps, Endoscopic .... GASTRO/UROLOGY
Forceps, Grasping, Atraumatic .... MIN. INV. SURGERY
Instrument, Dissecting, Laparoscopic .... MIN. INV. SURGERY
Kit, Cholecystectomy .... MIN. INV. SURGERY
Kit, Laparoscopy .... GASTRO/UROLOGY
Kit, Trocar .... MIN. INV. SURGERY
Peritoneoscope .... GASTRO/UROLOGY
Probe, Electrocauterization, Multi-Use .... MIN. INV. SURGERY
Probe, Suction, Irrigator/Aspirator, Laparoscopic .... MIN. INV. SURGERY
Scissors, Laparoscopy .... MIN. INV. SURGERY
Trocar, Abdominal .... GASTRO/UROLOGY
Trocar, Gastro-Urology .... GASTRO/UROLOGY

United Instrument Corp.
Tel: 215-635-4000
Tel: 800-426-5127
Fax: 215-635-4002
P.O. Box 20924
Philadelphia, PA 19141-0924
Advertising: Lee Borden, Advertising Mgr.
CEO: Lewis B. Udis
   Harry Barone, Controller
Marketing: Thomas Seward, Dir. Mktg. Mexico & South America
   Sam Wilson
   John Scott, Dir. Intl Mktg.
   James Wright, Distr. Sales
   Donald Weaver, V.P. Marketing
Production: Jack Pierce, Prod. Eng. & QC
   Dolores Hoff
   Bill Parker, Dir. Purchasing
Federal Procurement Eligibility: Small Business
Device Category:
Forceps, Grasping, Flexible Endoscopic................GASTRO/UROLOGY

United States Surgical Corp.
Tel: 203-845-1000
Fax: 203-847-0635
150 Glover Ave.
Norwalk, CT 06856-5080
CEO: Leon C. Hirsch, President
   Bruce S. Lustman, EVP & COO
Marketing: Turi Josefsen, EVP
   Robert A. Knarr, SVP
Research: David A. Saffir, Senior Dir.
Federal Procurement Eligibility: GSA Contract, VA Contract
Device Category:
Applier, Clip, Laparoscopic .... MIN. INV. SURGERY
Applier, Clip, Repair, Hernia, Laparoscopic........... MIN. INV. SURGERY
Bag, Specimen, Laparoscopic .... MIN. INV. SURGERY
Cannula with Inflatable Balloon (Distal Tip) .... MIN. INV. SURGERY
Cannula, Suprapubic, With Trocar .... GASTRO/UROLOGY
Equipment, Suction/Irrigation, Laparoscopic.....................SURGERY
Forceps, Endoscopic.. GASTRO/UROLOGY
Forceps, Grasping, Atraumatic........................... MIN. INV. SURGERY
Forceps, Grasping, Flexible Endoscopic............... GASTRO/UROLOGY
Forceps, Grasping, Traumatic............................ MIN. INV. SURGERY
Gauge, Thickness, Tissue .... MIN. INV. SURGERY
Instrument, Dissecting, Laparoscopic.................. MIN. INV. SURGERY
Kit, Laparoscopy .... GASTRO/UROLOGY
Needle, Endoscopic .... GASTRO/UROLOGY
Needle, Insufflation, Laparoscopic...................... MIN. INV. SURGERY
Obturator, Endoscopic .... GASTRO/UROLOGY
Peritoneoscope... GASTRO/UROLOGY
Retractor, Fan-Type, Laparoscopy .... MIN. INV. SURGERY
Retractor, Laparoscopy, Other .... MIN. INV. SURGERY
Stapler, Laparoscopic....................................... MIN. INV. SURGERY
Stapler, Surgical..SURGERY
Suture, Laparoscopy .... MIN. INV. SURGERY
Trainer, Laparoscopy.. MIN. INV. SURGERY
Trocar, Abdominal .... GASTRO/UROLOGY
Trocar, Gallbladder .... GASTRO/UROLOGY
Trocar, Laparoscopic ....SURGERY
Trocar, Other..GENERAL
Trocar, Short .... MIN. INV. SURGERY
Trocar, Thoracic .... CARDIOVASCULAR

Upsher Laryngoscope Co.
Tel: 415-341-2614
Fax: 415-341-1368
P.O. Box 4519
Foster City, CA 94404-4519
CEO: Michael Upsher
Production: Giles Wilson, Opers. Mgr.
Device Category:
Laryngoscope, Rigid... ANESTH/PUL MED

Uresil Corporation
Tel: 708-982-0200
Fax: 708-982-0106
5418 W. Touhy Ave.
Skokie, IL 60077-3232
CEO: Mark Filler, COO
   Bill Carpenter, CFO
Marketing: Barry Goldenberg, Mktg. Dir.
Production: Lev Melinyshyn, Operations Dir.
Federal Procurement Eligibility: Small Business
Device Category:
Catheter, Cholangiography ....SURGERY
Endoscope .... GASTRO/UROLOGY

Valley Forge Scientific, Inc.
Tel: 215-666-7500
Fax: 215-666-7565
P.O. Box 925
Valley Forge, PA 19482-0925
CEO: Thomas J. Gilloway, EVP
   Jerry L. Malis, President
Production: Robert Conrad, Production Mgr.
   Martin T. Mortimer, Eng. Mgr.
Federal Procurement Eligibility: Small Business
Device Category:
Generator, Power, Electrosurgical.................................SURGERY
Laparoscope, Gynecologic .... OBSTETRICS/GYN

Valleylab, Inc.
Tel: 303-530-2300
Tel: 800-255-8522
Fax: 303-530-6285
5920 Longbow Dr.
Boulder, CO 80301-3202
CEO: William D. Reichenberg, President & CEO
Marketing: William O'Connor, VP Sales & Mktg.
   William Hunter, Mktg. Dir.
   Mike Moore, Mktg. Dir. Adv. Poly. Tech.
   Karen Muhler, Mktg. Svcs. Mgr.
Production: John V. Scibelli, VP Oper.
   James Busse, VP RA & QA
Research: Clark Graham, VP Res. & Prod. Dev.
Federal Procurement Eligibility: GSA Contract
Device Category:
Coagulator, Laparoscopic, Unipolar .... OBSTETRICS/GYN
Coagulator/Cutter, Endoscopic, Unipolar .... OBSTETRICS/GYN
Cutter, Linear, Laparoscopic............................. MIN. INV. SURGERY
Electrocautery Unit, Endoscopic .... OBSTETRICS/GYN
Electrode, Electrosurgery, Laparoscopic .... MIN. INV. SURGERY
Equipment, Suction/Irrigation, Laparoscopic....................SURGERY
Forceps, Electrosurgical ....SURGERY
Generator, Power, Electrosurgical.................................SURGERY
Peritoneoscope... GASTRO/UROLOGY
Probe, Electrocauterization, Multi-Use .... MIN. INV. SURGERY
Probe, Electrocauterization, Single-Use .... MIN. INV. SURGERY
Probe, Suction, Irrigator/Aspirator, Laparoscopic .... MIN. INV. SURGERY

Veriflo Corporation
250 Canal Blvd.
P.O. Box 4034
Richmond, CA 94804-0034
Tel: 510-235-9590
Tel: 800-962-4074
Fax: 510-232-7396
CEO: Tom Bates, CEO
Marketing: Teresa Raymond, Nat'l Sales Mgr.
  Robin Luebker, Med. Sales Specialist
Production: Todd Steuteville, VP Mfg.
  Ken Seeber
Federal Procurement Eligibility: Small Business
Device Category:
Insufflator, Other .... SURGERY

Vermont Medical, Inc.
Industrial Park
P.O. Box 556
Bellows Falls, VT 05101-0556
Tel: 802-463-9976
Tel: 800-245-4025
Fax: 802-463-9228
CEO: Hurley J. Blakeney, President
Marketing: Patricia Trudo, Customer Service Mgr.
  Pam Sopczyk, Regulatory Affairs Mgr.
  Ed Herron, Dir. Mktg.
Production: Henry Gauthier, Plant Superintendent
  Bob Scoefman, Mats. Mgr.
Federal Procurement Eligibility: Small Business, VA Contract
Device Category:
Endoscope .... GASTRO/UROLOGY
Endoscope And Accessories, AC-Powered .... SURGERY

Vicom Systems
46107 Landing Parkway
Fremont, CA 94538-6407
Tel: 415-498-3200
Fax: 510-498-3225
Advertising: Sandy Staufenbiel, Mktg. Comm. Mgr.
CEO: Ron Cornell, CEO & President
  Nate Cammack, CFO & VP Finance
Marketing: Sandy Staufenbiel, Mktg. Comm. Mgr.
  Michael Piltoff, VP Domestic & Int'l Sales
  Frances Mann-Craik, Mktg. Programs Dir.
  Arun Taneja, VP Mktg.
Production: Samuel Tam, VP Eng.
  Joseph Marcianno, Field Support Dir.
  Doug Hagameier, Mfg. Dir.
Device Category:
Computer, Image, Endoscopic .... GENERAL

Visioneering, Inc.
3178 Pullman St.
Costa Mesa, CA 92626-3319
Tel: 714-549-2557
Fax: 714-549-4847
CEO: Anthony A. Nobles, Owner
Device Category:
Insufflator, Other .... SURGERY

Vital Signs, Inc.
20 Campus Rd.
Totowa, NJ 07512-1200
Tel: 201-790-1330
Tel: 800-932-0760
Fax: 201-790-3307
CEO: Terence D. Wall, President
  Barry Wicker, EVP

Marketing: Stuart Richter, VP sales & Mktg.
  Ronald Baum, Sales Dir.
  Paul Bennett, Int'l Sales & Mktg. Mgr.
  Kevin Schneider, Nat'l Sales Mgr.
  John Brown, Mktg. Dir.
  Gene Gadberry, Dir. Nat'l Accts.
  Alan Furler, Mktg. Dir.
Federal Procurement Eligibility: GSA Contract, VA Contract
Device Category:
Laryngoscope .... EAR/NOSE/THROAT
Laryngoscope, Rigid .... ANESTH/PUL MED

W.J. Medical Instruments, Inc.
3537 Old Conejo Rd.
Newbury Park, CA 91320
Tel: 805-499-8676
Tel: 800-832-8448
Fax: 805-499-9404
CEO: William Zinnanti, President
Marketing: William Zinnanti, Mkt. Res. Mgr.
  Jerry Case, Dir. Natl. Accounts
Federal Procurement Eligibility: Small Business
Device Category:
Accessories, Arthroscope .... ORTHOPEDICS
Cover, Laparoscope .... MIN. INV. SURGERY
Equipment, Suction/Irrigation, Laparoscopic .... SURGERY
Holder, Laparoscope .... OBSTETRICS/GYN
Holder, Needle, Laparoscopic .... MIN. INV. SURGERY
Instrument, Needle Holder/Knot Tying .... MIN. INV. SURGERY
Insufflator, Laparoscopic .... OBSTETRICS/GYN
Laparoscope, Gynecologic .... OBSTETRICS/GYN
Probe, Electrocauterization, Multi-Use .... MIN. INV. SURGERY
Probe, Electrocauterization, Single-Use .... MIN. INV. SURGERY

Wallach Surgical Devices, Inc.
P.O. Box 3287
291 Pepe's Farm Road
Milford, CT 06460-3671
Tel: 203-783-1818
Tel: 800-243-2463
Fax: 203-783-1825
CEO: Ronald Wallach, President
Marketing: Richard Bodnar, VP Sales
Production: Linda Cella, Prod. Mgr.
Federal Procurement Eligibility: Small Business, VA Contract
Device Category:
Colposcope .... OBSTETRICS/GYN

Waterloo Industries, Inc.
300 Ansborough Ave.
P.O. Box 2095
Waterloo, IA 50704-2095
Tel: 319-235-7131
Tel: 800-833-4419
Fax: 319-235-6849
CEO: William A. Happ
  John Trebel, President
Marketing: Patrick R. Stewart, Mktg. Mgr.
Production: Karen Burroughs, Prod. Mgr.
  K.F. Anderson, VP Mfg.
Federal Procurement Eligibility: VA Contract
Device Category:
Cart, Equipment, Video .... GENERAL

Weck & Co. Inc., Edward
1 Weck Dr.
P.O. Box 12600
Research Triangle Park, NC 27709
Tel: 919-544-8000
Tel: 800-334-9751
Fax: 908-359-9597
CEO: Dick Klein, President
Production: Michael Goffredo, EVP Techn. Oper.
Federal Procurement Eligibility: GSA Contract
Device Category:
Accessories, Cleaning, Endoscopic	GASTRO/UROLOGY
Anoscope, Non-Powered	GASTRO/UROLOGY
Endoscope	GASTRO/UROLOGY
Forceps, Electrosurgical	SURGERY
Forceps, Endoscopic	GASTRO/UROLOGY
Forceps, Grasping, Flexible Endoscopic	GASTRO/UROLOGY
Hysteroscope	OBSTETRICS/GYN
Laryngoscope, Flexible	ANESTH/PUL MED
Remover, Clip	SURGERY
Trocar, Abdominal	GASTRO/UROLOGY
Trocar, Gallbladder	GASTRO/UROLOGY

Wect Instrument Company, Inc.
5645 N. Ravenswood
Chicago, IL 60660-3922
Tel: 312-769-1944
Fax: 312-769-0982
Advertising: Rebecca Huba
CEO: Tom J. McManus III, General Manager
Marketing: David Dobbs, Prod. Dir.
Production: Bart Aiello, Asst. Plant Mgr.
Research: Stanley Welber, VP R&D
  Ernest Burke
Federal Procurement Eligibility: GSA Contract
Device Category:
Accessories, Photographic, Endoscopic	GASTRO/UROLOGY
Adapter, Bulb, Endoscope, Miscellaneous	GASTRO/UROLOGY
Arthroscope	ORTHOPEDICS
Bougie, Esophageal, ENT	EAR/NOSE/THROAT
Cannula, Suprapubic, With Trocar	GASTRO/UROLOGY
Forceps, Electrosurgical	SURGERY
Forceps, Endoscopic	GASTRO/UROLOGY
Hysteroscope	OBSTETRICS/GYN
Insufflator, Other	SURGERY
Laparoscope, General & Plastic Surgery	SURGERY
Laparoscope, Gynecologic	OBSTETRICS/GYN
Laryngoscope, Rigid	ANESTH/PUL MED
Obturator, Endoscopic	GASTRO/UROLOGY
Sheath, Endoscopic	GASTRO/UROLOGY
Teaching Attachment, Endoscopic	GASTRO/UROLOGY
Trocar, Abdominal	GASTRO/UROLOGY

Welch Allyn, Inc.
4341 State Street Rd.
P.O. Box 220
Skaneateles Falls, NY 13153-0220
Tel: 315-685-4100
Tel: 800-535-6663
Fax: 315-685-3361
Advertising: Tom Grant, Adv. Mgr.
CEO: Peter Soderberg, Bus. Dev. Mgr.
  Lew Allyn, President
  Dan Fisher, VP Personnel
  Bill Allyn, CEO
Marketing: Stephen Meyer, Mktg. Dir.
  John Moran, VP Sales
Production: Wolfgang Geihe, VP Mfg.
  Sue Overmann, Prod. Mgr.
  John Watkins, Reg. Affairs Mgr.
Device Category:
Accessories, Cleaning, Endoscopic	GASTRO/UROLOGY
Anoscope, Non-Powered	GASTRO/UROLOGY
Camera, Television, Endoscopic, Without Audio	SURGERY
Camera, Television, Surgical, Without Audio	SURGERY
Camera, Video, Endoscopic	GENERAL
Camera, Video, Multi-Image	MIN. INV. SURGERY
Endoscope, Electronic (Videoendoscope)	SURGERY
Endoscope, Flexible	GASTRO/UROLOGY
Endoscope, Rigid	SURGERY
Laparoscope, Flexible	SURGERY
Laparoscope, General & Plastic Surgery	SURGERY
Laparoscope, Gynecologic	OBSTETRICS/GYN
Laparoscope, Semi-Flexible	MIN. INV. SURGERY
Laryngoscope	EAR/NOSE/THROAT
Laryngoscope, Rigid	ANESTH/PUL MED
Light, Surgical, Endoscopic	SURGERY
Monitor, Video, Endoscope	GENERAL
Nasopharyngoscope (Flexible Or Rigid)	EAR/NOSE/THROAT
Power Supply, Endoscopic, Battery Operated	GENERAL
Power Supply, Endoscopic, Line Operated	GENERAL
Proctoscope	SURGERY
Proctosigmoidoscope	GASTRO/UROLOGY
Sigmoidoscope, Flexible	GASTRO/UROLOGY
Sigmoidoscope, Rigid, Electrical	GASTRO/UROLOGY
Sigmoidoscope, Rigid, Non-Electrical	GASTRO/UROLOGY
Thoracoscope	CARDIOVASCULAR

Wells Johnson Co.
8075 E. Research Ct., Ste. 101
Tucson, AZ 85710-6714
Tel: 602-298-6069
Tel: 800-528-1597
Fax: 602-885-1189
CEO: Ronald Boros
  John Wells, President
Marketing: Brad Miller, Sales & Mktg. Dir.
Production: Brenda Hunt, Reg. Affairs Mgr.
Federal Procurement Eligibility: Small Business
Device Category:
Camera, Television, Endoscopic, Without Audio	SURGERY
Endoscope	GASTRO/UROLOGY
Sheath, Endoscopic	GASTRO/UROLOGY

Westco Medical Corp.
7079 Mission Gorge Rd., Bldg. J
San Diego, CA 92120-2455
Tel: 619-286-1600
Tel: 800-543-5558
Fax: 619-286-8900
CEO: Avrom M. Shulman, President
Production: Wade C. Gilliland, Jr.
Federal Procurement Eligibility: Small Business
Device Category:
Colposcope	OBSTETRICS/GYN
Forceps, Electrosurgical	SURGERY

Wid-Med, Inc.　　　　　　　　　　　　Tel: 312-236-8586
111 N. Wabash Ave.　　　　　　　　　　Fax: 708-835-8880
Chicago, IL 60602-1903
CEO: Jerrold Widran, M.D., President
Marketing: Sanford Widran, Coord.
Production: Helmut Krebs, VP
Federal Procurement Eligibility: Small Business
Device Category:
Obturator, Endoscopic .... GASTRO/UROLOGY
Resectoscope .... GASTRO/UROLOGY
Sheath, Endoscopic .... GASTRO/UROLOGY
Telescope, Rigid, Endoscopic .... GASTRO/UROLOGY

Wild Microscopes　　　　　　　　　　Tel: 201-767-1100
24 Link Drive　　　　　　　　　　　　　Fax: 201-767-4196
Rockleigh, NJ 07647-2504
Advertising: John J. Ryan, Mgr.
CEO: Karl H. Hormel, President
  Edward Gallagher, VP
Marketing: Manfred Nahmmacher, VP Sales
Federal Procurement Eligibility: GSA Contract
Device Category:
Camera, Still, Endoscopic .... SURGERY

Wilson-Cook Medical, Inc.　　　　　　Tel: 919-744-0157
4900 Bethania Station Rd.　　　　　　　Tel: 800-245-4717
Winston-Salem, NC 27105-1203　　　　Fax: 919-744-1147
Advertising: Paula Almand, Adv. Mgr.
CEO: Woody Karr, Financial Mgr.
  Sue Knohl, Admin. Dir.
  Marsha Dreyer, PR Mgr.
  Don Wilson, President
Marketing: Scott Sewell, Natl. Sales Mgr.
  Glenn Hoskin, Mktg. & Sales Dir.
Production: Richard Marshall, VP Operations
  John Karpiel, VP Production
  Jack Calloway, Production Mgr.
  Clay Koon, QA Eng.
Research: Bruce McBrien, Research & Dev. Dir.
Federal Procurement Eligibility: Small Business
Device Category:
Bougie, Esophageal And Gastrointestinal .... GASTRO/UROLOGY
Brush, Cytology, Endoscopic .... GASTRO/UROLOGY
Catheter, Cholangiography .... SURGERY
Endoscope And Accessories, AC-Powered .... SURGERY
Kit, Gastrostomy, Endoscopic, Percutaneous .... MIN. INV. SURGERY
Needle, Endoscopic .... GASTRO/UROLOGY
Prosthesis, Esophageal .... EAR/NOSE/THROAT

Wisap Gesellschaft　　　　　　　　　Tel: 08104/1067
Rudolf Diesel Ring 20　　　　　　　　Fax: 08104/9664
D-82054 Sauerlach
Germany
CEO: Horst Semm
Marketing: Berthold Schwarz, Int'l Managing Sales Dir.
Device Category:
Coagulator, Laparoscopic, Unipolar .... OBSTETRICS/GYN
Coagulator/Cutter, Endoscopic, Bipolar .... OBSTETRICS/GYN
Coagulator/Cutter, Endoscopic, Unipolar .... OBSTETRICS/GYN
Hysteroscope .... OBSTETRICS/GYN
Insufflator, Hysteroscopic .... OBSTETRICS/GYN
Insufflator, Vaginal .... OBSTETRICS/GYN
Monitor, Video, Endoscope .... GENERAL
Teaching Attachment, Endoscopic .... GASTRO/UROLOGY

Wisap USA　　　　　　　　　　　　Tel: 713-351-2629
P.O. Box 324　　　　　　　　　　　　Tel: 800-233-8448
Tomball, TX 77377-0324　　　　　　　Fax: 713-255-6213
CEO: W. Przybyla, President
Federal Procurement Eligibility: Small Business
Device Category:
Arthroscope .... ORTHOPEDICS
Coagulator, Laparoscopic, Unipolar .... OBSTETRICS/GYN
Coagulator/Cutter, Endoscopic, Bipolar .... OBSTETRICS/GYN
Coagulator/Cutter, Endoscopic, Unipolar .... OBSTETRICS/GYN
Hysteroscope .... OBSTETRICS/GYN
Insufflator, Hysteroscopic .... OBSTETRICS/GYN
Insufflator, Vaginal .... OBSTETRICS/GYN
Trocar, Other .... GENERAL
Vaginoscope .... OBSTETRICS/GYN

WM Instrumente GmbH　　　　　　Tel: 07424/501310
Panoramastr. 6　　　　　　　　　　　Fax: 07424/501198
D-78604 Rietheim 1
Germany
CEO: Werner Martin
Marketing: Markus Hauser
Device Category:
Accessories, Arthroscope .... ORTHOPEDICS
Arthroscope .... ORTHOPEDICS
Camera, Videotape, Surgical .... SURGERY
Cannula, Drainage, Arthroscopy .... ORTHOPEDICS
Endoscope .... GASTRO/UROLOGY
Forceps, Endoscopic .... GASTRO/UROLOGY
Insufflator, Hysteroscopic .... OBSTETRICS/GYN
Insufflator, Laparoscopic .... OBSTETRICS/GYN
Laparoscope, General & Plastic Surgery .... SURGERY
Laparoscope, Gynecologic .... OBSTETRICS/GYN

Wolf Medical Instruments Corp., Richard
353 Corporate Woods Pkwy.
Vernon Hills, IL 60061-3110
Tel: 708-913-1113
Tel: 800-323-9653
Fax: 708-913-1488
Total Employees: 120
Ownership: Private
Distribution: Manufacturer Through Reps., Importer
Advertising: Peter Daut, Adv. Mgr.
CEO: Werner Mueller, COO
 Ingeborg Burkhard, CEO
 Britta Dickinson, VP Personnel
Marketing: Alfons Notheis, Mktg. Dir.
Production: Robert L. Casarsa, QA Mgr.
 Klaus Schilde, VP Mfg.
 Ed Cutler, Materials Mgr.
Research: Ulrich Obbarius, VP R&D
Device Category:

Accessories, Arthroscope	ORTHOPEDICS
Accessories, Cleaning, Endoscopic	GASTRO/UROLOGY
Accessories, Photographic, Endoscopic	GASTRO/UROLOGY
Amnioscope, Transabdominal (Fetoscope)	OBSTETRICS/GYN
Anoscope, Non-Powered	GASTRO/UROLOGY
Arthroscope	ORTHOPEDICS
Bronchoscope, Flexible	EAR/NOSE/THROAT
Bronchoscope, Rigid	EAR/NOSE/THROAT
Bronchoscope, Rigid, Non-Ventilating	ANESTH/PUL MED
Bronchoscope, Rigid, Ventilating	ANESTH/PUL MED
Brush, Cytology, Endoscopic	GASTRO/UROLOGY
Bulb, Inflation (Endoscope)	GASTRO/UROLOGY
Camera, Still, Endoscopic	SURGERY
Camera, Television, Endoscopic, With Audio	SURGERY
Camera, Television, Endoscopic, Without Audio	SURGERY
Camera, Television, Surgical, With Audio	SURGERY
Camera, Video, Endoscopic	GENERAL
Cannula, Drainage, Arthroscopy	ORTHOPEDICS
Cannula, Extraction, Appendix	MIN. INV. SURGERY
Cannula, Suprapubic, With Trocar	GASTRO/UROLOGY
Carrier, Sponge, Endoscopic	GASTRO/UROLOGY
Cart, Equipment, Video	GENERAL
Choledochoscope, Flexible Or Rigid	GASTRO/UROLOGY
Coagulator, Hysteroscopic (With Accessories)	OBSTETRICS/GYN
Coagulator, Laparoscopic, Unipolar	OBSTETRICS/GYN
Coagulator/Cutter, Endoscopic, Bipolar	OBSTETRICS/GYN
Coagulator/Cutter, Endoscopic, Unipolar	OBSTETRICS/GYN
Colposcope	OBSTETRICS/GYN
Cord, Electric, Endoscope	GASTRO/UROLOGY
Culdoscope	OBSTETRICS/GYN
Cystoscope	GASTRO/UROLOGY
Cystourethroscope	GASTRO/UROLOGY
Dilator, Blunt	MIN. INV. SURGERY
Dilator, Fascia, Umbilical	MIN. INV. SURGERY
Electrocautery Unit, Endoscopic	OBSTETRICS/GYN
Endoscope, Direct Vision	SURGERY
Endoscope, Electronic (Videoendoscope)	SURGERY
Endoscope, Flexible	GASTRO/UROLOGY
Endoscope, Rigid	SURGERY
Endoscope, Transcervical (Amnioscope)	OBSTETRICS/GYN
Equipment, Suction/Irrigation, Laparoscopic	SURGERY
Esophagoscope (Flexible Or Rigid)	EAR/NOSE/THROAT
Eyepiece, Lens, Prescription, Endoscopic	GASTRO/UROLOGY
Forceps, Electrosurgical	SURGERY
Forceps, Endoscopic	GASTRO/UROLOGY
Forceps, Grasping, Atraumatic	MIN. INV. SURGERY
Forceps, Grasping, Flexible Endoscopic	GASTRO/UROLOGY
Forceps, Grasping, Traumatic	MIN. INV. SURGERY
Gastroscope, General & Plastic Surgery	GASTRO/UROLOGY
Gastroscope, Rigid	GASTRO/UROLOGY
Generator, Power, Electrosurgical	SURGERY
Holder, Laparoscope	OBSTETRICS/GYN
Holder, Leg, Arthroscopy	ORTHOPEDICS
Holder/Scissors, Needle, Laparoscopic	MIN. INV. SURGERY
Hysteroscope	OBSTETRICS/GYN
Illuminator, Fiberoptic (For Endoscope)	GASTRO/UROLOGY
Instrument, Dissecting, Laparoscopic	MIN. INV. SURGERY
Instrument, Dissecting, Myoma, Laparoscopic	MIN. INV. SURGERY
Instrument, Knot Tying, Suture, Laparoscopic	MIN. INV. SURGERY
Instrument, Needle Holder/Knot Tying	MIN. INV. SURGERY
Instrument, Passing, Suture, Laparoscopic	MIN. INV. SURGERY
Insufflator, Carbon-Dioxide, Automatic (For Endoscope)	GASTRO/UROLOGY
Insufflator, Hysteroscopic	OBSTETRICS/GYN
Insufflator, Laparoscopic	OBSTETRICS/GYN
Insufflator, Other	SURGERY
Kit, Laparoscopy	GASTRO/UROLOGY
Kit, Pelviscopy	MIN. INV. SURGERY
Lamp, Endoscopic, Incandescent	SURGERY
Laparoscope, General & Plastic Surgery	SURGERY
Laparoscope, Gynecologic	OBSTETRICS/GYN
Laryngoscope, Rigid	ANESTH/PUL MED
Laryngostroboscope (Endoscope)	EAR/NOSE/THROAT
Light Source, Endoscope, Xenon Arc	SURGERY
Light, Surgical, Endoscopic	SURGERY
Mediastinoscope	SURGERY
Monitor, Video, Endoscope	GENERAL
Nasopharyngoscope (Flexible Or Rigid)	EAR/NOSE/THROAT
Needle, Aspiration, Cyst, Laparoscopic	MIN. INV. SURGERY
Needle, Endoscopic	GASTRO/UROLOGY
Needle, Insufflation, Laparoscopic	MIN. INV. SURGERY
Nephroscope, Flexible	GASTRO/UROLOGY
Nephroscope, Rigid	GASTRO/UROLOGY
Obturator, Endoscopic	GASTRO/UROLOGY
Peritoneoscope	GASTRO/UROLOGY
Probe, Electrocauterization, Multi-Use	MIN. INV. SURGERY
Probe, Suction, Irrigator/Aspirator, Laparoscopic	MIN. INV. SURGERY
Proctoscope	SURGERY
Pyeloscope	RADIOLOGY
Resectoscope	GASTRO/UROLOGY
Sheath, Endoscopic	GASTRO/UROLOGY
Sigmoidoscope, Rigid, Non-Electrical	GASTRO/UROLOGY
Snare, Endoscopic	SURGERY
Solution, Instrument, Laparoscopic, Anti-Fog	GENERAL
System, Camera, 3-Dimensional	MIN. INV. SURGERY
Tape, Television & Video, Endoscopic	GASTRO/UROLOGY
Teaching Attachment, Endoscopic	GASTRO/UROLOGY
Telescope, Rigid, Endoscopic	GASTRO/UROLOGY
Thoracoscope	CARDIOVASCULAR
Trainer, Laparoscopy	MIN. INV. SURGERY
Trocar, Abdominal	GASTRO/UROLOGY
Trocar, Amniotic	OBSTETRICS/GYN
Trocar, Gallbladder	GASTRO/UROLOGY
Trocar, Gastro-Urology	GASTRO/UROLOGY
Trocar, Laryngeal	EAR/NOSE/THROAT
Trocar, Other	GENERAL
Trocar, Short	MIN. INV. SURGERY

Trocar, Thoracic	CARDIOVASCULAR
Tube, Smoke Removal, Endoscopic	GASTRO/UROLOGY
Ureteroscope	GASTRO/UROLOGY
Urethroscope	GASTRO/UROLOGY
Vaginoscope	OBSTETRICS/GYN
Warmer, Endoscope	MIN. INV. SURGERY

Xenon Corp. Tel: 617-938-3594
20 Commerce Way Tel: 800-878-3594
Woburn, MA 01801 Fax: 617-933-8804
CEO: Louis R. Panico, CEO
　C. Richard Panico, VP
Federal Procurement Eligibility: Small Business
Device Category:
Light Source, Endoscope, Xenon Arc .... SURGERY

Ximed Medical Systems Tel: 408-945-4040
2195 Trade Zone Blvd. Fax: 408-945-3190
San Jose, CA 95131
CEO: A. Desai
Marketing: D. Sunil
Federal Procurement Eligibility: Small Business, Minority Owned
Device Category:
Bag, Specimen, Laparoscopic .... MIN. INV. SURGERY
Coagulator, Laparoscopic, Unipolar .... OBSTETRICS/GYN
Coagulator/Cutter, Endoscopic, Bipolar .... OBSTETRICS/GYN
Coagulator/Cutter, Endoscopic, Unipolar .... OBSTETRICS/GYN
Equipment, Suction/Irrigation, Laparoscopic .... SURGERY
Holder, Needle, Laparoscopic .... MIN. INV. SURGERY
Holder/Scissors, Needle, Laparoscopic .... MIN. INV. SURGERY
Kit, Cholecystectomy .... MIN. INV. SURGERY
Kit, Laparoscopy .... GASTRO/UROLOGY
Peritoneoscope .... GASTRO/UROLOGY
Probe, Electrocauterization, Multi-Use .... MIN. INV. SURGERY
Probe, Electrocauterization, Single-Use .... MIN. INV. SURGERY
Probe, Suction, Irrigator/Aspirator, Laparoscopic .... MIN. INV. SURGERY
Scissors with Removable Tips, Laparoscopy .... MIN. INV. SURGERY
Thoracoscope .... CARDIOVASCULAR

Xomed-Treace Tel: 904-296-9600
6743 Southpoint Drive N. Tel: 800-874-5797
Jacksonville, FL 32216-6218 Fax: 904-296-1004
CEO: W. P. Cusick, President
　John McCain, VP Human Res.
　David Grant, VP Fin.
Marketing: Waldron Palmer, VP Sales & Mktg. & Bus. Dev.
　Lisa Snyder, VP Mktg. Svcs.
Production: Marley Price, VP Oper.
　Don Bruce, Ophthalmology Mktg.
　Dan Treace, VP Tech. Affairs
Federal Procurement Eligibility: GSA Contract, VA Contract
Device Category:
Endoscope, Rigid .... SURGERY

Xomed-Treace Tel: 905-858-8588
Div. of Zimmer of Canada Ltd. Tel: 800-387-9632
2323 Argentina Rd. Fax: 905-858-0324
Missisauga, ONT L5N 5N3
Canada
Total Employees: 18
Distribution: Exclusive Distributor
Advertising: Gerry Pilon, Adv. Mgr.
CEO: Doug Thomson, President
Marketing: Johanne Touchette, Mgr. Professional Dev.
　Gerry Pilon, Mktg. Mgr.
　Doug Bremmer, Natl. Sales Mgr.
Production: Noel Baxter, Materials Mgr.
　Jim McDowell, Reg. Affairs
Device Category:
Anoscope, Non-Powered .... GASTRO/UROLOGY

Xylog Corp. Tel: 201-489-4040
83 Hobart St. Fax: 201-489-6745
Hackensack, NJ 07601-3948
CEO: Samuel Dickstein, VP
　Milton Frank, President
Marketing: Larry Doll, VP Marketing
Federal Procurement Eligibility: Small Business
Device Category:
Insufflator, Laparoscopic .... OBSTETRICS/GYN
Light Source, Endoscope, Xenon Arc .... SURGERY

Yagami International Trading Co. Tel: 052/9623811
3-2-29, Marunouchi, Naka-Ku Fax: 052/9711398
Nagoya 460
Japan
Medical Products Sales Volume: $2,400,000
Total Employees: 50
Distribution: Importer/Exporter, Manufacturer Direct & Through
　Distributors
Advertising: Takanari Kawamura
CEO: Nobuyuki Abe
Marketing: Tetsuya Matsumura
Research: Takako Yagami
Device Category:
Teaching Attachment, Endoscopic .... GASTRO/UROLOGY

Yole Company Tel: 516-757-9336
51 Boulevard Fax: 516-754-0468
Greenlawn, NY 11740-1401
CEO: J.C. Bryan, President
Federal Procurement Eligibility: Small Business
Device Category:
Cord, Electric, Endoscope .... GASTRO/UROLOGY
Forceps, Electrosurgical .... SURGERY

Zeiss Inc., Carl Tel: 914-747-1800
One Zeiss Dr. Tel: 800-442-4020
Thornwood, NY 10594-1939 Fax: 914-681-7409
CEO: Dieter Blennemann, President
Marketing: Joerg Schweizer, Mktg. Mgr.
Production: John C. Moore, VP Med. Products Div.
Federal Procurement Eligibility: GSA Contract
Device Category:
Colposcope .... OBSTETRICS/GYN
Endoscope .... GASTRO/UROLOGY

Zeiss, Carl Jena GmbH
Tel: 03641/588-0
Fax: 03641/588-2856
Tatzendpromenade 1a
D-07745 Jena
Germany
Advertising: Christa Schoder, Adv. Mgr.
Marketing: Holger Robberg, Mktg. Svc. Exec.
Device Category:
Colposcope .... OBSTETRICS/GYN

Zenith Medical Inc.
Tel: 619-535-0216
Tel: 800-747-0216
Fax: 619-535-9715
10064 Mesa Ridge Ct., Ste. 218
San Diego, CA 92121
CEO: Mark McGoothlin, President
Marketing: Stephanie Kramer, Nat'l Sales Mgr. & Mktg. Dir.
Federal Procurement Eligibility: Small Business
Device Category:
Bag, Specimen, Laparoscopic .... MIN. INV. SURGERY

Zibra Corp.
Tel: 508-374-9764
Fax: 508-374-0804
105 Ward Hill Ave.
Ward Hill, MA 01835-6928
CEO: Arthur C. McKinley
Device Category:
Endoscope .... GASTRO/UROLOGY

Zimmer, Patient Care Div.
Tel: 216-343-8801
Fax: 216-343-0995
200 W. Ohio Ave.
Dover, OH 44622-9642
Advertising: Gene Rugh, Mktg. Svcs. Dir.
CEO: Terry M. Egan, Sr. VP
   Charles L. Deeds, President
Production: Richard G. Betts, Mfg. VP
Device Category:
Insufflator, Hysteroscopic .... OBSTETRICS/GYN

Zinnanti Surgical Instruments
Tel: 818-700-0090
Tel: 800-223-4740
Fax: 818-700-0575
21540 B Prairie St.
Chatsworth, CA 91311-5886
CEO: Trish Villging, Reg. Affairs Mgr.
   Anthony Zinnanti Jr.
Marketing: Ken Mettler, VP Sales & Mktg.
Production: Mike Villanueva, Matls. Mgr.
   Anna Straight, VP Operations
Device Category:
Camera, Television, Endoscopic, With Audio .... SURGERY
Endoscope .... GASTRO/UROLOGY
Insufflator, Carbon-Dioxide, Automatic
   (For Endoscope) .... GASTRO/UROLOGY
Laparoscope, Gynecologic .... OBSTETRICS/GYN